Pathophysiology of Gastrointestinal Diseases

Pathophysiology of Gastrointestinal Diseases

Edited by

Sanjiv Chopra, M.D.
Assistant Professor of Medicine, Harvard Medical School;
Director of Clinical Hepatology and Physician,
Gastroenterology Division, Beth Israel Hospital, Boston

Roger J. May, M.D.
Instructor of Medicine, Harvard Medical School; Associate
Physician, Department of Medicine, Beth Israel Hospital,
Boston

Little, Brown and Company
Boston/Toronto/London

Library of Congress Catalog Card No. 89-83474

ISBN 0-316-13890-8

Printed in the United States of America

RRD VA

This book is dedicated to Amita,
Ratika, Kanika, and Bharat, and to
Louise and Channing for their
encouragement and understanding

Contents

Preface

There are many exhilarating moments in medicine. They can be a new observation of an old disease, the discovery of an entirely new syndrome, or the development of a successful treatment of a disabling illness. Understanding pathophysiology is the key to each of these insights and discoveries. With this understanding, one is able to translate the inexplicable into the comprehensible with the potential for preventing, treating, or curing disease. This understanding is also the foundation for the intelligent practice of clinical medicine. With comprehension of pathophysiology, one is able to transform symptoms, physical findings, and diagnostic results into a coherent model of disease and thus treat an illness rationally and specifically.

This book provides a scientific foundation for understanding the natural history, clinical features, and management of disorders of the gastrointestinal system. We also hope that this book communicates the joy of knowledge that we and our co-authors have derived from this study of pathophysiology. By understanding the diseases we treat, we find the practice of medicine truly exciting and fulfilling. We hope this zeal and excitement will also be shared by the reader and that the book will provide a framework through which medicine can be thoughtfully approached and patients can be intelligently managed.

In editing this book, we learned immeasurably from our contributors and each other. Our greatest source of learning, however, continues to be our patients and students, to whom we owe our sincere gratitude. In enlivening the readers' interest in our subspecialty, we hope to repay in some measure this debt of gratitude.

S. C.
R. J. M.

Contributors

Michael D. Apstein, M.D.
Assistant Professor of Medicine, Harvard Medical School,
Boston; Chief of Gastroenterology, Brockton/West Roxbury
Veterans Administration Medical Center, Brockton,
Massachusetts; Associate Physician, Brigham and Women's
Hospital, Boston

Sanjeev Arora, M.D.
Assistant Professor of Medicine, Tufts University School of
Medicine; Staff Physician, New England Medical Center,
Boston

George Benes, M.D.
Research Fellow in Gastroenterology, Harvard Medical School
and Beth Israel Hospital, Boston

Marvin D. Berman, M.D.
Assistant Professor of Medicine, Harvard Medical School,
Boston; Associate Chief of Gastroenterology, Brockton/West
Roxbury Veterans Administration Medical Center, Brockton,
Massachusetts

T. Edward Bynum, M.D.
Associate Professor of Medicine, Harvard Medical School;
Director of Clinical Gastroenterology, Brigham and Women's
Hospital, Boston

Sanjiv Chopra, M.D.
Assistant Professor of Medicine, Harvard Medical School;
Director of Clinical Hepatology and Physician,
Gastroenterology Division, Beth Israel Hospital, Boston

Jeffrey R. Crist, M.D.
Assistant Professor of Medicine, Harvard Medical School;
Assistant in Medicine, Gastroenterology Division, Beth Israel
Hospital, Boston

Yogeshwar Dayal, M.D.
Clinical Professor of Pathology, Tufts University School of
Medicine; Pathologist, New England Medical Center, Boston

Jules L. Dienstag, M.D.
Associate Professor of Medicine, Harvard Medical School;
Assistant Physician, Gastrointestinal Unit, Massachusetts
General Hospital, Boston

Z. Myron Falchuk, M.D.
Associate Professor of Medicine, Harvard Medical School;
Physician, Department of Medicine, New England Deaconess
Hospital, Boston

Karim A. Fawaz, M.D.
Associate Professor of Medicine, Tufts University School of
Medicine; Staff Physician, New England Medical Center,
Boston

Alexandra L. Gibas, M.D.
Research Fellow in Medicine, Harvard Medical School;
Clinical Fellow in Medicine, Gastrointestinal Unit,
Massachusetts General Hospital, Boston

John L. Gollan, M.D., Ph.D.
Associate Professor of Medicine, Harvard Medical School;
Physician, Brigham and Women's Hospital and The Children's
Hospital, Boston

Stephen Crane Hauser, M.D.
Assistant Professor of Medicine, Harvard Medical School;
Associate Physician, Department of Medicine, Brigham and
Women's Hospital, Boston

David E. Johnston, M.D.
Assistant Professor of Medicine, Tufts University School of
Medicine and New England Medical Center, Boston

Marshall M. Kaplan, M.D.
Professor of Medicine and Chief, Division of
Gastroenterology, Tufts University School of Medicine and
New England Medical Center, Boston

William D. Kasimer, M.D.
Instructor of Pathology, Tufts University School of Medicine
and New England Medical Center, Boston

J. Thomas Lamont, M.D.
Professor of Medicine, Boston University School of Medicine;
Chief of Gastroenterology, University Hospital, Boston

Roger J. May, M.D.
Instructor of Medicine, Harvard Medical School; Associate
Physician, Department of Medicine, Beth Israel Hospital,
Boston

Mark A. Peppercorn, M.D.
Associate Professor of Medicine, Harvard Medical School;
Associate Physician, Department of Medicine, Beth Israel
Hospital, Boston

James M. Richter, M.D.
Assistant Professor of Medicine, Harvard Medical School;
Assistant Physician, Medical Service, Massachusetts General
Hospital, Boston

Bernard F. Smith, M.D.
Assistant Professor of Medicine, Boston University School of
Medicine; Chief, Section of Gastroenterology, Boston City
Hospital, Boston

Stuart Jon Spechler, M.D.
Associate Professor of Medicine, Boston University School of
Medicine; Associate Chief of Gastroenterology, Boston
Veterans Administration Medical Center, Boston

Jerry S. Trier, M.D.
Professor of Medicine, Harvard Medical School; Co-Director,
Gastroenterology Division, Brigham and Women's Hospital,
Boston

John P. Vermeulen, M.D.
Instructor of Medicine, Harvard Medical School, Boston; Staff
Physician, Brockton/West Roxbury Veterans Administration
Medical Center, Brockton, Massachusetts; Associate
Physician, Brigham and Women's Hospital, Boston

M. Michael Wolfe, M.D.
Assistant Professor of Medicine, Harvard Medical School;
Senior Associate in Medicine, Gastroenterology Division, Beth
Israel Hospital, Boston

Jerome B. Zeldis, M.D., Ph.D.
Assistant Professor of Medicine, Harvard Medical School;
Associate Physician, Gastroenterology Division, Beth Israel
Hospital, Boston

Pathophysiology of
Gastrointestinal Diseases

Notice

The indications and dosages of all drugs in this book have been recommended in the medical literature and conform to the practices of the general medical community. The medications described do not necessarily have specific approval by the Food and Drug Administration for use in the diseases and dosages for which they are recommended. The package insert for each drug should be consulted for use and dosage as approved by the FDA. Because standards for usage change, it is advisable to keep abreast of revised recommendations, particularly those concerning new drugs.

1 : Motor Disorders of the Esophagus

Jeffrey R. Crist

The human esophagus is a hollow, tubular organ consisting of three major structural components — the upper esophageal sphincter, the esophageal body, and the lower esophageal sphincter (Fig. 1-1). These structures serve two primary functions: (1) during swallowing, they provide a mechanism by which a food bolus received from the pharynx is propelled into the stomach, and (2) between swallows, they prevent the retrograde flow of esophageal and gastric contents.

Abnormalities in the function of the esophagus are not uncommon and range from the very common entity of gastroesophageal reflux to such uncommon entities as achalasia. To properly diagnose and treat motor disorders of the esophagus, one must first understand the anatomy and physiology of the esophagus and the pathophysiology of esophageal disorders.

Anatomy and Physiology

Upper Esophageal Sphincter

Anatomy

The upper esophageal sphincter (UES) refers to an intraluminal high-pressure zone that exists between the pharynx and upper esophageal body (Figs. 1-1 and 1-2). In humans, the length of this high-pressure zone ranges between 2 and 4 cm and does not correlate with any distinct anatomically defined sphincter. Although there has been controversy as to which anatomic structures actually constitute the UES, most investigators now agree that this high-pressure zone is due to contraction of the cricopharyngeus and the most caudal (lowermost) portions of the inferior pharyngeal constrictor muscles. The cricopharyngeal muscle is only 1 cm in width and is believed to make up the most caudal portion of the UES. The inferior pharyngeal constrictor is believed to make up the remaining 1- to 3-cm segment. Both of these muscle groups are composed of striated muscle and are innervated by somatic nerves emanating from cranial nuclei (the nucleus ambiguus) located in the medulla oblongata of the brainstem.

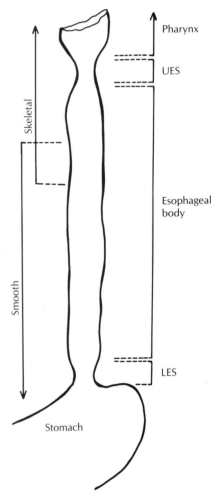

Composition
of
muscularis
externa

Fig. 1-1
Schematic diagram of the esophagus consisting of an upper esophageal sphincter (UES), esophageal body, and lower esophageal sphincter (LES). The muscularis externa of the UES is composed entirely of skeletal muscle, the LES of smooth muscle, and the esophageal body of both skeletal (uppermost portion) and smooth muscle (lowermost portion).

Physiology

In the intervals between swallows, the somatic nerves innervating the UES tonically stimulate the UES musculature. This continuous neural stimulation maintains muscle contraction and closure of the UES. This prevents esophageal contents from refluxing into the pharynx and respiratory tree, as well as entry of

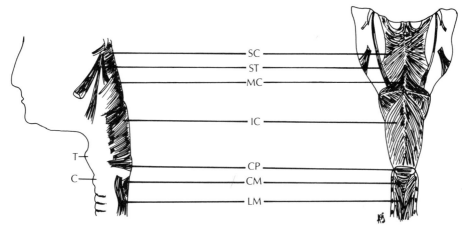

Fig. 1-2
Schematic diagram of the musculature of the oropharynx. The high-pressure zone comprising the upper esophageal sphincter is attributed to contraction of the cricopharyngeus (CP) and caudal portions of the inferior pharyngeal constrictor (IC) muscles. (SC = superior pharyngeal constrictor; ST = suprathyroid; MC = middle pharyngeal constrictor; CM = circular muscle layer of esophageal body; LM = longitudinal muscle layer of esophageal body; T = thyroid cartilage; C = cricoid cartilage)

air into the esophagus during inspiration. During swallows, this tonic nerve stimulation ceases and the muscles that constitute the UES abruptly relax. However, relaxation of the cricopharyngeus and inferior pharyngeal constrictor muscles alone is not capable of opening the UES. Opening of the sphincter requires associated contraction of the suprahyoid muscles. The UES remains open only long enough to allow the food bolus to pass rapidly from the pharynx into the upper esophagus before returning to its tonically contracted, closed state.

Esophageal Body **Anatomy**

The esophageal body extends from the lower border of the UES to the upper border of the lower esophageal sphincter (LES). The length of the esophageal body varies among individuals; it may be between 18 and 24 cm, generally being greater in men than in women. The wall of the esophageal body, like most other regions of the gastrointestinal tract, consists of layers (extending from inner to outer) of mucosa, muscularis mucosa, submucosa, and muscularis propria (Fig. 1-3). The muscularis propria in turn is made up of an inner circular muscle layer and an outer longitudinal muscle layer.

The mucosa throughout the esophageal body consists of stratified squamous epithelium. Only in the pathologic entity of Barrett's esophagus does columnar mucosa extend cephalad from the stomach into the esophageal body. Just external to the

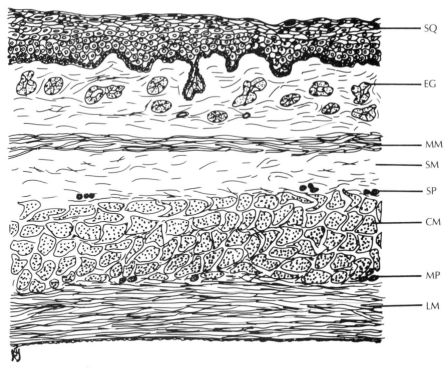

Fig. 1-3
Cross-sectional diagram of the esophageal wall. Note that the submucous plexus (SP, or Meissner's plexus) is located in the submucosa (SM) between the muscularis mucosa (MM) and the circular muscle layer (CM), whereas the myenteric plexus (MP, or Auerbach's plexus) is located between the CM and longitudinal muscle layers (LM). (SQ = squamous epithelium; EG = esophageal glands)

mucosa is a longitudinally oriented muscle layer known as the muscularis mucosa. This muscle layer is composed of smooth muscle throughout the length of the esophageal body.

Proximally, the esophagus is composed of striated muscle in both the inner circular and outer longitudinal muscle layers. Smooth muscle first begins to replace striated muscle in both layers at 4 to 5 cm from the most cephalad aspect of the esophageal body. A mixture of striated and smooth muscle exists from 4 to 5 cm to 11 to 12 cm from the most cephalad portion of the esophageal body. Caudal to this point, the circular and longitudinal muscle layers are composed entirely of smooth muscle. Hence, despite some minor variations among individuals, the most caudal half of the circular and longitudinal muscle layers of the human esophagus are composed entirely of smooth muscle (see Fig. 1-1).

The intrinsic nerves of the esophagus have their cell bodies in the submucosal (Meissner's) and myenteric (Auerbach's) plexuses. The submucous plexus is located between the muscularis mucosa and the circular muscle layer of the muscularis externa. Nerves of this plexus are believed to be primarily involved in the sensory innervation of the esophagus, as well as in the control of mucous secretion and vascular blood flow. The myenteric plexus is located between the circular and longitudinal muscle layers of the muscularis externa. Nerves of this plexus are believed to be primarily involved in the control of circular and longitudinal muscle contractions along the esophagus and play a key role in esophageal peristalsis.

The extrinsic nerves that serve to connect the central nervous system with the intrinsic nerves of the esophageal body run primarily within the vagus nerve. The cell bodies of vagal fibers that innervate the striated muscle of the esophagus are located in the nucleus ambiguus, whereas those vagal fibers that innervate the more caudal smooth muscle portion of the esophagus have their cell bodies located in the dorsal motor nucleus of the vagus. Both the nucleus ambiguus and the dorsal motor nucleus are located in the medulla oblongata of the brainstem (Fig. 1-4). The lower motor neurons whose cell bodies are located in the nucleus ambiguus project via the vagus nerve, directly to the striated musculature of the esophagus where they release acetylcholine at the neuromuscular junction. The vagal preganglionic fibers whose cell bodies are located in the dorsal motor nucleus do not directly innervate the smooth muscle of the esophagus but instead synapse with intrinsic neurons located in both the submucosal and myenteric plexuses of the esophagus. These intrinsic neurons send fibers that directly innervate the smooth muscle layers of the esophagus. Essentially all extrinsic motor fibers to the esophageal body run within the vagus nerve as it passes rostrally from the cranium. However, these fibers all leave the vagus trunk high in the neck to form an esophageal plexus at the level of the mid-esophageal body. This explains why a thoracic vagotomy performed for peptic ulcer disease has no effect on esophageal function.

Physiology
Primary and Secondary Peristalsis
The act of swallowing is associated with an orderly, progressive series of contractions throughout both the striated and smooth muscle portions of the esophageal body (Fig. 1-5). Peristalsis initiated by the conscious act of swallowing is termed *primary peristalsis,* whereas peristalsis initiated by intraluminal distention of the esophagus is known as *secondary peristalsis.* Secondary peristalsis is not accompanied by pharyngeal contractions or relaxation of the UES. Secondary peristalsis plays an important

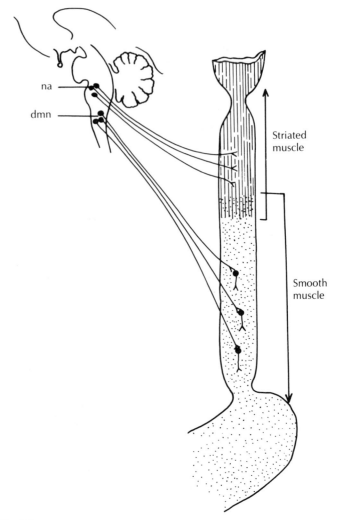

na

dmn

Striated
muscle

Smooth
muscle

Fig. 1-4
Vagal innervation to the esophagus. The striated muscle portion of the
esophagus is innervated by somatic lower motor neurons whose cell bodies
are located in the nucleus ambiguus (na) of the brainstem. The smooth
muscle portion is innervated by preganglionic vagal fibers whose cell bodies
are located in the dorsal motor nucleus (dmn) and synapse with intrinsic
neurons located within the wall of the esophagus.

role in the clearing of any food remaining in the esophagus
following primary peristalsis, as well as any gastric contents that
may have refluxed into the esophageal body. Both types of peristalsis have similar dimensions of amplitudes, duration, and
speed of propagation along the esophagus.

Deglutitive Inhibition
A phenomenon unique to the esophagus is *deglutitive inhibition*. This term is used to describe the finding that repetitive

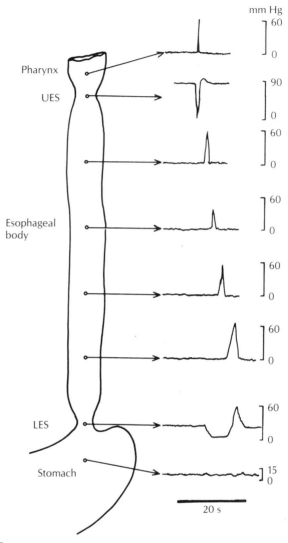

Fig. 1-5
Diagram of manometric recording of primary esophageal peristalsis. Swallowing is associated with contraction of the pharyngeal musculature, relaxation of the upper esophageal sphincter (UES), and a peristaltic wave along the esophageal body. As the peristaltic wave progresses along the esophageal body, the lower esophageal sphincter (LES) relaxes and remains relaxed until the peristaltic wave reaches the LES.

swallowing inhibits all esophageal body activity until after the last swallow, at which time a normal peristaltic wave progresses along the esophageal body (Fig. 1-6). This phenomenon occurs normally with drinking of fluids and is important in allowing only a single peristaltic wave to progress along the esophagus in response to multiple swallows.

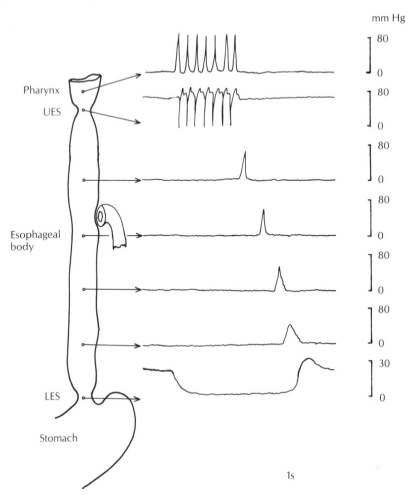

Fig. 1-6
Deglutitive inhibition as demonstrated in a manometric diagram of multiple successive swallows. Repetitive swallowing (as evidenced by repetitive pharyngeal contractions and upper esophageal sphincter [UES] relaxations) is associated with maintained relaxation of the lower esophageal sphincter (LES) and quiescence of the esophageal body. Following the final swallow, a peristaltic wave progresses along the esophageal body and the LES returns to baseline tone.

Control Mechanisms of Peristalsis

The neuromuscular mechanisms responsible for regulating peristaltic activity in the esophagus are located within the brain (central mechanisms), as well as within the wall of the esophagus itself (peripheral mechanisms).

Central Mechanisms. Primary peristalsis is initiated by activation of the "swallowing center" located in the brainstem. This activation occurs voluntarily by means of activating higher brain centers. Activation of the swallowing center results in the stimulation of brainstem vagal nuclei whose axons project to the esophagus.

1. *Striated muscle portion of the esophagus.* Vagal fibers innervating the striated muscle portion of the esophagus have their cell bodies in the nucleus ambiguus (see Fig. 1-4). During primary peristalsis, these motor neurons are sequentially activated by the swallowing center in such a way as to sequentially activate motor neurons destined for progressively more caudal levels of esophageal striated muscle; that is, motor neurons innervating the most cephalad portions of the esophagus are activated first, then activation sequentially spreads to neurons that innervate progressively more caudal portions of the striated musculature. Following bilateral high cervical vagotomy, both primary and secondary peristalsis in the striated muscle portion of the esophagus are abolished.

2. *Smooth muscle portion of the esophagus.* Vagal fibers innervating the smooth muscle portion of esophagus have their cell bodies in the dorsal motor nucleus of the vagus nerve (see Fig. 1-4). These preganglionic vagal fibers synapse with intramural neurons in the myenteric plexus of the esophagus, which directly innervate the smooth muscle fibers. During primary peristalsis, the preganglionic neurons located in the dorsal motor nucleus are activated by the "swallowing center," and these fibers in turn activate the intramural neurons in the esophagus. However, the cell bodies of vagal fibers innervating the smooth muscle portion of the esophagus do not appear to require sequential activation. This is evidenced by the ability to observe peristalsis in the smooth muscle portion by intraluminal distention following high cervical vagotomy (destruction of any possible sequential mechanism). Hence, most investigators now agree that activation of vagal nuclei in the dorsal motor nucleus by the swallowing center may be simultaneous rather than sequential in nature and that peristaltic behavior in the smooth muscle portion is due to a "peripherally located" mechanism.

Peripheral Mechanisms. As previously described, in the smooth muscle portion of the esophagus, central mechanisms of sequential stimulation are not needed for peristaltic behavior. This suggests that activation of neuromuscular mechanisms present within the wall of esophageal smooth muscle is capable of producing peristalsis. In vitro studies involving transmural nerve stimulation of isolated smooth muscle strips from different levels of the esophagus show that a significant latency period always occurs between the nerve stimulus and the onset of the

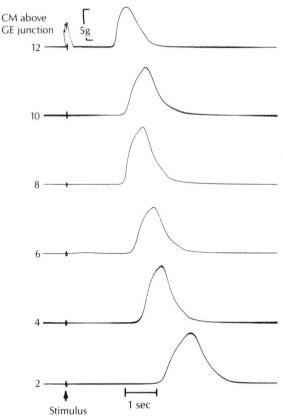

Fig. 1-7
Contractile responses of isolated circular muscle strips from different levels of the esophageal body to transmural nerve stimulation. All smooth muscle strips had a delay of greater than 1 second from the nerve stimulation before the onset of contraction. Strips from more caudal portions of the esophageal body had greater delays than strips from more proximal portions. (From N. W. Weisbrodt and J. Christensen. Gradients of contractions in the opossum esophagus. *Gastroenterology* 62(6):1159–1166, © by Williams & Wilkins, [1972].)

muscle contraction (Fig. 1-7). Moreover, these studies demonstrate that smooth muscle strips from more cephalad levels of the esophagus contract with a significantly shorter latency period than strips from more caudal levels. This latency gradient along the esophagus seen in vitro in many ways simulates primary peristalsis. It is clear that this gradient in latencies of contraction along the esophagus is of fundamental importance in the generation of a peristaltic contraction along the smooth muscle portion of the esophagus during either primary or secondary peristalsis. The basis for this latency period appears to be due to the release of inhibitory neurotransmitters from postganglionic nerves innervating the smooth muscle portion of the esophagus. Electrophysiologic studies of esophageal smooth muscle show a biphasic response of membrane potential following nerve stimulation. This biphasic response includes an initial period of membrane hyperpolarization followed by depolarization and spiking (the spiking is associated with smooth muscle contraction). The initial period of hyperpolarization is believed to be due to noncholinergic, nonadrenergic inhibitory neurotransmitter(s) and the ensuing depolarization resulting from a combination of myogenic rebound depolarization from the preceding hyperpolarization and the release of cholinergic and noncholinergic excitatory neurotransmitters. The noncholinergic, nonadrenergic inhibitory and excitatory neurotransmitters involved in the mechanism of esophageal peristalsis have yet to be identified.

Lower Esophageal Sphincter

The LES refers to an intraluminal high-pressure zone 2 to 4 cm in length that exists between the esophageal body and the stomach (see Fig. 1-1). This high-pressure zone does not correspond to a discrete thickened band of circular muscle and therefore is not a distinct histologic entity. The lower limit of the LES is typically marked by the junction between esophageal (squamous) mucosa and gastric (columnar) mucosa. The LES serves two primary functions: (1) by keeping the terminal portion of the esophageal lumen closed at rest, it forms a barrier preventing reflux of gastric acid and pepsin into the esophagus; and (2) by relaxing during a swallow, it allows a bolus to pass from the esophagus into the stomach.

The LES is composed entirely of smooth muscle and receives input from the central nervous system primarily through the vagus nerve. The extrinsic nerves that connect the central nervous system with the intrinsic nerves of the LES have their cell bodies in the dorsal motor nucleus of the brainstem (see Fig. 1-4). These preganglionic vagal fibers synapse with intrinsic neurons in the LES where they release acetylcholine. The cell bodies of the intrinsic neurons of the LES are located in the myenteric plexus and send projections to innervate LES smooth muscle.

Physiology

During the intervals between swallows, the LES remains closed because of the tonic contraction of the LES circular smooth muscle. LES smooth muscle remains tonically contracted owing to unique properties intrinsic to the muscle. This is quite different from the striated musculature of the UES, where continuous nerve stimulation is responsible for maintenance of muscle tone. Resting LES tone may be modulated by hormonal, myogenic, mechanical, and neural influences. Some of the sub-

Table 1-1
Substances that decrease LES pressure

Orally ingested substances
  Fat
  Chocolate
  Ethanol
  Nicotine (cigarette smoke)
  Theophylline
  Caffeine

Hormones
  Vasoactive intestinal polypeptide (VIP)
  Secretin
  Cholecystokinin (CCK)
  Progesterone, estrogens

Pharmacological agents
  Dopamine
  Anticholinergics
  Alpha-adrenergic antagonists

stances known to affect basal sphincter pressure are listed in Table 1-1. During pregnancy, a decline in LES pressure occurs; this is due to increased levels of sex hormones, most likely progesterone. A protein meal, intraduodenal installation of peptones, and gastric acidification cause an increase in LES pressure. This may be due to local effects of endogenous peptides such as pancreatic polypeptide, motilin, and bombesin or the activation of local neural reflex pathways.

Relaxation of the LES with swallows is due to activation of preganglionic vagal fibers that extend from the brainstem to the LES. These fibers synapse on and activate intramural inhibitory neurons located in the LES. These intramural nerves release an, at present, unidentified inhibitory transmitter that produces hyperpolarization of the cell membrane and associated relaxation of the smooth muscle.

Techniques of Studying Esophageal Motility

Methods of assessing esophageal motility that are currently available include standard barium x-rays, cinefluoroscopic x-rays, scintiscanning, and manometric techniques. The standard barium esophagogram (barium swallow) is generally the most readily available of these techniques. Such studies are useful in providing gross information about the movement of barium through the upper gastrointestinal tract but do not provide precise quantitative information concerning motility events. The more sophisticated technique of cinefluoroscopy allows one to examine the movement of barium by means of a rapid sequence of radiographic exposures. This technique is useful in the qualitative evaluation of the extremely rapid motility events that occur in the oropharynx with swallows; however, this study suffers in its inability to provide precise quantitative information concerning motility events.

Esophageal scintiscanning provides quantitative information concerning the emptying of swallowed radioactive particles from the esophagus. However, this information is not precise and therefore has proved to be of limited value in the assessment of esophageal motility.

At the present, esophageal motility is best studied using manometric techniques. These techniques use an assembly of pressure-sensing catheters to record intraluminal pressures at various sites along the esophagus. The catheter assembly typically consists of a number of individual tubes having recording orifices located at different sites along the length of the catheter assembly. Each of these tubes is continuously perfused with water and connected to a pressure transducer. The pressure transducer output is connected to an ink-writing polygraph. Occlusion of the recording orifice results in stoppage of the flow of water through the tube, which is translated to the force transducer and recorded as a contraction on the polygraph. The catheter assembly is passed into the esophagus so as to position the recording orifices at various sites along the esophagus. These sites should include the pharynx, UES, body (upper, middle, and lower portions), LES, and stomach. An example of a manometric recording of esophageal peristalsis using this technique is shown in Fig. 1-8.

Pharynx and Upper Esophageal Sphincter

The initial manometric event associated with the act of swallowing is contraction of the pharyngeal musculature. This contraction is abrupt in onset and lasts approximately 1 second. Associated with this pharyngeal contraction is an abrupt relaxation of the UES that is short-lived and generally followed by a brief after-contraction. Pharyngeal contraction and UES relaxation are synchronized such that the peak of pharyngeal contraction corresponds to maximum relaxation of the UES.

Esophageal Body

Shortly after relaxation of the UES is terminated, an abrupt contraction begins in the most cephalad portion of the esophageal body. This initial contraction is then followed by a series of contractions along the remainder of the esophageal body. The amplitudes and durations of these contractions vary at different sites along the esophagus. The amplitudes of contraction are greatest in the most caudal portions of the esophageal body and average 60 to 80 mm Hg. The amplitudes are slightly less in the most cephalad portions, averaging 50 to 70 mm Hg, and are lowest in the junctional zone between striated and smooth muscle, averaging 40 to 60 mm Hg. The duration of contraction at a

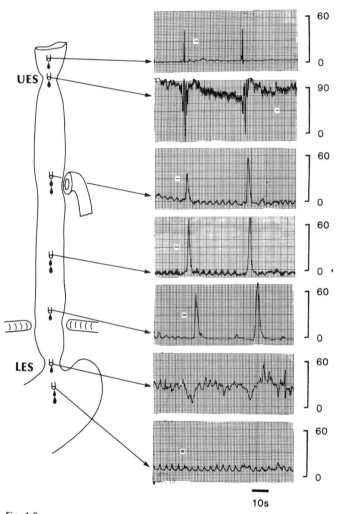

Fig. 1-8
Manometric tracings showing intraluminal pressures recorded concurrently along the upper gastrointestinal tract in an individual with normal esophageal motility. Each of the seven tracings depicts intraluminal pressures recorded concurrently from different sites along the pharynx, esophagus, and stomach. The uppermost tracing shows two distinct increases in pharyngeal pressure occurring in association with the act of swallowing. The two swallows are separated by an interval of approximately 30 seconds. Each pharyngeal contraction is associated with a brief relaxation of the upper esophageal sphincter (UES). Resting UES tone is approximately 90 mm Hg, and, with each swallow, the UES relaxes to atmospheric pressure (0 mm Hg, second tracing from top). Immediately after the UES pressure returns to baseline tone, a contraction begins in the most cephalad portion of the esophagus (third tracing from top). A peristaltic wave proceeds along the body of the esophagus at a speed of 3 to 4 cm per second (third, fourth, and fifth tracings from top). While this peristaltic wave progresses along the body of the esophagus, the lower esophageal sphincter (LES, sixth tracing from top) relaxes to gastric pressure (bottom tracing). As the peristaltic wave approaches the stomach, relaxation of the LES is terminated and LES pressure returns to baseline resting pressure (30 mm Hg).

particular site along the esophagus ranges between 2 and 6 seconds, being shortest at the more cephalad sites and becoming progressively longer at more caudal sites. The velocity of propagation of these contractions along the esophageal body is 3 to 4 cm per second and remains fairly constant throughout the length of the esophagus.

A number of factors have been shown to influence the amplitude, duration, and propagation velocity of the peristaltic wave. Primary peristalsis associated with a fluid bolus results in a decreased velocity of peristalsis and an increased amplitude and duration of contraction as compared with a "dry" or bolus-free swallow. Increasing the temperature of the bolus serves to further increase the amplitude and duration of contractions and the velocity of peristalsis. Increases in intraabdominal pressure tend to slow the velocity of peristalsis.

Lower Esophageal Sphincter

During the intervals between swallows, the LES maintains a mean pressure of 10 to 30 mm Hg. Swallowing causes relaxation of the LES, which usually begins 1.5 to 2.5 seconds after the initiation of the swallow. Normally, the LES slowly relaxes to a pressure equal to that of intragastric pressure and persists for a total of approximately 8 seconds. During LES relaxation, the peristaltic wave in the esophageal body progresses aborally toward the LES. As this peristaltic wave approaches the LES, the LES pressure begins to increase and may eventually rise above resting tone in continuity with the peristaltic contraction in the esophageal body. This "after-contraction" of the LES may last up to 7 seconds before returning to baseline resting tone.

Symptoms of Esophageal Disease

The patient with an esophageal abnormality may present with a variety of symptoms. In general, esophageal-related symptoms include dysphagia, odynophagia, pyrosis, angina-like chest pain related to esophageal spasm, and regurgitation.

Dysphagia

Dysphagia is a specific term referring to the subjective sensation of food being obstructed as it passes from the mouth toward the stomach. It may indicate (1) a neuromuscular dysfunction of the pharynx or esophagus during a swallow; (2) an obstructing lesion located in the oropharynx, esophagus, or gastric cardia; or (3) an inflammatory process in the esophagus. Diseases of the oropharynx and esophagus capable of producing dysphagia are listed in Table 1-2. It is important that the physician evaluating a patient with complaints suggestive of dysphagia obtain a detailed history. The history should be initially directed at determining whether the patient does indeed have true dysphagia. Patients experiencing only pain with swallowing and no sensa-

Table 1-2
Classification of dysphagia

Obstructing lesions
  Malignant tumors
  Benign tumors
  Strictures
  Webs and rings
  Diverticula

Neuromuscular dysfunction
  Neurologic diseases
  Myasthenia gravis
  Muscular dystrophy
  Polymyositis
  Cricopharyngeal dysfunction
  Achalasia
  Diffuse esophageal spasm
  Nonspecific motility disorders
  Pseudo-obstruction
  Systemic diseases

Inflammatory lesions
  Reflux esophagitis
  Infectious esophagitis

tion of obstruction do not have true dysphagia but rather odynophagia (described in greater detail in the following paragraphs). A clear distinction between the two symptoms is usually important in directing the physician to the correct diagnosis. It is also helpful to differentiate dysphagia from globus hystericus, which refers to the sensation of a permanent "lump" or "foreign body" in the throat.

If it is determined that the patient has true dysphagia, it should then be determined whether the difficulty is due to oropharyngeal or esophageal dysphagia. Oropharyngeal dysphagia refers to difficulty in either the initiation of swallowing or the transfer of food from the mouth into the upper esophagus. Most frequently, patients with oropharyngeal dysphagia have a neuromuscular disease. They usually complain of nasal or oral regurgitation or coughing immediately after swallowing. There may be associated dysphonia or dysarthria. Less commonly, patients with oropharyngeal dysphagia have a pharyngeal pouch, web, or fistula.

If solids and liquids leave the mouth without difficulty and immediate regurgitation does not occur, the problem is most likely esophageal dysphagia. It should next be determined whether the cause falls into the category of a mechanical obstruction or a neuromuscular dysfunction or whether it is related to esophageal inflammation. Patients with a mechanical obstruction will usually initially experience dysphagia for solids only. The dysphagia is usually persistent and frequently progressive as the

Table 1-3
Causes of esophageal inflammation that can produce odynophagia

Infections
Herpes virus
Candidiasis
Caustic agents
Lye ingestion
Pills
Dermatologic diseases
Bullous pemphigoid
Epidermolysis bullosa dystrophica
Gastroesophageal reflux
Esophagitis
Ulcers
Malignancies
Adenocarcinoma

lumen gradually narrows. An exception to this is the case of the lower esophageal ring (Schatzki's ring), in which dysphagia is typically episodic. Patients with a neuromuscular disorder usually complain of dysphagia to both liquids and solids. The dysphagia is usually episodic and progresses at a slower rate than that caused by mechanical obstruction. This group of patients may experience spontaneous angina-like chest pain during the course of their illness. Regurgitation may become a prominent symptom in the later stages of the disease process.

Odynophagia

Odynophagia refers to the sensation of pain distinctly associated with the act of swallowing. This is most commonly a sharp or searing pain located at the back of the throat or in the upper chest that is not present between swallows. Odynophagia is usually associated with disorders causing diffuse and severe inflammation of esophageal mucosa. Various causes of esophageal inflammation that commonly result in odynophagia are listed in Table 1-3.

Pyrosis

Pyrosis, or heartburn, is the most common symptom related to the esophagus and typically refers to a burning-like pain that radiates from the epigastrium toward the throat and sometimes culminates in regurgitation of acidic contents. Although pyrosis is rarely referred to as pain, it is almost never associated with the act of swallowing and therefore is usually easily distinguished from odynophagia. Pyrosis is usually the primary symptom of gastroesophageal reflux disease.

Chest Pain of Esophageal Origin

Pain arising from the esophagus as a result of motility abnormalities may closely mimic that of coronary artery disease. The pain is frequently described as a squeezing, pressure-like sensation located retrosternally in the xiphoid region that may radiate into the arm or jaw. Although it is sometimes impossible to distinguish between a cardiac and esophageal source prior to more invasive studies, including cardiac catheterization, distinctions should be sought. The chest pain of cardiac disease is more clear if it is related to exercise, relieved immediately by nitroglycerin, and associated with signs of cardiac failure and electrocardiographic (ECG) abnormalities. The chest pain of esophageal spasm is not typically exercise-related, is relieved more slowly with nitroglycerin, and may be associated with intermittent dysphagia.

Regurgitation, Vomiting, and Reflux

Most patients are familiar with the word *vomiting* and therefore use it as a catch-all in attempting to describe the various processes of regurgitation, reflux, and vomiting or retching. Hence, in evaluating a patient for possible esophageal disease, it is important for the physician to clearly distinguish from the patient's history whether his or her symptoms are those of regurgitation, retching or vomiting, or reflux of gastric contents.

Regurgitation refers to the sudden, effortless return of small volumes of gastric or esophageal contents into the pharynx. Reflux refers strictly to the effortless flow of gastric contents into the esophagus. Vomiting or retching, on the other hand, refers to the powered projection of gastric contents from the mouth and is always associated with vigorous contraction of the abdominal musculature. The importance of clearly distinguishing between these various symptoms in the evaluation of a patient with possible esophageal disease will become clear in the following discussion of various esophageal motor disorders.

Esophageal Motor Disorders

Esophageal motor disorders are clinical abnormalities in esophageal motility caused by a disruption in the neurohumoral or muscular control of peristalsis or esophageal sphincter function. These disorders may be primary to the esophagus or part of a systemic disease. Table 1-4 lists both primary and secondary motor disorders of the esophagus. Because there are remarkable differences in the neuromuscular mechanisms controlling esophageal function in the striated and smooth muscle portions of the esophagus, this list has been broken down into those primarily involving striated muscle and those primarily involving smooth muscle.

Disorders of Smooth Muscle

Achalasia

Achalasia is characterized by three primary abnormalities in the function of the LES and smooth muscle portion of the esophageal body: (1) an absence of peristaltic activity in the esophageal

Table 1-4
Esophageal motor disorders

Disorders of smooth muscle
  Achalasia
  Diffuse esophageal spasm
  Nonspecific motility disorders
  LES incompetence
  Scleroderma
  Chagas' disease
  Diabetes mellitus
  Muscular dystrophies
  Myopathies (thyrotoxicosis, alcoholism, etc.)
  Amyloidosis
Disorders of striated muscle
  Cerebrovascular accidents
  Central nervous system tumors
  Neurologic diseases
    Myasthenia gravis
    Parkinsonism
  UES achalasia
  Premature UES closure

body, (2) increased resting tone of the LES, and (3) absent or incomplete relaxation of the LES with swallows. These motility abnormalities are usually readily apparent on manometric recordings of the esophagus. Figure 1-9 is an esophageal manometric recording from a patient with achalasia. The UES in achalasia functions normally, maintaining normal tone between swallows and relaxing normally with swallows (marked by the pharyngeal contractions). The esophageal body displays a slightly elevated resting tone between swallows and fails to show peristaltic activity in association with swallowing. In most cases of achalasia, the esophageal body contractions are of low amplitude and short duration. The LES typically displays an elevated resting tone and either partially relaxes or shows no relaxation to swallows. The normal LES relaxes greater than 90 percent of its maintenance tone above gastric pressure; in achalasia, the LES relaxes less than 50 percent of its maintenance tone above gastric pressure.

Etiology and Pathophysiology
The cause of primary achalasia remains unknown. However, there are a number of disorders that can in many ways mimic primary achalasia and thereby provide some insight into the pathophysiology of achalasia. These disorders are believed to mimic the manometric and x-ray findings of primary achalasia through various mechanisms of damage to intramural nerves of the esophagus. The best example of this is Chagas' disease, which is caused by a trypanosoma prevalent in South America. The parasite is transmitted to humans by insect bites and prefer-

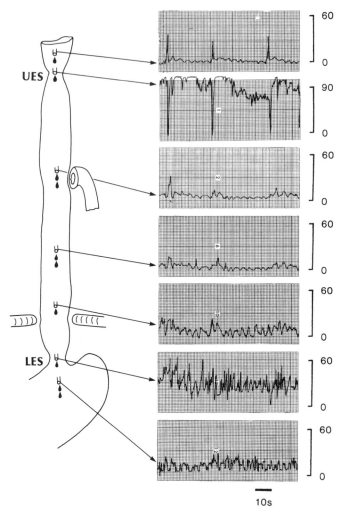

10s

Fig. 1-9

Manometric tracings showing intraluminal pressures recorded concurrently along the upper gastrointestinal tract in an individual with idiopathic achalasia. The uppermost tracing demonstrates three isolated increases in intraluminal pharyngeal pressure demarcating three swallows spaced at approximately 30-second intervals. There is normal baseline tone in the upper esophageal sphincter (UES) and normal relaxation with each swallow (second tracing from top). However, there is a marked decrease in the amplitudes and durations of contractions along the esophageal body in response to each of the three swallows (third, fourth, and fifth tracings from top). Moreover, these small amplitude contractions along the esophageal body are simultaneous in onset. As shown in the sixth tracing from the top, resting lower esophageal tone is somewhat elevated and does not show relaxation in response to any of the three swallows.

entially develops in smooth muscle cells. As it develops in the smooth muscle of the gastrointestinal tract, it releases a neurotoxic substance that damages intramural nerves. The destruction of nerves of the myenteric plexus of the esophagus results in a manometric and radiologic picture identical to that of primary achalasia.

Although the cause of primary achalasia remains unknown, there are several lines of evidence suggesting a defect in the intramural innervation of the esophagus. A number of pathologic studies have demonstrated a degeneration and diminution in the number of ganglion cells that make up the myenteric plexus. Moreover, physiologic studies have suggested a loss of intramural neurons in patients with achalasia. The loss of inhibitory neural input is believed to account for the elevated resting LES tone and impaired relaxation of the LES with swallows. In the body of the esophagus, the degeneration of intramural inhibitory and excitatory neurons is believed to lead to the low amplitude, short duration, and simultaneous contractions associated with swallowing.

Clinical Features
Primary achalasia is characteristically a disease of insidious onset that slowly progresses over a period of months or, more commonly, years. Dysphagia for both liquids and solids is the most common presentation and results from the absence of peristaltic contractions in the esophageal body and the incomplete relaxation of the LES. However, at times, the symptoms are so insidious in onset that a patient may present because of an abnormal chest x-ray demonstrating mediastinal widening. Unfortunately, once a dilated esophagus exists, therapy is less effective in allowing the esophagus to return to a semblance of its normal size and function. The symptoms of achalasia may vary during the course of the disease. Chest pain is not a feature of the disease once the disease is well established. However, many patients indicate episodic severe chest pain, which is often precipitated by cold liquids, early in the course of the disease. Regurgitation of food is generally not a feature of early disease, but as the esophagus becomes dilated and there is an increased retention of food in the esophagus, regurgitation readily occurs when the patient bends or assumes the supine position. Later in the disease, patients often awake to find food on their pillow. Since this food has never been in contact with gastric juices, it is rarely described as sour or bitter tasting. Predictably, asthma-like syndromes with nighttime wheezing and pneumonia may occur. Weight loss generally becomes significant as the obstruction to the passage of food worsens and increased retention and regurgitation occur.

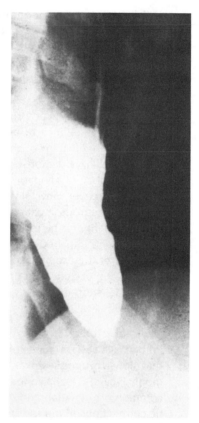

Fig. 1-10
Barium esophagram in a patient with idiopathic achalasia. The body of the esophagus is dilated (greater than 3 cm in diameter), and there is a distinct narrowing in the area of the lower esophageal sphincter (LES). The narrowing in the area of the LES is typically found in patients with achalasia and is described as "a bird-beak deformity."

Diagnosis

The diagnosis of primary achalasia is made by a combination of radiographic and manometric studies. A plain chest x-ray in a patient with achalasia may show a widened mediastinum (owing to dilatation of the esophagus) and an associated air-fluid level (owing to obstruction and retention of food). Barium swallow may reveal variable degrees of dilatation of the esophageal body. The normal barium-filled esophagus has a diameter of up to 3 cm. With increasing severity of disease, the barium swallow reveals a progressively more elongated, dilated (up to 10 cm), and tortuous esophagus. In addition to dilatation of the esophageal body, barium swallow typically reveals a bird-beak narrowing in the area of the hypertensive LES (Fig. 1-10). Upper endoscopy is useful only in ruling out disorders of the esophagus that may mimic achalasia, such as an infiltrating carcinoma. Esophageal motility studies are required to demonstrate the functional abnormalities characteristic of achalasia and provide quantitative information concerning the severity of the abnormality and response to treatment.

Treatment

Pneumatic dilatation and Heller myotomy remain the major modalities of treatment of achalasia. These procedures are aimed at relieving the obstruction to flow of esophageal contents by destroying the bands of circular smooth muscle fibers responsible for the hypertensive LES. Pneumatic dilatation involves the rupture of these bands of circular muscle fibers by means of various types of dilating devices positioned per os at the level of the LES. Heller myotomy consists of a thoracotomy and vertical incision extending along the serosal surface of the distal esophagus and transecting the circular muscle fibers that make up the LES. Approximately 80 percent of patients show marked improvement after surgical myotomy compared with 75 percent following dilatation. Unfortunately, successful destruction of the LES tone frequently gives rise to significant and sometimes disabling gastroesophageal reflux. For this reason, some surgeons prefer to perform some type of antireflux procedure (fundoplication) at the time of myotomy.

Medical pharmacologic therapy is less successful than surgical or pneumatic myotomy. Relieving the functional obstruction by decreasing resting LES pressure with long-acting nitrates or calcium channel blockers has been moderately successful in the earlier stages of the disease. These substances have been shown to produce relaxation of smooth muscle fibers making up the LES, thereby increasing esophageal clearance.

Diffuse Esophageal Spasm

Diffuse esophageal spasm (DES) is a rare motor disorder of the esophagus involving only the smooth muscle portion. This disorder is characterized by high amplitude, repetitive, nonperistaltic esophageal contractions often associated with chest pain. Although these abnormal contractions are frequently elicited by swallows, abnormal spontaneous contractions in the eosphagus also frequently occur in this disorder. DES is distinguished from achalasia by the normal function of the LES as well as by the intermittent presence of normal peristaltic sequences in DES.

Etiology and Pathophysiology

The cause of DES remains unknown. Because of the rarity of the disease, little information concerning the pathogenic mechanisms of DES is available. However, there are several disorders that partially mimic the esophageal manometric findings of DES.

These disorders, which include systemic lupus erythematosus (SLE), postradiation, and reflux esophagitis, may provide some insight into the pathogenesis of DES. Much like achalasia, DES appears to be due to damage of the esophageal nerves. The neural damage in DES appears to be far less extensive than that seen with achalasia. Some studies have suggested that myenteric ganglia are present but are infiltrated with inflammatory cells. It has also been hypothesized that the neural damage may be confined primarily to inhibitory nerves supplying the esophageal body and that this selective damage to inhibitory nerves might be due to intramural esophageal hypoxia. Such a decrease in inhibitory input along the smooth muscle portion would allow any excitatory input to the esophagus to become more apparent and could account for the simultaneous onset of large-amplitude, long-duration contractions seen with swallows and the occurrence of spontaneous and repetitive contractions.

Clinical Features

The criteria currently used for the diagnosis of DES include chest pain, dysphagia, and high-amplitude, long-duration, non-peristaltic contractions on esophageal motility study. The chest pain is often described as a pressure-like sensation in the retrosternal region that may closely mimic that of coronary artery disease. Both the chest pain and dysphagia are episodic in nature and tend to occur in association with ingestion of both liquids and solids. Interestingly, carbonated beverages and very hot or cold liquids may give rise to more severe symptoms. Since regurgitation is not a typical feature of DES, pulmonary symptoms and weight loss are rarely a problem.

Diagnosis

As mentioned previously, the diagnosis of DES is made by obtaining a history of episodic chest pain and dysphagia and by esophageal motility studies showing episodic nonperistaltic, long-duration, large-amplitude contractions of the distal esophagus (Fig. 1-11). Owing to the episodic nature of this disease, the esophageal motility study may be entirely normal in some persons. Provocative tests to increase the sensitivity of the esophageal motility in this group of patients include the intravenous administration of gastrin, bethanechol, and edrophonium as well as ice water swallows during the motility study.

The barium swallow in DES is usually normal. Less commonly, it may show segmental contractions of the distal esophagus, known as *tertiary contractions*. In extreme cases, these segmental contractions may produce a picture known as the *corkscrew esophagus*, which consists of deep asymmetric contractions,

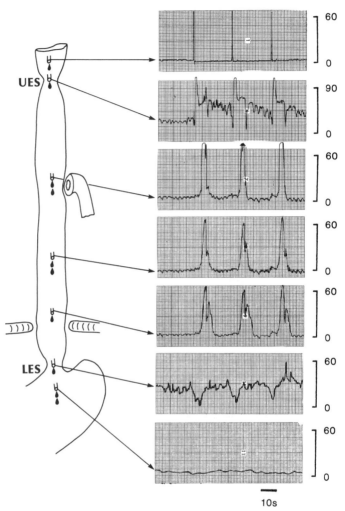

mm Hg

Fig. 1-11

Manometric tracings showing intraluminal pressures recorded concurrently along the upper gastrointestinal tract of an individual with diffuse esophageal spasm. The uppermost tracing demonstrates two isolated increases in intraluminal pharyngeal pressure associated with swallowing. There is normal upper esophageal sphincter (UES) tone and relaxation with swallowing (second tracing from top). The initial swallow demonstrates a normal peristaltic wave along the esophageal body (third, fourth, and fifth tracings) and normal relaxation of the lower esophageal sphincter (LES, sixth tracing from top). However, associated with the second swallow, there are large-amplitude, long-duration, simultaneous-onset contractions in the smooth muscle portion of the esophageal body (fourth and fifth tracings from the top).

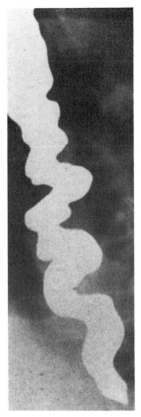

Fig. 1-12
Barium esophagram in a patient with diffuse esophageal spasm. There are multiple simultaneous segmental contractions in the body of the esophagus, known as *tertiary contractions*. This finding is often referred to as "a corkscrew esophagus."

separated by functional outpouchings, which may mimic diverticula (Fig. 1-12).

Treatment
Because reflux esophagitis may rarely be associated with esophageal spasm, patients are often treated initially for peptic esophagitis with the hope that treatment of acid reflux may resolve the spasm. This, however, is usually not successful, and most patients with spasm are therefore treated symptomatically. In approximately 25 percent of patients, nitrates are found to be effective in treating spasm. However, in the majority of patients, reassurance that the chest pain is not of cardiac origin is the most beneficial treatment. In some instances, rupturing some of the smooth muscle bundles of the distal esophagus by means of pneumatic dilatation has proved beneficial. Rarely, surgical my-

otomy has been required to relieve frequent and severe episodes of esophageal spasm.

Scleroderma (Progressive Systemic Sclerosis)
Scleroderma is a multisystem disorder characterized by fibrosis involving the skin and a variety of internal organs. The disease usually begins insidiously with tightness of the skin (sclerodactyly) and Raynaud's phenomenon. Raynaud's phenomenon refers to increased sensitivity of the fingers to cold and is characterized by pain and color changes in the distal portions of the fingers on exposure to cold. Although the hallmark of the disease is skin involvement, there may be internal organ involvement (most notably in the gastrointestinal tract, kidneys, heart, and lungs) in the absence of skin manifestations. Esophageal motility abnormalities occur in approximately 70 percent of patients with scleroderma.

Etiology and Pathophysiology
The primary event in the pathogenesis of scleroderma is postulated to be endothelial cell injury in blood vessels ranging from small arteries to capillaries. The cause of this endothelial damage is not known.

The prominent esophageal lesion in scleroderma is a patchy smooth muscle atrophy with fibrosis, which accounts for the decreased esophageal contractility and absence of resting LES tone. The predominant ultrastructural abnormalities in the esophagus are thickening of the basement membrane of capillaries along with a thickening of the dense bodies and plaques of smooth muscle fibers. Neural structures have been shown to be histologically normal with an abundance of neurosecretory granules. It is suggested that the basic abnormality is that of vascular insufficiency leading to smooth muscle atrophy and fibrosis. Additional support for this theory comes from the close association of Raynaud's phenomenon and esophageal dysfunction in sclerodermatous patients (see the following paragraph). This close association suggests a common pathogenic mechanism, such as the effect of ischemia.

Clinical Features
Patients with esophageal dysfunction owing to scleroderma almost always have Raynaud's phenomenon and generally have sclerodactyly. However, in some instances, the esophageal dysfunction and Raynaud's phenomenon may precede, by up to several years, the typical skin changes seen in scleroderma patients. In the earlier stages of the disease, the combination of LES incompetence and distal esophageal atony not only allows

free gastroesophageal reflux but deprives the esophagus of its usual mechanisms of acid clearance. Chronic esophagitis typically ensues and the symptom of heartburn becomes prominent. Persistence of this gastroesophageal reflux eventually leads to esophageal stricture formation. With increasing atony of the distal esophageal body and stricturing in the distal esophagus, heartburn may subside and dysphagia becomes the most prominent symptom.

Diagnosis

In the earlier stages of scleroderma, a normal diameter esophageal body, a slightly patulous LES, and a suggestion of a delay in the emptying of barium may be seen on barium swallow. However, as gastroesophageal reflux worsens, the barium swallow may show evidence of distal esophagitis, ulceration, and stricture formation. In the later stages of the disease, the barium swallow can give a picture identical to that of achalasia — namely, marked dilatation of the esophageal body and a bird-beak deformity in the area of the LES. However, unlike in achalasia where the bird-beak deformity is due to a hypertensive LES, this finding in scleroderma is due to the development of a stricture resulting from persistent gastroesophageal reflux.

Esophageal motility studies are much more reliable than radiologic studies in making the diagnosis of scleroderma. The characteristic finding on esophageal manometric studies is that of almost complete loss of any contractile activity in the smooth muscle portion of the esophagus, along with a marked decrease or absence of resting LES tone (Fig. 1-13). Function in the striated muscle portion, including the UES, remains entirely normal. The manometric findings of scleroderma in a patient with Raynaud's phenomenon are virtually diagnostic of the disease.

Treatment

Because the basic pathophysiologic process of scleroderma is not reversible, treatment becomes directed entirely toward attempting to control and treat the complications of gastroesophageal reflux disease (see Chap. 2).

Nonspecific Motility Disorders

Nonspecific motility disorders of the esophagus refers to a large group of motor abnormalities that do not fit into the classic descriptions of achalasia, DES, or scleroderma. The most frequently occurring of these abnormalities appears to be the normal peristaltic progression of high-amplitude, long-duration waveforms. Some investigators have labeled this motility ab-

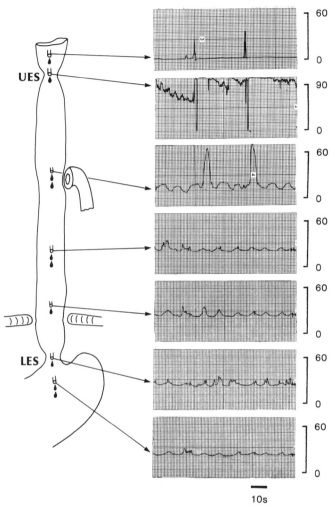

10s

Fig. 1-13

Manometric tracings showing intraluminal pressures recorded concurrently along the upper gastrointestinal tract in an individual with scleroderma. The uppermost tracing demonstrates two isolated increases in intraluminal pharyngeal pressure associated with the act of swallowing. There is normal baseline upper esophageal sphincter (UES) tone and relaxation with swallows (second tracing from top). In the body of the esophagus (third through sixth tracings from the top), resting tone is increased and equal to gastric pressure (bottom tracing). In the most cephalad (striated muscle) portion of the esophageal body (third tracing from top), there are normal contractions associated with swallows. However, in the more caudal (smooth muscle) portions of the esophageal body (fourth and fifth tracings from top), there are no contractions associated with swallows. Moreover, lower esophageal sphincter (LES) tone (sixth tracing from top) is markedly decreased and essentially identical to that of gastric pressure (bottom tracing).

normality as the "nutcracker esophagus," because the high-pressure squeezing of the esophageal body simulates that of a nutcracker.

Etiology and Pathophysiology
In most instances, the cause of the various nonspecific esophageal motility abnormalities is not known. The pathophysiology of this group of disorders is not well understood. This lack of understanding of the mechanisms responsible for producing these various motility abnormalities has most likely resulted in the grouping of widely different pathogenic disorders under the term *nonspecific motility disorders.*

The mechanism by which some of these motility abnormalities can produce symptoms of dysphagia or chest pain is not clear. For example, it is unclear how the normal peristaltic progression of high-amplitude, long-duration waveforms results in the symptoms of dysphagia or chest pain.

Clinical Features
The patient with a nonspecific motility abnormality most commonly presents with angina-like chest pain. In many instances, it is difficult to differentiate chest pain of esophageal origin from that of cardiac origin. For example, both types of chest pain can radiate into the arms or jaw and can be precipitated by emotional stress, relieved by nitroglycerin within 3 minutes, associated with vomiting and diaphoresis, and described as a tight, viselike pain.

Less commonly, the patient with a nonspecific motility abnormality may present with associated dysphagia or with dysphagia alone. The dysphagia is more commonly associated with solids but can occur with liquids.

Diagnosis
The diagnosis of a nonspecific motility abnormality is made by esophageal manometry studies. Barium swallow is most commonly normal but may show evidence of simultaneous contractions in the distal portion of the esophagus (tertiary contractions).

Treatment
Therapy for most nonspecific motility disorders is of unclear benefit. However, patients presenting with chest pain and dysphagia and demonstrating high-amplitude contractions on esophageal manometry studies may benefit from nitroglycerin, long-acting nitrates, or calcium channel blockers to decrease the force of smooth muscle contractions. In many instances,

confirmation that the pain is not cardiac, but probably esophageal in origin, is sufficient to allay patients' fears.

Disorders of
Striated Muscle

Oropharyngeal Paralysis

Disorders affecting the striated musculature of the esophagus also frequently involve the striated muscles of the pharynx and oral cavity. This is because the innervation of these structures has similar sites of origin in the central nervous system. In general, the primary clinical manifestations of this group of disorders is dysphagia localized to the neck and throat that is often associated with nasal regurgitation and tracheobronchial aspiration.

Etiology and Pathophysiology

A large number of neuromuscular diseases are known to cause motor disorders of the striated muscle portion of the esophagus and pharynx. These include disorders involving the central nervous system, the motor end-plate of somatic lower motor-neurons, and the striated musculature itself (see Table 1-3). A discussion of these various disorders is beyond the scope of this chapter.

Disorders causing paralysis of muscles of the oral cavity, including the tongue, generally produce difficulties in the initiation of a swallow. This is believed to occur because the tongue and lips are involved in the initial motor activities related to the act of swallowing. Disorders causing paralysis of pharyngoesophageal muscles generally produce dysphagia as well as a misdirection of the food bolus. This occurs because of a combination of weak and disordered pharyngeal contractions, poor opening and closure of the UES, and abnormal closure of the laryngeal and oropharyngeal musculature necessary to prevent intraluminal contents from passing into the respiratory tree and nasal passages.

Clinical Features

The clinical features of motor disorders of the striated muscle portion of the esophagus include dysphagia that is usually localized to the neck or upper chest and nasal regurgitation with tracheobronchial aspiration. In neurologic disorders involving a large degree of the oropharyngeal musculature, there is usually an inability, or refusal, to initiate a swallow.

Diagnosis

The diagnosis of a motor disorder involving the striated musculature of the upper gastrointestinal tract can usually be made by a detailed history of the patient and by physical examination. The characteristic history-taking and physical examination may reveal (1) a refusal, or inability, to initiate a swallow; (2) complaints of nasal or oral regurgitation or coughing immediately after swallowing; and (3) associated neurologic findings, such as dysphonia or dysarthria.

Owing to the rapidity of events in the pharyngoesophageal region during swallowing, radiologic studies of this area should include cinefluorography of the swallowing act with contrast material. The radiologic signs of neuromuscular disorders of this region include limited ascending movement of the hyoid bone or laryngeal cartilage, failure to develop a good pharyngeal stripping wave, poorly coordinated relaxation of the UES, spilling of barium into the airways, stasis of barium in the valleculae and pyriform sinuses, and absence of the primary peristaltic wave in the upper portion of the esophagus.

Manometric studies are helpful in showing a loss of contractility in the upper portion of the esophagus. However, because of the rapidity of events in the oropharyngeal region, currently available manometric recording systems are not capable of demonstrating subtle abnormalities in the coordination of events in this area.

UES Achalasia

The UES resting pressure normally falls to baseline pharyngeal pressure with swallows. Incomplete relaxation of the UES on swallowing is known as cricopharyngeal or UES achalasia. Although this entity is uncommon, it is believed to be one of several causes of dysphagia localized to the neck.

Etiology and Pathophysiology

Although UES achalasia has been described as an isolated phenomenon of unknown etiology, it occurs more commonly in association with other neurologic disorders such as bulbar paralysis, poliomyelitis, and recurrent laryngeal nerve paralysis.

The basis for the lack of complete relaxation of the UES is not fully understood. It may be due to impaired inhibition on swallowing of ongoing neural activity to the UES. Because the cell bodies of neurons innervating the UES are located in the brainstem, lesions of the brainstem could produce UES achalasia. Since such brainstem lesions are not well localized, other neurologic abnormalities should be present. It has been suggested that UES achalasia may also be due to spasm or fibrosis of the cricopharyngeus muscle.

Clinical Features

Dysphagia is the most prominent symptom of UES achalasia. In severe cases, an obstruction to the flow of substances from the

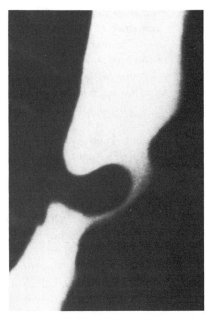

Fig. 1-14
Barium esophagram in a patient with upper esophageal sphincter (UES) achalasia. There is a maintained prominence of the cricopharyngeus muscle as recognized by the smooth contoured bar extending posteriorly into the esophageal lumen.

pharynx into the esophageal body may occur. In such instances, the bolus may be misdirected into the larynx, nasal cavities, and respiratory tree.

Diagnosis
The diagnosis of UES achalasia has been made mainly by a lateral x-ray of the hypopharynx revealing a partial obstruction to the barium bolus just above the cricopharyngeal muscle (Fig. 1-14). Manometric studies of this disorder using sophisticated low-compliance recording systems should be helpful in making the diagnosis but have not yet been described in UES achalasia. Motility studies using the more commonly available higher compliance systems are not helpful in making the diagnosis.

Treatment
In most cases of UES achalasia, treatment is not indicated because of the lack of a functional obstruction at the level of the cricopharyngeus muscle and the presence of more severe non-correctable associated neurologic abnormalities. However, in more severe cases in which there is complete obstruction at the level of the cricopharyngeal muscle, a cricopharyngeal myotomy may be indicated.

Premature Closure of the UES

Premature closure of the UES during the act of swallowing has been considered by some investigators to play an important role in the formation of a posterior pharyngeal pouch just above the cricopharyngeal muscle known as a Zenker's diverticulum. This view has been based primarily on radiologic studies suggesting an abnormal temporal relationship during the act of swallowing between pharyngeal contraction and UES relaxation and contraction. These studies have suggested that premature closure of the UES might result in an increased intraluminal pressure above the UES and the eventual formation of a posterior pharyngeal pouch, or Zenker's diverticulum. Supporting this view are reports that cricopharyngeal myotomy produces symptomatic relief as well as disappearance of the diverticulum in some patients. Recent low-compliance manometric recordings of the UES in patients with Zenker's diverticulum, however, have generally failed to show any abnormalities in the temporal relationship between pharyngeal contraction and UES relaxation and contraction. Further studies using high-quality manometric systems should be helpful in resolving this conflict in findings.

Study Questions

1. Are the following statements regarding achalasia true or false?
   a. The pressure in the lower esophageal sphincter (LES) is quite low and allows the severe gastroesophageal reflux often seen in this disease.
   b. Motility in the distal two-thirds of the esophagus is characterized by weak, simultaneous contractions following swallows.
   c. The abnormalities observed in LES function and esophageal motility are thought to be caused by the degeneration of inhibitory neurons.
   d. The dysphagia associated with this disease may respond to oral or sublingual administration of nitroglycerin and calcium channel blocking agents.
   e. The "birdbeak" narrowing of the distal esophagus, which is seen on radiographic barium studies in this disease, is due to reflux esophagitis with peptic stricture.

Answers

a. F
b. T
c. T
d. T
e. F

Achalasia is characterized by (1) a hypertensive LES that fails to relax with swallowing, and (2) absent peristalsis in the distal two-thirds of the esophagus. Swallows are associated with weak simultaneous contractions. These abnormalities are thought to be due to the degeneration of inhibitory neurons in the esophageal wall. The "birdbeak" narrowing of the distal esophagus observed on radiographic studies is caused by the hypertensive LES. Gastroesophageal reflux does not occur due to the hypertensive LES. In some patients, the dysphagia caused by the hypertensive LES may be ameliorated by nitroglycerin or calcium channel blockers, which produce relaxation of the LES.

2. A 53-year-old woman with scleroderma has a long history of Raynaud's phenomenon (vasoconstriction and blanching of the fingers with exposure to cold). Over the last 9 months she has experienced heartburn and the regurgitation of bitter and sour fluid into her mouth. Over the last 2 months she has noted increasing dysphagia to solid foods but is still able to swallow liquids easily. Which of the following statements is or are correct?
   a. A radiographic barium study will likely demonstrate a narrowing of the lumen in the distal esophagus.
   b. Esophageal manometry will demonstrate a very weak LES.
   c. The esophageal complications of scleroderma are associated with an increased risk of squamous carcinoma.
   d. Esophageal manometry will demonstrate weak, simultaneous contractions in the distal two-thirds of the esophagus.
   e. A full-thickness biopsy of the esophagus would demonstrate atrophy of the smooth muscle layer (muscularis externa).

Answers
a, b, d, e.
Sclerodermatous involvement of the esophagus results in marked atrophy of the smooth muscle in both the LES and the muscularis externa. These pathologic changes result in a hypotensive LES and weak, simultaneous contractions in the distal two-thirds of the esophagus. The clinical consequence of these changes would be severe gastroesophageal reflux with resulting peptic esophagitis and possibly a peptic stricture. The latter would be demonstrated as a narrowing of the esophageal lumen on radiographic studies. Squamous carcinoma of the esophagus is not a complication of either sclerodermatous involvement of the esophagus or peptic esophagitis.

References

Chey, W. Y. (ed.). *Functional Disorders of the Digestive Tract.* New York: Raven, 1983.

Clouse, R. E., Stenson, W. F., and Avioli, L. V. Esophageal motility disorders and chest pain. *Arch. Intern. Med.* 145:903, 1985.

Cohen, S. Motor disorders of the esophagus. *N. Engl. J. Med.* 301:191, 1979.

Crist, J. R. Dysphagia. In M. D. Aronson, and T. L. Delbanco (eds.), *Manual of Clinical Evaluation: Strategies for Cost-Effective Care.* Boston: Little, Brown, 1988. Pp. 143–150.

Goyal, R. K. Diseases of the Esophagus. In E. Braunwald, K. J. Isselbacher, R. G. Petersdorf, J. D. Wilson, et al. (eds.), *Harrison's Principles of Internal Medicine.* New York: McGraw-Hill, 1987. Pp. 1231–1239.

Hill, L., Kozarek, R., McCallum, R., et al. *The Esophagus: Medical and Surgical Management.* Philadelphia: Saunders, 1988.

Jones, B., and Donner, M. W. Examination of the patient with dysphagia. *Radiology* 167:319, 1988.

Ouyang, A., and Cohen, S. Motor Disorders of the Esophagus. In J. D. Berk (ed.), *Gastroenterology* (4th ed.). Philadelphia: Saunders, 1985. Pp. 690–704.

Vantrappen, G., and Hellemans, J. Treatment of achalasia and related motor disorders. *Gastroenterology* 79:144, 1980.

Wong, R. K. H., and Johnson, L. F. Achalasia. In D. O. Castell and L. F. Johnson (eds.), *Esophageal Function in Health and Disease.* New York: Elsevier, 1983. Pp. 99–117.

2 : Gastroesophageal Reflux Disease and Other Disorders of the Esophagus

Stuart Jon Spechler

Pathophysiology of Gastroesophageal Reflux Disease

Symptoms and Definitions

The reflux of noxious material from the stomach into the esophagus is sometimes accompanied by the symptom of heartburn, an unpleasant substernal burning sensation that moves up and down the chest in a wavelike fashion. If the refluxed material reaches the tongue, the patient may note a sour or bitter taste suggesting the presence of acid or bile, respectively. Regurgitation results when refluxed material appears in the mouth. Aspiration of this material into the airway can cause coughing, wheezing, and the sensation of choking. Laryngeal irritation by the aspirated fluid can cause hoarseness. Water brash, the sudden filling of the mouth with warm salty fluid, results when gastroesophageal reflux triggers reflex hypersecretion of saliva.

Refluxed material can damage the esophageal epithelium. The inflammatory injury so induced can progress to the point that areas of esophageal mucosa are destroyed. The resulting esophageal erosions and ulcerations may be manifested clinically by the symptom of painful swallowing (odynophagia). Mucosal erosions and ulcerations that injure esophageal blood vessels can cause hemorrhage. Ulceration into the submucosa may stimulate fibrous tissue production with esophageal stricture formation in some patients; dysphagia, the sensation that a swallowed bolus is impeded in its progress to the stomach, is a frequent complaint in these cases.

Reflux esophagitis is a nonspecific term used to refer to the symptoms or the esophageal injury (or both) that result from the reflux of noxious gastric contents into the esophagus. Pathologic gastroesophageal reflux and its manifestations are also called *gastroesophageal reflux disease*.

Pathophysiology of Gastroesophageal Reflux

Intragastric pressure ordinarily exceeds that in the thoracic esophagus. Therefore, gastroesophageal reflux would occur continuously in the absence of effective antireflux mechanisms. These mechanisms include the lower esophageal sphincter and,

Table 2-1
Mechanisms for gastroesophageal reflux

Lower esophageal sphincter (LES) mechanisms
  Weak basal LES pressure
  Inadequate LES response to increased abdominal pressure
  Inadequate LES response to gastric contraction
  Transient relaxation of the LES

Proposed anatomic abnormalities
  ? Hiatal hernia
  ? Short segment of esophagus subject to abdominal pressure

perhaps, some anatomic features of the gastroesophageal junction. Abnormalities in the antireflux mechanisms that might result in gastroesophageal reflux are listed in Table 2-1 and are discussed in the following paragraphs.

Lower Esophageal Sphincter
Normal Physiology
Manometric examination reveals a high pressure zone in the terminal 2 to 4 cm of the esophagus, which is called the *lower esophageal sphincter (LES)*. Tone in the specialized circular muscle that constitutes the LES maintains a resting pressure in this segment exceeding that in the stomach. The LES functions as the primary barrier to gastroesophageal reflux. With a swallow, the LES normally relaxes for 5 to 10 seconds to allow the bolus to enter the stomach. Secondary peristalsis (peristalsis induced by local esophageal stimulation rather than by swallowing) and esophageal distention also result in LES relaxation. With belching and vomiting, the LES relaxes to permit the egress of gas and other material from the stomach into the esophagus.

By routine anatomic dissection and histologic examination, the circular smooth muscle of the LES appears identical to that in the remainder of the esophagus. Functionally, however, LES muscle exhibits unique physiologic behavior that distinguishes it from adjacent esophageal muscle. Unlike circular muscle in the body of the esophagus, strips of LES circular muscle develop active tension with stretching, a property that is judged to contribute to the maintenance of sphincter pressure. Also, sphincter muscle is more sensitive to a variety of drugs, hormones, and other agents than is the adjacent esophageal muscle.

The innervation of the LES is complex. The vagus nerves supply the sphincter with preganglionic parasympathetic fibers from nerve cell bodies in the dorsal motor nucleus of the vagus. These preganglionic fibers synapse with postganglionic neurons in the wall of the esophagus. Sympathetic postganglionic fibers from the celiac ganglion and the thoracic greater splanchnic nerve also form synapses around neurons in the esophageal myenteric plexus. Axons from these intramural neurons are distributed to other neurons of the myenteric plexus and to the smooth muscle cells of the LES.

Some of the intramural neurons of the LES release an inhibitory neurotransmitter that causes relaxation of the sphincter muscle. The identity of this neurotransmitter is not clear. The inhibitory activity is not blocked by a variety of cholinergic and adrenergic antagonists, suggesting that the neurotransmitter is neither acetylcholine nor any of the adrenergic amines. One likely, but yet unproved, candidate for the role of inhibitory neurotransmitter is vasoactive intestinal peptide (VIP). The release of the inhibitory neurotransmitter from the postganglionic intramural neurons is engendered by the release of acetylcholine from the preganglionic vagal fibers. Thus, vagal stimulation can cause relaxation of the LES. Local stimuli such as esophageal distention can also cause sphincter relaxation by excitation of inhibitory neurons through extravagal pathways that involve other intramural neurons. This concept — that LES relaxation is caused by the stimulation of inhibitory neurons — is sometimes difficult to comprehend for those who are accustomed to regarding muscular excitation as the ultimate result of neural activity. There does appear to be excitatory cholinergic, adrenergic, and peptidergic innervation to the smooth muscle of the LES. These excitatory effects may be masked, however, by the release of the inhibitory neurotransmitter.

Pressure in the LES is generated by tone in its circular smooth muscle. In theory, basal LES pressure could be maintained by one, or a combination of two, mechanisms: (1) intrinsic tone in the circular muscle itself (i.e., tone independent neural stimulation), and (2) tonic neural stimulation of the sphincter muscle. In some animals, basal LES pressure is entirely the result of intrinsic tone in the sphincter muscle. In opossums, for example, basal sphincter pressure is unaffected by the administration of the antimuscarinic agent atropine and by chemical denervation of the LES with the nerve poison tetrodotoxin. Thus, tonic neural activity does not appear to contribute to basal LES pressure in this species. The human LES responds to the administration of atropine with a decrease in pressure, however. This implies that, in addition to intrinsic tone in the sphincter muscle, cholinergic neural activity contributes to the maintenance of resting LES pressure in humans.

LES pressure is affected by a variety of foods, drugs, hormones, and other agents in addition to the neural and muscular influences just discussed. For example, chocolate, nitrites, progesterone, and prostaglandin E_2 decrease sphincter pressure, whereas the administration of metoclopramide, prostaglandin $F_{2\alpha}$, and pharmacologic doses of gastrin increase pressure in the LES. An increase in intraabdominal pressure usually results in a simultaneous increase in LES pressure. This mechanism normally prevents gastroesophageal reflux during activities that increase intraabdominal pressure such as sneezing, coughing, and straining.

With all the endogenous and exogenous factors influencing the sphincter, it is not surprising that LES pressure fluctuates substantially throughout the day. The LES exhibits rhythmic pressure changes that occur at a rate of 3 to 4 per minute, as well as more dramatic phasic alterations in pressure that are related to myoelectrical phenomena in other parts of the gastrointestinal tract. In addition to these periodic alterations, LES pressure changes rapidly with body position and activities and with the ingestion of certain foods, drugs, and other agents. In clinical practice, it is common to record sphincter pressure during a brief esophageal manometric examination and to refer to the value so obtained as *the* LES pressure. It is important to realize, however, that no single value reflects the dynamic function of this sphincter, whose pressure can vary markedly from moment to moment.

Lower Esophageal Sphincter Mechanisms of Gastroesophageal Reflux

Weak Basal LES Pressure. A persistent notion, popularized in the early 1970s, attributes virtually all gastroesophageal reflux to weak basal LES pressure. This notion is based on early studies that suggested that subjects could be separated neatly into groups of symptomatic refluxers and asymptomatic nonrefluxers on the basis of sample LES pressure values. In some studies, all the symptomatic refluxers were found to have sample LES pressure values less than 10 mm Hg above gastric pressure, whereas asymptomatic nonrefluxers all had pressures exceeding 10 mm Hg. The weak LES was judged to pose an inadequate barrier to reflux and was therefore deemed "incompetent."

Other investigators did not observe such a neat distinction between refluxers and nonrefluxers on the basis of sample LES pressure values. Many patients with gastroesophageal reflux disease were found to have sample LES pressure values in the "normal" range. This finding cast doubt on the notion that all gastroesophageal reflux was the result of feeble resting LES pressure. In theory, furthermore, reflux should not occur so long as pressure in the LES exceeds that in the stomach by any increment, even a small one.

One possible explanation for the apparent disparities between these studies is the recent observation that LES pressure fluctuates dramatically throughout the day. Therefore, a single sample value may not be representative of a patient's true "basal" LES pressure. Differences in patient selection could also account for the differences in study results. Patients with endoscopic evidence of severe esophagitis tend to have lower sample LES pressure values than those with mild esophagitis on endoscopic examination. In studies limited to patients with severe esophagitis, one would expect to find weaker sphincter pressures than in studies that included patients with milder degrees of esophageal inflammation. Another explanation for the disparities is that weak basal LES pressure is not an important mechanism for gastroesophageal reflux in all subjects.

A group of investigators at the Medical College of Wisconsin studied the mechanisms of acid reflux in esophagitis patients using a technique that combined prolonged measurement of LES pressure with simultaneous monitoring of intraesophageal pH. For some patients, feeble resting LES pressure was the predominant mechanism of reflux. In these patients, there were extended periods of time during which LES pressure remained at or near zero; spontaneous reflux of acid was observed during these periods. For other patients in the study, weak LES pressure was not an important reflux mechanism. The mechanisms of reflux in these patients are discussed in the following paragraphs.

The following conclusions about basal LES pressure in patients with gastroesophageal reflux disease appear to be justified: (1) Mean values of LES pressure are lower in patients with gastroesophageal reflux disease than in healthy control subjects. (2) Because of the considerable overlap of values among individuals in those groups, sample LES pressure values do not reliably differentiate subjects with gastroesophageal reflux disease from those without pathologic reflux. (3) For some patients with reflux esophagitis, reflux occurs predominantly when basal LES pressure falls to or near 0 for extended periods of time. (4) Weak resting LES pressure alone does not account for reflux in all patients with gastroesophageal reflux disease.

Inadequate LES Response to Increased Abdominal Pressure. Contractions of the diaphragm and of the abdominal muscles (as occur with coughing, sneezing, straining, and leg raising) can cause sudden dramatic increases in abdominal pressure. Fortunately, these sudden pressure elevations in the abdomen are usually accompanied by simultaneous increases in LES pressure, which prevent the reflux of gastric contents that would otherwise attend every such episode. The mechanism of this LES response is not clear, and some experimental data are contradictory. Some investigators have proposed that the increased LES pressure is the result of a cholinergic reflex, mediated through the vagus nerves, that is triggered by increased abdominal pressure. In contrast, some recent investigations have not found evidence for such a cholinergic reflex mechanism. In these studies, it has been observed that increases in abdominal pressure cause commensurate increases in LES pressure that appear to be the result of a purely mechanical buttressing effect of the increased ambient pressure on the sphincter.

Sometimes, sudden increases in abdominal pressure are not attended by similar elevations in LES pressure. During these episodes, when intraabdominal pressure exceeds that of the sphincter, material in the stomach can be propelled into the esophagus by the resulting pressure gradient. This occurs occasionally in normal subjects. Furthermore, for some patients with reflux esophagitis, this inadequate LES response to sudden increases in abdominal pressure is the predominant mechanism of gastroesophageal reflux.

Inadequate LES Response to Gastric Contractions. A mechanism for reflux, similar to that associated with the sudden increases in abdominal pressure described in the preceding section, may be associated with increases in intragastric pressure caused by gastric contractions. LES pressure normally rises during gastric contractions — a response that appears to be mediated through the vagus nerves. An inadequate rise in LES pressure associated with gastric contractions could result in reflux when intragastric pressure exceeds that of the LES. It is not yet clear whether this is an important mechanism for gastroesophageal reflux.

Transient Relaxation of the LES. Both primary and secondary esophageal peristalsis are accompanied by relaxation of the LES, thus allowing esophageal contents to be propelled into the stomach. Recent studies involving extended monitoring of LES pressure have noted episodes of LES relaxation lasting 5 to 30 seconds that are not attended by esophageal peristalsis. Such episodes, called *transient LES relaxations,* are found both in normal subjects and in patients with gastroesophageal reflux disease. Studies in animals suggest that these isolated LES relaxations represent the incomplete expression of either the swallowing reflex or the reflex that mediates secondary peristalsis.

Transient complete relaxation of the LES unaccompanied by peristalsis provides an opportunity for the reflux of gastric contents into the esophagus. Episodes of gastroesophageal reflux can be found by extended intraesophageal pH monitoring in most normal subjects. In these subjects, more than 90 percent of such reflux episodes occur during periods of transient LES relaxation. Transient LES relaxation also appears to be the predominant mechanism of reflux for most patients with gastroesophageal reflux disease. These patients have more frequent episodes of transient LES relaxation and a higher prevalence of acid reflux associated with such episodes than do normal subjects. For some patients, reflux occurs almost exclusively during periods of transient LES relaxation.

Transient relaxation of the LES unaccompanied by peristalsis has only recently been identified as an important cause of reflux. This mechanism appears to explain some observations that puzzled earlier investigators. For example, it accounts for the reason that sample LES pressure values are normal in some patients with gastroesophageal reflux disease; transient LES relaxation could be the predominant reflux mechanism in these cases. Drugs that increase resting LES pressure may not affect transient LES relaxations; this could explain the failure of these medications to decrease reflux for some patients despite a significant increase in their resting LES pressure values. Also, the phenomenon of transient LES relaxation could explain the observation that 50 percent of patients with gastroesophageal reflux disease have no barium reflux seen in fluoroscopic examination. For patients who reflux by this mechanism, no barium reflux would be demonstrable unless a transient LES relaxation occurred during the brief period of the fluoroscopic examination. Despite the appeal of this recently discovered phenomenon, however, it is important to recognize that further studies are needed to confirm and elucidate the role of transient LES relaxation in the pathogenesis of gastroesophageal reflux disease.

In summary, three important LES mechanisms for gastroesophageal reflux have been identified: (1) weak basal LES pressure, (2) inadequate LES response to increased abdominal pressure, and (3) transient LES relaxation. These mechanisms are illustrated in Fig. 2-1. The relative importance of the three mechanisms varies among individual patients. For some patients, one mechanism predominates; for others, all three mechanisms are important. Transient LES relaxation appears to be the most prevalent of the three mechanisms and the predominant cause of gastroesophageal reflux in normal subjects.

Other Mechanisms for Gastroesophageal Reflux
The LES appears to be the major barrier to gastroesophageal reflux, and LES mechanisms are believed to account for most

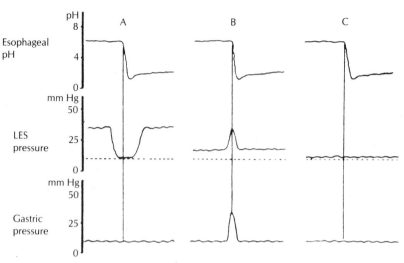

Fig. 2-1
Schematic representation of three different mechanisms for gastroesophageal reflux. Gastroesophageal reflux (shown as vertical lines) may accompany: (A) a transient LES relaxation, (B) an inadequate lower esophageal sphincter (LES) response to increased abdominal pressure, or (C) a period of feeble LES pressure. (From W. J. Dodds, J. Dent, W. J. Hogan, et al. Mechanisms of gastroesophageal reflux in patients with reflux esophagitis. Reprinted with permission from the *New England Journal of Medicine* 307:1547, 1982.)

reflux episodes. Other reflux mechanisms have been proposed, some of which are discussed in the following sections. The contribution of these mechanisms to the pathogenesis of gastroesophageal reflux is difficult to quantify, however, and their roles (if any) in the development of reflux esophagitis are not clear.

Hiatal Hernia and Anatomic Features of the Gastroesophageal Junction

It was once believed that anatomic features of the gastroesophageal junction (e.g., the angle with which the esophagus joins the stomach, compression of the esophagus by the diaphragm, or the gastric sling fibers) constituted a mechanical valve that functioned as the primary barrier to reflux. Herniation of the stomach into the chest through the esophageal hiatus of the diaphragm (hiatal hernia) was judged to disrupt these anatomic features and to result in gastroesophageal reflux. This notion that hiatal hernia was tantamount to reflux esophagitis prevailed for decades and was the rationale for hiatal herniorrhaphy in the treatment of gastroesophageal reflux disease. In the 1970s, at least three factors contributed to discredit the notion that hiatal hernia was the primary cause of reflux: (1) It was shown that many patients with reflux esophagitis had no demonstrable hiatal hernia and that many patients with hiatal hernia had no evidence of reflux esophagitis. (2) Simple hiatal herniorrhaphy had been found to be an ineffective therapy for many patients with reflux esophagitis. (3) With the availability of instruments capable of reliably recording esophageal pressures, investigators could better appreciate the importance of the physiologic LES as an antireflux mechanism.

Despite the many years of controversy, the role of hiatal hernia in the pathogenesis of gastroesophageal reflux disease remains unclear. There are data to suggest that the normal anatomic features of the gastroesophageal junction may augment the LES as an antireflux mechanism, and there is a strong association between severe reflux esophagitis and hiatal hernia. On the other hand, association is not proof of cause and effect, and most patients with hiatal hernia have no symptoms of reflux disease. If hiatal hernia does contribute to reflux, that contribution cannot be quantified precisely at the present time.

Short Segment of Esophagus Subject to Abdominal Pressure
The phrenoesophageal membrane is a segment of endoabdominal fascia that anchors the esophagus to the diaphragm. The membrane arises from the inferior surface of the diaphragm and normally extends upward across the hiatus to insert in the distal esophagus approximately 3 cm above the gastroesophageal junction. Thus, the phrenoesophageal membrane surrounds the distal esophagus in a tentlike fashion. Presumably, the segment of esophagus surrounded by phrenoesophageal membrane is subject to abdominal pressure. There are data to suggest that this esophageal exposure to abdominal pressure plays a role in the antireflux mechanism, with antireflux efficacy directly related to the length of the segment so exposed. An abnormally short segment of esophagus subject to abdominal pressure has been proposed as a mechanism for gastroesophageal reflux. The importance of this mechanism is controversial and difficult to quantify.

Gastric Volume
The presence of material in the stomach is a prerequisite for gastroesophageal reflux. Despite favorable pressure gradients, no reflux occurs when the stomach is empty. Furthermore, the frequency of gastroesophageal reflux episodes increases as gastric volume increases. This may be related to an increased frequency of transient LES relaxations, which has been observed in association with meals and with distention of the stomach.

Three processes contribute material to the gastric lumen: (1) ingestion, (2) gastric secretion, and (3) reflux of material from the duodenum. Gastric volume varies directly with the rates of these three processes. Increases in those rates might predispose to gastroesophageal reflux by increasing gastric volume. Conversely, gastric volume varies inversely with the rate of gastric emptying. Mechanical obstruction of the gastric outlet or abnormalities in gastric motor function can delay gastric emptying. These disorders may result in increased gastric volume and, consequently, increased gastroesophageal reflux. Also, gastric distention can stimulate gastric acid secretion, which further increases gastric volume. Delayed gastric emptying probably contributes to reflux disease in some patients, but the frequency of the disorder among the general population of patients with reflux esophagitis is not clear.

Factors Contributing to Esophageal Injury by Refluxed Material
The degree of esophageal injury induced by an episode of gastroesophageal reflux depends on the character of the refluxed material, the rate with which that material is cleared from the esophagus, and the ability of the esophageal mucosa to resist injury.

Character of the Refluxed Material
Reflux-induced injury is largely a function of the noxious properties of the refluxed material. For example, the reflux of gastric acid and pepsin is likely to be attended by more esophageal damage than is the reflux of water. Stomach contents available for reflux are a combination of ingested material, gastric secretions, and material refluxed from the small intestine. Little information is available on the effects of foods on the esophageal mucosa. Some studies have focused on the effects of acid, pepsin, bile salts, and pancreatic proteases on the esophagus.

The parietal and chief cells of the stomach secrete hydrochloric acid and pepsinogen, respectively. Hydrochloric acid at pH less than or equal to 2 causes denaturation of protein and demonstrable esophageal injury. Peptic digestion of protein in the esophageal epithelium can occur when hydrochloric acid activates pepsinogen to pepsin. Acid-pepsin injury to the esophagus is more severe than that caused by a similar concentration of hydrochloric acid alone. Small intestinal contents can also reflux into the stomach and, hence, into the esophagus. Noxious materials present in small intestinal contents include bile salts and pancreatic digestive enzymes. The combination of acid, pepsin, and bile salts has been shown to be particularly damaging to the esophageal mucosa. The pancreatic protease trypsin has also been found to cause esophageal injury. Other noxious substances such as lysolecithin are found in the lumen of the proximal small bowel, but few data are available concerning the role of these substances in producing esophageal injury. Acid and pepsin traditionally have received the most attention as injurious agents in gastroesophageal reflux disease, and medical therapy for this disorder often focuses on reduction of gastric acid. It is important to realize, however, that other noxious substances can be present in the stomach and that these substances may be important in the pathogenesis of esophagitis for some patients. For these patients, antacid therapy alone (e.g., with histamine H_2-receptor blockers) may not result in the healing of reflux esophagitis.

Esophageal Clearance
Esophageal injury increases with the duration of contact between the mucosa and the noxious refluxed material. This duration of contact is determined by the efficacy of esophageal clearance mechanisms. Effective clearance mechanisms may empty the esophagus of noxious material before injury results. Conversely, ineffective clearance mechanisms can result in prolonged contact between mucosa and noxious material, with consequent extensive esophageal damage.

Esophageal clearance mechanisms include gravity and peristalsis. In the upright posture, gravity enhances esophageal emptying, whereas in recumbency, gravity retards esophageal clearance. Both primary peristalsis (initiated by a swallow) and secondary peristalsis (initiated by local stimulation of the esophagus) are important mechanisms for esophageal clearance. Healthy subjects swallow approximately once a minute while awake. Thus, primary peristalsis occurs frequently in healthy individuals throughout the day. Swallowing, and hence primary peristalsis, decreases dramatically during sleep. Material refluxed during sleep may have prolonged contact with the esophagus because of recumbency and because of the decreased frequency of primary peristalsis. Therefore, nocturnal reflux episodes may be particularly damaging to the esophagus.

Some patients with reflux disease have esophageal motility disorders that interfere with esophageal clearance. It can be difficult to determine whether these motor abnormalities are a cause or an effect of the esophagitis. For some cases, the motility disorder improves with healing of the reflux disease, suggesting that the esophagitis caused or exacerbated the motor abnormality. For others, healing of the esophagitis has no apparent effect on the motility disorder; this suggests that the motor dysfunction antedated and perhaps contributed to the reflux esophagitis. For many patients with gastroesophageal reflux disease, no esophageal motility disorder is demonstrable. Furthermore, some patients with abnormal acid clearance have apparently normal esophageal motility on manometric examination.

The discussion on esophageal clearance has thus far pertained primarily to the emptying of a volume of material from the esophageal lumen. The restoration of normal esophageal pH involves more than the simple emptying of acid volume, however. The pH is a function of the concentration of hydrogen ions in a solution, not its volume. One drop of 0.1 N hydrochloric acid has the same pH as 1 liter of 0.1 N hydrochloric acid. Quantitative studies on esophageal emptying of radiolabeled material show that more than 95 percent of an acid bolus injected into the esophagus is cleared rapidly by peristalsis, but intraesophageal pH does not rise until the small amount of residual acid is either neutralized or diluted. Even if gravity and peristalsis clear the bulk of refluxed acid from the esophageal lumen, the small amount of acid left behind in contact with the mucosa may cause injury.

Salivation appears to be an important mechanism for clearing acid from the esophagus. While awake, healthy individuals secrete approximately 0.5 ml of saliva per minute; salivary secretion virtually ceases during sleep. The pH of saliva under basal conditions is approximately 7. Both its pH and its capacity to neutralize acid increase during the stimulated salivary flow that occurs with sucking on a lozenge or with the administration of a cholinergic drug. Swallowed saliva can neutralize small amounts of acid in the esophageal lumen. Following the administration of an acid bolus, esophageal pH has been shown to return to normal in a series of step increases (Fig. 2-2). Each step increase in pH is associated with a primary peristaltic sequence during which swallowed saliva neutralizes a portion of the residual acid. Although it is conceivable that abnormalities in salivation leading to ineffective neutralization of esophageal acid may contribute to gastroesophageal reflux disease in some patients, few data are available on this subject.

In summary, it appears that the bulk of refluxed acid volume is emptied from the esophagus by peristalsis and that swallowed saliva neutralizes the small amount of residual acid. Delayed esophageal clearance can result in prolonged contact of noxious refluxed material with the esophageal mucosa. Abnormalities in esophageal emptying and acid clearance may contribute to gastroesophageal reflux disease for some patients.

Mucosal Resistance
Examination of esophageal biopsy specimens from patients with chronic reflux esophagitis often reveals increased thickness of

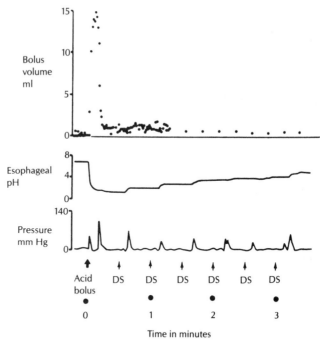

Fig. 2-2

Relations of esophageal volume clearance, esophageal acid clearance, esophageal motor activity, and swallowing. Only peristaltic pressure complexes from the distal esophagus are shown. Despite clearance of an injected acid bolus volume to less than 1 ml by a secondary peristaltic sequence, esophageal pH does not begin to rise until the first dry swallow (DS) 30 seconds after bolus injection. Esophageal pH returns to normal in a series of step increases associated with swallowing. (From J. F. Helm, W. J. Dodds, L. R. Pelc, et al. Effect of esophageal emptying and saliva on clearance of acid from the esophagus. Reprinted with permission from the *New England Journal of Medicine* 310:284, 1984.)

the basal cell layer, the proliferative zone for the stratified squamous epithelium. This histologic finding suggests a proliferative response of the mucosa to chronic irritation. Further evidence for increased cellular proliferation in response to reflux injury comes from organ culture studies on esophageal biopsy specimens from patients with reflux disease. These studies show increased uptake of radiolabeled thymidine by the cells of the basal layer. Severe esophagitis results when the proliferative capacity of the epithelium is overwhelmed by injurious factors.

Healthy individuals regularly experience brief episodes of gastroesophageal reflux but do not develop signs or symptoms of esophagitis. Apparently the normal esophageal mucosa can temporarily resist the injurious effects of refluxed material. The mechanisms whereby the esophageal epithelium resists injury are not completely understood.

Normally, the esophageal mucosa is impermeable to hydrogen ions and to a variety of other molecules. This property is referred to as the *esophageal mucosal barrier*. Disruption of the esophageal mucosal barrier — that is, increased permeability to hydrogen ions and other molecules — has been observed in the early phases of esophageal injury induced by noxious agents in a variety of animal models. Mucosal barrier disruption by these agents can occur in the absence of demonstrable histologic damage and may play a role in potentiating esophageal injury. It is conceivable that some patients with gastroesophageal reflux disease have abnormalities of the mucosal barrier or other mucosal defects that decrease resistance to injury by gastric juice. Proof for this hypothesis, however, is not yet available.

Heterogeneity of Gastroesophageal Reflux Disease

As discussed previously, the development of gastroesophageal reflux disease appears to be a multifactorial process. Factors that play a major pathogenetic role for some patients may have no importance for others. Thus, reflux esophagitis is the common clinical manifestation of a heterogeneous group of disorders. This explains why treatments that are used to correct a specific pathophysiologic defect may not be effective for all cases. Appreciation of the heterogeneity of gastroesophageal reflux disease allows for flexibility in treating individual patients.

Complications of Gastroesophageal Reflux Disease

Ulceration and Stricture of the Esophagus

Often, the histologic changes of reflux esophagitis are limited to the mucosa of the esophagus. In some patients, the esophageal inflammation erodes through the muscularis mucosa into the submucosa and muscularis propria. The resulting ulcer may cause hemorrhage if it damages large blood vessels or, uncommonly, may perforate the esophagus. The submucosal inflammation may also result in the production of fibrous tissue with subsequent esophageal stenosis. Such stenoses are often called *peptic* strictures because they are presumed to be the result of peptic injury to the esophagus. Thus, erosive esophagitis and ulceration are judged to be the precursors of esophageal stricture.

Strictures complicate approximately 10 percent of cases of reflux esophagitis evaluated by gastroenterologists. It is unclear why only the minority of these patients develop esophageal ulcerations and strictures. Very weak LES pressures and nonspecific disorders of esophageal motility have been observed in patients with peptic strictures, but these same abnormalities can be found for patients with uncomplicated reflux esophagitis. Esophageal strictures are discussed further in the section entitled Mechanical Causes of Dysphagia.

Barrett's Esophagus

Barrett's esophagus is the condition wherein the squamous mucosa that normally lines the distal esophagus is replaced by a columnar epithelium resembling that of the stomach and intestines. Barrett's epithelium can be found in 8 to 20 percent of patients who undergo endoscopic examinations for evaluation of gastroesophageal reflux disease. The aberrant columnar mucosa appears to be acquired through the process of metaplasia (the replacement of one adult cell type by another). The pathogenesis of Barrett's epithelium is judged to involve reflux-induced ulceration of the squamous epithelium, followed by reepithelialization of the ulcer with multipotential, undifferentiated stem cells. In the abnormal milieu of chronic gastroesophageal reflux, it is believed that these stem cells differentiate into columnar cells.

Three types of aberrant columnar epithelia have been found in patients with Barrett's esophagus (Fig. 2-3): (1) a distinctive specialized columnar epithelium that has a villiform surface and crypts lined by goblet cells, mucus-secreting columnar cells, enteroendocrine cells, and Paneth cells; (2) a junctional-type epithelium similar to that of the normal gastric cardia in which the surface, pits, and glands are lined by mucus-secreting cells; and (3) an atrophic gastric fundic-type epithelium, whose glands contain parietal and chief cells in addition to mucus-secreting cells. Zonation is often observed when two or more types of Barrett's epithelia occur together, with specialized columnar epithelium adjacent to squamous mucosa in the proximal segment, followed by junctional type mucosa, with atrophic gastric fundic-type epithelium in the most distal zone. Specialized columnar epithelium is the most common of the three epithelial types in adults with Barrett's esophagus.

Barrett's esophagus has clinical importance because of its association with esophageal cancer. For patients with Barrett's esophagus, the risk of developing an esophageal carcinoma is increased 30- to 40-fold above that of the general population. Although squamous cell carcinoma is the most common histologic type of esophageal cancer in the general population, adenocarcinoma is the histologic type of malignancy associated with Barrett's epithelium. Most adenocarcinomas of the esophagus are judged to have arisen from Barrett's epithelium.

Pulmonary Problems

Refluxed gastric material can be aspirated into the airway, resulting in coughing, wheezing, and even aspiration pneumonia. The mechanism whereby the refluxed material traverses the up-

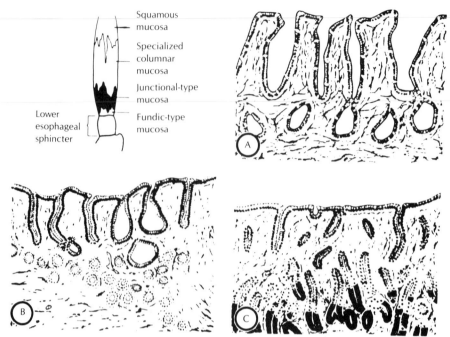

Fig. 2-3
Distribution (top left panel) and morphologic features (A, B, and C) of the three types of epithelia in Barrett's esophagus. In A, specialized columnar epithelium is shown; both the villiform surface and the crypt-like glands are lined by goblet cells (clear and oval) and by cells that resemble small intestinal absorptive cells but that contain mucous granules similar to those in gastric foveolar cells. In B, gastric junctional-type epithelium is shown, in which the surface, pits, and glands are lined by mucus-secreting cells. In C, gastric fundic-type epithelium is seen, in which the pitted surface is lined by mucus-secreting cells. The glands contain parietal cells (large, clear) and chief cells (dark), as well as mucus-secreting cells. (From S. J. Spechler and R. K. Goyal. Barrett's esophagus. Reprinted with permission from the *New England Journal of Medicine* 315:362, 1986.)

per esophageal sphincter in such cases is not known. Even without aspiration, acid infused into the esophagus has been found to cause wheezing and changes in small airway resistance in some asthmatics, presumably through a reflex mechanism. The prevalence of gastroesophageal reflux is high among children with asthma and among adult asthmatics in whom skin tests for common allergens are negative. Furthermore, radioisotopes instilled into the stomachs of some patients with asthma have been detected in their lungs, suggesting pulmonary aspiration of gastric contents in these cases. The association of reflux and asthma does not prove cause and effect, however. The true frequency and importance of gastroesophageal reflux disease in patients with pulmonary disorders is unclear.

Table 2-2
Pathophysiologic defects demonstrated by diagnostic
tests for gastroesophageal reflux disease

Diagnostic test	Reflux	Acid reflux	Mucosal damage	Association of esophageal acid and chest pain
Barium swallow	+		+	
Radionuclide scan	+			
pH probe		+		+
Esophagoscopy	+		+	
Esophageal biopsy			+	
Acid perfusion test				+

Diagnostic Tests for Gastro-esophageal Reflux Disease

The basic pathophysiology of gastroesophageal reflux disease is as follows: Noxious material refluxed from the stomach into the esophagus causes injury to the esophageal mucosa and chest pain. Diagnostic tests for gastroesophageal reflux disease exploit these pathophysiologic features. Tests are available to ascertain the presence of gastroesophageal reflux, to document the occurrence of acid reflux, to estimate the degree of reflux-induced damage to the esophageal mucosa, and to provide evidence that the patient's chest pain is the result of acid reflux. Some common diagnostic tests for gastroesophageal reflux disease and the pathophysiologic defects they reveal are summarized in Table 2-2.

Barium Swallow
The barium swallow is often the first diagnostic test used to evaluate the patient with suspected gastroesophageal reflux disease. It is an insensitive test for demonstrating reflux, however. Reflux of barium is observed fluoroscopically in fewer than 50 percent of patients with verified reflux esophagitis. For patients who reflux by the mechanism of transient LES relaxation, no reflux would be demonstrable unless such relaxations occur during the brief period of the fluoroscopic examination. This might account for the insensitivity of the barium swallow, because transient LES relaxation appears to be the predominant reflux mechanism for many patients. The frequent failure to demonstrate reflux fluoroscopically may also be related to the physical properties of barium, which differ in some respects from those of gastric juice (e.g., weight, viscosity).

In addition to its role in demonstrating reflux, the barium swallow can reveal reflux-induced esophageal abnormalities such as thickened folds, ulcerations, and strictures. These abnormalities are not specific for gastroesophageal reflux disease, however. In addition, these abnormalities are usually associated only with severe disease; the barium swallow is normal for many patients with mild or moderate reflux esophagitis. Because of these problems with sensitivity and specificity, other diagnostic tests, in addition to the barium swallow, are required for many patients.

Radionuclide Imaging Techniques

Radionuclide imaging techniques appear to be more sensitive than the barium swallow for demonstrating gastroesophageal reflux. Patients ingest a known quantity of a radionuclide such as ^{99m}Tc sulfur colloid, after which the areas of the esophagus and stomach are scanned for evidence of radioactivity. Gastroesophageal reflux results in persistent radioactivity in the area of the esophagus. Because the amount of radionuclide ingested is known, a quantitative estimate of the amount of reflux can be made.

Intraesophageal pH Monitoring

Intraesophageal pH monitoring is a sensitive technique for detecting acid reflux. A pH electrode is passed into the esophagus through the nose or mouth, and acid reflux is manifested by a sudden drop in intraesophageal pH. One modification of this technique involves the instillation of a quantity of 0.1 N hydrochloric acid into the stomach, followed by the performance of a variety of movements designed to elicit gastroesophageal reflux (e.g., leg raising, Valsalva's maneuver). Acid reflux is detected by the esophageal pH electrode.

Holter monitoring of intraesophageal pH for periods of 24 hours or longer has recently become available. This technique provides a quantitative estimate for the number and duration of reflux episodes occurring during daily activities and during sleep. Often, an episode of acid reflux is recognized as a drop in esophageal pH to less than or equal to 4. Symptoms can be correlated with acid reflux episodes. Unfortunately, "alkaline" reflux of bile and pancreatic fluid is not reliably detected by this technique. This is because these fluids are not strongly alkaline, particularly after mixing with gastric acid. For example, the reflux of bile and pancreatic juice at a pH of 6 would not be recognized as an abnormal event by intraesophageal pH monitoring.

Esophagoscopy

Reflux-induced damage to the esophageal mucosa can be visualized directly by esophagoscopy. The endoscopic findings of erosions and ulcerations in the distal esophagus strongly support the diagnosis of reflux esophagitis. Barrett's epithelium also has a characteristic endoscopic appearance. The endoscopist can obtain biopsy specimens through the instrument to confirm the presence of esophagitis or Barrett's esophagus.

Esophagoscopy can be an insensitive test for reflux esophagitis in patients with disease that does not produce gross erosions or ulcerations of the esophageal mucosa. The endoscopic diagnosis of lesser degrees of esophagitis is based on the subjective findings of mucosal hyperemia and fold thickening. Biopsy specimens obtained from such cases often have no histologic evidence of esophagitis. Conversely, the endoscopic examination can be normal for some patients with symptoms and histologic changes characteristic of reflux esophagitis. Other tests for gastroesophageal reflux disease may be required in such cases.

Esophageal Biopsy

Normally, the basal cell layer comprises less than 15 percent of the total thickness of the esophageal squamous epithelium. Esophageal biopsy specimens from patients with chronic gastroesophageal reflux disease often show thickening of this layer, judged to represent a cellular proliferative response to injury. In normal subjects, the papillary projections of the lamina propria extend less than two thirds of the distance to the epithelial surface. In patients with reflux esophagitis, these papillae frequently appear to extend almost to the surface. This is judged to be caused primarily by reflux-induced sloughing of the surface epithelial cells rather than by true hypertrophy of the papillae. The decrease in the absolute thickness of the epithelium results in a relative lengthening of the papillae. Finally, the findings of polymorphonuclear leukocytes and ulceration in esophageal biopsy specimens provide strong support for the diagnosis of acute esophagitis. Esophageal biopsy is a relatively insensitive test for gastroesophageal reflux disease, however, with normal results obtained in many patients.

Acid Perfusion (Bernstein) Test

Some patients with gastroesophageal reflux disease experience chest discomfort with features not typically those of heartburn. For these patients, other causes of chest pain, such as myocardial ischemia or musculoskeletal disorders, must be considered. The acid perfusion (Bernstein) test has been used in these cases to ascertain that the chest pain is the result of acid in the esophagus. A tube is placed in the esophagus, then either saline perfusion or 0.1 N hydrochloric acid perfusion takes place. Reproduction of the chest pain with acid perfusion, but not with saline perfusion, supports acid-reflux as the cause of the symptoms. Although this test is conceptually appealing, its interpretation is necessarily subjective and often difficult. False-positive findings are common. Furthermore, one study found that esophageal acid perfusion in some patients with coronary artery disease can result in angina pectoris with electrocardiographic (ECG) evidence of myocardial ischemia. This finding suggests that the acid perfusion test may not be a reliable indicator in differentiating patients with pain of esophageal origin from those with pain of cardiac origin.

Treatment of Gastroesophageal Reflux Disease

Medical Treatment

Some of the pathophysiologic features of gastroesophageal reflux disease are amenable to medical treatment. Measures can be implemented to reduce the number of reflux episodes, to render the gastric contents less harmful, to improve gastric emptying, and to enhance mucosal resistance. When treating patients with reflux esophagitis, it is important to consider the heterogeneity of the disorder. Pathophysiologic features that are important for some patients may not be important for other patients; therefore, treatments that benefit some patients may be ineffective for others.

General Antireflux Measures

General antireflux measures involve life-style modifications designed to minimize gastroesophageal reflux. The simple maneuver of elevating the head of the bed on 4- to 6-in. blocks exploits the influence of gravity on esophageal clearance and has been shown to be effective in reducing the duration of esophageal acid exposure during recumbency for patients with reflux esophagitis. Bedtime snacks can stimulate gastric acid production as well as reflux and therefore should be avoided. Patients should be instructed not to eat large meals, because reflux is related to gastric volume. Patients should not wear tight garments; these might predispose to reflux by increasing intraabdominal pressure. Agents that decrease LES pressure such as chocolate, coffee, alcohol, fat, cigarette smoke, and a variety of medications may predispose to reflux in susceptible individuals. Patients should avoid these agents whenever possible.

Antacids

Antacids have two verified salutary effects for patients with gastroesophageal reflux disease: (1) They neutralize gastric acid so that any gastric material subsequently refluxed may be less injurious to the esophageal mucosa, and (2) they result in gastric alkalinization, which increases LES pressure. Sucking on tablet antacids may also stimulate salivation and primary peristalsis, both of which can enhance esophageal acid clearance. Antacids traditionally have been the backbone of medical therapy for reflux esophagitis.

Histamine H₂-Receptor Blocking Agents

Histamine H_2-receptor blocking agents such as cimetidine and ranitidine decrease acid production by the gastric parietal cells. Use of these agents has been shown to result in relief of symptoms and reduction in antacid consumption for patients with gastroesophageal reflux disease. The results of some studies show significant histologic improvement of esophagitis for patients treated with these medications, whereas such an effect has not been documented in other studies. The H_2-receptor blocking agents appear to have no beneficial mechanism in gastroesophageal reflux disease other than reduction of gastric acidity. Thus, for patients whose esophagitis is caused by the reflux of bile or pancreatic juice, these agents may not be effective.

Gaviscon

Gaviscon is a mixture of alginic acid and antacid found to be effective in relieving reflux symptoms. The beneficial action of Gaviscon is judged to be due to mechanical effects rather than to its antacid content, which is negligible. Gaviscon forms a viscous gel on contact with saliva and gastric acid that coats the esophagus. This gel also floats on top of the gastric contents, where it is alleged to function in a corklike fashion as a mechanical barrier to reflux.

Bethanechol

Bethanechol, a choline ester with muscarinic actions, has been found to decrease symptoms for some patients with gastroesophageal reflux disease. The beneficial effect in these cases has been ascribed primarily to bethanechol's ability to increase LES pressure. Stimulation of salivation may also contribute to the drug's efficacy in treating reflux disease.

Metoclopramide

Metoclopramide has been shown to be effective in relieving the symptoms of reflux esophagitis. Metoclopramide is a dopamine antagonist that has substantial muscarinic effects on the smooth muscle of the proximal gastrointestinal tract. Its salutary effect in gastroesophageal reflux disease has been attributed to its ability to increase LES pressure and to accelerate gastric emptying. Use of the drug is often limited by its frequent neurologic side effects.

Sucralfate

Sucralfate is an aluminum hydroxide salt of sucrose sulfate that has been found to prevent esophagitis induced by several injurious agents in animal models. The drug appears to work by a local protective effect on the esophageal mucosa. Reported clinical experience with sucralfate for the treatment of esophagitis is still limited, however.

Experimental Agents

Experimental agents that have shown promise for the treatment of esophagitis in preliminary investigations include some of the synthetic prostaglandins and omeprazole, a substituted benzimidazole. The prostaglandins both inhibit acid secretion and exert an incompletely understood protective effect called *cytoprotection* on some epithelia. Omeprazole, by irreversibly inhibiting the proton pump on the secretory membrane of parietal cells, causes a marked and extended reduction in gastric acid secretion. These drugs may become available in the future for treatment of gastroesophageal reflux disease.

Surgical Treatment

The modern surgical treatment of gastroesophageal reflux usually involves one of three procedures: (1) the Belsey cardioplasty, (2) the Nissen fundoplication, and (3) the Hill posterior gastropexy. All three procedures incorporate hiatal hernia reduction and creation of an intraabdominal segment of esophagus around which a variable portion of the gastric fundus is plicated.

The Belsey cardioplasty is performed through a left thoracotomy. It entails mobilization of the esophagus up to the aortic arch, return of the distal esophagus to the abdomen, and plication of the gastric fundus around approximately 270 degrees of the esophageal circumference.

With the Nissen fundoplication, an abdominal approach is usually used, although the procedure may be performed transthoracically. In this procedure, the gastric fundus is wrapped completely around the intraabdominal esophagus.

The Hill posterior gastropexy requires a transabdominal approach. The Hill procedure involves suturing the phrenoesophageal membrane and esophagogastric junction to the median arcuate ligament of the aortic hiatus, with plication of a small segment of the gastric fundus around the intraabdominal esophagus.

Each of these procedures has its proponents, and each has been used successfully as primary surgical treatment for patients with gastroesophageal reflux disease. In most large series, more than 80 percent of surgically treated patients experienced good relief of symptoms, although relatively few reports describe objective tests confirming a decrease in gastroesophageal reflux episodes. At the present time, antireflux surgery is recommended primarily for patients with symptoms or complications of reflux esophagitis that are unresponsive to medical therapy.

The precise mechanisms whereby antireflux surgery inhibits gastroesophageal reflux are not completely understood. For reasons that remain unclear, these operations result in significant increases in LES pressure above preoperative values for most patients. Some investigators have attributed the beneficial effects of fundoplication to this postoperative increase in LES pressure. In many reports, however, there are descriptions of patients who had relief of symptoms after the operation without concomitant increases in LES pressure. Furthermore, antireflux surgery has been found to inhibit reflux in patients who had surgical resections of the LES and in an experimental model involving cadavers. These observations suggest that in some cases factors other than an increase in LES pressure may be responsible for the beneficial effects of antireflux surgery. Some prominent esophageal surgeons believe strongly that the establishment of a segment of esophagus exposed to intraabdominal pressure is a key feature of antireflux surgery and that the resultant mechanical buttressing of the distal esophagus by intraabdominal pressure is an important antireflux mechanism.

Caustic Injury to the Esophagus and Stomach

The esophagus and stomach are vulnerable to injury by a variety of caustic agents. Those agents most often responsible for serious esophageal and gastric damage are the strongly alkaline household cleaning products such as drain cleaners and lye soaps. Less often, esophageal and gastric injuries are seen with ingestions of strong acids (e.g., some toilet bowl and swimming pool cleaners) or household bleaches (5% solutions of sodium hypochlorite). Accidental ingestions of these products occur most frequently in children younger than 5 years of age. Adults may ingest caustic substances with suicidal intent. Also, many medications taken in pill form can cause caustic esophageal injury if the pills linger in the esophagus. The severity and extent of damage induced by a caustic agent vary directly with its corrosive properties, its concentration, the quantity ingested, and the duration of contact with the esophagus and stomach.

Pathophysiology

Alkali
Liquefactive necrosis, the complete destruction of entire cells and their membranes, is the acute lesion that results from contact of the esophagus and stomach with strong alkali such as lye.

These agents penetrate and destroy tissue until the alkali is rendered less harmful by dilution with tissue fluid. In the esophagus and stomach, concentrated lye solutions can cause transmural necrosis within seconds. Thus, perforations of these organs with resultant mediastinitis and peritonitis are frequent complications of lye ingestion. In dogs, lye that enters the stomach is violently ejected back into the esophagus from where it is again propelled into the stomach. This to-and-fro activity lasts several minutes, after which the alkali passes into the duodenum.

Liquid preparations of lye cause severe esophageal and gastric injury more often than the granular preparations. The granules tend to adhere to the mucous membranes of the oropharynx, where they cause pain and induce expectoration. Children who accidentally ingest such preparations often spit out the granules before they can enter the esophagus. Serious esophageal injury is found in fewer than 25 percent of patients who ingest granular lye products. In contrast, liquid lye preparations tend to be swallowed quickly into the esophagus, where they commonly cause severe damage.

Three phases of injury and healing have been observed following lye injury to the esophagus in animals: (1) an acute inflammatory phase, lasting 1 to 4 days, characterized by intense inflammation, edema, vascular thrombosis, and progressive necrosis; (2) a subacute phase, lasting approximately from day 4 to day 15, during which the necrotic tissue sloughs off, granulation tissue develops, fibroblasts proliferate, and collagen is deposited; and (3) a cicatrization phase, beginning on about day 15, during which the mucosa is reepithelialized and scar tissue retraction can result in a fibrous stricture of the esophagus.

Acid

Histologic examination of esophageal and gastric mucosae exposed to strong acid reveals coagulation necrosis, that is, clumping and opacification of the cell cytoplasm with preservation of the cell outline. This coagulation necrosis results in the rapid formation of an eschar, which is judged to limit the depth of penetration and injury produced by the acid. Although strong acids clearly can cause severe esophageal injury resulting in perforation and stricture formation, the esophagus is often only minimally damaged in cases of acid ingestion. The more severe injuries tend to involve the stomach, frequently with subsequent stricture formation in the gastric antrum. Pylorospasm induced by the acid with subsequent pooling of the caustic agent in the antrum may contribute to the gastric injury.

It is not entirely clear why acid ingestion often spares the esophagus. Perhaps the eschar formed during coagulation necrosis prevents the deep injury that is so common with alkali ingestion. Factors other than intrinsic corrosive properties may be more important in limiting damage induced by acid substances, however. Acids usually cause immediate pain in the oropharynx; this might limit the amount ingested, particularly in cases of accidental ingestions. Furthermore, strong alkalis generally are more readily available than strong acids for ingestion. Liquid drain cleaners and lye soaps are common household items; highly concentrated acid solutions are not.

Clinical Features

Agents that cause immediate pain and injury in the oropharynx may be expectorated before being swallowed. Other agents that cause extensive esophageal and gastric injury may cause little damage to the oropharynx. Therefore, during the early phase following caustic ingestion, neither symptoms nor signs of injury to the oropharynx reliably indicate the severity of the damage done to the esophagus and stomach. Patients with extensive injury to these organs may have only minimal early complaints. Conversely, patients with no esophageal or gastric damage may have intense discomfort caused by caustic burns of the oropharynx.

With esophageal injury, patients often experience early dysphagia, odynophagia, and drooling. Epigastric pain, retching, and vomiting frequently accompany gastric injury. Damage to the larynx and upper airway may be manifested by hoarseness and stridor. These acute symptoms usually subside within 2 weeks. Severe esophageal and gastric injuries can be accompanied by shock. With perforation of these organs, mediastinitis and peritonitis may ensue. Stricture formation is a common late sequela. In most such cases, the development of the stricture is apparent by the eighth week following injury. Esophageal strictures are manifested by dysphagia. With strictures in the stomach, gastric outlet obstruction can occur; it may be characterized by early satiety, postprandial vomiting, and weight loss. Finally, lye strictures of the esophagus are associated with a dramatically increased risk for developing esophageal carcinoma.

Treatment

The treatment of caustic ingestion is based largely on empirical and pathophysiologic data, not on the results of controlled therapeutic trials. Thus, there is much uncertainty as to what constitutes appropriate therapy for these patients. Supportive care is clearly indicated to correct hypotension and to treat respiratory difficulties that may result from pulmonary aspiration of the caustic agent. Esophageal and gastric perforations are usually treated surgically. If the patient is seen soon after the ingestion, attempts to neutralize the caustic substance have been recommended by some authorities and condemned by others. Neutralization of strong acids and alkalis can generate substantial heat, which may further damage tissues. Passage of a tube into the stomach to remove any retained caustic material is also a controversial issue. Both tube passage and neutralization attempts carry the risk of inducing emesis, which reexposes the esophagus to the caustic agent and increases the chance of pulmonary aspiration.

Because early symptoms and physical findings do not reliably predict the severity of esophageal and gastric damage following caustic ingestion, endoscopic examination of the upper gastrointestinal tract is recommended for most cases. Tissue injury is recognized endoscopically as areas of erythema, hemorrhage, exudate, blistering, and ulceration. If these lesions are present, therapy is usually implemented. If the endoscopic examination reveals no esophageal or gastric lesions, no further medical treatment is necessary.

In animal models of caustic ingestion, the early administration of corticosteroids has been shown to decrease collagen deposition and subsequent stricture formation. These data have been extrapolated to support the use of corticosteroids in the treatment of caustic ingestion in humans. This practice entails the risk of masking signs and symptoms of mediastinitis and peritonitis and of increased infectious complications. In animal models, septic complications are decreased by the concomitant administration of antibiotics with corticosteroids. These data have also been extrapolated to support the administration of antibiotics in addition to steroids for patients who have ingested caustic agents. Total parenteral nutrition has been recommended by some authorities as a means of providing nutrition without the physical trauma to the esophagus that could be inflicted by eating; data to support this practice are unconvincing. Esophageal stents and early esophageal dilatations have been used prophylactically in an attempt to prevent severe stricture formation. In the absence of controlled studies, the efficacy of any of these therapeutic modalities in preventing strictures is questionable. Finally, agents that interfere with some physicochemical properties of collagen such as N-acetylcysteine and penicillamine have been found to be effective in preventing stricture formation following lye injury in animals. At the present time, few data are available concerning the use of these agents in humans.

Pill-Induced Esophageal Injury

Radiographic and scintigraphic techniques have documented that pills swallowed without water by subjects in both the upright and supine positions frequently remain in the esophagus for more than 10 minutes. In contrast, pills taken with water by subjects in the upright position are rapidly cleared from the esophagus. Water ingestion does not markedly hasten esophageal pill clearance for subjects in the supine position, however.

A variety of medications taken in pill form are capable of inflicting caustic injury if they linger in the esophagus. Those agents most often responsible include antibiotics (particularly some tetracycline preparations), potassium chloride tablets, ferrous sulfate, quinidine, and some nonsteroidal anti-inflammatory medications. When these pills are taken without water, prolonged contact with the esophagus is possible. The practice of taking a pill at bedtime may result in especially prolonged esophageal retention, both because of recumbency and because of the dramatic reduction in swallowing and primary peristalsis associated with sleep.

In most reported cases, pill injury has involved the esophagus approximately at the level of the aortic arch. Factors that may contribute to pill retention at this level include esophageal compression by the arch and the low amplitude of the contraction wave in this area of transition from striated to smooth esophageal muscle.

For most patients with pill-induced injury, there is no prior history of esophageal disease. Patients often admit to taking the pills with little or no water just before retiring. Odynophagia and persistent retrosternal pain are the most frequent complaints. Dysphagia occurs in approximately one fifth of cases. Esophageal perforation, stricture, and hemorrhage are uncommon complications. When the offending medication is withdrawn, the lesions heal without sequelae in the majority of cases.

Because of the danger of pill-induced esophageal injury, patients should be instructed to take pills while in an upright position with a full glass of water. Also, patients should be advised not to ingest pills immediately before going to bed. For patients with known esophageal motility disorders, it seems prudent to avoid particularly caustic pills such as doxycycline and slow-release potassium chloride tablets.

Infectious Esophagitis

Three infections most often responsible for important esophageal infections include candidiasis, herpes simplex virus (HSV), and cytomegalovirus (CMV). Esophageal infection resulting from these organisms is seen most frequently in patients who are immunocompromised by malignancy, the acquired immunodeficiency syndrome (AIDS), debilitation, or the administration of corticosteroids and immunosuppressive agents. All three infections occasionally occur in patients who have no demonstrable disorders of immunity, however. Typically, patients with infectious esophagitis complain of the acute onset of odynophagia. Dysphagia and fever are also frequent symptoms. Symptoms do not invariably accompany infectious esophagitis, however, and some cases are discovered unexpectedly during endoscopic or postmortem examinations in patients who had no complaints of esophageal disease.

Candida
Esophagitis

The Candida species that causes esophagitis most often is *Candida albicans,* an organism that can be cultured from the oropharynx or stool of most healthy subjects. In addition to the immunodeficiency disorders listed previously, Candida esophagitis has been associated with a variety of endocrinopathies (e.g., diabetes mellitus, hypothyroidism, hypoparathyroidism, Addison's disease) and with the administration of broad-spectrum antibiotics, which may eliminate the bacteria that ordinarily inhibit fungal growth.

On endoscopic examination, the esophagus infected by Candida is typically coated with creamy white plaques. Barium filling the interstices between these plaques creates a characteristic shaggy outline of the esophageal wall on barium swallow. These endoscopic and radiographic findings are not specific for Candida infection, however, and other tests are required to confirm the diagnosis. Because Candida is such a common commensal organism in the gastrointestinal tract, proof of infection requires more than just culture of the fungus from the esophagus. The diagnosis of Candida esophagitis is usually confirmed by the finding of fungal mycelia in endoscopic brush cytology specimens of the esophageal lesions; this mycelial form of Candida reflects tissue invasion and is not commonly found in healthy individuals. Esophageal biopsy is an insensitive test for Candida esophagitis, but the histologic finding of tissue invasion by the fungus is diagnostic of infection. The clinical utility of the many serologic tests for Candida infection is limited by their lack of sensitivity and specificity.

Treatment of Candida esophagitis involves correction of the underlying immunodeficiency disorder whenever possible and the administration of antifungal agents. Oral nystatin is often the first-line drug. For infections that do not respond to oral nystatin, other antifungal medications that may be effective include imidazole derivatives (e.g., ketoconazole, clotrimazole, miconazole), 5-fluorocytosine, and amphotericin B.

Herpes Simplex Virus Esophagitis

Esophageal infection by HSV can be the result of: (1) herpes simplex viremia, (2) direct extension of active HSV infection from the oropharynx, or (3) reactivation of latent HSV infection with migration of the virus to the esophagus by way of the vagus nerves. Esophagoscopic examination in patients with HSV esophagitis typically reveals superficial punched-out ulcers covered by a white pseudomembrane. These ulcers can also be seen on barium swallow, but neither the endoscopic nor the radiographic findings are specific for HSV esophagitis. Knowledge of the characteristic histologic and cytologic changes of HSV infection can be used clinically. The diagnosis of HSV esophagitis is often confirmed by the examination of esophageal biopsy and cytology specimens, which reveals multinucleated giant cells and eosinophilic intranuclear inclusion bodies in the epithelial cells. Isolation of HSV in tissue culture of these specimens establishes the diagnosis of HSV esophagitis unequivocally. Serologic tests for HSV are of little clinical value because of problems with their sensitivity and specificity in acute infections. Systemic antiviral chemotherapy with acyclovir and vidarabine has been used to treat severe HSV esophagitis, but there have been no controlled studies to document the efficacy of these agents in this setting.

Cytomegalovirus Esophagitis

Cytomegalovirus is a herpesvirus that can cause esophagitis after reactivation of endogenous latent infection or during the primary infection that may occur with exposure to exogenous CMV in blood products and organ allografts. Esophageal infection with CMV can cause ulcerations that appear similar to those of HSV esophagitis on endoscopic and radiographic examination. Cytomegalovirus gets its name from the characteristic enlargement it elicits in infected cells. The finding of these enlarged cells with characteristic intranuclear and cytoplasmic inclusions on examination of esophageal biopsy and cytology specimens confirms the diagnosis. Because of CMV's predilection for endothelial cells, the yield of biopsy specimens obtained from the granulation tissue in the ulcer crater may be higher than that obtained from the epithelium at the ulcer's edge. Isolation of CMV in tissue culture of these specimens also supports the diagnosis of CMV esophagitis. A rising antibody titer to CMV may be additional supportive evidence for infection, but such a rise may not occur for weeks following onset of the acute illness. No specific treatment has proved effective for CMV infection.

Mechanical Causes of Dysphagia

The esophagus is a relatively distensible organ. Because of its elasticity, circumferential involvement of the esophageal wall is often required for a mechanical lesion to produce dysphagia.

One must be cautious about attributing dysphagia to lesions that have caused less than extensive luminal narrowing. Partial mechanical obstruction typically causes dysphagia for solid foods only; meat and bread are particularly common offenders. Dysphagia for liquids occurs with complete obstruction of the lumen, which may result from the impaction of a solid bolus with the esophageal lesion. Pulmonary aspiration of retained esophageal material can occur. Characteristic clinical features related to the pathophysiology of some common mechanical causes of dysphagia are discussed in the following sections.

Cancer of the Esophagus

Squamous cell carcinoma is the most common histologic type of esophageal cancer, accounting for more than 70 percent of cases. Adenocarcinoma constitutes most of the remaining cases; other histologic types of esophageal cancer are rare. Alcoholism and cigarette smoking are important risk factors. Squamous cell carcinoma affects men more often than women, and blacks more often than whites. Male predominance is also a feature of adenocarcinoma, but whites are affected more frequently than blacks. Adenocarcinoma is associated with Barrett's epithelium in most cases.

Patients with esophageal cancer typically complain of rapidly progressive dysphagia and weight loss over a period of months. Other symptoms are related to the tumor's extent and location in the esophagus. For example, cancer of the cervical esophagus may invade the recurrent laryngeal nerve and cause hoarseness. An esophagotracheal or esophagoaortic fistula may result from mediastinal invasion by a lesion of the midesophagus. Characteristically, barium swallow reveals an abrupt narrowing of the esophageal lumen by a mass with irregular borders (Fig. 2-4A). Esophagoscopy and examination of biopsy and cytology specimens from the lesion confirm the diagnosis.

The esophagus has an extensive lymphatic system that provides opportunity for both longitudinal and lateral spread of malignancies. Because of this unique lymphatic drainage and because the tumor must achieve substantial size before it causes symptoms, most patients have disseminated disease at the time of diagnosis. These features of esophageal cancer are judged to account for its dismal prognosis. Treatments include surgery, radiotherapy, and chemotherapy. Despite treatment, the overall 5-year survival rate is only 5 percent.

Fig. 2-4
Barium esophagogram showing esophageal cancer (A), peptic esophageal stricture (B), and a Schatzki ring (C). (Radiographs provided by Dr. Miriam E. Vincent.)

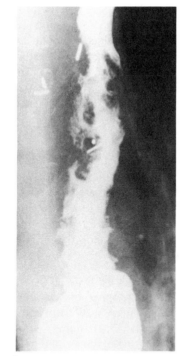

A

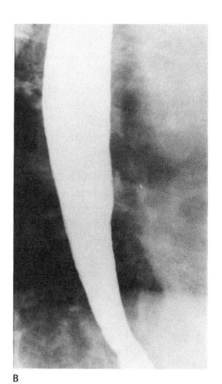

B

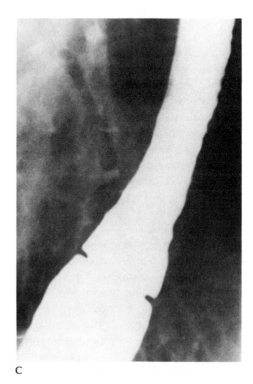

C

Benign Strictures
of the Esophagus

Benign strictures of the esophagus are most often complications of gastroesophageal reflux disease. Such esophageal stenoses are frequently called *peptic strictures,* although factors other than acid and pepsin may be involved in their pathogenesis, as discussed previously. Benign fibrotic strictures can also result from caustic ingestions, radiation exposure, and esophageal infections. Patients suspected of having a benign stricture of the esophagus should be questioned in order to get a history of these predisposing conditions.

Peptic strictures are located most often in the distal esophagus. Approximately one half of all cases of peptic stricture are associated with Barrett's epithelium. Strictures in Barrett's esophagus occur frequently at the junction of squamous and columnar mucosae. Patients with exceptionally long segments of Barrett's epithelium, therefore, may have strictures involving the middle or even the proximal esophagus.

Peptic esophageal strictures typically result in dysphagia that is insidious in onset and slow in progression. Frequently, the patient will reveal a gradual change in diet to semisolid foods. Profound weight loss is unusual. The barium swallow characteristically reveals a smooth tapering of the esophageal lumen (Fig. 2-4B). Fluoroscopically, subtle degrees of esophageal narrowing may be visualized more easily if the patient swallows a solid bolus (e.g., a barium-soaked marshmallow) whose passage is seen to be impeded by the stricture. Endoscopic examination is useful to rule out a malignant obstruction of the esophagus. Treatment usually involves dilatation of the stricture by passage of a series of mercury-filled bougies of progressively increasing diameter. Other devices used for esophageal dilatation include a variety of metal sounds and balloons that are guided fluoroscopically or endoscopically into the stricture, where they are inflated to a predetermined pressure and diameter. Surgical treatment is required in some cases. This usually includes antireflux surgery, often with either intraoperative dilatation of the stricture or resection of the stenosed segment of esophagus.

Rings and Webs

The terms *rings* and *webs* are usually used to refer to thin projections of mucosa and submucosa that encroach upon the lumen of the esophagus. The term *ring* is commonly reserved for such a projection that involves the most distal esophagus; synonyms include Schatzki ring and B ring. Mucosal projections found elsewhere in the esophagus are usually called *webs.* Thus, the distinction between a ring and a web is primarily one of location in the esophagus.

Mucosal rings and webs can cause mechanical obstruction of the esophageal lumen with dysphagia. The pathogenesis of these mucosal structures is unclear. Webs of the cervical esophagus are sometimes found in women with iron deficiency anemia, an association known as Patterson-Kelly syndrome or Plummer-Vinson syndrome. Such patients are at increased risk for developing cancer of the esophagus. The role, if any, of iron deficiency in the pathogenesis of the webs is not known.

Schatzki rings are often associated with distinctive clinical features sometimes called the *steak-house syndrome*. Affected patients are usually older than 40 years of age and experience intermittent dysphagia for solids, often meat, and often during periods of emotional excitement or hurried eating, as may occur in the steak-house setting. Some patients are seen initially with acute meat impaction that results in total esophageal obstruction. Typically, the symptoms are not progressive; the episodes of dysphagia are widely separated. The Schatzki ring is often apparent on barium swallow as a symmetric lesion less than 5 mm in thickness (Fig. 2-4C). Dysphagia occurs frequently with rings that narrow the lumen to less than 13 mm. Endoscopic examination is useful to rule out the presence of a thin peptic stricture that can mimic a ring. Schatzki rings usually have squamous mucosa lining their proximal surfaces, with gastric columnar mucosa on the distal side. Treatment usually involves passage of a large-diameter bougie in order to fracture the ring, rather than the progressive dilatation used for peptic strictures.

Study Questions 1. A 48-year-old man complains of heartburn and dysphagia. Abnormal esophageal acid exposure is demonstrated by 24-hour esophageal pH monitoring. All of the following could contribute to his gastroesophageal reflux disease except:
  a. A weak lower esophageal sphincter
  b. Delayed esophageal clearance
  c. Failure of relaxation of the lower esophageal sphincter
  d. Delayed gastric emptying

Answer
Choice "c" is correct. The lower esophageal sphincter is the major barrier to the reflux of gastric contents. Failure of that sphincter to relax could cause dysphagia but would prevent gastroesophageal reflux. In contrast, a weak lower esophageal sphincter may not pose an adequate barrier to the reflux of gastric material. Delayed esophageal clearance can result in prolonged exposure of the esophagus to injurious refluxed material, thus contributing to gastroesophageal reflux

disease. Delayed gastric emptying can cause gastric distention, which predisposes to reflux.

2. For patients with gastroesophageal reflux disease, ingestion of any of the following might exacerbate symptoms except:
   a. Chocolate
   b. Fatty foods
   c. Amitryptiline (a tricyclic antidepressant)
   d. Bethanechol (a cholinergic agent)

Answer
Choice "d" is correct. Cholinergic agents tend to increase lower esophageal sphincter pressure, thus increasing the barrier to gastroesophageal reflux. Ingestion of substances that decrease lower esophageal sphincter pressure such as chocolate, fatty foods, and amitryptiline (a medication with anticholinergic activity) can result in increased reflux and, consequently, an exacerbation of symptoms.

References

Dodds, W. J., Hogan, W. J., Helm, J. F., Dent J. Pathogenesis of reflux esophagitis. *Gastroenterology* 81:376, 1981.

Dodds, W. J., Dent, J., Hogan, W. J., et al. Mechanisms of gastroesophageal reflux in patients with reflux esophagitis. *N. Engl. J. Med.* 307:1547, 1982.

Goldman, L. P., and Weigert, J. M. Corrosive substance ingestion: A review. *Am. J. Gastroenterol.* 79:85, 1984.

Goyal, R. K., and Rattan, S. Neurohumoral, hormonal, and drug receptors for the lower esophageal sphincter. *Gastroenterology* 74:598, 1978.

Helm, J. F., Dodds, W. J., Pelc, L. R., et al. Effect of esophageal emptying and saliva on clearance of acid from the esophagus. *N. Engl. J. Med.* 310:284, 1984.

Kikendall, J. W., Friedman, A. C., Oyewole, M. A., et al. Pill-induced esophageal injury. Case reports and review of the medical literature. *Dig. Dis. Sci.* 28:174, 1983.

Mathieson, R., and Dutta, S. K. Candida esophagitis. *Dig. Dis. Sci.* 28:365, 1983.

Spechler, S. J., and Goyal, R. K. Barrett's esophagus. *N. Engl. J. Med.* 315:362, 1986.

3 : Peptic Ulcer Disease

Sanjiv Chopra

Functional Gastric Anatomy

The stomach is a sac-shaped organ connected superiorly with the esophagus and inferiorly wih the first part of the duodenum. There is considerable individual variation in the shape and capacity of the stomach. It is most frequently J-shaped and has a capacity of 1500 ml. The anatomic regions of the stomach consist of the cardia, fundus, body, antrum, and pylorus and are schematically depicted in Fig. 3-1. The stomach is composed of four tissue layers: mucosa, submucosa, muscularis propria, and serosa. The muscularis propria, as its name implies, is the major muscular component and consists of outer longitudinal, middle circular, and inner oblique muscle layers. The arterial blood supply to the stomach is provided by branches of the celiac artery: left gastric artery, right gastric artery, short gastric arteries, and left and right gastroepiploic arteries. The innervation of the stomach is both sympathetic and parasympathetic. The preganglionic sympathetic fibers arise from the sixth through eighth thoracic segments of the spinal cord, whereas the postganglionic sympathetic fibers arise from the celiac plexus. The parasympathetic nerve supply is derived from the left and right vagus nerves and their branches. Vagal nerve fibers connect with gastric ganglion cells, both in the submucosa (Meissner's plexus) and in the muscularis propria (Auerbach's plexus) from which postganglionic fibers innervate secretory and motor components of the stomach. Thus, acid-secreting parietal cells, gastrin-secreting cells, and zymogen cells are all innervated by postganglionic vagal fibers.

Functions of the Stomach

The stomach performs the following diverse functions: (1) storing of ingested food, (2) grinding of food and mixing with gastric secretions, (3) gastric emptying, and (4) gastric secretion. These functions will be discussed in the following paragraphs.

Storage of Ingested Food

The proximal stomach is the principal reservoir and accommodates food by a process called *receptive relaxation*, during which the stomach "relaxes" to accommodate a large volume of food and secretions without a concomitant increase in intragastric pressure. During the fasted state, the volume of the stomach

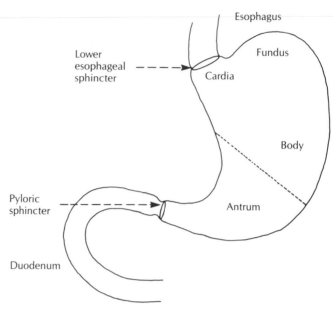

Esophagus

Lower
esophageal   — — — —▶
sphincter

Cardia

Fundus

Body

Pyloric   — — — — — — — —▶
sphincter

Antrum

Duodenum

Fig. 3-1
Anatomic regions of the stomach.

is 50 ml or less; following a meal, it is often 1500 ml. The phenomenon of receptive relaxation is mediated via the vagus nerve. It is not surprising that early satiety and postprandial epigastric fullness is a common symptom experienced by patients after a vagotomy.

Grinding of Food and Mixing with Gastric Secretions

This process occurs in the distal stomach and results in the conversion of the ingested food into a homogeneous chyme regardless of whether it started as a delicious French gourmet offering or a typical not-so-palatable hospital cafeteria meal. Mixing occurs as a consequence of phasic myogenic contractions. In the body of the stomach, contractions of low amplitude knead solid food and propel food and secretions to the antrum, where stronger contractions coupled with a narrower lumen result in jetlike streams proceeding antegradely through the pylorus and also retrogradely into the body. This process is strikingly efficient and results in a "sieving," such that only particles that are a millimeter or less in size enter the duodenum. Grinding and mixing of food is believed to be regulated primarily via the vagus nerve. Additionally, several hormones can affect motility in the distal stomach. Thus, gastrin, cholecystokinin, and motilin enhance motility, whereas secretin, glucagon, somatostatin, gastric inhibiting polypeptide (GIP), and vasoactive intestinal polypeptide (VIP) inhibit contractions in the distal stomach. The physiologic importance of these hormones in regard to gastric motility in humans is not known.

Gastric Emptying   The orderly gastric emptying of solids and liquids from the stomach is an important function (see Chap. 9). When the antrum contracts against an open pylorus, food is propelled into the duodenum. The pylorus then contracts despite continued antral contraction, causing food to be propelled retrogradely into the antrum or body of the stomach. The antrum then relaxes, and the cycle is repeated. Thus, the antrum and pylorus help to regulate gastric emptying. Gastric emptying of a solid meal in humans is usually complete in 4 hours. In contrast to the emptying of solid foods, which depends on strong antral contractions, emptying of liquids depends on the amount of fluid within the stomach. Thus, the larger the gastric volume, the faster the rate of emptying. The nature of chyme (chemical composition, pH, particle size, and osmolarity) also influences gastric emptying. For example, inhibition of gastric emptying is seen with products of fat digestion, by chyme that has a pH less than 3.5, or by chyme that has particles of a large size or a high osmolarity. This process is probably mediated via sensitive receptors in the duodenum. Neural and humoral factors may also be important. Following vagotomy in humans, gastric emptying of solids is retarded, whereas that of liquids is accelerated. The role of different peptide hormones such as motilin, gastrin, cholecystokinin, somatostatin, and neurotensin is not clear at the present time. Gastric motility is also affected by heat, cold, and emotional stimuli.

Gastric Secretion   Specialized cells in the stomach secrete a variety of substances into the gastric lumen (Table 3-1). Some of these cells secrete more than a single product, whereas others secrete only one known substance. A precise function is known for some of the secreted products, whereas for others, it is speculative or unknown. In this section, we focus on gastric acid secretion. As a generalization, any circumstance that decreases or increases

Table 3-1
Gastric secretory products and their cell(s) of origin

Product	Cell(s) of origin
Hydrochloric acid	Parietal (oxyntic) cell
Intrinsic factor	Parietal (oxyntic) cell
Pepsinogens	Chief cells and mucous cells
Mucus	Mucous cells
Gastrin	G cell
Bicarbonate	Unknown

gastric acid secretion has a similar parallel effect on the secretion of intrinsic factor and of pepsinogen. An exception is juvenile pernicious anemia, in which, although secretion of gastric acid is normal, that of intrinsic factor is either deficient or a biologically inert kind of intrinsic factor is secreted. Another exception is the effect of the hormone secretin, which decreases gastric acid secretion but increases pepsinogen secretion.

Other substances secreted into the gastric lumen include mucoproteins, such as the blood group substances, and immunoglobulin A. Approximately 80 percent of normal individuals secrete blood group substances A, B, and H and are categorized as secretors, whereas the remaining 20 percent do not and are referred to as nonsecretors. Blood group O nonsecretor individuals have an increased risk of development of duodenal ulcer.

Gastric Acid
Secretion

Hydrochloric acid is secreted by parietal or oxyntic cells located in the fundus and body of the stomach. Secretion of acid by the stomach serves two purposes in humans: (1) Together with secretion of pepsinogen, which is catalyzed by acid to active pepsin, it facilitates digestion of ingested protein; and (2) the acid milieu of the stomach provides a protective mechanism against ingested bacteria, viruses, and parasites. In the unstimulated state, the average basal acid output (BAO) is 2.5 mM/hour. However, there is considerable variation between normal individuals, who may secrete virtually no acid to greater than 10 mM/hour. Indeed, even the same individual may secrete strikingly different amounts of hydrochloric acid on different days. Several factors, including histamine, gastrin, and vagal tone, probably contribute to basal acid secretion. A circadian rhythm is present for acid secretion with high rates in the evening and low rates in the morning. The cause for this is not known, and the changes in acid secretion are not accompanied by parallel changes in serum gastrin concentrations.

Maximal acid output (MAO) refers to the maximal amount of acid that the parietal cells can secrete in response to the maximal effective dose of a potent secretagogue such as histamine or gastrin. Maximal acid output is a function of gender (greater in men than in women), age, and lean body mass and correlates well with parietal cell mass. Although there is considerable difference in peak acid output (PAO) between normal individuals, ranging from 8.0 to 80.0 mM/hour, it is strikingly constant in a particular individual (PAO is calculated by multiplying the sum of the two highest consecutive 15-minute acid outputs by 2). Peak acid output also correlates very well with levels of serum group I pepsinogen. Maximal acid output is usually markedly

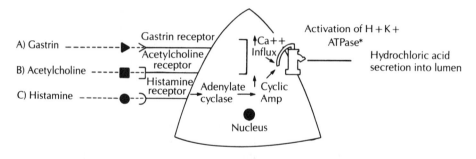

Fig. 3-2
Physiology of parietal cell receptors.

Type of receptor	Kind of physiologic function exemplified	Blocked by
A) Gastrin	Endocrine	Proglumide
B) Acetylcholine	Neurocrine	Atropine, pirenzepine
C) Histamine	Paracrine	H₂ receptor antagonists

* Blockade of H + K + ATPase gastric proton pump achieved by Omeprazole

increased in patients with Zollinger-Ellison syndrome or gastrinoma in whom endogenous gastrin is very likely exerting a trophic effect on parietal cells. Maximal acid output decreases within 24 hours following vagotomy. Secretion of hydrogen ion into the gastric lumen is an active energy-dependent process occurring against a 3 million to 1 concentration gradient. The enzyme H^+K^+ ATPase located on the surface of the parietal cell is activated by intracellular cyclic AMP and calcium and results in the luminal secretion of hydrogen ion in exchange for potassium. Omeprazole is a synthetic substituted benzimidazole that potently inhibits gastric acid secretion by virtue of its ability to block H^+K^+ ATPase (Fig. 3-2).

Phases of Gastric Acid Secretion
Cephalic Phase
The cephalic phase of acid secretion refers to the component of acid secretion evoked via the central nervous system in response to the sight, smell, or taste of appetizing food. It is conventionally studied by sham feeding (food is chewed but not swallowed) and can also be initiated by inducing hypoglycemia with 2-deoxy-D-glucose, a very potent agent in this regard, producing a maximal response equivalent to that produced by gastrin. In contrast, sham feeding (food but not water is effective) produces a maximal response that is about 40 to 50 percent of

the maximal response to exogenous gastrin. The cephalic phase is thought to be mediated via the vagus nerve and is abolished by vagotomy. Vagal stimulation of parietal cells occurs by means of two pathways: (1) a direct action of vagal efferents releasing acetylcholine in the vicinity of the parietal cell, and (2) an indirect action mediated by means of vagally stimulated release of gastrin from G cells in the antrum. The former is blocked by anticholinergic agents such as atropine, whereas the latter is not. The nature of the neurotransmitter responsible for the vagal-gastrin component of the cephalic phase is not known, although it has been suggested that the tetradecapeptide bombesin is responsible.

Gastric Phase
The gastric phase of acid secretion is mediated by events occurring within the stomach. Two mechanisms initiate acid secretion by the parietal cell in the gastric phase: gastric distention and the chemical composition of food. The former is mediated by two neural reflexes: long vagovagal reflexes (distention of antrum) and short intramural reflexes. The latter depends on the nature of the food constituents ingested. For example, amino acids, particularly tryptophan and phenylalanine, act directly on G cells, causing release of gastrin and subsequent acid secretion. Commonly ingested food items that are fairly potent secretagogues include coffee (caffeinated and decaffeinated), ethanol, and calcium-containing foods such as milk.

Intestinal Phase
The intestinal phase of acid secretion is initiated by two factors: intestinal distention and products of protein digestion. The hypothetical hormone mediating the intestinal phase of acid secretion by the parietal cells has tentatively been designated entero-oxyntin. The salient features of the various phases of acid secretion are summarized in Table 3-2.

Intrinsic Factor Secretion

The secretion of intrinsic factor by the parietal cells located in the fundus and body of the stomach is essential for life. Intrinsic factor is a glycoprotein with a molecular weight of 48,000 to 60,000 daltons. It binds with dietary vitamin B_{12} to form a complex that is then absorbed at specific receptor sites in the terminal ileum. Vitamin B_{12} (cobalamin) is crucial for normal division and viability of human cells. Vitamin B_{12} analogs synthesized by microorganisms are structurally similar but biologically inactive. Agents that augment gastric acid secretion also cause an increase in intrinsic factor secretion. Intrinsic factor deficiency occurs in patients with gastric atrophy and achlorhydria or following gastric resection and leads to vitamin B_{12} deficiency.

Table 3-2
Gastric acid secretion: Factors stimulating acid secretion and pathway involved

Phase	Stimulant	Percentage of total acid secretion[a]	Pathway	Mediator at parietal cell
Cephalic	Sight, smell, or taste of food	30	Direct vagal	Acetylcholine
			Vagal-antral-gastrin	Gastrin[b]
Gastric	Distention	50	Long vagal-vagal, short intramural	
	Food in stomach (amino acids, calcium)		Gastrin released from G cells	Gastrin[b]
Intestinal	Distention	5	Unidentified hormone not dependent on vagal integrity	Entero-oxyntin
	Food in intestines (amino acids, peptides)		Amino acids in blood	Amino acids

[a]15% is accounted for by basal or interdigestive acid secretion.
[b]Following gastric acid secretion, the luminal pH in the stomach falls. At pH 3.0, gastrin release from the antrum is markedly inhibited, and, at pH 1.5, it is virtually abolished.

Pepsinogen
Secretion

Pepsinogens are secreted by chief cells located in the fundus and body and by mucous cells located in the cardia, fundus, body, antrum, and pylorus. In the presence of gastric acid, the inactive pepsinogens are autocatalytically transformed into the active proteolytic enzyme pepsin. The optimum pH for different pepsins ranges from 1.8 to 3.5. Pepsinogens have been classified into two groups on the basis of immunologic reactions. Group I (pepsinogens 1–5) and group II (pepsinogens 6–8) pepsinogens can be measured in the serum by specific radioimmunoassays. There is a positive correlation between serum group I pepsinogen levels and PAO. High serum group I pepsinogen levels appear to be inherited in an autosomal dominant manner in some families whose members have duodenal ulcer disease. The strongest stimulus for pepsinogen secretion is by cholinergic neural pathways. As mentioned previously, agents that augment acid secretion also increase pepsinogen secretion, the one notable exception being secretin, which, while inhibiting acid secretion, acts as a potent stimulus for pepsinogen secretion. Histamine and gastrin stimulate pepsinogen secretion, whereas H_2 receptor antagonists, anticholinergics, and vagotomy lead to a fall in pepsinogen secretion.

Mucus Secretion

Mucus is secreted by mucous cells situated in all regions of the stomach. Gastric mucus consists of glycoproteins and mucopolysaccharides, including the blood group substances mentioned previously. The bulk (95 percent by weight) of mucus is water. Gastric mucus forms a thin viscoelastic gel that lines the entire mucosal surface and lubricates the stomach. It protects the stomach from mechanical abrasion by the onslaught of diverse foods eaten by humans. Mucus may also form an unstirred water layer that "traps" secreted bicarbonate and retards the back diffusion of hydrogen ion from the luminal surface into the mucosa. Factors regulating mucus secretion are not well understood. Prostaglandin E_2 and carbenoxolene augment mucus gel thickness, whereas aspirin, nonsteroidal anti-inflammatory drugs, and N-acetyl-L-cysteine reduce its thickness. A recent study suggested that patients with peptic ulcer have more soluble and degradable mucus than do non-ulcer controls.

Pathophysiology of Peptic Ulcer

Definition

In contrast to an erosion, which is a superficial lesion that extends into the mucosa but does not penetrate through the muscularis mucosa, an ulcer is a hole that extends through the muscularis mucosa into the submucosa or deeper. The word *peptic* signifies that peptic proteolysis involving acid and pepsin is important in the development of whatever lesion to which this term is being applied (Fig. 3-3). Experimental studies in animals have demonstrated that the combined action of acid and pepsin is more injurious to vulnerable mucosa than that of either agent alone.

Epidemiology and Prevalence of Peptic Ulcer

Approximately 10 percent of Americans develop peptic ulcer disease during their lifetime. Duodenal ulcers occur much more commonly than gastric ulcers in the United States and in most countries. In contrast, gastric ulcers are more common than duodenal ulcers in Japan, Peru, and Norway. In the United

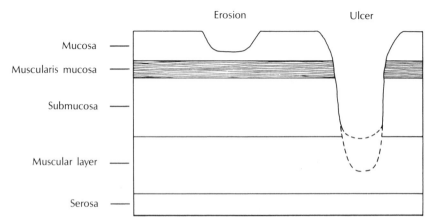

Fig. 3-3
Schematic depiction of erosion and ulcer.

States, 350,000 new cases of peptic ulcer disease are diagnosed each year, and 4 million Americans suffer from an active ulcer each year. The annual cost from absenteeism, loss of wages, and health care in the United States exceeds 3 billion dollars. The onset of symptoms for duodenal ulcer occurs most commonly between the ages of 25 and 55 years of age, whereas gastric ulcer symptoms are most common between the ages of 40 and 65 years.

Hereditary factors appear to play a role in some patients with ulcer disease. For example, there is an increased risk of ulcer disease (site-specific) in first-degree relatives of patients with peptic ulcer disease. Additionally, there is a greater likelihood of concordance for peptic ulcer disease in identical than in fraternal twins. Some members of families with multiple endocrine neoplasia type 1 (MEN-I) syndrome develop ulcers because of the presence of gastrinomas, which secrete the hormone gastrin, leading to increased serum level of gastrin and, in turn, increased acid secretion.

Environmental factors associated with the development of ulcer disease include cigarette smoking, aspirin and nonsteroidal anti-inflammatory drugs, steroids, and psychological stress.

Pathophysiology of Duodenal Ulcer

Acid is important in the pathogenesis of duodenal ulcer (DU) disease. Acid in itself can damage the mucosa, and an acid milieu is necessary for activation of pepsin. In an example of sustained and pronounced acid hypersecretion of gastric acid, namely, gastrinoma or Zollinger-Ellison syndrome, approximately 90 percent of patients have peptic ulcer disease. Since 10 percent of patients with this condition do not develop ulcer disease, abnormalities in mucosal defense are also probably important. Nevertheless, most studies have focused on physiologic alterations in regard to acid production. The physiologic defects described in some, but certainly not all, patients with duodenal ucler include the following:

1. Increased parietal cell mass
2. Increased capacity to secrete acid and pepsin (basal)
3. Increased parietal cell sensitivity to gastrin
4. Increased rate of gastric emptying
5. Decreased acid-induced inhibition of gastrin release

The pH in the duodenum is lower in DU patients as a group than in normal subjects because of increased acid production and more rapid gastric emptying. These individual defects occur in 25 to 50 percent of patients with DU; some patients with DU have none of these defects.

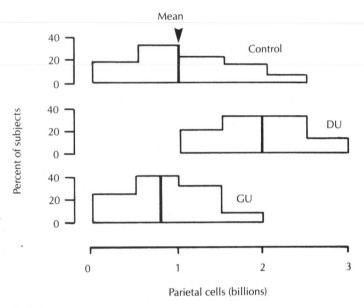

Fig. 3-4
Parietal cell mass in normals, patients with duodenal ulcer (DU), and gastric ulcer (GU). (From A. H. Soll and J. I. Isenberg. Duodenal ulcer diseases. In M. H. Sleisenger and J. S. Fordtran (eds.), *Gastrointestinal Disease*. Philadelphia: Saunders, 1983.)

The old adage "no acid, no ulcer" (Schwarz, 1910) is rightly honored. Duodenal ulcers are virtually unknown in subjects who have a PAO of less than 10 mM/hour, which corresponds to about 0.5 billion parietal cells. Thus, it is reasonable to state that no matter how weak mucosal defense mechanisms may be, a DU will not occur unless sufficient acid is present.

The mean parietal cell mass in normal subjects is 1 billion, whereas the mean for DU patients is 2 billion (Fig. 3-4). However, there is marked overlap. Thus, normal subjects occasionally have greater than 2 billion parietal cells and yet do not develop an ulcer, whereas other individuals with only 1 billion parietal cells develop a DU. An increased capacity to secrete acid and pepsin in the basal state has been postulated to occur on the basis of an increase in vagal tone, but this hypothesis remains unproven, as there is no method for measuring vagal tone.

The concept of a heightened parietal cell sensitivity to gastrin is based on the observation that a significantly lower dose of exogenous gastrin or pentagastrin is needed to produce one half the maximal acid secretory response in DU patients than in normal subjects (Fig. 3-5). Likewise, patients with DU are more sensitive than non-ulcer controls in regard to the release of endogenous

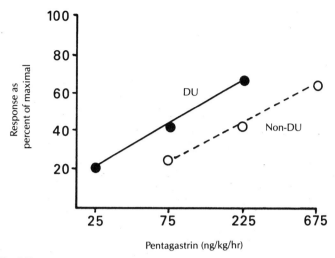

Fig. 3-5
Increased sensitivity to pentagastrin in patients with duodenal ulcer (DU).
(Modified from J. I. Isenberg, et al. Increased sensitivity to stimulation of acid
secretion by pentagastrin in duodenal ulcer. *J. Clin. Invest.* 55:330, 1975.)

gastrin following ingestion of a protein meal. An increased rate
of gastric emptying of liquids and solids has been shown in
patients with DU, but the reason for this abnormality is not
known. Another abnormality found in some patients with DU is
decreased acid-induced inhibition of gastrin release. Normally,
instillation of an acidified (pH 2.5) protein meal into the stomach
produces little or no release of gastrin and stimulates little or no
acid secretion. However, in DU patients, instillation of such a
meal produces a significant increment in gastrin release and in
acid secretion. Thus, the normal autoregulatory negative feedback mechanism for acid inhibition is missing in some patients
with DU disease. A net consequence of many of these physiologic abnormalities is an increased load or delivery of acid to the
duodenum. Neutralization of acid is achieved by salivary secretions and by pancreatic bicarbonate secretion. Patients with
DU have normal pancreatic bicarbonate output following secretin injection, and, currently, there is no evidence that secretin release or pancreatic bicarbonate output is impaired in
DU patients. Patients with Sjögren's syndrome or with chronic
pancreatic insufficiency who have decreased pancreatic bicarbonate secretion do not have an increased incidence of DU
disease.

Duodenal ulcer has often been viewed as a condition in which
aggressive factors (increased acid and pepsin) overwhelm the
mucosal defense mechanisms. However, it is worth reiterating
that only one third of patients have *increased* acid secretion.
Thus, two thirds of patients with proven DU disease have acid

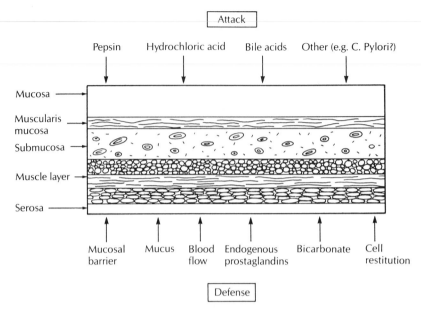

Fig. 3-6
Normal mucosa. A healthy balance exists between injurious and protective mechanisms.

secretion well within the normal range. Alterations in mucosal defense mechanisms are probably important in many patients. The precise nature and contributory role of various factors in modulating mucosal defense, such as blood flow, DNA synthesis and cell turnover, mucus production, and cytoprotective factors (endogenous prostaglandins and perhaps other agents) remain to be elucidated.

In summary, DU is a heterogeneous group of disorders; in some patients, acid hypersecretion is present. The reason that an individual develops a DU is not known. Genetic, psychological, and environmental factors probably have a complex interacting role. Some factors — for example, stress — are difficult to accurately quantify. When an imbalance between aggressive factors and defense mechanisms occurs, it can result in the expression of a mucosal lesion characterized by a hole extending through the muscularis mucosa into the submucosa or deeper — an ulcer (Figs. 3-6 and 3-7).

Pathophysiology of Gastric Ulcer

The pathophysiology of gastric ulcer (GU) is not completely understood. For decades, students of physiology and medicine have asked the question: Why doesn't the stomach, which contains acid, pepsin, and occasionally bile and pancreatic secretions, digest itself? Certainly, acid and pepsin are noxious agents that are quite injurious to the skin or certain parts of the

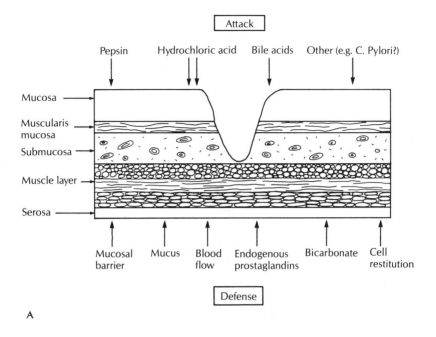

A

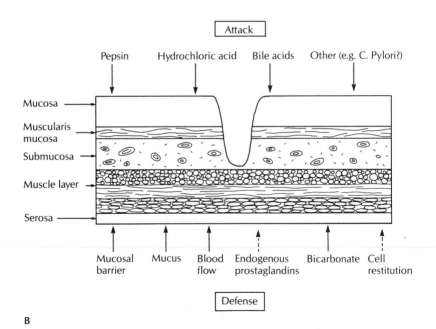

B

Fig. 3-7
A. Peptic ulcer. Although the defense is normal, the attacking forces are overwhelming and the delicate balance is disrupted. Example: Zollinger-Ellison syndrome (gastrinoma). B. Peptic ulcer. Although the attack is normal, the defense mechanisms are inadequate and the delicate balance is disrupted. Examples: aspirin, nonsteroidal anti-inflammatory drugs, smoking.

gastrointestinal system such as the esophagus and small intestine. Factors postulated to play a defensive role in this regard include mucus, the gastric mucosal barrier, production of endogenous bicarbonate and prostaglandins, rapid gastric epithelial renewal, and alterations in gastric mucosal blood flow. Some acid is indeed necessary for the development of gastric ulcers. Gastric ulcers occurring in the setting of achlorhydria are rare. Gastric ulcers almost always occur at the junction of non–acid-secreting gastric mucosa and acid-secreting mucosa and are most often located on the lesser curvature near the angulus of the stomach. The reason for this site predilection is not known, although the peculiar sling arrangement of gastric smooth muscle underlying the mucosa at this site has been advanced as a predisposing factor. Physiologic defects found in some patients with gastric ulcer include the following:

1. Decreased pyloric sphincter pressure
2. Increased reflux of duodenal contents into the stomach
3. Chronic atrophic gastritis
4. Decreased acid output
5. Mildly elevated serum gastrin levels

Pyloric sphincter dysfunction has been observed in patients with gastric ulcer. In some patients, pyloric sphincter pressure is abnormally low at rest, whereas in others, although the baseline resting pressure is normal, the pyloric sphincter pressure fails to rise in the presence of acid or fat in the duodenum. This had led to the belief that the pyloric sphincter fails to respond appropriately to endogenously released secretin or cholecystokinin. Pyloric sphincter dysfunction could, in turn, lead to increased amounts of duodenal contents (bile, lysolecithin, and pancreatic secretions) entering the stomach. It is postulated that these agents either alter the composition of the protective gastric mucus or damage the gastric mucosal barrier or both, permitting back-diffusion of hydrogen ion, which, over a prolonged period of time, leads to chronic gastritis. Although chronic gastritis is often present in patients with non–drug-related gastric ulcers, it is not evident why many patients with this histologic lesion never develop gastric ulcers, whereas others (albeit rarely) appear to develop gastric carcinoma. Chronic gastritis usually involves the antrum, but occasionally, the extent can be more widespread and can result in destruction of parietal cells. Consequently, some patients with gastric ulcers produce less gastric acid than do controls. Despite the presence of antral gastritis, the function of G cells in the antrum is preserved and antral gastrin content in patients with gastric ulcer is normal. The combination of decreased acid secretion and preserved antral G cell function explains the increased fasting and postprandial serum gastrin levels observed in many patients with gastric ulcer. Although gastric emptying is decreased in patients with gastric ulcers located in the body and increased in patients with prepyloric gastric ulcers, the importance of this defect in the pathogenesis of gastric ulcer disease is negated by the observation that gastric emptying usually reverts to normal following healing of the ulcer.

Causes of Peptic Ulcers

The use of aspirin and nonsteroidal anti-inflammatory agents is associated with an increased incidence of gastric ulcers. Approximately 25 percent of patients ingesting 3 gm or more of aspirin per day for 3 or more months will develop gastric ulcers. A noteworthy feature of aspirin-induced ulcers is the lack of gastritis in the surrounding or adjacent mucosa. Inhibition of prostaglandin production is believed to be important in the pathogenesis of aspirin and nonsteroidal anti-inflammatory drug–induced gastric ulceration.

Smoking

Recently, several studies have shown that not only do smokers have an increased likelihood of developing peptic ulcers but that once formed, these ulcers heal more slowly, and, once healed, they tend to recur sooner than in nonsmokers. Some of the physiologic effects related to smoking include decreased gastric mucosal blood flow and prostaglandin synthesis as well as decreased pancreatic bicarbonate secretion.

Stress

The role of stress in the pathogenesis of ulcer disease remains controversial. Many patients and some physicians ascribe significant importance to the role that stressful life events play in producing symptomatic exacerbations of peptic ulcer disease. The classic studies of two patients with gastric fistulas by Beaumont and Wolff demonstrated alterations in gastric physiology at the time of emotional disturbances. Feelings of anxiety, resentment, and hostility led to an augmentation of gastric mucosal hyperemia and gastric acid secretion. The observation of an increased incidence of perforated ulcers during air raids in London during World War II and the recent report of two patients with symptomatic gastric ulcer disease occurring shortly after severe emotional stress lends credence to the hypothesis that stress may cause or aggravate peptic ulcer disease. According to the latter report, both patients had markedly increased gastric acid secretion rates (one patient had a BAO level like that typically seen in patients with Zollinger-Ellison syndrome) that decreased to normal with abatement of the stressful situation.

Heredity

Relatives of patients with gastric ulcers have a threefold increased prevalence of gastric ulcers compared to that of the general population. The increased risk is site-specific, so the prevalence of duodenal ulcers is not increased in these subjects. Studies in twins, as mentioned previously, support the concept that the tendency to develop an ulcer is inherited.

Campylobacter pylori

In recent years, there has been considerable interest in the possible relationship between this S-shaped rod and gastrointestinal disease. Several studies have now confirmed the positive association of this bacterium with the presence of duodenal ulcer, gastric ulcer, and non-ulcer dyspepsia. It is found only in gastric epithelium, and its presence is strongly correlated with an active antral gastritis. This organism evokes both a local (IgA and IgM antibodies to *C. pylori* are present in gastric juice) and a systemic response (IgG or IgA antibodies or both to *C. pylori* are present in the serum). Koch's postulates have been fulfilled in volunteers who developed symptoms of epigastric discomfort, nausea, bloating, vomiting, and halitosis together with histologic evidence of gastritis following ingestion of live *C. pylori*. Although it has not been proved that this organism is pathogenetically causative of peptic ulcer disease, it raises the intriguing possibility that an infectious agent may be the cause of peptic ulceration in some patients. Bismuth salts in combination with an antimicrobial agent (erythromycin or metronidazole) may prove to be of considerable value in the treatment of such individuals.

Pathophysiology of Zollinger-Ellison Syndrome

In 1955, Zollinger and Ellison described two patients with the triad of severe peptic ulcer disease, strikingly increased gastric acid secretion, and non-beta islet cell tumors of the pancreas (see Chap. 21). A few years later, Gregory and colleagues conclusively demonstrated that the biologically potent acid secretagogue in the tumors of patients with this syndrome was the hormone gastrin. The predominant form of gastrin in the tumor tissue is G 17 or heptadecapeptide gastrin, whereas the major form in the circulation of these patients is G 34 or "big gastrin." Since approximately 10 to 15 percent of these gastrin-producing tumors are present outside the pancreas and since 5 to 10 percent of patients with this syndrome do not have ulcer disease, the currently preferred term is *gastrinoma*. The gastrinomas in patients with Zollinger-Ellison syndrome are most often located in the head and tail of the pancreas. They vary in size from 0.2 cm to 20 cm in diameter, 50 percent are multiple, and 60 to 70 percent are malignant. Sites of metastases include regional lymph nodes, liver, spleen, bone, mediastinum, and peritoneum. Extrapancreatic gastrinomas are most often located in the stomach, spleen, liver, mesenteric lymph nodes, parathyroid glands, or ovaries. Approximatley 20 percent of patients with gastrinomas have the MEN-I syndrome present concomitantly. This syndrome consists of tumors or hyperplasia of the three "P's" — pituitary, parathyroid, and pancreas.

The marked acid hypersecretion leads to several pathophysiologic consequences. Peptic ulcer disease is present in most patients (90–95%) and may express itself as garden-variety ulcer disease or a very virulent process with one or more complications of obstruction, hemorrhage, perforation, intractable pain, poor healing, or high recurrence. Esophagitis with ucleration and stricture formation may be present. Acid hypersecretion also leads to diarrhea and steatorrhea. Multiple mechanisms are operative, including sheer volume overload, mucosal damage to the small bowel, inactivation of pancreatic lipase, and precipitation of bile salts. In addition, high levels of circulating gastrin may contribute to diarrhea, since it has been shown that intravenous infusion of a large amount of gastrin directly increases intestinal secretion of potassium and reduces jejunal absorption of sodium and water. It is noteworthy that the diarrhea is usually ameliorated by removing acid from the stomach by nasogastric suction or by effective antisecretory (an H_2 receptor antagonist or a proton pump blocker) therapy. In normal human subjects, gastrin decreases the rate of gastric emptying of liquids. However, patients with gastrinoma have an increased rate of gastric emptying of liquids. The reason for this paradoxical increase in gastric emptying of liquids is unknown but probably explains the limited efficacy of orally administered antacids in patients with this syndrome.

Another consequence of hypergastrinemia is pepsin secretion by gastric zymogen cells. Pepsin is activated in the acid milieu of the jejunum of these patients and is believed to contribute to ulceration in the small intestine. Patients with gastrinomas may also develop vitamin B_{12} malabsorption that is not corrected by oral administration of intrinsic factor. Gastric secretion of intrinsic factor is probably normal in these patients, and the mechanism by which a low intraluminal pH adversely affects distal ileal absorption of vitamin B_{12} remains undefined at the present time. Gastrin is probably also responsible for the large gastric rugae or folds in patients with gastrinoma by virtue of its trophic qualities on gastric mucosa. The diagnosis and treatment of gastrinoma are discussed in Chapter 2.

Clinical Features of Peptic Ulcer

The classic teaching is that ulcer pain is "epigastric, gnawing, or burning; relieved by food or antacids; recurs 2 to 3 hours after eating; awakens the patient at 2:00 A.M., but is virtually never present on first awakening in the morning." In fact, ulcer pain, in many patients, bears no relationship to meals; it may occur within an hour of eating or worsen after eating. Additionally, although 85 to 90 percent of ulcer patients report nocturnal pain and relief by antacids, more than 30 percent of patients with chronic abdominal pain not caused by an ulcer also report nocturnal pain and relief by antacids.

Distinction between a duodenal ulcer and gastric ulcer based on symptoms is, likewise, not possible in most patients. Studies have also demonstrated that resolution of a patient's symptoms when the patient is on active antiulcer treatment does not necessarily mean that the ulcer crater has healed. Similarly, patients may have continued symptoms despite endoscopic documentation of ulcer healing.

Diagnostic Studies for Peptic Ulcer Disease

Barium contrast studies are conventionally used in patients suspected of having active peptic ulcer disease. These studies have a 60 to 80 percent accuracy rate in detecting ulcers. Demonstration of an ulcer crater is necessary for diagnosing a gastric ulcer, whereas demonstration of an ulcer niche, or deformity, spasm, and "irritability" of the duodenal bulb or second portion of the duodenum suffices in diagnosing a duodenal ulcer. Improved accuracy in the detection rate of ulcers is achieved by the use of double-contrast techniques; the skill of the radiologist performing the examination is also an important factor in accuracy of detection. Figure 3-8 illustrates the important criteria for benignity of gastric ulcers. Ulcers in the duodenum are almost always benign, whereas gastric ulcers that appear "benign" radiographically are malignant approximately 5 percent of the time. The latter represent malignant lesions of the stomach such as gastric adenocarcinoma or lymphoma that are ulcerated, hence simulating a gastric ulcer and *not* malignant transformation of a previously benign gastric ulcer.

Fiberoptic upper gastrointestinal *endoscopy* is considered the "gold standard" for evaluation of active ulcer disease. Endoscopy is indicated if one or more of the following conditions applies to the patient: (1) persistent dyspepsia with a normal upper gastrointestinal tract study on examination with barium (UGI); (2) a gastric ulcer seen on UGI so as to rule out a cancer; (3) previous gastric surgery, since the UGI series is insensitive in distinguishing active ulcer disease from surgical deformity; or (4) certain complications of ulcer disease — for example, hemorrhage and obstruction. Endoscopy is not indicated in patients with uncomplicated duodenal ulcer disease.

Acid secretory studies have a minimal role in clinical medicine. As mentioned earlier, there is considerable overlap between normal subjects, patients with gastric ulcers, and those with duodenal ulcers; hence, acid secretory values have no diag-

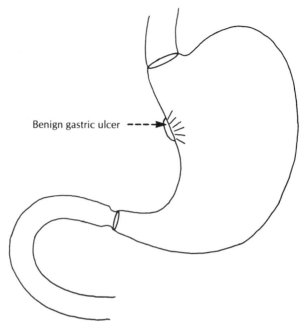

Fig. 3-8
Schematic depiction of criteria for benignity in gastric ulcer. Criteria for benignity: (1) smooth margins and projection beyond wall of stomach; (2) luminal margin of ulcer demarcated by a thin radiolucent line — Hampton's line — which represents collar of edema surrounding ulcer; (3) gastric folds radiate to the ulcer.

Benign gastric ulcer

nostic or prognostic significance. In those patients in whom an acid-reducing surgical procedure is being considered, the preoperative level of acid secretion does not clearly dictate the type of acid-reducing operation that should be performed. Lastly, the level of acid secretion and the ratio of BAO : MAO is not a sensitive enough screening test for patients with gastrinomas and has been effectively replaced by gastrin assays and the secretin test (discussed later).

Serum gastrin determinations can be readily made using a sensitive radioimmunoassay. Indications for measuring serum gastrin include the following: (1) suspected gastrinoma (Zollinger-Ellison syndrome; see Chap. 21); (2) suspected G cell hyperplasia; (3) suspected retained antrum syndrome; (4) anastomotic ulcer; and (5) prior to elective surgery for patients with peptic ulcer disease. It is important to note that cimetidine and ranitidine do not influence fasting serum gastrin levels; hence, discontinuation of these drugs is not necessary prior to obtaining fasting serum gastrin levels.

Increased serum gastrin levels may be considered "appropriate" or "inappropriate." "Appropriate" hypergastrinemia refers

Table 3-3
Causes of hypergastrinemia

Normal or decreased gastric acid secretion	Increased gastric acid secretion
Pernicious anemia	Gastrinoma
Chronic gastritis	G cell hyperplasia
Gastric carcinoma	Retained antrum syndrome
Gastric ulcer	Gastric outlet obstruction
Postvagotomy	Renal failure
Pheochromocytoma	Massive small bowel resection

to the situation in which achlorhydria or marked hypochlorhydria coupled with the presence of a functionally intact antrum (and hence antral G cells) results in elevated serum gastrin levels. "Inappropriate" hypergastrinemia is associated with excessive gastric acid secretion and is most commonly due to gastrinomas (Table 3-3).

Complications of Peptic Ulcer Disease

Complications occur most frequently in patients with gastric ulcer. It should be noted that clinicians are unable to predict accurately which patients will develop complications such as hemorrhage, perforation, and obstruction, which occur in approximately 20 percent, 5 to 10 percent, and 5 percent, respectively.

Medical Treatment of Peptic Ulcer Disease

Diet

In the past, patients with peptic ulcer disease were advised to adhere to "bland" diets that were quite restrictive and unpalatable. Currently, such dietary therapy is no longer recommended, since patients with uncomplicated peptic ulcers heal as readily on a diet of their own choosing as on a strictly "bland" dietary regimen. Patients are advised to avoid foods that have caused abdominal symptoms in the past and to curtail the use of coffee and alcohol, which are known to stimulate acid secretion. Both regular and decaffeinated coffee stimulate acid secretion to an equivalent degree, since they contain peptides derived from the roasted coffee beans, which presumably produce similar increments in the release of the hormone gastrin. Milk in small amounts is permissible. Large amounts of whole milk may be detrimental, because the protein and calcium content of milk is sufficient to produce stimulation of acid secretion.

Table 3-4
Potential medical strategies for treating peptic ulcer

Objective	Pharmacologic agent
Suppression of gastric acid secretion	H_2 receptor antagonists, e.g., cimetidine, ranitidine, famotidine
	Anticholinergics, e.g., Pro-Banthine, pirenzepine
	H^+K^+ ATPase inhibitor, e.g., omeprazole
Neutralization of gastric acid	Antacids
Shielding of mucosa and provision of cytoprotection	Sucralfate Prostaglandins Bismuth Carbenoxolone

Pharmacologic Therapy

Potential pharmacologic strategies for treating peptic ulcer are predicated on the role of aggressive factors and defense mechanisms in the pathogenesis of an ulcer; these are summarized in Table 3-4. The objectives of treatment include the relief of pain, acceleration of healing of the ulcer, and prevention of recurrences and complications.

H_2 Receptor Antagonists

Histamine stimulates gastric acid secretion by acting on a receptor (histamine H_2 receptor) located on the gastric parietal cell. Since histamine is the messenger involved in the final pathway leading to stimulation of gastric acid secretion, H_2 receptor antagonists inhibit acid secretion in response to a variety of secretagogues. Cimetidine was the first H_2 receptor antagonist to become commercially available. It is a powerful inhibitor of basal and nocturnal acid secretion and is more effective than placebo in healing duodenal ulcers. Ranitidine and famotidine are more potent than cimetidine and are currently available for use.

Anticholinergics

The traditional anticholinergics are weak inhibitors of acid secretion at the recommended doses, reducing basal acid secretion by 50 to 60 percent and meal-stimulated acid secretion by 30 to 50 percent. Reduction of acid secretion occurs by the ability of these drugs such as propantheline bromide (Pro-Banthine) to block the acetylcholine receptor on gastric parietal cells. However, these drugs also block muscarinic receptors on other parts of the body, resulting in a number of undesirable side effects such as dry mouth, blurred vision, and urinary retention. For this reason, these drugs are not currently favored for the treatment of peptic ulcer disease except as adjunctive therapy in combination with an antacid or a H_2 receptor antagonist. Pirenzepine is a selective muscarinic M_1 receptor antagonist that has promise of healing peptic ulcers without the side effects common to the nonselective antimuscarinic drugs.

Omeprazole

Omeprazole is a substituted benzimidazole derivative that irreversibly blocks the proton pump (hydrogen potassium ATPase enzyme) located on the luminal surface of parietal cells and results in profound inhibition of gastric acid secretion, far greater than that achieved by the currently available H_2 receptor antagonists. It is capable of healing severe peptic esophagitis as well as gastric and duodenal ulcers. Additionally, omeprazole is capable of healing ulcers in the setting of profound and sustained acid hypersecretion seen in patients with Zollinger-Ellison syndrome (gastrinoma). This drug causes an elevation in fasting serum gastrin in humans and has been linked to the development of gastric carcinoid tumors in rats.

Antacids

Antacids vary in their ability to neutralize gastric acid. Most antacids contain various combinations of aluminum hydroxide, magnesium hydroxide, and calcium salts. Reduction in gastric acidity occurs when an antacid constituent chemically reacts with hydrochloric acid. Antacids are superior to placebo in healing duodenal ulcers but are not clearly superior to placebo in healing gastric ulcers.

Sucralfate

This drug is a basic aluminum salt of sucrose octasulfate, which forms a viscous adhesive gel that adheres to the ulcer crater, thereby shielding the ulcer from acid and pepsin. Additionally, recent studies suggest that sucralfate may enhance mucosal defense by stimulating gastric mucosal prostaglandin synthesis. Prostaglandins may have unique cytoprotective properties. Sucralfate has been shown to be significantly better than placebo and as effective as cimetidine in healing duodenal ulcers.

Gastrinoma (Zollinger-Ellison Syndrome)

As mentioned earlier, in 1955, Zollinger and Ellison defined this syndrome, named after them, as a triad consisting of "primary peptic ulcerations in unusual locations," "gastric hypersecretion of gigantic proportion," and the presence of "nonspecific islet cell tumor of the pancreas." Currently, none of these three criteria are necessary for the diagnosis of this syndrome, which is more aptly referred to as gastrinoma. Some patients are

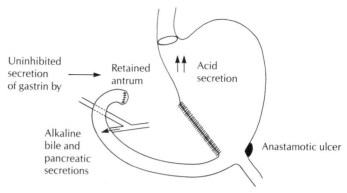

Fig. 3-9
Pathophysiology of retained antrum syndrome.

asymptomatic and are discovered on the basis of screening performed in family members of a patient with the syndrome. Gastrinoma is rare, being estimated to occur in 0.1 to 1.0 percent of all patients with duodenal ulcer. It may occur in early childhood or manifest in the tenth decade, although it appears most commonly in patients between 30 and 50 years of age. The clinical manifestations, pathophysiology, and management of gastrinoma are discussed in Chapter 21.

Retained Gastric Antrum Syndrome

Retained gastric antrum syndrome is an extremely rare condition that develops in patients who undergo a partial gastric resection with a Billroth II gastroenterostomy and in whom a cuff of antral tissue is inadvertently left attached to the excluded proximal duodenal stump. The pathophysiology of this syndrome is easily appreciated by realizing that the excluded antrum is totally isolated from the gastric acid stream (Fig. 3-9). Consequently, the G cells in the antrum are constantly bathed by alkaline secretions (bile and pancreatic juice) and are not subject to the normal inhibition of gastrin release that occurs by gastric acid. Patients present with a syndrome clinically indistinguishable from gastrinoma, namely, recurrent ulcer disease, increased basal serum gastrin levels, and acid hypersecretion. The possibility of the presence of this syndrome should always be considered in patients with recurrent ulcer disease following a Billroth II anastomosis. The diagnosis may be suggested by a careful review of the original resected specimen (distal stomach margin lacks a generous cuff of duodenal mucosa) and ^{99m}Tc-pertechnetate scanning (uptake by antral tissue in the duodenal stump). The secretin test is used to distinguish this syndrome from that found in gastrinoma patients. In contrast to patients with gastrinoma who show a significant increment in serum gastrin values following intravenous secretin administration, patients with this syndrome do not show a rise in serum gastrin values above baseline.

G Cell Hyperplasia

G cell hyperplasia is a rare disorder that has confusingly been termed *pseudo Zollinger-Ellison syndrome* as well as *Zollinger-Ellison syndrome type I*. Patients have peptic ulcer disease, increased serum gastrin levels, and acid hypersecretion, thus mimicking gastrinoma patients. There are increased numbers of antral G cells in these patients, who have no evidence of a gastrin-secreting tumor. The diagnosis is suggested by the aforementioned findings coupled with a negative secretin test (i.e., following intravenous secretin, the serum gastrin falls or rises minimally) and an exaggerated positive response to a standard meal, that is, greater than a 100 percent increment in serum gastrin. Following antrectomy, fasting and postprandial gastrin values return to normal.

Study Questions

1. Answer true or false:
   a. Patients with duodenal ulcer are more likely to have increased gastric acid secretion than patients with gastric ulcer.
   b. Ninety percent of all patients with hypergastrinemia will have peptic ulcer disease.
   c. Patients with chronic pancreatic insufficiency who have decreased pancreatic bicarbonate secretion are at increased risk for developing duodenal ulcer.
   d. Increased gastric acid secretion and increased serum gastrin levels are seen in patients with gastrinoma as well as G cell hyperplasia.

   Answers
   a. True
   b. False. There are many causes of hypergastrinemia. Increased serum gastrin levels can be seen in patients with *increased* gastric acid secretion (e.g., gastrinoma) as well as in patients with *decreased* gastric acid secretion (e.g., pernicious anemia). Among patients with hypergastrinemia secondary to gastrinoma, approximately 90 percent will develop ulcer disease.
   c. False
   d. True

2. For each of the diagnoses in List I, select the appropriate feature from List II.

   List I
   a. Gastric ulcer
   b. Duodenal ulcer
   c. Both
   d. Neither

List II
A. Bland diet is effective treatment.
B. Must be differentiated from an ulcerating malignancy.
C. Is caused by *Campylobacter pylori* infection.
D. Is associated with chronic gastritis.
E. May be a cause of gastrointestinal bleeding.
F. Is a premalignant condition.

Answers
A:d
B:a
C:d
D:a
E:c
F:d

References

Allen, A. Structure and Function of Gastrointestinal Mucus. In L. R. Johnson (ed.), *Physiology of the Gastrointestinal Tract*. New York: Raven, 1981. Pp 617–639.

Feldman, M., and Richardson, C. T. Gastric Acid Secretion in Humans. In L. R. Johnson (ed.), *Physiology of the Gastrointestinal Tract*. New York: Raven, 1981. Pp 693–707.

Ganguli, P. C., Polak, J. M., Pearse, A. G. E., et al. Antral-gastrin-cell hyperplasia in peptic ulcer disease. *Lancet* I:583, 1974.

Grossman, M. I. Regulation of Gastric Acid Secretion. In L. R. Johnson (ed.), *Physiology of the Gastrointestinal Tract*. New York: Raven, 1981. Pp 659–671.

Grossman, M. I. (ed.). *Peptic Ulcer: A Guide for the Practicing Physician*. Chicago: Year Book, 1981.

Grossman, M. I., Guth, P. H., Isenberg, J. I., et al. A new look at peptic ulcer. UCLA conference. *Ann. Intern. Med.* 84:57, 1976.

Grossman, M. I., Kurata, J. H., Rotter, J. I., et al. Peptic ulcer: New therapies, new diseases. UCLA conference. *Ann. Intern. Med.* 95:609, 1981.

Isenberg, J. I. Peptic ulcer. *Disease a Month* 28:6, 1981.

Isenberg, J. I., and Johansson, C. (guest eds.). Peptic ulcer disease. *Clin. Gastroenterol.* 13:2, 1984.

Jensen, R. T., Gardner, J. D., Raufman, J., et al. Zollinger-Ellison syndrome: Current concepts and management. *Ann. Intern. Med.* 98:59, 1983.

Malagelada, J. R. Medical versus surgical therapy for duodenal ulcer. Making the right choices. *Mayo Clin. Proc.* 55:25, 1980.

McArthur, K. A., Collen, M. J., Maton, P. N., et al. Omeprazole: Effective, convenient therapy for Zollinger-Ellison syndrome. *Gastroenterology* 88:939, 185.

McCarthy, D. M. Smoking and ulcers — time to quit. *N. Engl. J. Med.* 311:726, 1984.

Rathbone, B. J., Wyatt, J. I., and Heatley, R. V. Campylobacter pyloridis — a new factor in peptic ulcer disease? *Gut* 27:635, 1986.

Richardson, C. T. Gastric Ulcer. In M. H. Sleisenger and J. S. Fordtran (eds.), *Gastrointestinal Diseases* (3rd ed.). Philadelphia: Saunders, 1983. Pp 672–693.

Rotter, J. I. Genetic aspects of ulcer disease. *Compr. Ther.* August 1981, Pp. 16–25.

Soll, A. H. The Parietal Cell and Regulation of Gastric Acid Secretion. In H. J. Binder (ed.), *Viewpoints on Digestive Diseases* (Vol. 16). Thorofare, NJ: Slack, 1984. Pp. 1–4.

Soll, A. H., and Isenberg, J. I. Duodenal Ulcer Disease. In M. H. Sleisenger and J. S. Fordtran (eds.), *Gastrointestinal Disease* (3rd ed.). Philadelphia: Saunders, 1983. Pp. 625–672.

Taylor, I. L. Gastrointestinal hormones in the pathogenesis of peptic ulcer disease. *Clin. Gastroenterol.* 13:355, 1984.

Van Heenden, J. A., Bernatz, P. E., and Rovelstad, R. A. The retained antrum — clinical considerations. *Mayo Clin. Proc.* 46:25, 1971.

Walsh, J. H., and Grossman, M. I. Gastrin. *N. Engl. J. Med.* 292:1324–1334 and 1377–1384, 1975.

Zollinger, R. M., and Ellison, E. H. Primary peptic ulcerations of the jejunum associated with islet cell tumors of the pancreas. *Ann. Surg.* 142:709, 1955.

4 : Gastritis and Gastric Neoplasia

William D. Kasimer
Yogeshwar Dayal

Histology of the Normal Gastric Mucosa

The entire luminal surface of the gastric mucosa is lined by a single layer of tall columnar mucus-producing epithelial cells whose chief function is to protect the deeper layers from the injurious effects of the acidic pH of the gastric luminal contents. This epithelial layer dips down every so often to form small tubular crevices called *gastric pits*, or *foveolae*. In the body-fundic region of the stomach, these pits are rather shallow, extending only into the superficial third of the mucosal thickness, whereas in the cardiac, antral, and pyloric regions, they extend deeper, reaching midway into the mucosal thickness. In the body-fundic region, the gastric pits communicate at their base with compactly packed straight-tubular–type glands in which four morphologically and functionally distinct cell types — mucus cells, parietal cells, chief cells, and endocrine cells — can be identified. Since the lumen of these glands is continuous with that of the pits, gastric juices (the aggregate secretion of these cell types) can easily reach the gastric lumen. The mucus cells, most numerous in the area where the gastric glands open into the gastric pits, have a clear or foamy cytoplasm and basally located nuclei. This appearance of the cytoplasm is due to its abundant mucin content, which is best seen by the periodic acid–Schiff (PAS) stain. The parietal cells produce hydrochloric acid and intrinsic factor, are most numerous in the middle third of the mucosal thickness, and are seen in hematoxylin-eosin (H&E) stains as oval- or triangular-shaped cells with abundant pink cytoplasm and a dark centrally placed nucleus. The chief cells, most numerous in the lower third of the mucosa, produce pepsinogen and are characterized by a granular, pale blue cytoplasm and a basally oriented nucleus. The endocrine cells, relatively sparse in number, are dispersed randomly between the parietal and chief cells in the middle and lower third of the mucosa. These triangular, pyramidal, or pear-shaped cells with a clear or faintly pink granular cytoplasm are difficult to identify in H&E stains but can easily be visualized by certain silver stains because of their affinity for silver salts (agent affinity) and their ability to reduce them to metallic silver (argyrophilia).

In the cardiac and antropyloric areas, the gastric pits communicate with simple tubular mucus-producing glands. Parietal and chief cells are absent, whereas the endocrine cells, interspersed between the mucus cells lining the glands, are almost exclusively confined to the lower third of the mucosal thickness. It should be noted that although the endocrine cells in the body-fundic and the antral mucosa are morphologically similar, the endocrine cell population of the stomach (as also in the remainder of the gastrointestinal tract) is actually a constellation of several functionally distinct cell types, each of which produces a specific biogenic amine or peptide hormone such as histamine, serotonin, gastrin, and somatostatin. Each cell type is normally distributed in a specific anatomic location in numbers that are tailored to meet physiologic requirements pertinent to that site.

Acute Gastritis

Acute gastritis is a term that has been applied to a broad spectrum of disorders ranging from vague gastrointestinal discomfort following the ingestion of certain agents to the life-threatening "stress ulceration" that may complicate many major medical illnesses. When discussing the pathogenesis of acute gastric mucosal injury, it is useful to consider the stomach in terms of "protective" factors (those that prevent mucosal injury) and "aggressive" factors (those that promote injury).

Protective Factors

Despite the hostile intraluminal environment of the stomach, the normal gastric mucosa is well protected under normal circumstances by several mechanisms.

The first "line of defense" consists of the material that covers the gastric mucosal cells, consisting primarily of mucus and bicarbonate. Mucus is derived from glycoproteins and is secreted by the surface epithelial cells of the gastric mucosa by a combination of exocytosis, apical expulsion, and exfoliation forming a fairly continuous layer over the mucosa. In order for glycoproteins to form this mucus "gel," they must be secreted at a sufficiently high rate to produce a concentration of 30 to 50 mg/ml. The two important mechanisms by which mucus acts as a protective barrier are (1) the prevention of mechanical abrasion to the mucosal cells, and (2) the provision of a surface for the neutralization of hydrogen ions by bicarbonate. Although bicarbonate is constantly secreted by the surface epithelial cells at a rate sufficient to saturate the mucus gel, elevations in intraluminal acid concentration are accompanied by a concomitant increase in bicarbonate secretion.

The gastric mucosa is further protected by certain properties of the epithelial cells themselves. One feature is their rapid "turnover." The surface epithelial cells have a very short life span, and exfoliated cells are rapidly replaced by proliferating cells from the gastric glands below the surface. Prior to their migration to the mucosal surface, immature cells in the regenerative zone lose their potential for DNA synthesis (replicative ability) and undergo gradual maturation and differentiation into cells capable of synthesizing glycoproteins. In addition, mucosal cells themselves constitute a mechanical "barrier" that prevents hydrogen ions and other substances from penetrating the deeper layers of the stomach wall. A vital component of this barrier is the presence of tight junctions between the mucosal cells, which, by complex electrophysiologic mechanisms, maintain the high pH gradient across the mucosa, and thus across the barrier. The rate at which hydrogen ions cross the mucosa is an important factor in the development of gastric injury.

Mucosal blood flow is another crucial protective mechanism. The lamina propria of the stomach contains a complex capillary network that constantly exchanges ions between the blood and the interstitial fluid, thereby preventing their accumulation.

Recent experimental evidence indicates that prostaglandins exert a strong protective influence on the integrity of the gastric mucosa. Prostaglandins are a group of hormones that act locally at their site of synthesis. All are 20-carbon, unsaturated fatty acids. In many diverse organs, prostaglandins have been shown to have a wide variety of effects, especially as secondary mediators of inflammation. Prostaglandins E, A, and I have been shown to be potent inhibitors of both basal and stimulated gastric acid secretion, but all prostaglandins appear to have cytoprotective effects. The exact mechanisms underlying these cytoprotective effects remain undefined but are distinct from prostaglandins' inhibition of acid secretion. Prostaglandins may not only prevent and slow the disruption of the gastric mucosal barrier but may also stimulate the formation of both mucus and bicarbonate. Furthermore, because of their important vasoactive effects, prostaglandins may also serve to increase mucosal blood flow. Other postulated effects include increased cell synthetic activity (of DNA, RNA, protein, sulfhydryl compounds, and surface-active phospholipids) and transport processes, as well as production of gross architectural changes in gastric mucosa. Specific prostaglandin receptors have been identified on gastric epithelial cells.

Aggressive Factors

After the preceding brief discussion of the protective factors of the gastric mucosa, it will come as no surprise that the presence of acid is necessary for the production of acute gastric injury. There is no evidence, however, that *increased* acid secretion is necessary to produce acute gastritis, and, although hyperacidity may play an important role under certain circumstances, many of the conditions that predispose to acute gastritis are accompanied by normal or decreased acid secretion. The control of acid secretion will be discussed only as it pertains to the pathogenesis of acute gastritis in specific circumstances. The role of pepsin is similar; its presence is necessary to produce injury, but increased secretion is not. The primary pathogenetic role of pepsin in acute gastritis is its ability to break down gastric mucus by dissolving the disulfide bonds between glycoprotein subunits. The importance of histamine lies in its ability to stimulate gastric acid secretion by means of H_2 receptors. Histamine is also an important secondary mediator of gastric mucosal injury, since it is released in mucosa damaged by any mechanism, and its effects on blood flow and capillary permeability contribute to bleeding.

In patients with "acute stress ulceration," mucosal ischemia secondary to splanchnic vasoconstriction is an important pathogenetic factor. This may occur despite the maintenance of normal systemic blood pressure and has been postulated to produce deleterious effects by at least two mechanisms. First, it may decrease the rate at which hydrogen ions, which have crossed the mucosal barrier into the lamina propria and have been buffered by bicarbonate, can be removed; tissue ischemia also produces acidosis with a concomitant decrease in bicarbonate, thus diminishing the capacity for buffering of hydrogen ions. Second, mucosal ischemia causes tissue hypoxia and thereby reduces the synthesis of cellular ATP. This in turn leads to a reduction of active transport processes and compromises cellular functioning vital for mucosal integrity.

Under normal circumstances, bile acids do not produce mucosal injury because there is a compensatory increase in mucosal blood flow to enhance the buffering capacity. Under experimental conditions, however, bile salts do disrupt the mucosal barrier and permit back-diffusion of hydrogen ions. The role of bile salts in the pathogenesis of gastric mucosal injury in conditions such as drug-induced gastritis and acute stress ulceration is not clear at the present time.

Specific Etiologic Agents

Alcohol

In the outpatient setting, alcohol is a common cause of acute gastritis. Investigations have shown that ingestion of alcohol produces both gross and microscopic evidence of acute gastric mucosal injury. In experimental models, the extent of injury depends on the volume and concentration of ethanol ingested, as well as on whether the animals were fasted prior to the administration of ethanol. Several pathogenetic mechanisms may be responsible for alcohol-induced injury. Ethanol appears to disrupt the tight junctions between epithelial cells, allowing back-diffusion of hydrogen ions, and may cause an increase in gastric acid secretion. Ethanol also causes a decrease in both intracellular and extracellular mucin.

Aspirin

Acetylsalicylic acid has been studied extensively with regard to its role in the development of acute gastritis. It appears that a pharmacologic dose causes gross and microscopic gastric injury within an hour of ingestion, although most patients do not complain of symptoms. Aspirin has been reported to cause mucosal injury by several mechanisms. Because of its biochemical properties, the acidity of gastric contents favors its absorption in the stomach, where it causes rapid back-diffusion of hydrogen ions by disrupting the mucosal barrier (either tight junctions or the cell membranes themselves); damage and bleeding are compounded by the effects of histamine. In addition, acid stimulates gastric motility, and, since venous drainage is impaired during contraction, this factor may cause further blood loss from damaged blood vessels. Inhibition of prostaglandin synthesis by aspirin may also play an important role in mucosal injury, because prostaglandins are cytoprotective in nature. Parenterally administered salicylate also causes damage to the gastric mucosa. Aspirin and alcohol appear to have synergistic effects in producing gastritis.

Other Pharmacologic Agents

Other nonsteroidal anti-inflammatory compounds, such as indomethacin, phenylbutazone, and ibuprofen, also cause acute gastric injury. The exact pathogenetic mechanism(s) are not known but may be related to their inhibition of prostaglandin synthesis. Although steroids do alter gastric mucus, there is no evidence that steroids cause acute gastritis. Cytotoxic agents given as chemotherapy for tumors may also be responsible for gastric mucosal damage because of their inhibition of cell regeneration.

Foods

Despite common folklore, there is little evidence that consumption of certain foods causes acute gastric injury. Although caffeine produces gastritis in animals, its effect in humans is not clear.

Major Illness

Acute gastritis may be a life-threatening complication of many diverse illnesses; in this clinical setting, it is often termed *acute stress ulceration* or *acute hemorrhagic gastritis*. Although almost any major illness may predispose to stress ulceration, some of the more common clinical settings include major trauma, extensive burns (Curling's ulcers), sepsis, respiratory failure, renal failure, jaundice, and diseases of the central nervous system (Cushing's ulcers). A common denominator in most of these conditions is hypotension, often prolonged, and the resultant mucosal ischemia appears to be the primary pathogenetic mechanism in the production of stress ulcers. The autonomic nervous system and various hormonal substances may also be involved. Patients with Cushing's ulcers appear to represent a distinct group in that these patients show increased secretion of gastrin, acid, and pepsin, possibly mediated by increased vagal activity. In contrast, patients with non-neurologic diseases invariably have normal acid secretion.

Pathology

Despite its diverse causes, the morphologic changes seen in acute gastritis are fairly constant. Grossly, the appearance of the stomach is often not particularly impressive, showing only areas of petechial hemorrhage and minute erosions. Microscopically, there is necrosis of the surface epithelial cells with acute inflammation and focal loss of mucosa, thus exposing the lamina propria. Red cell extravasation or frank hemorrhage is a prominent feature both histologically and clinically. Damage may be extensive and deep enough to cause erosion in a major vessel or perforation of the stomach.

Treatment

From the previous discussion of pathogenic factors and etiologic agents, the primary modalities of treatment follow logically. Mere avoidance of the identifiable precipitating agents may be adequate in some cases. Similarly, maintenance of blood pressure in major illnesses may prevent or minimize mucosal injury. Finally, measures directed at decreasing intraluminal acidity are also beneficial. In patients with active bleeding, treatment should consist of supportive measures. If hemorrhage is life-threatening or cannot be controlled by conservative measures, surgical intervention is often necessary.

Acute Phlegmonous Gastritis

Acute phlegmonous gastritis is a rare, often fatal illness characterized by localized or diffuse bacterial infection of the stomach wall. It appears to be more common in patients whose gastric mucosa is already compromised in some fashion, such as by an underlying carcinoma or alcohol abuse. The source of bacteria is usually the oropharynx, and some patients give a history of recent pharyngitis; alpha-hemolytic Streptococcus is the most common etiologic agent. Although aggressive antibiotic treatment may be successful, standard treatment has been total or subtotal gastrectomy.

Hyperplastic Gastropathy ("Ménétrier's Disease")

Despite its rare occurrence, many colorful terms have been used to describe this condition. The macroscopic appearance of this disease is striking. There is marked thickening of the gastric wall with giant, inelastic rugal folds, which resemble cerebral convolutions. Both diffuse and localized forms of mucosal involvement have been described; in the latter form, the involved mucosa is sharply demarcated from and stands out in sharp contrast to the surrounding normal mucosa. Microscopically, it is characterized by extreme hyperplasia of the gastric epithelium, which forms broad folds, often with projections of the muscularis mucosa into these folds. The mucosal hyperplasia has been divided into three types: (1) mucous cell type, in which the hyperplasia involves the surface and foveolar cells; (2) glandular cell type, which shows hyperplasia of the gastric glands, including chief and parietal cells; and (3) mixed mucous-glandular type, in which both elements are hyperplastic. The gastric pits and glands are elongated. The relative proportions of the various mucosal cells may be normal; in some cases, there is depletion of parietal and chief cells. Cystic dilation of glands, intestinal metaplasia, and inflammatory changes are often present.

The etiology and pathogenesis of hyperplastic gastropathy are unknown; many possible factors have been suggested. Clinically, common symptoms include pain, vomiting, and hemorrhage. In addition, the abnormal gastric mucosa releases an excessive amount of protein into the lumen, where it is degraded and lost (protein-losing gastropathy). The resultant hypoproteinemia often produces weight loss and peripheral edema. Levels of gastric acid may be high (usually in the glandular cell type), low (usually in the mucous cell type), or normal.

Several pharmacologic agents, such as steroids, anticholinergic drugs, and cimetidine, have been used with variable success in its treatment; surgical resection is sometimes necessary if hemorrhage or protein loss are prominent. Because of the rarity of this disease, its prognosis is unclear and there is little tendency toward spontaneous regression. There appears to be an association between this condition and gastric carcinoma, often a difficult diagnosis to make in the presence of such marked hypertrophy.

Chronic Gastritis

Unlike the situation with acute gastritis, the etiology and pathogenesis of chronic gastritis are largely unknown.

Pathology

Chronic gastritis has been differentiated into types A, B, and AB. Type A is associated with parietal cell antibodies and vitamin B_{12} deficiency (pernicious anemia) and shows diffuse involvement of the body of the stomach, usually with sparing of the antrum. Type B is not associated with parietal cell antibodies or pernicious anemia and shows primarily involvement of the antrum with little or no disease in the body. In type AB, in which parietal cell antibodies and vitamin B_{12} deficiency are again lacking, there is patchy involvement of both antrum and body.

The histologic changes in these three types are similar and have been further subdivided into chronic superficial gastritis, atrophic gastritis, and gastric atrophy. The macroscopic appearance is usually not impressive; in severe cases, there may be loss of the normal mucosal architecture.

In *superficial gastritis,* the pathologic changes are limited to the superficial one third of the mucosa. The lamina propria is infiltrated by lymphocytes, plasma cells, and a few eosinophils. Active disease is accompanied by a neutrophilic infiltrate, sometimes with aggregation in dilated foveolar pits, producing an appearance similar to the crypt abscesses seen in inflammatory bowel disease. The surface epithelial cells are abnormal and appear flattened with loss of mucin. There are also degenerative and regenerative changes, consisting of necrosis, nuclear enlargement and hyperchromaticity, increased mitotic rate, and occasionally thickening of the epithelium to form a layer several cells thick.

Atrophic gastritis (Fig. 4-1) differs primarily in the extent of disease and involves the full mucosal thickness. As its name sug-

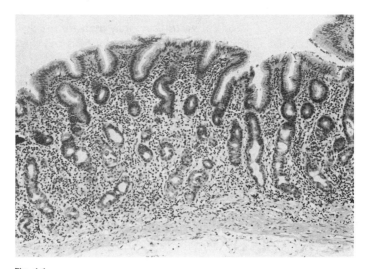

Fig. 4-1
Chronic atrophic gastritis. This low-magnification photomicrograph shows a thinning (atrophy) of the mucosa, increase in the inflammatory cell infiltrates in the lamina propria, and an almost total loss of parietal and chief cells.

gests, this extensive involvement produces atrophy of gastric glands, with loss of chief and parietal cells. The inflammatory infiltration is similar in composition to that of superficial gastritis but appears more prominent, in part, as a result of the dropout of glands. When inflammation is a prominent feature, lymphoid follicles may form, sometimes with germinal centers ("follicular gastritis"). In addition to the epithelial abnormalities seen in superficial gastritis, the normal cellular elements of the tubules are gradually replaced by mucous neck cells, a process that in its advanced stages, produces a mucosa closely resembling that of the pylorus and is thus termed *pseudopyloric metaplasia.*

In *gastric atrophy,* the pathologic changes are more severe and irreversible. The chronic inflammatory infiltrate is usually not prominent, although a few lymphoid follicles may remain. The normal epithelium is almost entirely obliterated, with a few clusters of chief and parietal cells scattered throughout the mucosa. The tubules are elongated and almost entirely composed of darkly staining mucous cells. In its most advanced form, the mucosa is identical to that of the small or large bowel, including villous architecture and the presence of a brush border; ultrastructurally, these epithelial cells are indistinguishable from normal enterocytes. This "intestinal metaplasia" may involve the entire gastric mucosa and has important consequences, both functionally and regarding the relationship between chronic gastritis and gastric cancer. The metaplastic epithelium may mimic either small intestinal or colonic mucosa. There may also be proliferation of neuroendocrine cells within the metaplastic glands; studies have shown the presence of the same hormones as are normally seen in the small intestine.

Etiology and Pathogenesis

Many diverse etiologic factors have been implicated in the causation of chronic gastritis, and the evidence in favor of some of these hypotheses appears convincing. The manner in which these factors actually produce chronic gastritis and intestinal metaplasia, however, remains a mystery. Etiologic factors may be separated into three groups: constitutional, environmental, and immunologic.

Constitutional Factors
Genetic factors are among the most important, particularly in those patients with pernicious anemia (a condition always accompanied by atrophic gastritis) whose first-degree relatives have a 20-fold increase in the incidence of atrophic gastritis. In fact, an autosomal dominant gene, called factor A, has been suggested for type A chronic gastritis. Further evidence of genetic predisposition is derived from studies showing that types

A, B, and AB tend to "breed true"; that is, these types aggregate in separate families.

Age is another important constitutional factor. Atrophic gastritis is rare in people younger than 40 years of age but is common in those older than 50 years. Males and females are equally affected.

Reflux of duodenal contents, including bile acids, which has been implicated in the pathogenesis of acute gastritis, has also been suggested as a mechanism of chronic gastritis, although this hypothesis remains unproven.

Environmental Factors

Although there is no evidence that acute gastritis per se is a precursor of atrophic gastritis, some of the same agents that cause acute gastritis may, with chronic use, produce atrophic gastritis. Alcohol is the best documented of these agents; chronic alcoholics often have antral gastritis (type B). Aspirin and other drugs have been suggested, but evidence is lacking. Heavy smokers, however, do have a greater incidence of chronic gastritis (also type B). Low socioeconomic status is also associated with chronic gastritis, even when corrected for alcohol and tobacco consumption.

Immunologic Factors

Antibodies to intrinsic factor (IF) and to parietal cells are present in the gastric juice or serum of most patients with pernicious anemia, all of whom have chronic atrophic gastritis (type A). Although parietal cell antibodies are often found in type B gastritis, IF antibodies are rarely found in the absence of vitamin B_{12} deficiency. Although these antibodies are clearly associated with chronic gastritis, their role in its pathogenesis is unknown. Although most investigators agree that they play a causal role, some have suggested that they merely represent a secondary response to mucosal injury.

It should be noted that chronic gastritis (as well as pernicious anemia) is associated with several immunologically mediated diseases, such as Hashimoto's thyroiditis, thyrotoxicosis, and Addison's disease; there is no association, however, with the collagen-vascular diseases.

Postgastrectomy Gastritis

Although chronic gastritis in the gastric remnant is extremely common in the late postoperative period (as high as 100 percent), it may occasionally occur quite rapidly. Histologically, it is identical to chronic gastritis occurring in the absence of surgery.

Immunologic mechanisms do not appear to play a role, since these patients do not have an incidence of parietal cell antibodies higher than that in the general population. Surgical loss of the gastrin-secreting cells of the antrum may play a role, since gastrin has a trophic effect on parietal cells. Reflux of intestinal contents has also been suggested as a pathogenetic mechanism.

Consequences of Chronic Gastritis

Under normal circumstances, the stomach serves primarily a secretory role and is among the most important sites of digestion (as opposed to absorption) of food. Clearly, a stomach with advanced chronic gastritis, with its loss of parietal and chief cells and their subsequent replacement by metaplastic intestinal epithelium, is not able to fulfill this function. Although secretory function may remain relatively intact in chronic superficial gastritis, it is lost as an increasing degree of atrophy supervenes.

Acid secretion is usually decreased, producing hypochlorhydria or achlorhydria. Even when there is maximal stimulation of acid secretion, the pH of the stomach may remain high. The maximal acid secretion correlates quite well with the severity and extent of atrophic changes. Pepsin and pepsinogen levels parallel acid levels in most gastric diseases; this remains true in chronic gastritis. Likewise the level of IF correlates well with parietal cell mass. It should be noted, however, that since only a small amount of IF is needed to absorb an adequate amount of vitamin B_{12}, few patients with chronic gastritis develop pernicious anemia.

The situation with gastrin is somewhat complex. In type A gastritis (associated with autoantibodies and pernicious anemia), the gastrin-secreting antral mucosa is uninvolved. Since acid, which normally has an inhibitory effect on gastrin secretion, is lacking, these patients usually have extremely high serum gastrin levels, and the degree of elevation correlates well with the severity of disease. In type B gastritis, on the other hand, the extent of antral involvement is quite variable, and serum gastrin levels may therefore be high, low, or normal.

Surprisingly, however, the symptomatology of chronic gastritis is ill defined, and some studies have shown no correlation between the state of the mucosa and symptoms. In fact, the incidence of chronic gastritis in the general population is quite high, with as many as 60 percent of asymptomatic subjects showing morphologic evidence of gastritis. Certain symptoms such as abdominal pain or discomfort, bloating, nausea, vomiting, belching, and flatulence appear to be associated with chronic gastritis. These symptoms are usually made worse by the ingestion of foods and, as one might expect, are usually not relieved by antacids, since these patients are already hypochlorhydric. Similar symptoms, however, are often found in peptic ulcer disease and, in fact, in normal individuals. Thus, a specific complex of symptoms cannot be ascribed to chronic gastritis.

Bacterial overgrowth in the gastrointestinal tract is an important sequela of chronic gastritis and occurs secondary to decreased acid secretion, which permits unrestricted bacterial proliferation in the upper gastrointestinal tract.

The most feared consequence of chronic gastritis, however, is the development of gastric carcinoma; the relationship between these two entities will be discussed later in this chapter.

Benign Gastric Neoplasms

Little is known about the etiology and pathogenesis of the benign tumors of the stomach. Based on their histogenesis, they may be divided into epithelial and nonepithelial types. Although all types may appear grossly polypoid, the term *polyp* is used here to denote a space-occupying lesion of epithelial origin.

Gastric Mucosal Polyps

In sharp contrast to the colon, where polyps are frequently encountered, the stomach appears to be an uncommon site for polyps to develop. Although their incidence in autopsy series is near 1 percent, gastric polyps have been observed in approximately 6 percent of patients who undergo gastroscopy for various indications. This higher incidence of gastric polyps in the clinical series most likely reflects a selection bias weighted toward symptomatic patients. Gastric polyps may be histologically classified into neoplastic and non-neoplastic types:

NEOPLASTIC	NON-NEOPLASTIC
Adenoma	Hyperplastic polyp (Syn:
Tubular adenoma	regenerative polyp)
Villous adenoma	Hamartomatous polyp
Carcinoma	

Hyperplastic polyps are by far the most common (>90%) type of gastric polyp and result from an exaggerated regenerative (hyperplastic) response to mucosal injury (Fig. 4-2). Because it often reflects a field effect, these polyps are usually mutiple and occur as smooth, slow-growing mucosal elevations that rarely exceed 1 cm in size. Histologically, they are composed of branching and cystically dilated glands lined by benign epithelium identical to that of the normal surface epithelium. The stroma may show edema, inflammation, and irregular bundles of smooth muscle. There is usually no atypia of the surface epithelium, and malignant change is a rare occurrence (<1%). When atypia is present, it is usually related to regenerative activity secondary to inflam-

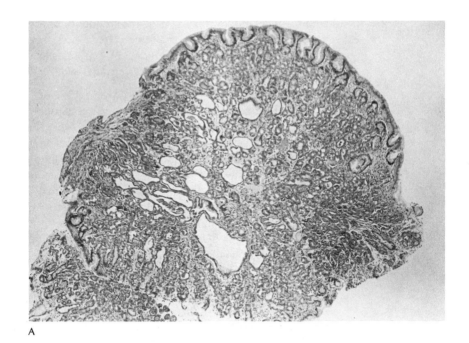

A

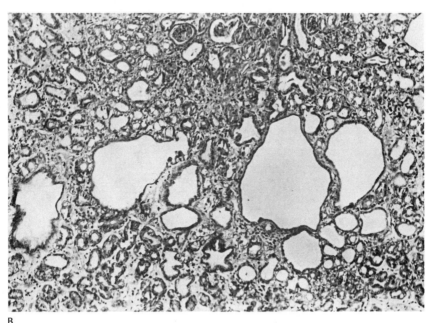

B

Fig. 4-2
Hyperplastic polyp. This endoscopically removed gastric polyp is composed
predominantly of epithelial elements forming gland-like structures with only
a minimal amount of supporting connective tissue stroma in between (A).
Although these glandular structures show considerable variation in size and
shape, all of them are lined by normal gastric epithelium without any cytologic abnormalities (B).

mation or ulceration at the surface. The frequency of a coexistent carcinoma elsewhere in the same stomach is significantly high (20 to 28%). Hence, the finding of hyperplastic polyps should prompt a search for carcinoma elsewhere in the stomach.

Although more common in the colon, hamartomatous polyps also occur in the stomach. Like hyperplastic polyps, they are composed of cystically dilated glands lined by normal-appearing gastric epithelium. The difference lies in the abundant amount of connective tissue between the glands in hamartomatous polyps. Although hamartomatous gastric polyps may occur sporadically, they are commonly observed in patients with the Peutz-Jeghers syndrome, familial juvenile polyposis, Cowden's disease, and Cronkhite-Canada syndrome. Hamartomatous gastric polyps have no malignant potential per se but serve as markers for such syndromes.

Adenomatous polyps or adenomas (Figs. 4-3 and 4-4) are true neoplasms and account for about 10 percent of all gastric polyps. In contrast to the hyperplastic polyps, these polyps are invariably single and larger lesions, which may grow up to 4 cm or more in size. Usually pedunculated (stalked), these polyps have a lobulated surface that is frequently ulcerated. Histologically, they are composed of closely packed, uniform-sized

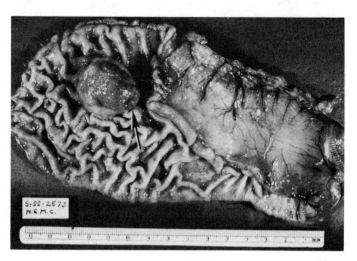

Fig. 4-3
Adenomatous polyp. Gastrectomy specimen showing a large pedunculated polyp in the body. Note the large size and the faintly lobulated contour that is so commonly seen in polyps of this type. A small depression on the surface (*arrow*) indicates an area of ulceration. The patient had no symptoms until he suddenly developed chronic iron deficiency, presumably from chronic blood loss from this site.

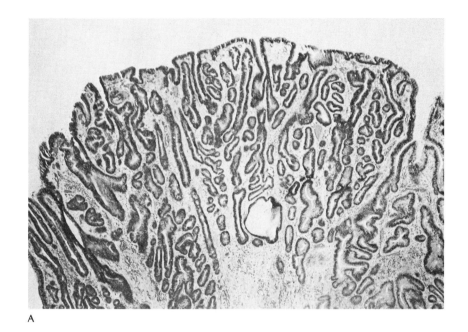

A

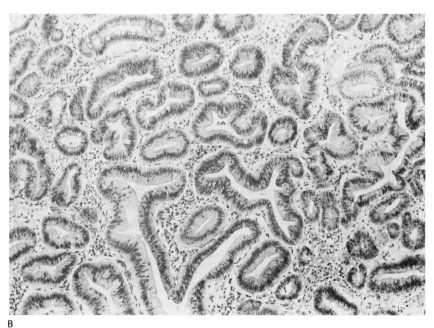

B

Fig. 4-4
Adenomatous polyp. The low-power photomicrograph shows the neoplastic glands embedded in the connective tissue stroma (A). Although this may bear some resemblance to a hyperplastic polyp, it can be easily differentiated from it on the basis of the cytologic atypia and pleomorphism of the cells lining these glands, as seen under higher magnification (B).

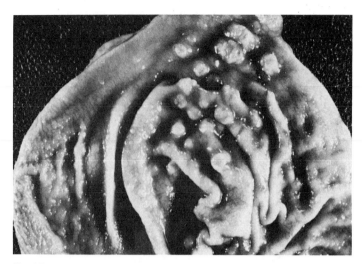

Fig. 4-5
Diffuse polyposes. Note that in this gastrectomy specimen, the mucosa is studded with multiple polyps of varying sizes. All these polyps were diagnosed to be of the hyperplastic variety.

glands lined by benign, atypical epithelium. Like their counterpart in the colon, gastric adenomas are subclassified into tubular and papillary (villous) types. As their names suggest, the former is composed of branching glands, the latter of papillary fronds. Atypia is more common and severe in the papillary adenoma, and this type has a higher incidence of being transformed into carcinoma. The overall risk of malignant change in an adenomatous polyp of the stomach is about 40 percent; the risk of a coexistent gastric carcinoma is also close to 40 percent.

Diffuse polyposis (Fig. 4-5) refers to the presence of multiple polyps involving a large portion of the stomach. The polyps may be either hyperplastic or adenomatous in nature. Patients with diffuse polyposis are at increased risk for the development of gastric carcinoma. The hereditary polyposes, such as familial polyposis, Gardner's syndrome, and Peutz-Jegher's syndrome, may also involve the stomach to a greater or lesser extent; in general the incidence of primary gastric malignancy is low in these syndromes, although much higher elsewhere.

Most gastric polyps, irrespective of histologic types, are asymptomatic and are discovered incidentally at autopsy or during a radiologic, endoscopic, or surgical procedure for an unrelated cause. However, the larger polyps may ulcerate, bleed, or prolapse into the pylorus, leading to outlet obstruction. Asymptomatic hyperplastic polyps, diagnosed at biopsy, can be left alone, whereas adenomatous polyps, because of their propensity for malignant change, should be completely excised and evaluated for possible malignancy. Since both adenomatous and hyperplastic polyps are markers for a malignancy (or pre-malignant change) elsewhere in the stomach, a thorough search for a coexistent (or incipient) gastric carcinoma must be undertaken. Similarly, hamartomatous polyps should prompt evaluation for other stigmata of the various syndromes with which such polyps are associated.

Connective Tissue Tumors

The nonepithelial tumors constitute a much more diverse group of neoplasms. The only common tumor in this group is the leiomyoma, so-called because of the popular belief that it is derived from the smooth muscle cells of the stomach wall. This tumor is a common incidental finding at autopsy. It is composed of interlacing bundles of elongated spindle cells that resemble smooth muscle. Grossly, they may appear as intramural nodules or intraluminal space-occupying lesions or may project by means of a stalk into the peritoneum. Other tumors of mesen-chymal origin, such as lipomas, angiomas, granular cell tumors, and neurofibromas, are much less common and have gross and histologic characteristics similar to their counterparts elsewhere in the body.

Like gastric polyps, leiomyomas, too, may remain asymptomatic and be detected incidentally or may cause clinical symptoms. The most common symptoms are pain and bleeding owing to ulceration of the overlying mucosa. This may occasionally be extensive and life-threatening. In other patients, bleeding may be insidious and produce an iron deficiency anemia. Pedun-culated tumors in the antrum may prolapse through the pylorus, producing gastric outlet obstruction. Obstruction may also be produced by sessile tumors if they are large or cause intussus-ception. Vomiting is a prominent symptom in patients with ob-struction. Rarely, proximally located tumors may prolapse through the gastroesophageal junction, producing dysphagia. In the body of the stomach, benign tumors are often entirely asymptomatic and, particularly in the case of mesenchymal tumors, may grow to enormous size. All benign tumors are treated surgically; those that protrude into the lumen and have stalks can sometimes be removed endoscopically. If malignancy is detected on pathologic examination, further surgery is dic-tated by the type and extent of malignancy.

Carcinoma of the Stomach

Gastric carcinoma is a relatively uncommon tumor and accounts for approximately 3 percent of all malignancies. As recently as 1945, however, it was the most common fatal cancer in the United States; for reasons unknown, its incidence in this country has fallen precipitously, although it remains common in other parts of the world.

As is the case with most neoplasms, some etiologic and epidemiologic factors have been identified, but the actual pathogenesis remains obscure. Consumption of certain foods and chemicals such as starches, smoked foods, and nitrates (found in processed foods) has been implicated in the development of gastric carcinoma. Nitrates produced endogenously by bacteria in the stomach of patients with chronic atrophic gastritis and high intraluminal pH may also play a significant role in its development. Consumption of fresh vegetables appears to be a protection against gastric cancer; this effect may be mediated through vitamin C, which interferes with nitrosation in vivo. Asbestos exposure increases the risk of gastric cancer, probably because of the swallowing of such fibers present in the environment. Heredity appears to be an important factor, at least in some families, although the mode of transmission has not been elucidated. Finally, since blood type A is more common in patients with gastric cancer than in the general population, patients with this blood type are said to be at increased risk for gastric cancer.

Although all the aforementioned factors are important, there are a number of conditions that strongly predispose one to the development of gastric cancer. Because it is so common, the most important factor is chronic gastritis. Intestinal metaplasia, which commonly accompanies chronic gastritis, appears to be the crucial element in this predisposition. The metaplastic epithelium, which is primarily absorptive, perhaps facilitates the absorption of carcinogens. Chronic gastritis, in fact, shows a continuum of dysplastic changes (Fig. 4-6), ranging from minimal to severe, the latter almost indistinguishable from carcinoma in situ. Disorders of maturation have been demonstrated clearly in atrophic mucosa. Normally, the proliferating, dividing cells are located within the gastric pit, and the mature surface epithelial cells are unable to divide. In atrophic mucosa, on the other hand, the surface epithelial cells retain their ability to synthesize DNA and RNA and thus can divide; they accumulate in the mucosa rather than being exfoliated into the gastric lumen. It is this uncontrolled proliferative activity that leads to carcinoma. Although both small intestinal and colonic metaplasia are seen in association with carcinoma, some authors believe that the colonic type is more closely linked to the development of malignancy.

Pernicious anemia also predisposes to gastric carcinoma, but its relative rarity makes it less important. It is likely that the risk in pernicious anemia is due to the inevitable development of

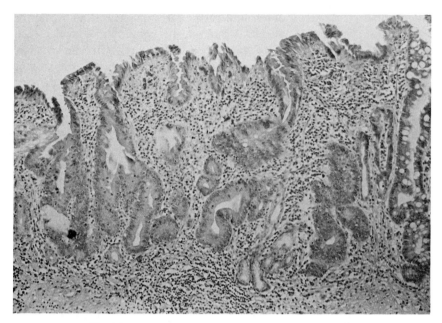

Fig. 4-6
Intestinal metaplasia and dysplasia in chronic gastritis. Compared to the features seen in Fig. 4-1, this gastric mucosa shows more diffuse distribution of the inflammatory cells. Cytologic abnormalities seen in the epithelial cells included increased size of the nucleus, stratification of nuclei, atypia, and increased nuclear cytoplasmic ratio. A focus of intestinal metaplasia is present along the right border of the photomicrograph and is readily identified because of the goblet cells.

chronic gastritis, since cancer develops in the body and fundus of the stomach in these patients rather than in the antrum, which corresponds to the involvement by gastritis. Similarly, patients who have had a subtotal gastrectomy have an increased incidence of cancer; this again appears to be related to the high rate of development of chronic gastritis, since cancer and chronic gastritis tend to develop in the same place — namely, the anastomotic site. As mentioned previously, gastric polyps are also associated with the development of cancer. Gastric polyps are more common in patients with atrophic gastritis (with or without pernicious anemia), as well as following gastrectomy. Finally, atrophic gastritis with pernicious anemia is seen in some patients with immunoglobulin deficiency; a few of these patients have later developed gastric cancer.

The common feature of all the aforementioned conditions is the development of chronic gastritis, lending further proof that this change is an important precursor of gastric cancer. In fact, atrophic changes and intestinal metaplasia are present in about 90 percent of stomachs resected for carcinoma.

Pathology

About one half of gastric carcinomas occur in the antrum; the remainder are located in the body, fundus, and cardia, most commonly along the lesser curvature. Many classifications have been proposed, based on gross characteristics, microscopic appearance, or combinations thereof. We will divide carcinoma into four groups: superficial spreading, ulcerative, fungating (polypoid), and diffuse. For practical purposes, all gastric carcinomas should be considered to arise from mucus-secreting cells; tumors of specialized cells (such as parietal or chief cells) are rare.

Superficially spreading gastric carcinoma (see Fig. 4-10) is confined to mucosa or submucosa. It may be manifested by severe cytologic abnormalities within the glands (carcinoma in situ) or by invasion of the lamina propria or muscularis mucosae. In the former case, the glands appear well oriented, but their cells display such marked dysplasia that they must be considered malignant. When there is superficial invasion, the glands also show architectural abnormalities: They are irregular in size and shape; they show branching and generally appear haphazard in arrangement; individual cells and clusters may lie outside the basement membrane. Grossly, these tumors are usually seen as flat irregular plaques with ill-defined borders. They may be slightly raised or depressed and occasionally show superficial ulceration. They may extend over a large area and, in some cases, are multifocal. These tumors pose certain diagnostic difficulties. Because they are flat and do not involve muscle or cause thickening of the stomach wall, they may be undetectable by radiographic techniques. Endoscopically, they may also be quite subtle; when ulcerated, they may mimic benign ulcer disease. Fortunately, their superficial location makes them quite accessible to biopsy and cytologic examination, both of which are quite accurate in diagnosing this type of cancer. If resected, superficial spreading carcinoma, even in the presence of nodal metastases, has a much better prognosis (95 percent overall 5-year survival rate) than advanced invasive gastric carcinoma that has extended to involve the muscle coats (12 percent overall 5-year survival rate). Unfortunately, few tumors are diagnosed while still limited to the mucosa and submucosa.

As their name implies, ulcerated carcinomas (Figs. 4-7 and 4-8) appear grossly as ulcers. In the typical case, they differ from benign ulcers by having a necrotic base and heaped-up edges, which overhang the ulcer crater and interrupt the normal rugae at the edges of the lesion. Microscopically, they appear qualitatively similar to superficial spreading carcinomas (i.e., in glandular architecture) but differ in quantity and extent of tumor. They may penetrate deeply into or through the muscularis propria;

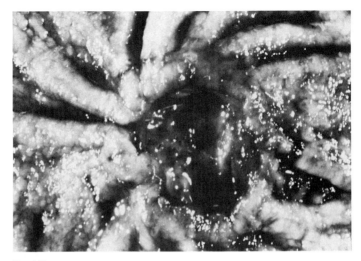

Fig. 4-7
Malignant gastric ulcer (ulcerated carcinoma). This close-up picture of an ulcerated gastric carcinoma highlights some of the features that help differentiate it from a benign gastric ulcer. This large-sized carcinoma eroded deep into the wall of the stomach. Both the overhanging margins and the thickened rolled-up edges, so characteristic of malignant ulcers, can be appreciated. The latter is due to infiltration by malignant cells in the underlying tissues.

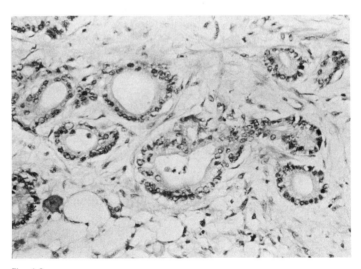

Fig. 4-8
Well-differentiated adenocarcinoma of the stomach. This area shows well-formed neoplastic glands infiltrating the submucosal connective tissues.

the bulk of the tumor is usually found in the heaped-up margin of the ulcer. This type of tumor presents a different set of diagnostic problems. Radiographically and endoscopically, the lesion is usually easily visible. In some cases, however, it may mimic a benign peptic ulcer. Microscopically, tumor may be present only at one margin of the ulcer. The ulcer base may be entirely composed of necrosis or granulation tissue. For this reason, multiple biopsies should be performed at several points along the margin of the ulcer.

Polypoid carcinomas are similar microscopically to the two types previously mentioned. They are readily detected by radiographic and endoscopic techniques. Diagnostic problems in this type of cancer occur in its differentiation from adenomatous polyps. The latter, as discussed previously, always show some degree of cytologic or architectural atypia, sometimes difficult to distinguish from carcinoma. In addition, carcinoma often arises within an adenomatous polyp, a process that may be quite focal and is thus liable to be undetected unless the polyp is thoroughly sampled. Polypoid carcinoma invades locally by means of its stalk into the deep layers of the stomach wall.

Finally, the diffuse form of gastric carcinoma is quite different both grossly and microscopically. No clearly visible mass is formed; rather, the entire wall is infiltrated by tumor cells that may elicit a florid inflammatory and fibrous reaction (desmoplasia), producing marked thickening of the stomach, which is seen to contract poorly by radiographic techniques. This inelastic, rigid appearance is often referred to as *linitis plastica,* or *leather-bottle stomach.* The tumor cells sometimes assume a "signet ring" shape (Fig. 4-9). Although there may be focal ulcerations, the mucosa is usually intact. This entity produces diagnostic difficulty for other reasons. Because the superficial mucosa is not involved, biopsy and cytology, which only sample the most superficial layers of the wall, may not reveal the presence of tumor. Even in resected stomachs, the extensive inflammatory and fibrotic (desmoplastic) reaction may mask the presence of the individual tumor cells. Because the symptomatology of these tumors is often minimal, they are usually far advanced by the time they are diagnosed, with extension through the serosa and nodal or distant metastases or both; the latter often represent the first clinical manifestation of an occult carcinoma. Fortunately, this type of carcinoma is rare compared with the ulcerative and fungating types. However, recent evidence indicates that its incidence may be rising.

Signs and Symptoms

The stomach is able to expand fairly easily to accommodate a mass, whether it is food or tumor. Because of this distensibility,

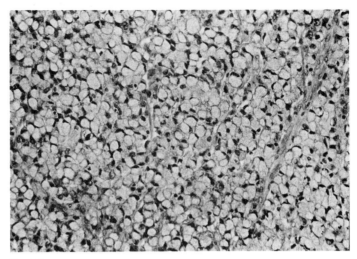

Fig. 4-9
Diffusely infiltrating carcinoma (signet ring–type) of the stomach. Note that here the diffusely infiltrating tumor cells do not form any glands and show abundant mucin within their cytoplasm, which renders the cells somewhat amphophilic. This intracellular accumulation of mucin pushes the nucleus to the periphery of the cell to produce the characteristic signet ring appearance.

most of the signs and symptoms of gastric carcinoma are those of far-advanced disease. Anorexia and weight loss are common; for unknown reasons, there is a selective distaste for beef products. Tumors in the distal portion of the stomach may cause gastric outlet obstruction with pain, nausea, and vomiting after eating. These symptoms cause patients to further decrease their food intake, contributing to the weight loss; patients also complain of constipation, since little food passes through the pylorus. Bleeding is also common and may be seen either in the vomitus or in the stool. Often bleeding is chronic, producing anemia and its symptoms. Bleeding occurs both in the early stages of cancer as well as in more advanced disease.

Carcinomas in the cardia may cause dysphagia by extension into the esophagus. In patients with total obstruction of the esophageal lumen, aspiration is common. In addition, tumor may extend into the submucosal neural plexus of the esophagus, mimicking achalasia. Extension outside the stomach to the colon may produce large bowel obstruction. We have seen a patient whose only complaint was malodorous belching, resulting from a gastrocolic fistula produced by a gastric carcinoma eroding into the transverse colon. Occasionally, metastatic disease may produce the first manifestations, such as bilateral ovarian masses (Krukenberg tumor; Fig. 4-10), ascites owing to peri-

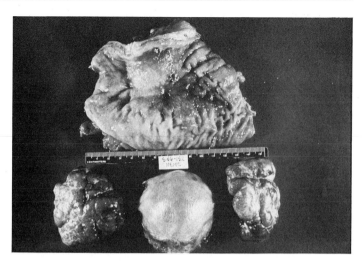

Fig. 4-10
Gross picture portion of a stomach with infiltrative type of carcinoma (upper-most specimen) along with a uterus flanked by bilaterally enlarged ovaries. Both ovaries showed metastatic tumor (Krukenberg tumors).

toneal seeding, or jaundice owing to either massive hepatic metastases or biliary obstruction caused by enlarged porta hepatis lymph nodes.

Other Malignant Neoplasms

Compared with gastric adenocarcinoma, other malignant tumors of the stomach are rare. Squamous cell carcinomas occasionally occur in the cardia, where they may represent either extension from a distal esophageal cancer or an origin from congenital rests of squamous epithelium. Squamous cell carcinoma of the distal stomach is extremely unusual, since this part of the stomach does not normally contain squamous epithelium. More common is a combination of both glandular and squamous components, a tumor called an *adenocanthoma*. Both squamous cell carcinoma and adenocanthoma are similar to adenocarcinoma in all respects other than their histology.

Another rare tumor of epithelial origin is the carcinoid tumor. Gastric carcinoids account for 2 to 3 percent of all carcinoid tumors. They occur as solitary or multicentric tumors and may be distributed anywhere in the stomach. Usually small and clinically silent, they may occasionally produce bleeding. Like gastric carcinoma, carcinoids of the stomach most often arise in patients with a background of chronic gastritis and pernicious anemia and are derived from a hyperplasia of the gastric endocrine cells that occurs secondarily in chronic gastritis. Gastric carcinoids are potentially malignant tumors with a slow rate of growth.

The most common nonepithelial malignancy of the stomach is malignant lymphoma, accounting for 3 to 8 percent of all gastric malignancies. The stomach may be the site of primary origin or may be involved secondarily. Clinically and radiologically, the presentation is similar to that of carcinoma. Primary gastric lymphomas are usually of the non-Hodgkin's type. Their subclassification is a complex subject that does not require discussion here; suffice it to say that any type may be seen in the stomach. Hodgkin's disease is rare in the stomach and is almost always part of diffuse organ involvement.

A variety of sarcomas are occasionally seen in the stomach, the most common of which is leiomyosarcoma. Metastatic carcinoma to the stomach is occasionally encountered; the most common primary sites are breast, melanoma, and lung.

Study Questions   1. Which of the following factors are essential in the development of acute gastric mucosal injury?
   a. Ischemia
   b. Pepsin
   c. Reflux of bile into the stomach
   d. Hydrochloric acid
   e. Ingestion of gastric irritants

   Answers
   b, d.
   The presence of hydrochloric acid and pepsin is essential to produce acute gastric injury. Although ischemia, bile reflux, and the ingestion of certain substances (such as alcohol) may be important in some cases, acute gastritis may occur in the absence of any of these three factors.

   2. Consequences of chronic atrophic gastritis include:
   a. Hypochlorhydria
   b. Development of carcinoma
   c. Perforation
   d. Gastric outlet obstruction
   e. Intestinal metaplasia

   Answers
   a, b, e.
   Hypochlorhydria is present in most cases of atrophic gastritis, and intestinal metaplasia is also quite common. The development of gastric carcinoma is much rarer, but its incidence is much higher in the presence of atrophic gastritis. Perforation is a feature of other conditions (e.g., peptic ulcer), and gastric outlet obstruction does not occur unless another condition (e.g., carcinoma) is also present.

References

Allen, A., and Gardner, A. Mucus and bicarbonate secretion in the stomach and their possible role in mucosal protection. *Gut* 21:249, 1980.

Antonioli, D. A. Current Concepts in Carcinoma of the Stomach. In H. D. Appelman (ed.), *Contemporary Issues in Surgical Pathology*, Vol 4. New York: Churchill Livingstone, 1984.

Bordi, C., and Ravazzola, M. Endocrine cells in the intestinal metaplasia of gastric mucosa. *Am. J. Pathol.* 96:391, 1979.

Brooks, J. J., and Enterline, H. T. Primary gastric lymphoma. *Cancer* 51:701, 1983.

Correa, P. et al. Diet and gastric cancer: Nutrition survey in a high risk area. *J. Natl. Cancer Inst.* 70:673, 1983.

Edwards, F. C., and Coghill, N. F. Aetiological factors in chronic atrophic gastritis. *Br. Med. J.* 2:1409, 1966.

Edwards, F. C., and Coghill, N. F. Clinical manifestations in patients with chronic atrophic gastritis, gastric ulcer, and duodenal ulcer. *Q. J. Med.* 37:337, 1968.

Eklof, O. Benign tumors of the stomach and duodenum. *Acta Chir. Scand.* Suppl. 291:14, 1962.

Fieber, S. S., and Rickert, R. R. Hyperplastic gastropathy. *Am. J. Gastroenterol.* 76:321, 1981.

Fromm, D. Drug-induced gastric mucosal injury. *World J. Surg.* 5:199, 1981.

Glass G. B. J., and Pitchumoni, C. S. Atrophic gastritis. *Hum. Pathol.* 6:219, 1975.

Gurll, N. J., and Damianos, A. J. The role of histamine and histamine receptors in the pathogenesis and treatment of erosive gastritis. *World J. Surg.* 5:181, 1981.

Ivey, K. J., and Roth, J. L. A. Drug and Chemical-induced Injuries of the Stomach. In J. E. Berk (ed.), *Bockus Gastroenterology* (4th ed.). Philadelphia: Saunders, 1985. Pp. 975–1003.

Joossens, J. V., and Geboers, J. Epidemiology of Gastric Cancer: A Clue to Etiology. In P. Sherlock, B. C. Morson, L. Barbara, et al. (eds.), *Precancerous Lesions of the Gastrointestinal Tract.* New York: Raven, 1983.

Kurtz, R. C., and Sherlock, P. Carcinoma of the Stomach. In J. E. Berk (ed.), *Bockus Gastroenterology* (4th ed.). Philadelphia: Saunders, 1985. Pp. 1278–1304.

Lipkin, M. In "defense" of the gastric mucosa. *Gut* 12:599, 1971.

Lucas, C. E. Stress ulceration: The clinical problem. *World J. Surg.* 5:139, 1981.

Menguy, R. Role of gastric mucosal energy metabolism in the etiology of stress ulceration. *World J. Surg.* 5:175, 1981.

Miller, A. I., Smith, B., and Rogers, A. I. Phlegmonous gastritis. *Gastroenterology* 68:231, 1975.

Miller, T. A. Protective effects of prostaglandins against gastric mucosal damage: Current knowledge and proposed mechanisms. *Am. J. Physiol.* 245:G601, 1983.

Moody, F. G., Cheung, L. Y., Simons, M. A., and Zalewsky, C. A. Stress and the acute gastric mucosal lesion. *Dig. Dis. Sci.* 21:148, 1976.

Moody, F. G., Zaslewsky, C. A., and Larsen, K. R. Cytoprotection of the gastric epithelium. *World J. Surg.* 5:153, 1981.

Nelson, R. S., and Lanza, F. L. Benign and Malignant Tumors of the Stomach (Other than Carcinoma). In J. E. Berk (ed.), *Bockus Gastroenterology* (4th ed.). Philadelphia: Saunders, 1985. Pp. 1255–1277.

Olearchyk, A. S. Gastric carcinoma: A critical review of 243 cases. *Am. J. Gastroenterol.* 70:25, 1978.

Ranieri, R., and Weisburger, J. H. Reduction of gastric carcinogens with ascorbic acid. *Ann. N.Y. Acad. Sci.* 258:181, 1975.

Ritchie, W. P., Jr. Role of bile and reflux in acute hemorrhagic gastritis. *World J. Surg.* 5:189, 1981.

Silen, W., Merhav, A., and Simson, J. N. L. The pathophysiology of stress ulcer disease. *World J. Surg.* 5:165, 1981.

Skillman, J. J., and Silen, W. Stress ulceration in the acutely ill. *Ann. Rev. Med.* 27:9, 1976.

Sipponen, P. Intestinal metaplasia and gastric carcinoma. *Ann. Clin. Res.* 13:139, 1981.

Strickland, R. G., and Mackay, I. R. A reappraisal of the nature and significance of chronic atrophic gastritis. *Dig. Dis. Sci.* 18:426, 1973.

Tomasulo, J. Gastric polyps: Histologic types and their relationship to gastic carcinoma. *Cancer* 27:1346, 1968.

Varis, K. Family behavior of chronic gastritis. *Ann. Clin. Res.* 13:123, 1981.

Vilardell, F. Gastritis. In J. E. Berk (ed.), *Bockus Gastroenterology* (4th ed.). Philadelphia: Saunders, 1985. Pp. 941–974.

Whitehead, R. *Mucosal Biopsy of the Gastrointestinal Tract.* Major Problems in Pathology, Vol. 3. Philadelphia: Saunders, 1985. Pp. 33–115.

Wilander, E., El-Salhy, M., and Pitkanen, P. Histopathology of gastric carcinoids: A survey of 42 cases. *Histopathology* 8:183, 1984.

5 : Diarrhea and Malabsorption

Sanjiv Chopra
Jerry S. Trier

Diarrhea is a symptom that is probably experienced at some point in time by every person. It can be annoying to varying degrees, embarrassing, subject to unhealthy introspection, and even life-threatening. It may serve a useful purpose in that it represents in many instances a physiologic phenomenon whereby the body rids itself of infectious or toxic foreign substances by purging them through the gastrointestinal tract. Indeed, in some instances, such a natural response on the part of the body should not be inhibited by pharmacologic agents that impair intestinal transit. Diarrhea is a common symptom among patients with malabsorption in whom there is impairment of normal digestion or absorption of one or more dietary nutrients. Diarrhea and malabsorption may be responsible for significant morbidity and even mortality, as exemplified by epidemics of cholera or invasive enteric or colonic infections, diseases that produce severe inflammation of the small or large intestine, and by diseases that result in prolonged perturbation of nutrient absorption by the small intestine.

Definitions

Diarrhea

A precise definition of diarrhea is elusive, since there is considerable variation in normal bowel habits in the population at large and from day to day in some individuals. Stool mass is considered the best objective gauge of diarrhea. It is influenced by the amount of dietary fiber intake and is normally greater in those who consume modest or large amounts of fiber. People in the United States and Great Britain normally excrete less than 200 gm of stool per day, of which 65 to 85 percent is water. When the stool weight is in excess of 250 gm and the stool contains 70 to 95 percent water, it is usually perceived by the patient as diarrhea. This is far from a pragmatic definition, as patients will not be able to provide such information. A useful working approach is to first establish the normal bowel pattern for that particular individual when he or she is in good health. Some healthy people will pass two stools a day, whereas others may normally pass two stools per week. When individuals have an increase in the frequency and fluidity of the stool, they often complain of having diarrhea. Diarrhea implies a greater than normal fecal mass consisting predominantly of water. Visual inspection of the patient's stool is often sufficient to determine that diarrhea is present.

Malabsorption

Malabsorption results from diseases that impair one or more of the processes involved in the normal digestion and absorption of dietary nutrients. These processes include (1) intraluminal digestion, (2) mucosal absorption, and (3) subsequent transport of nutrients from the mucosa to the systemic circulation for utilization in all body organs and tissues. Malabsorption may be generalized as, for example, in celiac sprue, in which diffuse disease of the mucosa of the small intestine may impair absorption of virtually all nutrients. On the other hand, malabsorption may be highly selective, as, for example, in pernicious anemia, in which deficiency of intrinsic factor secretion by the gastric mucosa selectively impairs ileal cobalamin absorption.

Normal Physiology

Intestinal Water and Ion Absorption

The human gastrointestinal tract normally handles approximately 9 liters of fluid on a daily basis (Fig. 5-1). Most of this fluid is absorbed by the small bowel so that only 1 to 1.5 liters normally enters the colon. The colon then absorbs most of the remaining fluid so that only 100 to 150 ml is normally excreted in

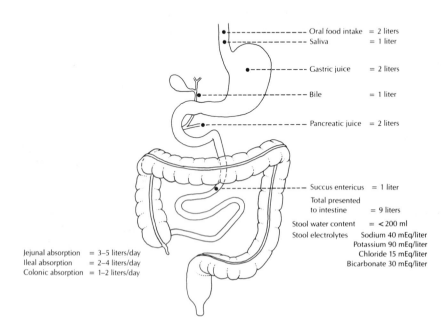

Oral food intake = 2 liters
Saliva = 1 liter
Gastric juice = 2 liters
Bile = 1 liter
Pancreatic juice = 2 liters
Succus entericus = 1 liter
Total presented to intestine = 9 liters
Stool water content = < 200 ml
Stool electrolytes   Sodium 40 mEq/liter
Potassium 90 mEq/liter
Chloride 15 mEq/liter
Bicarbonate 30 mEq/liter

Jejunal absorption = 3–5 liters/day
Ileal absorption = 2–4 liters/day
Colonic absorption = 1–2 liters/day

Fig. 5-1
Normal daily intestinal fluid balance.

the feces during a 24-hour period. Under normal circumstances, the secretory and absorptive processes shown in Fig. 5-1 proceed simultaneously. Whereas the normal colon usually absorbs only 1 to 2 liters of fluid per day, it is capable of absorbing almost 6 liters of water and 800 mEq of sodium per day if challenged by excessive secretions or impaired small bowel absorption. This adaptive capacity is impaired in certain colonic diseases (e.g., ulcerative colitis) and by an excess of a variety of some constituents in the ileal effluent, such as bile salts, fatty acids, and carbohydrates. Patients who have diarrhea secondary to a primary small bowel mucosal disorder such as extensive Crohn's disease or celiac sprue often have three or four large-volume bowel movements. In contrast, patients with disease limited to the distal colon as occurs in ulcerative proctosigmoiditis may have more than six bowel movements per day, but these usually consist of one or two formed stools and several movements consisting of small volumes of fluid, mucus, and blood.

The primary mechanism of absorption of various nutrients is accomplished by two major transport mechanisms: passive diffusion and active transport. Substances absorbed by passive diffusion require neither energy nor a membrane carrier, and absorption follows either a chemical gradient from high to low concentration or an electrical gradient. Examples of nutrients absorbed by passive diffusion include water; the products of triglyceride hydrolysis; potassium; and vitamins A, D, E, and K. Fructose is absorbed by the process of facilitated diffusion, which is similar to passive diffusion but is more rapid, presumably because a carrier is present. Substances absorbed by active transport require energy and selective carriers or pumps. Examples of substances absorbed by active transport include glucose, amino acids, sodium, chloride, bicarbonate, iron, calcium, and vitamin B_{12}.

A final transport mechanism is endocytosis, in which large molecules such as intact proteins are absorbed by way of bulk or receptor-mediated pathway. Initially, small regions of the apical plasma membrane indent the cytoplasm of the absorptive cell. These regions then pinch off, forming small membrane-bounded vesicles containing luminal contents. These vesicles may then help form or be incorporated into organelles of the lysosomal system, or their contents may leave the cell cytoplasm by fusion of the vesicle membrane with the basolateral membrane. Although endocytosis and vesicular transcytosis are important in the intestinal transport of colostral immunoglobulins in some neonatal mammals, they are of questionable significance in the direct intestinal transport of nutrients in humans.

However, receptor-mediated endocytosis of vasoactive intestinal polypeptide (VIP) and possibly other peptide mediators by the basolateral membrane of intestinal epithelial cells appears to be important in the regulation of intestinal electrolyte transport.

Water transport in the intestine is a passive phenomenon. Water transport occurs secondary to osmotic and hydrostatic gradients across the intestine. Osmotic gradients can be generated by the active transport of electrolytes or by nonelectrolytes such as sugars and amino acids. There is evidence that in health, crypt epithelial cells secrete water and ions, whereas villous epithelial cells absorb water and ions.

It is proposed but has not been proved that active secretion by the small intestine serves several important functions. It may help to maintain the fluidity of the bowel content, rendering its passage through the small bowel easier than if it were of a more solid consistency. Active fluid secretion may serve to dilute potentially injurious (e.g., cytotoxic or carcinogenic) substances present within the lumen. Finally, fluid secretion emanating from the crypt cells may help propel secreted macromolecules such as secretory IgA and lysozyme out of the crypts toward the villi.

Net water and ion transport in the gastrointestinal tract reflects the balance between net secretion and absorption. Absorption predominates under normal circumstances; however, in a number of diarrheal disorders such as certain toxigenic enteric infections and with certain hormone-secreting tumors, fluid secretion by the gastrointestinal tract greatly exceeds absorption with dire consequences.

There are two pathways by which water and various ions may cross the intestinal mucosa. Transport by way of the paracellular pathway requires penetration of the "tight junctions" that connect adjacent epithelial cells at the apex of the lateral membrane, followed by diffusion along the intercellular space. The junctions in the jejunum are somewhat more permeable than those in the ileum. In addition to water, some sodium, chloride, and potassium transport also occurs through the tight junctions. Transport by way of the paracellular pathway is a passive phenomenon and follows hydrostatic, osmotic and electrochemical gradients. In addition, some sodium, potassium, chloride, and other small solutes are transported across the tight junction passively following water flow by a process termed *solvent drag*, which accounts for a significant component of solute movement in the small intestine. The paracellular shunt pathway is cation selective; it is more permeable to K^+ and Na^+ than to Cl^-, presumably because it presents predominantly a negatively

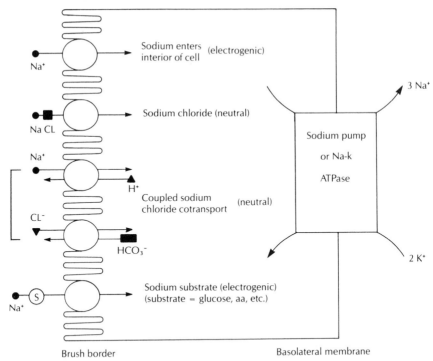

Fig. 5-2
Schematic depiction of intestinal sodium absorption.

charged surface to diffusing ions. Transport by way of the *trans-cellular* pathway requires the passage of ions through both the apical and basolateral plasma membranes as well as through the cytosol. Since plasma membranes are predominantly lipoidal, diffusion of hydrophilic molecules is limited and transcellular transport is dependent upon membrane carriers and pumps.

Sodium is the major ion actively absorbed. An important requisite for this process is the "sodium pump" (Na-K-ATPase) located in the basolateral plasma membrane of the cell. This pumps sodium out of the cell into the interstitial space, lowering the intracellular concentration of sodium. Three Na ions are pumped out for every two K ions that enter the cell (Fig. 5-2). Consequently, the interior of the cell becomes electrically negative. Thus, both electrical and chemical gradients may drive sodium from the intestinal lumen into the cell. Movement of Na into the cell may occur by means of electrogenic or neutral mechanisms (see Fig. 5-2). In the former, when one ion of Na moves from the lumen into the cell, it results in the lumen becoming negatively charged in relation to the serosal surface. In the neutral mechanism, movement of Na into the cell either occurs coupled to a negatively charged ion such as chloride or

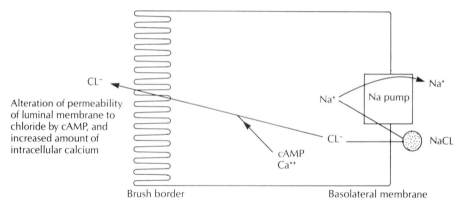

Brush border   Basolateral membrane

Fig. 5-3
Proposed cellular model of electrogenic chloride secretion.

by a more complex mechanism that involves the parallel ex-change of Na^+ for H^+ and Cl^- for HCO_3^-. Consequently, there is no change in charge on the luminal side following entry of sodium from the lumen into the cell. Sodium absorption follow-ing ingestion of a meal occurs principally by "sodium substrate" transport proteins. In this "co-transport" mechanism, sodium is transported linked in a 1:1 ratio with D-glucose or D-galactose, with amino acids, dipeptides, or tripeptides.

Sodium absorption by the colon is primarily electrogenic and is very efficient, with the resultant concentration of sodium in stool water being considerably less than in ileal effluent, as ex-emplified by sodium losses of 30 to 50 mEq/day in patients with an ileostomy contrasted to virtually no sodium loss in the stool of patients on a diet containing almost no sodium. Aldosterone is the hormone responsible for avid sodium absorption and sig-nificant potassium secretion by the colon.

Chloride is the major ion that is actively secreted. Chloride se-cretion, like sodium absorption, requires the presence of the Na-K-ATPase pump in the basolateral membrane. In a proposed model of the cellular basis of active chloride secretion, sodium and chloride enter the epithelial cell across the basolateral bor-der via a coupled process (Fig. 5-3). Sodium extrusion from the cell occurs by the sodium pump while the cell accumulates chloride ion. Cyclic AMP or an increase in the intracellular con-centration of calcium (calmodulin, a Ca^{2+}-dependent regulator protein, may be the critical mediator) increases chloride se-cretion. A number of bacterial enterotoxins, detergents (bile acids, fatty acids, commercial laxatives), and hormones have been demonstrated to stimulate active chloride secretion.

Potassium transport in the small intestine appears to be passive, but both active potassium absorption and secretion can be demonstrated in mammalian colonic mucosa, with the latter predominating. Control of colonic potassium transport is complex; cholinergic and adrenergic neurotransmitters, ecosanoids and mineralocorticoids, and glucocorticoids appear to participate in the process. Bicarbonate is largely secreted by the duodenum, ileum, and colon, whereas this ion is usually absorbed in the jejunum.

Carbohydrate Absorption

Dietary carbohydrates include polysaccharides such as starch, disaccharides such as lactose and sucrose, and monosaccharides such as glucose and fructose. The two components of starch, amylose (glucose residues linked by α-1, 4 bonds) and amylopectin (glucose residues linked by α-1, 4 bonds with α-1, 6 linkages forming branch points), are digested in the alimentary tract lumen by salivary and pancreatic amylases. The products of digestion include α limit dextrans, which consist of 4 to 10 glucose molecules and the di- and trisaccharides maltose and maltotriose.

The products of intraluminal starch digestion and dietary disaccharides must then be digested to their constituent monosaccharides before they can be transported across the epithelial barrier of the small intestine. This occurs at the level of the absorptive cell microvillus membrane in which the enzymes limit dextrinase, glucoamylase, isomaltase, sucrase, and lactase are located. Absorption of monosaccharides is generally the rate-limiting step, since hydrolysis of oligosaccharides and most disaccharides is more rapid than uptake of monosaccharides. Lactose is an exception and is hydrolyzed at a slower rate than its constituent monosaccharides — glucose and galactose — are absorbed.

The dietary monosaccharides — glucose, galactose, and fructose — are absorbed at rates that are more rapid than those expected from passive diffusion. Glucose and galactose are actively transported across the absorptive cell brush border by a transporter, presumably a membrane protein that cotransports Na^+ with the monosaccharide. The energy required for this process is derived from the Na^+, K^+-ATPase at the basolateral membrane. The accumulated monosaccharide then exits from the absorptive cell along the basolateral membrane by facilitated diffusion. Fructose transport across the brush border occurs by facilitated diffusion and does not require Na^+.

The amount of amylase secreted normally by the salivary glands and the pancreas greatly exceeds what is needed for the normal digestion of dietary polysaccharides. As a result, malabsorption of carbohydrates in disease usually involves defective digestion or transport by the intestinal mucosa. Such malabsorption can result from (1) primary disaccharidase deficiency as occurs in lactase deficiency, (2) congenital absence of the brush border membrane carrier protein for glucose and galactose (glucose-galactose malabsorption), or (3) a reduction in or damage to the absorptive surface, resulting in secondary disaccharidase deficiency and impaired monosaccharide transport (extensive intestinal resection or celiac sprue).

Carbohydrates not absorbed in transit through the small intestine are metabolized, in part, to short-chain fatty acids by the colonic bacterial flora. Although the colonic mucosa cannot absorb monosaccharides, it can absorb short-chain acids and thus salvage calories from malabsorbed dietary carbohydrates.

Protein
Absorption

Protein to be absorbed by the small intestine includes that ingested as food and endogenous protein from secretions such as saliva, bile, and pancreatic juice and from exfoliated alimentary tract epithelial cells. It has been estimated that in humans, endogenous proteins constitute approximately 40 percent of the total protein processed in the intestinal lumen. Digestion of protein begins in the stomach, where a small fraction is hydrolyzed by gastric pepsin. The polypeptides and amino acids that result play an important role in releasing cholecystokinin, the major stimulus for secretion of pancreatic proteases, from duodenal and jejunal endocrine epithelial cells. These small peptides and amino acids are also potent stimuli for the release of gastrin from the antral mucosa and, hence, the secretion of gastric acid from the oxyntic mucosa. Pancreatic proteases are secreted as inactive proenzymes, and each enzyme molecule must be activated by hydrolysis of a peptide bond. Enterokinase, an enzyme located in the microvillus membrane of duodenal absorptive cells, is released by bile salts and converts trypsinogen to trypsin by cleaving a hexapeptide from its amino terminus. Trypsin then autocatalytically activates additional trypsinogen as well as all other pancreatic proteases, including endopeptidases (trypsin, chymotrypsin, and elastase), which hydrolyze bonds in the interior of the proteins, and exopeptidases (carboxypeptidases), which hydrolyze bonds at the protein's carboxyl terminus. The products of pancreatic protease digestion within the intestinal lumen are amino acids and peptides composed of two to six amino acid residues.

A large number of peptidases are located in the absorptive cell microvillus membrane where they are, like disaccharidases, integral membrane proteins. These hydrolyze extracellularly all peptides that are larger than three amino acid residues and some tri- and dipeptides. Unlike disaccharides, which must be hydrolyzed to monosaccharides for absorption, certain tri- and dipeptides (including diglycine, glycyl-leucine, and triglycine) are efficiently absorbed by sodium-dependent energy-requiring active transport. These then serve as substrates for additional peptidases located within the absorptive cells, where they are largely hydrolyzed to amino acids before delivery to the portal circulation.

The transport mechanisms for absorption of amino acids are complex in that they are multiple and may interact with one another. All appear to be selective for the L-stereo isomers, require energy, and are at least partially sodium-dependent. There is evidence for separate carriers for neutral, basic, and dicarboxylic amino acids. The multiplicity of amino acid transport mechanisms is emphasized by the selective defects of amino acid absorption that occur in genetic disorders of amino acid transport. In these diseases, there is defective transport of only those amino acids that utilize the specific carrier that is absent or defective. For example, neutral, but not basic or acidic amino acids, are poorly transported by intestinal absorptive and renal tubular cells in Hartnup's disease.

Some dipeptides such as glycyl-leucine are absorbed more efficiently by the small intestine than are equimolar mixtures of their constituent amino acids. The number of transport systems present in absorptive cells for specific di- and tripeptides is not known. Since dipeptide solutions present less of an intraluminal osmotic load than comparable amino acid solutions, their efficient absorption has important nutritional implications in patients with diseases that severely compromise the available effective intestinal absorptive surface.

Fat Digestion and Absorption

Most dietary fat consists of long-chain triglycerides, which are poorly absorbed by the small intestine unless they are hydrolyzed and dispersed. Fat digestion begins in the stomach (Fig. 5-4), where peristalsis grinds dietary fat into a fine emulsion of triglyceride droplets. In the stomach, the fat droplets are mixed with a lipase secreted by cells in von Ebner's glands, which surround the circumvallate papillae of the tongue. Since this lingual lipase is acid stable with an optimum pH 5, it releases some fatty acids from triglyceride in the stomach. Although its quantitative contribution to triglyceride hydrolysis in adults is probably small, it is of considerable importance in newborns, where it may account for up to 50 percent of dietary lipid hydrolysis. Even in adults, lingual lipase may be physiologically important, since the fatty acids it releases facilitate triglyceride emul-

STOMACH

INTESTINAL LUMEN

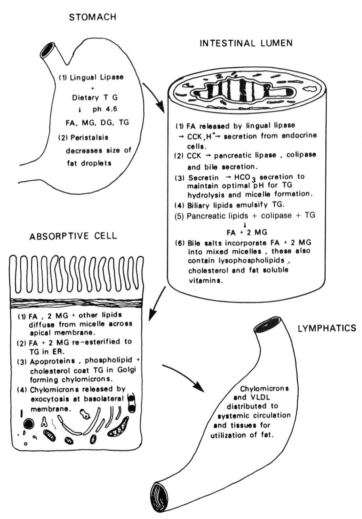

ABSORPTIVE CELL

(1) Lingual Lipase
+
Dietary T G
↓ ph 4.6
FA, MG, DG, TG

(2) Peristalsis
decreases size of
fat droplets

(1) FA released by lingual lipase
→ CCK,H$^+$→ secretion from endocrine
cells.
(2) CCK → pancreatic lipase , colipase
and bile secretion.
(3) Secretin → HCO$_3$ secretion to
maintain optimal pH for TG
hydrolysis and micelle formation.
(4) Biliary lipids emulsify TG.
(5) Pancreatic lipids + colipase + TG
↓
FA + 2 MG
(6) Bile salts incorporate FA + 2 MG
into mixed micelles , these also
contain lysophospholipids ,
cholesterol and fat soluble
vitamins.

(1) FA , 2 MG + other lipids
diffuse from micelle across
apical membrane.
(2) FA + 2 MG re-esterified to
TG in ER.
(3) Apoproteins , phospholipid +
cholesterol coat TG in Golgi
forming chylomicrons.
(4) Chylomicrons released by
exocytosis at basolateral
membrane.

LYMPHATICS

Chylomicrons
and VLDL
distributed to
systemic circulation
and tissues for
utilization of fat.

Fig. 5-4
Schematic depiction of major events of dietary fat absorption. (FA = fatty
acid; MG = monoglyceride; DG = diglyceride; TG = triglyceride; CCK =
cholecystokinin; ER = endoplasmic reticulum; VLDL = very low-density
lipoprotein.) (From J. S. Trier. Intestinal Absorption. In J. H. Stein (ed.),
Internal Medicine (2nd ed.). Boston: Little, Brown, 1987.)

sification and stimulate cholecystokinin release from the
duodenal mucosa. Cholecystokinin then stimulates delivery of
bile and pancreatic lipase into the duodenum. Lingual lipase is
inhibited by bile salts and by high pH; hence, it is normally not
effective in the intestinal lumen. Although a gastric lipase has
been described, its characteristics resemble closely those of lingual lipase, and there is question as to whether this is a separate
enzyme or lingual lipase adsorbed to the gastric mucosa.

Hydrogen ion–containing gastric contents enter the duodenum,
where they stimulate secretin release, which stimulates pancre-

atic and bile duct bicarbonate secretion. The resulting intraluminal pH of approximately 6.5 is optimal for fat digestion and dispersion. The detergent action of bile salts facilitates further emulsification of dietary fat; bile salts also interact with pancreatic lipase to reduce its optimum pH from 8.0 to that of luminal contents. Pancreatic lipase hydrolyzes long-chain triglycerides at the surface of the fat droplets to a mixture of free fatty acids, 2-monoglycerides, and glycerol. Colipase, a small protein secreted by the pancreas, is necessary for this process; it binds stochiometrically to pancreatic lipase at a 1:1 ratio, facilitates lipase attachment to the surface of triglyceride droplets, and prevents bile salt inhibition of pancreatic lipase. Dietary and biliary phospholipids are hydrolyzed in the lumen at their 2-ester linkage by phospholipase A2; cholesterol esters are hydrolyzed by pancreatic cholesterol esterase, adding additional fatty acids, 1-lysophospholipids, and cholesterol to the intraluminal chyme.

The complex mixture of lipolytic products is solubilized for intestinal absorption by bile salts originally synthesized in the liver and secreted largely as glycine and taurine conjugates of cholic and chenodeoxycholic acid. Since bile salts are amphipathic molecules with both hydrophilic and hydrophobic domains, they function as detergents and, at their normal intraluminal concentrations of 5 to 10 nM, form water-soluble micelles. Bile salt micelles incorporate the products of fat digestion and other lipids, including fat-soluble vitamins, to form mixed micelles. Larger aggregates, termed *liposomes*, also form during fat digestion. Liposomes require less bile salts for solubilizing lipolytic products than do micelles and may be of great importance for maintaining fat absorption in patients deficient in bile salts.

The lipid components of mixed micelles and liposome then cross the lipid-rich absorptive cell microvillus membrane, probably by diffusion. The bulk of the unconjugated bile salts remain in the lumen until they reach the ileum, where they are absorbed by an efficient Na^+-dependent active transport mechanism. They are returned to the liver by the portal circulation and are again secreted into the bile, resulting in an efficient enterohepatic circulation (Fig. 5-5). The major portion of the 3 to 4 gm bile salt pool recirculates four to six times daily with great efficiency so that only 0.2 to 0.6 gm are normally excreted daily in the stool (see Fig. 5-5).

Having entered the absorptive cell cytoplasm, fatty acids bind to a fatty acid–binding protein, which transports them to the smooth endoplasmic reticulum. Fatty acids are then activated to acyl CoA, which is esterified either with α-glycerophosphate to triglyceride and phospholipid or with monoglyceride to triglyceride. Next, chylomicrons are assembled largely in the Golgi

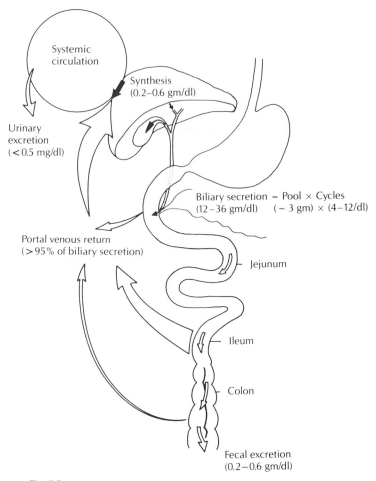

Fig. 5-5
Enterohepatic circulation of bile salts. (From M. C. Carey and S. J. Robins.
Bile Production and Secretion. In J. H. Stein (ed.), *Internal Medicine* (2nd
ed.). Boston: Little, Brown, 1987.)

region from resynthesized triglyceride, phospholipid, cholesterol esters, and apoproteins. The chylomicrons migrate in vesicles to the basolateral membrane, where they leave the cell by
exocytosis. The chylomicrons then enter the mucosal lymphatic
lacteals for distribution to the general circulation. Medium-
chain triglycerides (containing fatty acids composed of 6 to 10
carbons) are more readily hydrolyzed in the intestinal lumen by
pancreatic lipase and, to some degree, can be absorbed intact by
the small intestine. In contrast to long-chain fatty acids, medium-
chain fatty acids traverse the absorptive cells without resynthesis
to triglycerides and enter the portal circulation directly as free fatty
acids. As a result of this simpler absorptive process, medium-chain
triglycerides are useful dietary supplements in patients with diseases that produce impaired fat digestion and absorption.

Localization of Intestinal Nutrient Absorption

Under normal circumstances, absorption of the digestion products of the major calorie-containing nutrients (fats, protein, and carbohydrates) is so efficient that absorption is virtually completed in the proximal half of the small intestine, although these substances could be absorbed by the ileal mucosa. On the other hand, a few nutrients are selectively absorbed by specific regions of the small intestine.

Iron absorption is a highly regulated process. Whereas the average diet of a person living in the western hemisphere contains about 20 mg of iron per day, the average adult male requires only 1 mg/day, and the average adult female in her reproductive years requires only 2 mg/day. Dietary iron is absorbed predominantly by the duodenum and proximal jejunum. Similarly, calcium is absorbed most avidly by the proximal intestine. Calcium absorption occurs by two mechanisms: (1) a saturable, transcellular route that takes place largely in the duodenum and proximal jejunum; and (2) a nonsaturable, concentration-dependent process that occurs along the length of the small intestine. The selectivity of dietary iron and calcium absorption is underscored by the high prevalence of iron deficiency and osteopenia among patients in whom the duodenum has been surgically bypassed or in whom mucosal lesions decrease the absorptive surface of the duodenum and proximal jejunum.

Cobalamin (vitamin B_{12}), like conjugated bile salts, is selectively absorbed by the mucosa of the distal ileum. After ingestion, cobalamin binds to glycoproteins, termed *R-binders*, in saliva, gastric juice, and bile. Pancreatic proteases hydrolyze the R-binders, releasing the cobalamin, which then binds to intrinsic factor (IF), a protein secreted in humans by gastric parietal cells. The IF-cobalamin complex is resistant to intraluminal proteolysis and ultimately binds to a specific receptor on the microvillus membrane of distal ileal absorptive cells. Cobalamin subsequently traverses the absorptive cells and appears in several hours in the circulation complexed to transcobalamins. The selectivity of absorption of bile salts and cobalamin are of clinical relevance, because extensive resections of the distal ileum result in steatorrhea owing to depletion of the bile salt pool and, upon depletion of cobalamin stores in the liver, cobalamin deficiency, which leads to megaloblastic anemia and significant neurologic manifestations.

Laboratory Tests and Diagnostic Procedures

A wide array of laboratory tests are available for the evaluation of patients with diarrhea or suspected malabsorption (Table 5-1). These tests include studies of formed blood elements, serum levels of various substances, stool and urine determinations, breath tests, radiologic contrast examinations of the gastrointestinal tract, oral absorption tests, and histologic examination of

Table 5-1
Useful laboratory tests in evaluation of intestinal malabsorption

Test	Impaired intraluminal digestion	Mucosal disease	Lymphatic obstruction	Limitations
Stool fat (qualitative, quantitative)	Increased	Increased	Increased	False-negative if inadequate ingestion of dietary fat or recent barium ingestion; false-positive with castor oil or mineral oil ingestion
^{14}C-triolein absorption breath test	Decreased $^{14}CO_2$ excretion	Decreased $^{14}CO_2$ excretion	Decreased $^{14}CO_2$ excretion	Impaired gastric emptying or obesity may produce false-positive results
Serum carotene	Decreased	Decreased	Decreased	Low values may occur in normal subjects who ingest little dietary carotene
Serum cholesterol	Decreased	Decreased	Decreased	May be normal or increased in patients with untreated lipoprotein abnormality
Serum albumin	Usually normal, except with bacterial overgrowth	Often decreased	Often decreased	
Prothrombin time	Decreased if severe	Decreased if severe	Decreased if severe	May also be decreased in liver disease, but parenterally administered vitamin K should induce normalization if caused by malabsorption
Serum iron	Normal	Often decreased	Normal	

Test				Comments
Serum folate	Normal	Often decreased	Normal	
Xylose absorption	Normal, except with bacterial overgrowth	Abnormal, unless disease confined to distal small intestine	Normal	Requires normal gastric emptying and renal function
Lactose absorption (lactose tolerance test or breath hydrogen after lactose load)	Normal, except in some instances of bacterial overgrowth	Decreased serum lactose, increased breath H_2	Normal	May be abnormal in all categories if patient has isolated intestinal lactase deficiency
Vitamin B_{12} (Schilling test)	Decreased in bacterial overgrowth and exocrine pancreatic insufficiency	Decreased in extensive ileal disease	Normal	Requires good renal function
^{14}C-cholylglycine breath tests	Increased $^{14}CO_2$ excretion in bacterial overgrowth	Increased $^{14}CO_2$ excretion in ileal disease	Normal	Requires normal gastric emptying
Lactulose breath test	Early appearance of H_2 in breath in bacterial overgrowth	Normal	Normal	Requires normal gastric emptying; false-positives may occur in patient with rapid small intestinal transit
Secretin/cholecystokinin stimulation tests	Abnormal in chronic pancreatic disease	Normal	Normal	Relatively low sensitivity
Peroral intestinal biopsy	Normal except in severe bacterial overgrowth	Often abnormal	Often abnormal	May miss patchy mucosal disease

Source: J. S. Trier. Intestinal Absorption. In J. H. Stein (ed.), *Internal Medicine.* Boston: Little, Brown, 1987.

the small bowel and colon. The judicious use of these tests is based on a proper understanding of the pathophysiology of diarrhea and of malabsorption.

The patient's history and findings on physical examination can often provide a logical framework on which appropriate diagnostic considerations can be based. The tests carried out may corroborate a clinical suspicion, establish that a feature such as malabsorption is indeed present, or actually provide a definitive diagnosis. For example, a patient may present with diarrhea consisting of large, greasy stools of a rancid odor and weight loss, despite an apparent normal caloric intake. Such a history is suggestive of malabsorption. A quantitative or perhaps qualitative stool fat determination showing excessive fecal fat excretion will establish that the patient has steatorrhea. In order to help distinguish pancreatic insufficiency from small bowel mucosal disease (both can cause steatorrhea) a D-xylose absorption test can be performed. If abnormal, this indicates the possibility of a mucosal disorder; the clinician is likely to proceed to a small bowel biopsy, which may reveal histologic features characteristic (e.g., celiac sprue) or even diagnostic (e.g., Whipple's disease) of a specific primary small bowel mucosal malabsorptive disorder. A brief discussion of the various tests follows. A more thorough explanation can be found in standard texts of gastrointestinal disorders.

Studies of Formed Blood Elements

Anemia can accompany a number of disorders causing diarrhea or malabsorption. Knowledge of the type of anemia can be helpful. If the patient has a microcytic iron deficiency anemia, this suggests the possibility of malabsorption of iron (common with diffuse mucosal lesions, which involve most severely the proximal small bowel such as celiac sprue or Whipple's disease) or chronic blood loss secondary to idiopathic inflammatory bowel disease or neoplasia. Macrocytic anemia may be secondary to folate or cobalamin deficiency. Folate deficiency is a common feature of celiac sprue, tropical sprue, and Whipple's disease (diseases with severe proximal lesions), whereas cobalamin deficiency may accompany bacterial overgrowth syndromes or ileal disease or may occur in patients following ileal resection.

Leukocytosis is not a feature of viral gastroenteritis or drug-induced diarrhea but is often present in patients with mucosally invasive bacterial infections (campylobacter, salmonella, shigella, yersinia), severe idiopathic inflammatory bowel disease, amebic dysentery, and pseudomembranous enterocolitis. Peripheral eosinophilia accompanies eosinophilic gastroenteritis, Addison's disease, vasculitides, and certain parasitic infestations such as round worms and tapeworms. Lymphopenia is a common feature of disorders characterized as having protein-losing enteropathy and is seen characteristically in intestinal lymphangiectasia. Thrombocytosis is occasionally seen in patients with severe idiopathic inflammatory bowel disease or celiac sprue.

Serum Levels of Various Substances

Abnormal serum electrolyte concentrations are observed in a number of conditions causing acute or chronic diarrhea. Severe hypokalemia, for example, may be present in patients with villous adenomas or pancreatic cholera syndrome or in those with chronic laxative abuse. Hypoalbuminemia may be seen in patients with malnutrition, malabsorption with or without excessive leakage of plasma protein into the gastrointestinal tract, or coexistent liver disease. If the globulin fraction of the total protein concentration in the serum is also decreased, this suggests severe protein-losing enteropathy. Hypogammaglobulinemia occurs in some patients with benign lymphonodular hyperplasia of the gastrointestinal tract, often with associated giardiasis, and rarely with celiac sprue and idiopathic inflammatory bowel disease. In patients with severe malabsorption, there are increased fecal losses of calcium, magnesium, and zinc, which may result in decreased serum concentrations of these cations. The prothrombin time is prolonged in patients with vitamin K deficiency secondary to malabsorption of this fat-soluble vitamin. The prothrombin time corrects to normal with parenteral, but often not with oral, administration of vitamin K. Correction of this and other possible coagulation defects is necessary before performing a biopsy of the small intestine for histologic assessment. In patients with malabsorption, the serum cholesterol and carotene concentrations are often decreased. The serum alkaline phosphatase value may be increased in malabsorption, reflecting osteopenic bone disease.

Determinations of serum levels of certain hormones can be useful in evaluating patients with diarrhea or malabsorption. Examples include serum cortisol (Addison's disease), serum thyroxine (hyperthyroidism), serum gastrin (gastrinoma, or Zollinger-Ellison syndrome), serum vasoactive intestinal polypeptide (pancreatic cholera syndrome, or WDHA syndrome, see Chap. 21), and serum calcitonin levels (medullary carcinoma of the thyroid).

Stool Examination

Examination of the stool can provide important diagnostic information leading to a specific diagnosis or in support of a clinical suspicion. For example, a stool suspension stained with methylene blue or Wright's stain that demonstrates polymorphonuclear leukocytes in a patient with diarrhea suggests a mucosally invasive infectious process that is characteristic of salmonella, shigella, campylobacter, or amebic colitis. Pus cells are also present in the stool in patients with idiopathic inflammatory bowel disease and pseudomembranous enterocolitis but are not present in patients with viral gastroenteritis, most drug-induced diarrheas, hormone-mediated diarrhea, celiac sprue, and lactase deficiency. Similarly, a positive Sudan stain of the stool provides evidence that a patient has steatorrhea but does not distinguish pancreatic insufficiency (e.g., in an alcoholic patient with chronic pancreatitis) from a primary small bowel mucosal malabsorptive disorder (e.g., a patient with celiac sprue). If properly performed, a Sudan stain of the stool will detect approximately 90 percent of patients with clinically significant steatorrhea. Quantitative determination of fat in a complete 72- to 96-hour stool collection is more accurate but is also a more cumbersome and expensive test to perform.

Stool examination for ova and parasites, stool cultures, and a stool assay that is positive for *Clostridium difficile* toxin can provide precise and accurate diagnostic information. Determination of stool volume in a 24-hour period and of stool electrolytes and osmolarity can be helpful in distinguishing secretory diarrhea from osmotic diarrhea. In secretory diarrheas (discussed later), the 24-hour stool volume usually exceeds 1 liter, diarrhea does not significantly abate on fasting, and the stool osmolarity is approximately twice the concentration of stool sodium and potassium. In contrast, in patients with osmotic diarrheas (e.g., diarrhea secondary to magnesium-containing antacids, severe lactase deficiency, sorbitol ingestion), the stool osmolarity is substantially greater than twice the sum of stool sodium and potassium concentration, and the diarrhea will cease if the patient is fasted and is, hence, not ingesting the offending poorly absorbed solute. A simple test that indicates that the patient is ingesting a phenolphthalein-containing laxative involves addition of sodium hydroxide to a sample of the patient's diarrheal stool; alkalinization of the stool results in the dramatic appearance of a pink or red color. Surreptitious laxative abuse in adults and "laxative abuse by proxy" in children are being increasingly recognized as important causes of unexplained refractory diarrhea in many referral centers.

Urine Tests

Alkalinization of urine like that of stool may detect laxative abuse. Increased urinary excretion of 5-hydroxyindoleacetic acid is seen in patients with carcinoid syndrome. Determination of the amount of D-xylose and radiolabeled vitamin B_{12} excreted in the urine is discussed in the section entitled Oral Absorption Tests.

Breath Tests

Recently introduced breath tests can be helpful in screening for steatorrhea and in diagnosing lactase deficiency, ileal disease, idiopathic bile salt malabsorption, and bacterial overgrowth. Idiopathic bile salt malabsorption refers to a condition characterized by chronic watery diarrhea in patients with no other recognized ileal dysfunction (hence, vitamin B_{12} absorption is normal) and a normal small bowel radiographic study. Bile salt malabsorption is suggested by increased $^{14}CO_2$ excretion in the breath following oral administration of ^{14}C-cholylglycine and by an unequivocal response to cholestyramine (a bile salt–sequestering agent) therapy. This disorder appears to be more prevalent than was previously recognized and merits consideration in patients with chronic watery diarrhea.

Radiographic Studies

A plain x-ray of the abdomen may disclose pancreatic calcification. In a patient with a history of heavy ethanol abuse, steatorrhea, and a normal D-xylose test, this would suggest that the patient's malabsorption is secondary to pancreatic insufficiency. Confirmation of this can be sought by measuring pancreatic bicarbonate or enzyme secretion after secretin or cholecystokinin administration, by obtaining a serum trypsin determination, or by administering exogenous pancreatic enzymes to the patient and observing whether a therapeutic response is obtained. Barium contrast studies of the gastrointestinal tract may provide important information in patients with diarrhea or malabsorption or both. Barium studies should not be carried out in patients with suspected infectious or parasitic causes of diarrhea until appropriate stool examination has been performed, because barium will interfere with the detection of many pathogens. Barium enema examination can disclose characteristic findings in patients with idiopathic ulcerative colitis or Crohn's disease.

In patients with diarrhea, an upper gastrointestinal contrast study showing large gastric rugae and evidence of increased gastric secretions with or without gastroduodenal ulceration suggests the possibility of gastrinoma. Barium contrast studies may disclose evidence of gastrocolic or enterocolic fistulae — rare causes of severe malabsorption. Diffusely thickened and coarse folds of the small bowel mucosa are evident in many patients with infiltrative disease such as celiac sprue, Whipple's disease, lymphoma, amyloidosis, and eosinophilic gastroenteritis. Multiple jejunal diverticula may be seen and should raise the possibility of bacterial overgrowth. Computed tomography examination may show a pancreatic mass in patients with gastrinoma or the pancreatic cholera syndrome.

Oral Absorption Tests

Oral absorption tests are useful in patients with suspected malabsorption. The D-xylose absorption test helps to distinguish malabsorption caused by small bowel mucosal disease from that caused by impaired intraluminal digestion. After ingestion of a 25-gm dose of this nonmetabolized 5-carbon sugar by a fasted but well-hydrated subject, blood levels at 2 hours should exceed 25 mg/dl, and 5 gm or more of D-xylose should be excreted in the urine in 5 hours. Since D-xylose requires no intraluminal digestion, low blood levels and urinary excretion suggest mucosal disease such as celiac sprue. D-xylose excretion is normal in most patients with pancreatic insufficiency. Abnormal values can be encountered in patients with marked gastric retention, bacterial overgrowth of the proximal small intestine (some strains of enteric bacteria metabolize D-xylose), and ascites. In patients with renal impairment, urinary excretion will be low, whereas serum levels will be higher than expected. The lactose absorption test consists of the administration of 50 gm of lactose to a fasting subject and measurement of blood glucose 2 hours later. In normal individuals, the blood glucose concentration should increase 20 to 30 mg/dl. The test does not distinguish between primary and secondary lactase deficiency (discussed later in this chapter).

The mechanism of vitamin B_{12} (cobalamin) absorption is unique and has already been discussed. Urinary excretion of radiolabeled vitamin B_{12} is measured after its oral administration both alone and with IF. In patients with pernicious anemia, free vitamin B_{12} is malabsorbed, but there is normal absorption of the IF-B_{12} complex. In patients with bacterial overgrowth, the malabsorption of vitamin B_{12} can be corrected by administering antibiotics that will surpress the overgrowth of bacteria in the small intestine. In patients with severe pancreatic insufficiency, malabsorption of vitamin B_{12} can be corrected by administration of exogenous pancreatic enzymes. Absorption of oral vitamin B_{12} alone or combined with IF will be abnormal in patients with severe infiltrative ileal disease or in those with ileal resection and will not correct itself despite administration of antibiotics or pancreatic enzymes. Since there is substantial storage of vitamin B_{12} in the liver, abnormal B_{12} absorption is often present for a number of years before the appearance of low vitamin B_{12} blood levels or abnormal blood cell morphology.

Endoscopy and Histologic Assessment

Proctosigmoidoscopy should be performed in all patients with chronic diarrhea and in selected patients with acute diarrhea. Examples of the latter category include those patients with bloody diarrhea or prominent tenesmus. Proctosigmoidoscopy may identify a rectosigmoid neoplasm such as a villous adenoma or reveal mucosal abnormalities characteristic of inflammatory bowel disease, ischemic colitis, or pseudomembranous colitis.

Colonoscopy can be helpful in detecting neoplasms, in gauging the extent of inflammatory bowel disease, in possibly distinguishing Crohn's colitis from ulcerative colitis, in diagnosing pseudomembranous enterocolitis in those patients with normal proctosigmoidoscopic examination, and in diagnosing microscopic colitis and collagenous colitis. Patients with the last two disorders have normal radiographic and endoscopic appearance but microscopic examination discloses inflammatory cell infiltration with or without deposition of a band of collagen in the subepithelial layer. Unexplained watery diarrhea of months to years duration is the usual presentation in patients with these two disorders.

Suction biopsy of the small intestine can be performed on an outpatient basis and is particularly valuable in the evaluation of patients with malabsorption. Information provided by peroral small bowel biopsy is summarized in Table 5-2.

Pathophysiology of Diarrhea

Normally, the absorptive processes predominate over the secretory processes. If the gastrointestinal tract is converted from a predominantly absorptive organ into a predominantly secretory organ, diarrhea ensues. All diarrheal disorders studied to date have revealed net intestinal secretion in some part of the gastrointestinal tract. The secretory process may be localized to or originate in the jejunum, ileum, or colon. From a pathophysiologic standpoint, diarrhea may be classified as a consequence of a process that is: (1) secretory, (2) osmotic, (3) characterized by abnormal gastrointestinal motility, (4) exudative, or (5) malabsorptive. In some instances, more than one pathophysiologic process is operative.

Secretory Diarrhea

Secretory diarrhea refers to a large group of disorders in which there is active intestinal secretion of electrolytes with a concomitant flow of water. The stool of patients with secretory diarrhea is occasionally isotonic with plasma and can resemble an ultrafiltrate of plasma. The disease process may emanate within or outside the gastrointestinal tract; active secretion may be mediated by a hormone such as VIP, bacterial toxin (e.g., *Escherichia coli* toxin), or a chemical drug; and excess secretion may involve the entire intestine or be localized to the jejunum, ileum, or colon. The absorptive and secretory capacities of the colon are not significantly affected in most types of secretory diarrheas. Exceptions to this rule are seen in patients with diarrhea secondary to bile salt or fatty acid malabsorption and in patients with villous adenomas of the colon. Small bowel morphology is most often normal, even in the dramatic prototypic example of secretory diarrhea caused by the enterotoxin of *Vibrio cholerae*, a

Table 5-2
Information provided by peroral small bowel biopsies and diagnosis

I. Disorders in which biopsy is diagnostic: diffuse lesions
  A. Whipple's disease
    1. Lamina propria infiltrated with PAS-positive macrophages
    2. Characteristic bacilli in mucosa
  B. Agammaglobulinemia and severe hypogammaglobulinemia
    1. Mucosal architecture from normal to flat
    2. Plasma cells absent or markedly diminished in lamina propria
    3. Giardia trophozoites often present
  C. Abetalipoproteinemia
    1. Mucosal architecture normal
    2. Lipid-laden absorptive cells appear vacuolated
II. Disorders in which biopsy may be diagnostic: patchy lesions
  A. Intestinal lymphoma
    1. Villi widened, shortened, or absent
    2. Malignant lymphoma cells in lamina propria and submucosa
  B. Intestinal lymphangiectasia
    1. Mucosal architecture normal
    2. Dilated lymphatics in lamina propria and submucosa
  C. Eosinophilic enteritis
    1. Mucosal architecture from normal to flat
    2. Patchy infiltration of lamina propria with eosinophils and neutrophils
  D. Mastocytosis
    1. Mucosal architecture from normal to flat
    2. Patchy infiltration of lamina propria with mast cells, eosinophils, and neutrophils
  E. Amyloidosis
    1. Mucosal architecture normal
    2. Amyloid in lamina propria and submucosa shown with Congo red stain
  F. Crohn's disease
    1. Mucosal architecture variable
    2. Sarcoid granulomata and inflammation in lamina propria and submucosa
  G. Giardiasis
    1. Mucosal architecture from normal to flat
    2. Trophozoites in lumen and on surface of absorptive cells
    3. Minimal to severe inflammation in lamina propria
  H. Coccidiosis
    1. Villi shortened
    2. Crypts hyperplastic
    3. Coccidial forms on surface of (cryptosporidosis) or within (*Eimeria, Isospora*) absorptive cells
    4. Inflammation of lamina propria
III. Disorders in which biopsy is abnormal but not diagnostic
  A. Celiac sprue
    1. Villi shortened or absent
    2. Crypts hyperplastic
    3. Severe absorptive cell damage
    4. Inflammation of lamina propria
  B. Unclassified sprue: indistinguishable from celiac sprue
  C. Tropical sprue
    1. Mucosal architecture from nearly normal to flat mucosa (like celiac sprue)
    2. Absorptive cell damage mild
    3. Inflammation of lamina propria
  D. Viral gastroenteritis: indistinguishable from mild to moderate tropical sprue lesion
  E. Intraluminal bacterial overgrowth: may be normal or indistinguishable from mild to moderate tropical sprue lesion
  F. Folate and/or B_{12} deficiency, acute radiation enteritis
    1. Shortened villi
    2. Hypoplastic crypts
    3. Megalocytic epithelium
    4. Diminished mitoses
    5. Inflammation of lamina propria

Source: J. S. Trier. Evaluation of Intestinal Diseases. In J. H. Stein (ed.), *Internal Medicine*. Boston: Little, Brown, 1987.

Table 5-3
Causes of secretory diarrhea

Infectious causes
  Enterotoxin-mediated
    *Vibrio cholerae**
    Escherichia coli
    Bacillus cereus
    Clostridium perfringens

Neoplastic causes
  Hormone-mediated
    Medullary carcinoma of thyroid (calcitonin, prostaglandin)
    Carcinoid (serotonin, ? prostaglandins)
    Pancreatic cholera (VIP, others [e.g., GIP, PP, secretin, prosta-
    glandins])
    Ganglioneuroma, ganglioneuroblastoma, neurofibroma (VIP,
    prostaglandins)

  Nonhormone-mediated
    Villous adenoma

Miscellaneous causes
  Bile salt malabsorption
  Hydroxy fatty acid diarrhea
  Idiopathic secretory diarrhea
  Lethal familial protracted diarrhea

*Cholera is the classic prototypic example of a toxin-mediated secretory
diarrhea (see text).
Key: VIP = vasoactive intestinal polypeptide; GIP = gastric inhibitory peptide; PP = pancreatic polypeptide.

situation in which the rate of intestinal fluid loss may exceed 1
liter/hour. Secretory diarrhea should be suspected if the following criteria are present: (1) large-volume diarrhea (stool volume
greater than 1 liter/24 hours), and (2) diarrhea persists during
fasting. Table 5-3 lists the causes of secretory diarrhea.

In many other diarrheal disorders (e.g., osmotic diarrhea, some
primary malabsorptive syndromes [to be discussed later]), specific dietary manipulations can aggravate or ameliorate the diarrhea. For example, a high-lactose diet in a patient with lactose
intolerance will result in worsening of the diarrheal problem,
whereas a low-fat diet will significantly ameliorate the diarrhea
in many patients with steatorrhea. Exceptions to the rule stating
that in secretory diarrheas the diarrhea persists during fasting
include cases of fatty acid– and bile acid–induced secretory diarrhea, in which the diarrhea will subside while the patient is
fasting.

Cholera

V. cholerae is a short, comma-shaped gram-negative bacterium
that has a single polar flagellum and is actively motile. It is oxi-
dase-positive, grows in the presence of bile and bismuth salts,
and produces a neuraminidase. There are three serotypes:

Ogawa (AB), Inaba (AC), and Hikojima (ABC). Each of these has two major biotypes, classic and El Tor.

Cholera has wreaked havoc for many centuries in the Indian subcontinent, considered by many to be the "cradle of cholera." Since 1817, there have been seven cholera pandemics. The most recent one started in 1961, in the Celebes Island in Indonesia and subsequently spread to other parts of Asia, Africa, Europe, and the Gulf Coast of the United States. In endemic areas such as Bangladesh, cholera is a disease of children, whereas in the epidemic form, adults and children are at equal risk of contracting the disease. Sporadic cases have been seen in recent years in the United States along the Gulf Coast. The current dominant biotype is the El Tor strain, a hardier strain that is excreted in the stool for a longer period of time than the classic variety. Waterborne fecal-oral spread is the predominant mode of transmission of this disease, which has a ratio of asymptomatic to hospitalized patients ranging from 35:1 to 100:1 in different surveys. Although the disease has been produced experimentally in animals, humans are the only natural hosts for cholera vibrios. A chronic carrier state (site of harboring the organism is the gallbladder) is estimated to occur in 3 to 5 percent of individuals following acute infection.

Clinically, the disease varies from mild diarrhea to a severe secretory diarrhea, leading to severe volume depletion, dehydration, acidosis, and death if fluid and ion losses are not promptly replaced. Patients may have severe "rice-water" diarrhea. Abdominal pain, bloody diarrhea, and high fever are notably absent. Shock may supervene within a few hours of the illness, and victims of this disease may succumb rapidly. Malpighi described it as "a disease which begins where other diseases end, with death," illustrating the fact that the patient with cholera may be dead within a few hours of the onset of symptoms. Other patients are often desperately ill, conscious but gaunt and apathetic, with no obtainable blood pressure, barely audible heart sounds, and marked wrinkling of the skin on the dorsum of the fingers ("washer woman's hands"). Metabolic acidosis and muscle cramps are not unusual findings. Laboratory evaluation reveals hemoconcentration, hypoglycemia, hyperchloremic metabolic acidosis, and hyperkalemia. If fluid losses are not adequately replaced, azotemia and acute tubular necrosis may follow. Untreated, the typical course lasts 4 to 7 days and carries a mortality rate in excess of 50 percent.

The entire clinical syndrome develops as a consequence of the interaction of the cholera toxin with the small bowel mucosal cells. Before this can happen, the ingested vibrios have to survive passage through the acid milieu of the stomach. In human volunteer studies, it has been shown that ingestion of 10^6 vibrios is needed to produce clinical illness in 50 percent of challenged subjects in whom gastric acid has been neutralized by administration of sodium bicarbonate. This contrasts with the 50 percent attack rate seen after ingestion of only 10^4 *Salmonella typhimurium* or 10^2 *Shigella dysenteriae* under similar conditions. Thus, many organisms are needed to produce the clinical illness. The seminal protective role of gastric acid is exemplified by the following observations: (1) ingestion of 10 billion cholera microorganisms does not produce clinical illness in healthy adult male volunteers with intact gastric acid secretion; (2) significant numbers of patients with cholera have hypochlorhydria or achlorhydria; and (3) in an experimental canine model of cholera, prior neutralization of gastric acid is necessary for production of the disease.

In the alkaline milieu of the small intestine, the cholera microorganisms multiply and elaborate a protein enterotoxin with a molecular weight of 84,000 daltons. The enterotoxin is composed of two moieties: (1) a binding (B) moiety, consisting of five identical subunits of 11,000 daltons each; and (2) activating (A) moiety, consisting of a large A_2 subunit of 23,000 daltons linked by a single disulfide bond to a small A_1 subunit of 5,000 daltons. The sequential steps starting from binding of the enterotoxin to the receptor on the mucosal cell and culminating in active secretion are depicted in Fig. 5-6.

Cholera stool is characterized by a mean sodium value of 128 mEq/liter, potassium of 16 mEq/liter, bicarbonate of 48 mEq/liter, and chloride of 90 mEq/liter. The toxin has no known effect on gastric or colonic function, and it is noteworthy that there are no histologic alterations of the small bowel mucosa. Mucosal invasion does not occur, and bacteremia is virtually unknown. Of considerable therapeutic importance is the observation that absorptive function remains normal; this provides a sound and logical basis for the efficacy of oral fluid replacement therapy.

The cornerstone of therapy consists of appropriate fluid replacement, a modality that was accepted by the medical profession only around the mid-twentieth century, despite a proposal for such therapy a century earlier and the description of lifesaving effects of "copious injections of aqueous and saline solutions" as early as 1832. Recognition of the enhancing effects of glucose on sodium absorption by the small intestine has led to the development of glucose-containing electrolyte solutions and represents a significant advance in the treatment of this disease. Enteric glucose absorption and glucose-facilitated

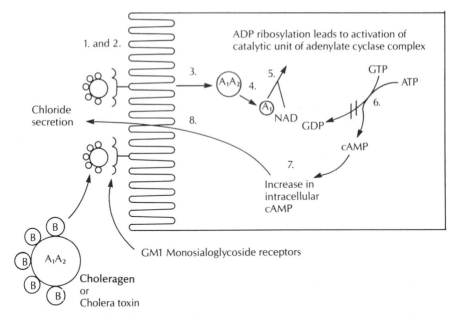

ADP ribosylation leads to activation of
catalytic unit of adenylate cyclase complex

1. and 2.

Chloride
secretion

GM1 Monosialoglycoside receptors

Choleragen
or
Cholera toxin

Fig. 5-6
Schematic representation of putative mechanism of action of cholera toxin.
Steps 1 to 8: 1 and 2. Rapid and irreversible binding of choleragen to GM_1
receptors followed by a conformational change, allowing hydrophobic regions in A component to interact with hydrophobic regions in the membrane. 3. A component separates from B component and penetrates membrane to enter cell. 4. Reduction of disulfide bond generating active A_1
peptide. 5. A_1 peptide catalyzes cleavage of NAD to nicotinamide and ADP-
ribose. 6. Transfer of ADP-ribose to adenylate cyclase complex and its activation by inhibition of GTPase. 7. Increase in intracellular cAMP levels.
8. Active chloride secretion. (B = binding moiety; A = activating moiety [A_1
and A_2 subunits].)

sodium absorption is intact in patients with cholera. Oral hydration therapy does not decrease the rate of intestinal fluid loss,
but absorption of water and ions occurs at a rate sufficient in
most cases to counterbalance the continuing fluid losses.

Treatment with the antimicrobial agent tetracycline results in
about a 60 percent reduction in fluid losses. Fluid losses are not
significantly reduced for the first 12 hours following administration of the drug; thereafter, however, it has a striking effect —
within 2 days, the secretory process is virtually abolished. Although tetracycline treatment results in the rapid killing of the
culprit vibrios, the gradual cessation of fluid loss is explained by
the fact that enterotoxin already bound to the receptors in the
mucosal cells is biologically active at the time of antimicrobial
administration. Indeed, it has been well demonstrated that all
the manifestations of the natural disease can be produced by
administration of the cholera enterotoxin. Agents capable of
reducing fluid loss after binding of toxin to the receptor, by

reversing the secretory process, include chlorpromazine, nicotinic acid, and berberine.

Pancreatic Cholera Syndrome

In 1958, Verner and Morrison described two patients with profuse watery diarrhea, hypokalemia, and non–β cell islet cell adenomas of the pancreas. The pancreatic cholera syndrome (see Chap. 21) has since then been known by a variety of terms, including Verner-Morrison syndrome, WDHA syndrome (watery diarrhea, hypokalemia, achlorhydria syndrome), and VIPoma.

Features of this syndrome include profuse watery diarrhea (intermittent or constant), hypokalemia, achlorhydria (60%), hypercalcemia (75%), glucose intolerance (50%), and flushing (20%). A dilated gallbladder containing stones and an urticarial skin rash are other noteworthy features in some patients. Steatorrhea is absent or minimal.

Pathologically, the pancreas may display hyperplasia, microadenomatosis, or a malignant tumor of the endocrine islets. In recent series, less than 40 percent of subjects have a malignant neoplasm of the pancreas. An identical syndrome with excess VIP production has been reported in patients with nonpancreatic neoplasms, particularly neural crest tumors such as ganglioneuromas. In fact, in children with this syndrome who are younger than 10 years of age, ganglioneuromas are often discovered. Although VIP formation by the tumor and high serum levels of VIP are present in most patients with this syndrome, several other hormones or candidate hormones, including gastric inhibitory peptide (GIP), prostaglandins, calcitonin, pancreatic polypeptide, substance P, secretin, glucagon, neurotensin, and enkephalins, have been isolated from such patients. Vasoactive intestinal polypeptide has received the most attention, because it has been shown to suppress gastric acid secretion and stimulate pancreatic and small bowel secretion. This 28 amino acid polypeptide occurs in large amounts in the pancreas, jejunum, and colon. In the intestine, it is predominantly located in nerve cells. Large amounts are also present in the cerebral cortex. Vasoactive intestinal polypeptide stimulates the adenylate cyclase-cyclic AMP system, thus producing diarrhea by a mechanism very similar to that produced by *V. cholerae* infection.

Medical treatment with somatostatin analogs may dramatically ameliorate the diarrhea. Chemotherapeutic agents such as combination streptozotocin and 5-fluorouracil may benefit patients with metastatic disease. Surgical treatment consists of removal of any grossly evident tumor or total or subtotal pancreatectomy if no tumor is discernible.

Osmotic Diarrhea

Osmotic diarrhea occurs when poorly absorbed solutes are present within the lumen of the gastrointestinal tract. This may occur following: (1) ingestion of a nonabsorbable or poorly absorbed solute (e.g., divalent ion such as Mg^{2+}), commonly present in some laxatives and antacids; (2) ingestion of selected foods such as lactose-containing foods in patients with lactase deficiency; or (3) failure to transport an osmotically active dietary nonelectrolyte such as glucose, which is normally absorbed by a special mechanism. The unabsorbed solute draws water into the lumen, since the intestinal mucosa is freely permeable to water in order to establish an osmotic equilibrium between the intestinal lumen and plasma. When the intraluminal water load exceeds the capacity of the small intestine and colon to absorb water, diarrhea ensues. Characteristic features of osmotic diarrhea include (1) volume of stool is generally greater than 1 liter/day; (2) diarrhea abates when the patient fasts or no longer ingests the poorly absorbed solute; (3) an osmotic gap is present in the stool (i.e., stool osmolality — stool $[Na^+ + K^+] \times 2 = > 50$ mOsm); and (4) in patients with carbohydrate malabsorption, the stool is often acidic — stool pH = 5.0 or 6.0 (normally around 7.0). The acid pH of the stool occurs as a consequence of colonic bacteria fermenting in absorbed nutrients to short-chain organic and fatty acids. Table 5-4 provides a list of some of the important causes of osmotic diarrhea.

Lactase Deficiency

Malabsorption of a specific dietary constituent leading to osmotic diarrhea is best exemplified by the condition of lactase

Table 5-4
Causes of osmotic diarrhea

Disaccharidase deficiency; e.g., lactose intolerance
Lactulose therapy (used for hepatic encephalopathy, constipation)
Gut lavage solutions commonly used for colonoscopy (GoLYTELY — contains sodium sulfate as the predominant salt and polyethylene glycol)
Sodium sulfate (Glauber's salt, carlsbad salt), sodium phosphate
Magnesium sulfate (Epsom salt), magnesium-containing antacids
Glucose-galactose malabsorption
Fructose malabsorption
Mannitol
Sorbitol ingestion ("chewing gum diarrhea," "dietetic food diarrhea")
Generalized malabsorption caused by small intestinal mucosal disease

deficiency. Decreased intestinal brush border lactase levels are found in most of the world's adult population. Lactase deficiency is present in 10 to 20 percent of adult North American Caucasians, 80 percent of North American and African blacks, and 95 percent of Orientals. This condition is referred to as primary lactase deficiency and is, in fact, so prevalent that it has been remarked that lactase deficiency is normal and that the abnormal persons are those who are lactase sufficient. In affected individuals, levels of lactase are adequate in infancy and decline during childhood or adolescence. Secondary lactase deficiency may occur in patients with a variety of intestinal disorders, including Crohn's disease, gluten-sensitive enteropathy, tropical sprue, lymphoma, acute gastroenteritis, and short-bowel syndrome. The pathophysiology of lactase deficiency leading to gastrointestinal symptomatology is depicted in Fig. 5-7. Symptoms consist of abdominal distention, bloating, cramps, borborygmi, flatulence, and diarrhea and develop whenever a certain threshold ingestion of lactose (e.g., milk, cream, cheese, ice cream) is achieved.

The diagnosis is suggested by relief of the classic symptoms on a lactose-free diet and reappearance of symptoms upon rechallenge. Definitive diagnosis may be made by biochemically assay-

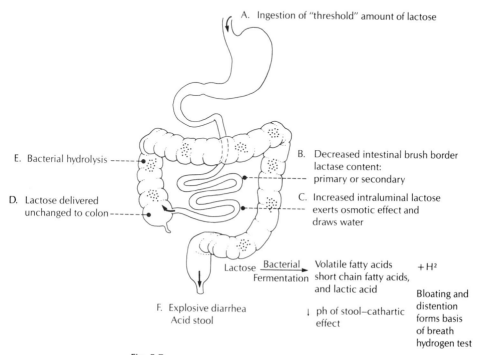

A. Ingestion of "threshold" amount of lactose

E. Bacterial hydrolysis

B. Decreased intestinal brush border lactase content: primary or secondary

D. Lactose delivered unchanged to colon

C. Increased intraluminal lactose exerts osmotic effect and draws water

Lactose $\xrightarrow[\text{Fermentation}]{\text{Bacterial}}$ Volatile fatty acids short chain fatty acids, and lactic acid $+ H^2$

F. Explosive diarrhea Acid stool

↓ ph of stool—cathartic effect

Bloating and distention forms basis of breath hydrogen test

Fig. 5-7
Diagrammatic representation of pathophysiology of lactose intolerance.

ing the lactase content of small intestinal mucosa obtained by a peroral biopsy technique or by the lactose tolerance test. In the latter test, if the blood sugar rises less than 20 mg/dl during the 2 hours following a 50-gm oral lactose challenge and symptoms appear, the test is considered diagnostic. The diagnosis can also be made in most instances by a breath hydrogen test. The rate of breath hydrogen excretion is roughly proportional to the quantity of carbohydrate reaching the colon. Thus, in patients with lactase deficiency, there is increased breath hydrogen excretion after a 50-gm oral lactose challenge. Treatment consists of a reduction or near total abstinence of lactose intake. Some patients are sensitive to as little as 3 gm of lactose intake and need to scrupulously avoid almost all milk and dairy products. Enzyme replacement (a yeast lactase preparation added to milk at 4°C results in 70 percent hydrolysis of lactose in 1 day and 90 percent hydrolysis in 2 to 3 days) is beneficial in people who wish to ingest milk. A recent study demonstrated that ingestion of yogurt resulted in a decreased reported incidence of diarrhea or flatulence than with a similar quantity of lactose ingestion with milk or water. Breath hydrogen excretion in these lactase-deficient subjects was also significantly reduced following ingestion of lactose in yogurt compared with a similar amount of lactose in milk or water. It is believed that this benefit derives from the incubation of concentrated milk with *Lactobacillus bulgaricus* and *Streptococcus thermophilus* (two organisms that contain β-galactosidase, a lactase) during the manufacture of yogurt. The bacterial lactase survives passage through the stomach. Perhaps this "autodigesting" feature of yogurt explains its popularity in India and the Middle East, where lactase deficiency is so prevalent.

Motility Disorders

Motility or motor disorders of the small bowel or colon are often associated with diarrhea. Both rapid and delayed transit of chyme through the gastrointestinal tract can result in diarrhea. In the former instance, this presumably occurs because of reduced exposure time of the chyme to the surface absorptive epithelium. Patients with diarrhea caused by rapid intestinal transit time include those with pyloroplasty, hemigastrectomy, irritable bowel syndrome, hyperthyroidism, and carcinoid syndrome. Examples of diarrhea owing to delayed transit time include patients with intestinal strictures, scleroderma, and amyloid and intestinal pseudo-obstruction. In such situations, bacterial overgrowth is often present and results in diarrhea and steatorrhea. The precise contribution of disordered motility in mediating diarrhea is not always known. For example, in patients with carcinoid syndrome in which hypermotility is believed to cause diarrhea, other factors such as active intestinal secretion induced by serotonin are probably also operative. Recent studies have also suggested that altered motility may play a role in the pathogenesis of certain acute infectious diarrheal disorders.

Motor abnormalities have perhaps been best demonstrated in patients with irritable bowel syndrome (IBS; see Chap. 9). Patients with this syndrome have been shown to have (1) a greater frequency of high-amplitude pressure contractions, often in long segments, in the subgroup with pain predominant symptoms; (2) normal or low-amplitude contractions in patients with diarrhea-predominant IBS; (3) alterations in colonic motility in response to stress; (4) induction of colonic hypermotility following food ingestion; (5) induction of diffuse spastic contractions in the rectosigmoid following balloon distention; (6) an exaggerated colonic hypermotility response to prostigmine, a cholinergic agent; and (7) abnormalities in the basal and postprandial myoelectric rhythm of the colon. Since myoelectric activity originates from muscle rather than nerve, it has been suggested that the pathophysiologic abnormality in IBS resides in the smooth muscle. Interestingly, peppermint oil, which has a smooth muscle relaxant effect, has been found to be beneficial in patients with IBS in a recently reported study.

Exudative
Diseases

Diarrhea can occur as a consequence of outpouring of serum proteins, blood, mucus, and pus from sites of mucosal inflammation and ulceration. Examples of such diarrhea include idiopathic inflammatory bowel disease (ulcerative colitis and Crohn's disease) and certain infectious diarrhea such as those produced by shigella, salmonella, campylobacter and *Entamoeba histolytica*. Although the number of bowel movements with infectious diarrhea is often in excess of six per day, the amount of stool passed each time is small, so that the total daily volume of stool is usually less than 1 liter. Tenesmus, which is passage of a very small amount of stool or no stool at all preceded by a sense of rectal urgency, is a noteworthy feature in patients with significant rectal involvement. Long-standing exudative diarrhea can lead to hypoalbuminemia and anemia from cumulative protein and blood loss. Intestinal inflammatory disease may produce significant alterations in absorptive capacity and may result in excessive loss of water and electrolytes and, if the small intestine is involved, other nutrients in the stool, thus producing diarrhea. This feature is well exemplified by patients with active ulcerative colitis who have been shown to have significant impairment of colonic absorption of water and electrolytes. If the ileal flow is diverted in the patients, the amount of fluid discharge from the colon decreases significantly despite the persistence of the inflammatory process in the colon. Pathophysiologic mechanisms of diarrhea such as alterations in intestinal secretion and in gastrointestinal motility may also contribute to the diarrhea seen in exudative disorders.

Malabsorption

Classification

Malabsorption of dietary nutrients may occur in any of the many diseases in which one or more of the processes involved in normal digestion and absorption are perturbed. For purposes of classification, there are three major categories of malabsorption. First, there may be defective intraluminal digestion of nutrients owing to impaired delivery to the intestine of digestive enzymes and bile salts needed for intraluminal processing of dietary lipids. This occurs in pancreatic diseases such as chronic pancreatitis, pancreatic carcinoma, and cystic fibrosis and in hepatobiliary disease, ileal disease, ileal resection, and intraluminal bacterial overgrowth. Second, there may be defective uptake and transport of nutrients by the absorptive epithelium as a result of intestinal mucosal disease as occurs in celiac sprue or abetalipoproteinemia. Third, there may be defective transport of dietary nutrients from the mucosa to the systemic circulation, as occurs when the lymphatics draining the intestine are obstructed.

Such classification is most useful for diseases in which there is a single, clear-cut abnormality as occurs in abetalipoproteinemia, in which lack of synthesis of apoprotein B prevents formation of chylomicrons and impairs the exit of absorbed lipid from intestinal absorptive cells. However, in many malabsorptive diseases, a defect in one pathophysiologic process predominates, but others may contribute. Such rigid classification is an oversimplification. For example, in conditions that produce small intestinal intraluminal bacterial overgrowth, the major defect results from bacterial deconjugation and dehydroxylation of bile salts in the proximal small intestine. The more lipid-soluble deconjugated bile acids are then readily absorbed in the proximal intestine by passive nonionic diffusion, whereas conjugated bile salts normally remain in the lumen until they reach the distal ileum, where they are absorbed by a specific receptor-mediated transport process. This results in intraluminal bile salt deficiency. Additionally, deconjugated bile acids are less effective detergents at the normal pH of the intestinal lumen. As a result, there is impaired incorporation of the products of lipid digestion into micelles. Thus, fat absorption is impaired and steatorrhea results. However, both enzymes produced by the bacteria and altered bile acids may be cytotoxic to intestinal epithelial cells and produce a mucosal lesion characterized by shortened villi, crypt hyperplasia, and lamina propria inflammation. This then compromises nutrient absorption by the mucosa. Thus, in many instances, both defective intraluminal digestion and impaired mucosal absorption contribute to the malabsorption observed in patients with intestinal intraluminal bacterial proliferation. In addition, there is binding of both free and intrinsic factor–bound vitamin B_{12} by the excessive bacterial flora in the proximal intestine, impairing its normal absorption by the ileal mucosa, which eventually may lead to megaloblastic anemia and neurologic abnormalities.

Clinical Features (Table 5-5)
Weight loss is common in patients with generalized malabsorption and steatorrhea, but its assessment requires a thorough

Table 5-5
Features of malabsorption

Organ system	Clinical feature	Cause
Gastrointestinal tract	Diarrhea	Nutrient malabsorption; small intestinal secretion of fluid and electrolytes: action of unabsorbed bile acids, hydroxy fatty acids, and short-chain fatty acids on the colonic mucosa
	Weight loss	Nutrient malabsorption
	Flatus	Bacterial fermentation of unabsorbed dietary carbohydrates
	Abdominal pain	Distention of bowel, muscle spasm, serosal and peritoneal involvement by disease process
	Glossitis, stomatitis, cheilosis	Iron, riboflavin, niacin deficiency
Hematopoietic system	Anemia, microcytic	Iron, pyridoxine deficiency
	Anemia, macrocytic	Folate, vitamin B_{12} deficiency
	Bleeding	Vitamin K deficiency
Musculoskeletal system	Osteopenic bone disease	Calcium, vitamin D, protein malabsorption
	Osteoarthropathy	Not known
	Tetany	Calcium, magnesium, and vitamin D deficiency
Endocrine system	Amenorrhea, impotence, infertility	Generalized malabsorption and malnutrition
	Secondary hyperparathyroidism	Protracted calcium and vitamin D deficiency
Epidermal system	Purpura and petechiae	Vitamin K deficiency
	Follicular hyperkeratosis and dermatitis	Vitamin A, zinc, essential fatty acids, niacin deficiency
	Edema	Protein-losing enteropathy, malabsorption of dietary protein
Nervous system	Peripheral neuropathy	Vitamin A deficiency Vitamin B_{12}, thiamine deficiency

Source: Modified from J. S. Trier. Intestinal Absorption. In J. H. Stein (ed.), *Internal Medicine* (2nd ed.). Boston: Little, Brown, 1987. P. 129.

dietary history. Most patients with malabsorption will lose weight if caloric intake is normal or decreased. However, some individuals with significant malabsorption have a ravenous appetite and are able to compensate for excessive fecal wastage by consuming excessive calories, resulting in little or no weight loss.

Diarrhea is common but not a universal complaint. Depending on the severity of the absorptive defect, individuals may have up to 10 or more watery stools per day or as few as one stool per day, but that stool is generally voluminous and putty-like. Thus, stool mass is invariably more than 200 gm per day in persons with clinically significant malabsorption and steatorrhea. Osmolarity of the stool is usually increased owing to unabsorbed nutrients. Unabsorbed fatty acids, when delivered to the colon, are converted by bacteria to hydroxy fatty acids, which in turn, impair absorption and stimulate secretion of water and electrolytes. If ileal disease is present or the ileum has been resected, unabsorbed bile acids also impair water and ion absorption and induce colonic secretion. Excessive flatus commonly occurs with malabsorption, especially if primary or secondary disaccharidase deficiency is present. Unabsorbed carbohydrates that enter the colon are fermented by the bacterial flora, producing both excessive gas and short-chain fatty acids. The short-chain fatty acids also impair water and ion transport by colonic mucosa.

Not surprisingly, the effects of nutrient malabsorption may produce symptoms and signs related to dysfunction of organ systems other than the gastrointestinal tract. These symptoms may overshadow gastrointestinal symptoms. It is important to be aware that these extraintestinal manifestations may be the presenting feature of malabsorption so that the diagnosis of the primary disease process causing malabsorption is not unduly delayed or totally undetected. Fatigue and lassitude may reflect anemia, which may be microcytic as a result of iron deficiency, macrocytic owing to folate or cobalamin deficiency, or dimorphic because of combined deficiencies. Purpura or hemorrhage may reflect hypoprothrombinemia resulting from impaired absorption of fat-soluble vitamin K. Skeletal pain may be caused by osteopenic bone disease toward which impaired absorption of calcium and vitamin D may contribute. Occasionally, pathologic fractures may be the presenting feature of malabsorption. If malabsorption of calcium and magnesium is severe, tetany may occur; if protracted, secondary hypoparathyroidism may develop. Other endocrine manifestations occasionally associated with severe malabsorption include amenorrhea, infertility, and impotence. Edema and ascites may reflect decreased plasma oncotic pressure caused by leakage of albumin and other circulating proteins into the gastrointestinal lumen. This occurs in patients with severe mucosal damage or lymphatic obstruction in such diverse diseases as celiac sprue, Whipple's disease, Crohn's disease, and intestinal lymphangiectasia. Follicular hyperkeratosis and dermatitis may result from vitamin A, zinc, essential fatty acid, or niacin deficiency. Peripheral neuropathy may reflect cobalamin or thiamine deficiency.

Etiology

Defective Intraluminal Digestion of Nutrients

Pancreatic insufficiency caused by primary pancreatic disease such as chronic pancreatitis or cystic fibrosis is a common cause of malabsorption in this category and is discussed in detail in Chap. 20. Impaired delivery of bile salts to the proximal intestine results in malabsorption of fat and fat-soluble vitamins, but protein and carbohydrate digestion and absorption are not generally impaired. Steatorrhea commonly accompanies jaundice in patients with acute viral hepatitis and acute toxic liver disease. Steatorrhea is also seen in jaundiced patients with primary biliary cirrhosis, posthepatitic cirrhosis, and cirrhosis caused by hepatotoxins such as alcohol. Both impaired hepatic synthesis and hepatic secretion of conjugated bile salts may contribute. Diseases that obstruct the extrahepatic biliary tree such as sclerosing cholangitis and ductular carcinoma impair delivery of bile salts to the gastrointestinal tract and produce clinically significant steatorrhea.

Resection or extensive disease of the distal small intestine as occurs in Crohn's disease involving the ileum may cause serious diarrhea and steatorrhea. Reduction or complete removal of the active absorptive sites for conjugated bile salts and for cobalamin in the ileum disrupts the enterohepatic circulation of bile salts and prevents cobalamin absorption. The bile acid breath tests are abnormal in such patients, with increased excretion in the breath of $^{14}CO_2$ following oral administration of a test dose of ^{14}C-cholylglycine. Also, cobalamin is malabsorbed when administered alone or with intrinsic factor. These two tests, together with radiologic barium contrast studies, are of value in assessing the severity of ileal disease and the extent of ileal resection.

If less than 100 cm of distal ileum has been resected or its equivalent is unable to absorb bile salts owing to disease, watery diarrhea with little or no steatorrhea usually results. Increased bile salts reach the colon in this *cholerheic diarrhea* and not only impair water and ion absorption by the colonic mucosa but actually stimulate their secretion. However, hepatic synthesis of bile acids increases sufficiently to maintain adequate concentrations in the lumen of the proximal intestine to permit normal digestion and absorption of fat. Administration of agents that bind bile salts intraluminally such as the basic anion exchange resin cholestyramine usually reduces cholerheic diarrhea.

If more than 100 cm of distal ileum has been resected or if ileal disease is sufficiently severe and extensive to cause fecal loss of bile salts in excess of 2 gm/day, even maximal hepatic synthesis will be unable to maintain a sufficient bile salt pool for normal intraluminal processing of dietary fat. As a result, fat absorption is impaired and steatorrheic diarrhea results, with the stool containing not only excess water, ions, and bile acids but also excess fat. Dilution resulting from the large intraluminal volume entering the colon coupled with the low stool pH that accompanies steatorrhea reduces the concentration of bile salts in the aqueous phase of colonic contents to low levels. As a result, they have little effect on colonic mucosal function, and bile salt binding agents such as cholestyramine produce little benefit and may aggravate already severe steatorrhea by further depleting the bile salt pool. Patients who have had extensive ileal resection require periodic injection of cobalamin to maintain their vitamin B_{12} stores.

As discussed previously, bacterial overgrowth also produces steatorrhea by depleting the intraluminal concentration of conjugated bile salts.

Defective Mucosal Absorption

Celiac Sprue. Celiac sprue (also termed gluten sensitive enteropathy) is one of the more commonly encountered diseases caused by a primary lesion of the mucosa of the small intestine. Patients with this disease have a characteristic, although not specific, mucosal lesion that, if extensive, can result in malabsorption of virtually all dietary nutrients and that improves on withdrawal from the diet of the cereal grains wheat, barley, rye, and oats. Celiac sprue has been estimated to occur in 1 to 6 per 10,000 individuals in the western world but is more common in western Ireland, where a prevalence as high as 3 per 1,000 individuals has been reported. The disease may present at any age, but it is most frequently diagnosed during the first 6 years of life and during the third to fifth decades.

In patients with celiac sprue gluten, the water-insoluble protein of the offending cereal grains interacts with the mucosa to produce the characteristic lesion. Villi are markedly shortened or absent, resulting in a mucosal surface that often is flat and presents a substantially reduced surface area to the intraluminal products of digestion. Moreover, the remaining absorptive surface is lined by damaged absorptive cells, which are often vacuolated, are decreased in height, have shortened microvilli, and are infiltrated by many lymphocytes. Since the life span of absorptive cells is reduced considerably in this disease as a result of their interaction with noxious glutens, crypts show a regenerative response with hyperplasia and increased mitoses. In severe lesions, the crypts extend to the flat absorptive surface. There is inflammation of the lamina propria with increased plasma cells and lymphocytes; in some instances, neutrophils are present but the underlying submucosa is usually not involved. The lesion is consistently most severe in the proximal intestine but may involve the entire small bowel. Involvement of the distal small intestine with sparing of the duodenum and proximal jejunum does not occur. Although characteristic and invariably present in the proximal intestine of symptomatic patients with this disease, the lesion is not specific in that virtually identical lesions are observed in several other diseases in which absorptive cells are damaged and exfoliate into the lumen prematurely, including tropical sprue, severe gastric acid hypersecretion associated with gastrinoma, severe intraluminal bacterial overgrowth, and viral enteritis.

The precise reason for damage to the mucosa by toxic glutens in celiac sprue is not known. Several possible mechanisms have been incriminated. Although it has been suggested that deficiency of a brush border peptidase results in production of a toxic product through incomplete digestion of gluten, there is no evidence supporting such a specific metabolic defect. The activity of all brush border hydrolases that have been measured, including peptidases and disaccharidases, is reduced in mucosa with an active lesion and this, no doubt, contributes to the observed malabsorption. However, activity of these enzymes reverts toward normal following successful treatment and parallels healing of the mucosal lesion. If such a defect was to be the specific primary cause, it should persist despite withdrawal of gluten from the diet.

Dietary lectins such as phytohemagglutinin from red kidney beans have been shown to interfere with absorption in experimental animals. Such lectins damage villus absorptive cells after binding to specific sugar residues on the microvillus membrane glycocalyx. It has been suggested that there is a distinctive abnormality in the surface glycoproteins on microvilli of patients with celiac sprue and that gluten fractions may bind to and damage these cells. There is, however, little evidence that gluten has lectin-like activity against either normal intestinal absorptive cells or those of patients with celiac sprue.

There is no doubt that genetic factors play a role in celiac sprue. The histocompatibility antigens HLA-B8 and HLA-DR3 are present in 60 to 90 percent of patients with celiac sprue compared with 20 percent or less in normals. Recently, HLA-DQW2 has been observed in 80 to 100 percent of patients with celiac sprue. Those who lack HLA-B8 and HLA-DR3 often have the IgG immunoglobulin heavy-chain phenotype, G2m(n). Moreover, a polymorphic 4.0 kb DNA fragment was detected with a DQ B chain cDNA probe in lymphoblastoid B cell lines of 90 percent of HLA-DQW2 patients with celiac sprue but only 20 percent of HLA-DQW2 controls. In addition to the presence of these genetic markers, it is well established that celiac sprue is present, often in subclinical latent form, in 5 to 10 percent of first-order relatives of patients with overt disease.

Immune mechanisms have been implicated in the pathogenesis. Plasma cells and lymphocytes are abundant in the involved mucosa. Circulating antibodies to gluten fractions are often present in the serum. Intestinal mucosal biopsies from patients with active disease have been shown to make antibodies directed against gluten fractions. A lymphokine-like substance that inhibits migration of leukocytes is produced in the mucosa when it is exposed to gluten fractions. However, it is not known whether these immunologic features represent primary abnormalities or secondary phenomena, possibly reflecting increased mucosal permeability of the diseased mucosa to gluten peptides.

The clinical features of celiac sprue parallel the extent of the mucosal lesion. Devastating malabsorption of virtually all nutrients with flagrant diarrhea, steatorrhea, weight loss, and symptoms reflecting involvement of many body systems (see Table 5-5) occurs in individuals whose entire small intestine is involved. At the other extreme, isolated microcytic or macrocytic anemia may be the only clinical feature in patients whose disease is confined to the proximal small intestine, where iron and folate acid are most avidly absorbed, and even this feature may be absent in asymptomatic persons with a mild proximal lesion. Thus, patients who present with typical clinical symptoms may reflect only the tip of the iceberg in the spectrum of celiac sprue.

Diarrhea reflects more than malabsorption of nutrients in celiac sprue; in addition, the damaged intestine secretes water and ions, further increasing stool volume. Secondary lactose deficiency can also contribute if dairy products are ingested. Moreover, with severe lesions, mucosal content and release of cholecystokinin is decreased, reducing delivery of pancreatic enzymes and bile salts into the gastrointestinal lumen, possibly compromising intraluminal digestion.

The diagnosis is established by (1) documenting malabsorption by demonstrating steatorrhea (often absent in mild disease) and impaired absorption of xylose, (2) demonstrating the presence of the characteristic mucosal lesion by peroral biopsy of the mucosa of the proximal intestine, and (3) documenting a clinical response and histologic improvement of the mucosal lesion following withdrawal of noxious dietary glutens. The structure of surface absorptive cells improves within a few days, but restoration of mucosal architecture to normal may take months or years and fails to occur if small amounts of gluten are ingested inadvertently. The gluten-free diet should be maintained for life. Initially, treatment for specific deficiencies with vitamins, iron, folate, calcium, magnesium, and so on may be needed, but these can be reduced or eliminated once the patient is repleted.

The incidence of malignant disease, especially lymphoma, is somewhat higher among patients with celiac sprue. A few patients become refractory to the beneficial effects of a gluten-free diet. Some refractory patients respond to treatment with orally administered corticosteroids. For the vast majority of patients with celiac sprue who are maintained on a gluten-free diet, the long-term prognosis is excellent.

Defective Transport of Nutrients from Mucosa to the Systemic Circulation

Obstruction of the mesenteric, retroperitoneal, or main thoracic lymphatics interferes with the transport of chylomicrons formed in the intestinal mucosa to other tissues by way of the systemic circulation. Such obstructions produce dilatation of mucosal and submucosal lymphatics, which has been termed *intestinal lymphangiectasia*. Intestinal lymphangiectasia may be primary owing to congenital malformations of intestinal and more proximal lymphatic channels or secondary as a result of acquired obstruction of mesenteric or more proximal lymphatics resulting from traumatic injury or diseases such as neoplasm, Whipple's disease, or tuberculosis, which produce mesenteric or retroperitoneal lymphadenopathy.

Consumption of a meal containing animal fats, shortening, or most vegetable oils, which consist primarily of long-chain triglycerides and fatty acids, results in increased intestinal lymph flow. If lymphatics are hypoplastic or obstructed, not only is there no pathway through which to transport absorbed fat to the circulating blood, but pressure in the lymphatics increases, resulting in their ectasia and rupture. Lymph then leaks into the intestinal lumen, carrying with it serum proteins. This results in a condition that has been termed *protein-losing enteropathy*. Concomitantly, lymphocytes are also lost into the gastrointestinal lumen. The characteristic histopathology of intestinal segments involved with intestinal lympangiectasia reveals normal mucosal architecture, but mucosal and submucosal lymphatics are dilated. If intestinal protein loss is severe, edema of the bowel wall, including the mucosal villi, is often present.

The clinical findings in lymphangiectasia are predictable; fat malabsorption results in diarrhea, weight loss, or growth failure, whereas loss of serum proteins results in peripheral edema, chylous ascites, and pleural effusions. In congenital lymphangiectasia, clinical findings are usually evident soon after birth and edema is often asymmetric since lymphatics in the extremities may be involved. Acquired defects present later in life, often with a history of clinical features that suggest the underlying etiologic process — neoplastic, infectious, or posttraumatic. Laboratory findings include steatorrhea if an extensive intestinal segment is involved; lymphopenia; and striking reduction in serum proteins, including albumin, immunoglobulins, transferrin, ceruloplasmin, and α_1-antitrypsin. D-xylose absorption, which, unlike fat, is not transported by lymphatics, is usually normal. Excessive fecal clearance of α_1-antitrypsin or loss of radiolabeled chromium in the stool following intravenous administration of $^{51}CrCl_3$, which binds to transferrin, establishes the intestine as the site of protein loss. Small intestinal mucosal biopsies are useful if they demonstrate lymphangiectasia, but normal biopsies do not rule out the disorder since mucosal involvement may be patchy.

Substitution of medium-chain triglyceride supplements for dietary long-chain triglycerides reduces intestinal lymph flow. Unlike long-chain triglycerides, medium-chain triglycerides are transported directly by way of mucosal blood capillaries to the portal blood following their absorption. This reduces steatorrhea and exudation of serum proteins and lymphocytes into the intestinal lumen since lymphatic flow and intralymphatic pressure are reduced.

Treatment of Diarrhea

Clinical Approach

Formulation of a logical approach to the patient with diarrhea is predicated on a sound understanding of the pathophysiology of diarrhea (Table 5-6). The following questions are posed, and the answers received dictate a focused work-up in order to elucidate the cause of diarrhea in that particular individual.

Table 5-6
Approach to patient with chronic diarrhea

Suspect irritable bowel syndrome if:	Suspect organic pathology if:	If malabsorption suspected:	If secretory diarrhea suspected:	If diarrhea remains unexplained:
No weight loss	Weight loss	Distinguish maldigestion from mucosal malabsorption	Quantify 24-hr stool volume and ascertain what happens to diarrhea with fasting	Rule out the following: Surreptitious laxative abuse
No blood noted in stool	Blood in stool	Check KUB for pancreatic calcification		Idiopathic bile salt malabsorption
No fecal incontinence	Fecal incontinence	Perform US, CT, ERCP	Perform appropriate studies as per clinical context (see text).	Collagenous colitis
No nocturnal diarrhea	Nocturnal diarrhea	Perform D-xylose test		
Normal physical examination	Systemic manifestations (e.g., fever, joint symptoms, skin rash)	Perform Schilling test		
Normal proctosigmoidoscopy		Perform small bowel biopsy		
Normal hematocrit, sedimentation rate, K$^+$	Check the following: Hematocrit			
Rule out:	Sedimentation rate			
Drug-induced diarrhea	Serum electrolytes			
Dietary indiscretion (e.g., sorbitol, excess caffeine, alcohol)	Stools for O and P*			
	Stools for C and S*			
Lactase insufficiency	Stool for *Clostridium difficile* toxin			
	Stool for fat (Sudan stain)			
	If stool studies are negative, perform the following:			
	Proctosigmoidoscopy			
	Barium enema			
	Barium contrast study of small intestine			

*Must be obtained prior to any barium contrast studies of the gastrointestinal tract.
Key: O and P = ova and parasites; C and S = culture and sensitivity; KUB = kidney, ureter, and bladder; US = ultrasonography; CT = computed tomography; ERCP = endoscopic retrograde cholangiopancreatography.

1. *Is it acute or chronic?* Diarrhea lasting less than 3 weeks is considered acute. Common causes of acute diarrhea include drugs (antacids, antibiotics, alcohol, digitalis, quinidine, propranolol, colchicine, lactulose, laxatives, diuretics, and many others) and infectious agents (viral, bacterial, parasitic infestations). Common causes of chronic diarrhea include lactose intolerance, irritable bowel syndrome, and idiopathic inflammatory bowel disease.

2. *Is it functional or organic?* Four key features differentiate these two categories: weight loss, bloody diarrhea, nocturnal diarrhea, and incontinence. The presence of any of these features in a patient with diarrhea should behoove the physician to find an organic explanation for the diarrhea. Patients with functional diarrhea (irritable bowel syndrome) may have disabling or even incapacitating diarrhea but may lack any of these features.

3. *Is it bloody or nonbloody?* Patients with bloody diarrhea often require hospitalization. A concerted and thorough work-up should include the appropriate stool studies (stool for ova and parasites, stool cultures, stool for *C. difficile* toxin assay) and proctosigmoidoscopy. A rectal biopsy and serologic tests (e.g., to diagnose *E. histolytica*) may be indicated. Causes of bloody diarrhea include infectious causes (shigella, salmonella, campylobacter, hemorrhagic *E. coli* — *E. coli* 0157:H7, schistosomiasis, *E. histolytica*), idiopathic inflammatory bowel disease (ulcerative colitis, Crohn's disease), ischemic colitis, radiation-induced damage, and colonic neoplasms.

4. *Is it of small bowel or large bowel origin?* Certain historical clues may indicate the origin. For example, small bowel diarrhea usually occurs less than six times per day, is bulky, and is unaccompanied by tenesmus. Pain, if present, is often periumbilical. In contrast, large bowel diarrhea, particularly if emanating from left-sided colonic disease, characteristically occurs more than six times per day, is small in amount, and is often accompanied by tenesmus. Pain, if present, is most often situated in the left lower quadrant. These distinctions are not absolute and only serve as a guide to the appropriate initial work-up.

5. *Does the patient have steatorrhea?* Patients with steatorrhea often have stools that are greasy, may contain recognizable oil, are extremely offensive in odor, and may necessitate "repeated flushing" because of adherence to the toilet bowl. Historical clues to steatorrhea may exist in the form of xerophthalmia and nyctalopia (vitamin A deficiency), osteopenia and bone fractures (vitamin D and calcium malabsorption), and purpura, easy bruisability, nosebleeds, and gumbleeds (vitamin K deficiency). Other features of malabsorption include weight loss, stunted

growth, anemia, glossitis, stomatitis and cheilosis (iron, riboflavin, and niacin deficiency), and edema.

6. *Does the patient have secretory diarrhea?* Patients with chronic secretory diarrhea pose a formidable diagnostic challenge. The important causes of secretory diarrhea are listed in Table 5-3. Diarrhea that is of large volume and persists during fasting is likely to be secretory. A frequently discovered cause of chronic secretory diarrhea in referral centers is surreptitious laxative abuse.

The aforementioned six categories have considerable overlap but are clinically useful in the evaluation of patients with diarrhea — a symptom that can pose considerable discomfort to the patient and a formidable challenge to the physician.

Study Questions

1. Answer true or false:
   a. Cholera has a high mortality rate because of the organism's ability to invade the mucosa with subsequent bloodborne spread to many vital organs.
   b. Mechanisms of diarrhea that may be operative in patients with gluten-sensitive enteropathy (celiac sprue) include:
      i. Decrease in mucosal absorptive surface
      ii. Secondary lactase insufficiency
      iii. Secretion rather than absorption of water and electrolytes by the damaged intestine
   c. The lesion of gluten-sensitive enteropathy is characteristically more severe in the distal small intestine than in the proximal small intestine.
   d. Examples of malabsorption in which there is malabsorption of a specific nutrient include pernicious anemia, primary lactase deficiency, and abetalipoproteinemia.

   Answers
   a. False. There is no mucosal invasion or bacteremia. The high mortality of cholera is a consequence of the severe secretory diarrhea that is toxin-mediated.
   b. True
   c. False. Since celiac sprue is caused by the dietary ingestion of gluten, the lesion begins first and is most severe in the proximal small intestine.
   d. True. In pernicious anemia there is selective malabsorption of cobalamin (vitamin B_{12}); in primary lactase deficiency, of lactose; and in abetalipoproteinemia, of fat.

2. Match items in List I with the most appropriate one in List II.
   List I
   a. Bile salt malabsorption

b. Voluminous watery diarrhea in a patient with hypokalemia.

c. Patient with malabsorption, fever, and joint pains.

d. Diarrhea responsive to H_2-receptor antagonist treatment.

e. Steatorrhea in a 40-year-old alcoholic patient with a normal D-xylose absorption test.

List II

i. Vasoactive intestinal peptide (VIP) producing tumor

ii. Gastrinoma (Zollinger-Ellison syndrome)

iii. Extensive Crohn's ileitis

iv. Calcification of the pancreas seen on CT scan

v. Small bowel biopsy is diagnostic. Patient responds favorably to antibiotic treatment.

Answers
a:iii
b:i
c:v (Whipple's disease)
d:ii
e:iv

References

Alpers, D. H. Digestion and Absorption of Carbohydrates and Proteins. In L. R. Johnson (ed.), *Physiology of the Gastrointestinal Tract*. New York: Raven, 1987. Pp. 1469–1487.

Binder, H. J. Net Fluid and Electrolyte Secretion: The Pathophysiological Basis for Diarrhea. In H. J. Binder (ed.), *Mechanisms of Intestinal Secretion*. New York: Liss, 1979. Pp. 1–5.

Carpenter, C. C. J. The pathophysiology of secretory diarrhea. *Med. Clin. North Am.* 66:597, 1982.

Debongnie, J. C., and Philips, S. F. Capacity of the human colon to absorb fluid. *Gastroenterology* 74:698, 1978.

Drossmann, J. P., Powell, D. W., and Sessions, J. T., Jr. The irritable bowel syndrome. *Gastroenterology* 73:811, 1977.

Field, M., Fordtran, J. S., and Schultz, S. G. (eds.), *Secretory Diarrhea*. Bethesda, Maryland: American Physiological Society, 1980.

Fordtran, J. S. Speculation on the pathogenesis of diarrhea. *Fed. Proc.* 26:1405, 1967.

Frizzell, R. A., Field, M., and Schultz, S. G. Sodium-coupled chloride transport by epithelial tissues. *Am. J. Physiol.* 236:F_1, 1979.

Gooptu, D., Truelove, S. C., and Warner, G. T. Absorption of electrolytes from the colon in cases of ulcerative colitis and in control subjects. *Gut* 10:555, 1969.

Harris, J., and Shields, R. Absorption and secretion of water and electrolytes by the intact human colon in diffuse untreated proctocolitis. *Gut* 11:27, 1970.

Kolars, J. C., Levitt, M. D., Aouji, M., and Savaiano, D. A. Yogurt — an autodigesting source of lactose. *N. Engl. J. Med.* 310:1, 1984.

Fine, K. D., Krejs, G. J., and Fordtran, J. S. Diarrhea. In M. H. Sleisenger and J. S. Fordtran (eds.), *Gastrointestinal Disease* (4th ed.). Philadelphia: Saunders, 1988. Pp. 290–316.

Perera, D. R., Weinstein, W. M., and Rubin, C. E. Small intestinal biopsy. *Hum. Pathol.* 6:157, 1975.

Philips, S. F. Diarrhea: A current view of the pathophysiology. *Gastroenterology* 63:495, 1972.

Powell, D. W. Intestinal Water and Electrolyte Transport. In L. R. Johnson (ed.), *Physiology of the Gastrointestinal Tract*. New York: Raven, 1987. Pp. 1267–1305.

Ravry, M. J. R. Dietetic food diarrhea. *J.A.M.A.* 244:270, 1980.

Read, N. W., Krejs, G. J., Read, M. G., et al. Chronic diarrhea of unknown origin. *Gastroenterology* 78:264, 1980.

Schwartz, C. J., Kimberg, D. V., Sheerin, H. E., et al. Vasoactive intestinal peptide stimulation of adenylate cyclase and active electrolyte secretion in intestinal mucosa. *J. Clin. Invest.* 54:536, 1974.

Shia, Y. F. Lipid Digestion and Absorption. In L. R. Johnson (ed.), *Physiology of the Gastrointestinal Tract*. New York: Raven, 1987. Pp. 1527–1556.

Simar, G. L., and Gorbach, S. L. Intestinal flora in health and disease. *Gastroenterology* 86:174, 1984.

Summers, R. W. Role of motility in infectious diarrhea. *Gastroenterology* 80:1070, 1981.

Trier, J. S. Diseases of Intestinal Absorption. In J. H. Stein (ed.), *Internal Medicine*. Boston: Little, Brown, 1987. Pp. 129–141.

Trier, J. S. Celiac Sprue. In M. H. Sleisenger and J. S. Fordtran (eds.), *Gastrointestinal Disease* (4th ed.). Philadelphia: Saunders, 1988. Pp. 1134–1152.

Trier, J. S., and Lipskey, M. The Short Bowel Syndrome. In M. H. Sleisenger and J. S. Fordtran (eds.), *Gastrointestinal Disease* (4th ed.). Philadelphia: Saunders, 1988. Pp. 1106–1112.

6 : Intestinal Infections

Bernard F. Smith

J. Thomas Lamont

Gastrointestinal tract infections are a leading cause of human morbidity and mortality on a global scale. In industrialized countries, enteric infections are a leading cause of loss of time from the workplace. However, in underdeveloped countries, these infections are a major cause of infant and childhood mortality. In this chapter, we will discuss the pathophysiology of gastrointestinal tract infections with particular reference to the syndromes and diseases seen commonly in clinical practice. Our initial discussion will focus on host defense mechanisms and the pathophysiology of bacterial pathogens. Specific clinical syndromes and common human pathogens will then be discussed separately.

Host Defense Mechanisms

The mucosal surface of the gastrointestinal tract provides the largest surface area for interaction of the human host with the external environment. The mammalian gastrointestinal tract has evolved to provide maximum absorptive potential for the host while providing an effective barrier to invasion by microorganisms. Immediately following birth, the gastrointestinal tract is colonized with aerobic and anaerobic bacterial populations, which provide each individual with a unique internal milieu. Variations in gastrointestinal flora exist between individuals, but little variation occurs in a single individual over time. This unique internal milieu is maintained by complex host-bacterial and bacterial-bacterial interactions; these, in turn, prevent colonization of the gastrointestinal tract by pathogenic microorganisms. The normal physiology of the gastrointestinal tract appears to regulate the distribution and relative quantity of bacteria therein as well as provide important defense mechanisms against enteric infection (Table 6-1).

Gastric acid secretion is primarily responsible for killing swallowed bacteria and preventing colonization of the proximal gastrointestinal tract. Reduction of gastric acidity by peptic ulcer surgery, atrophic gastritis, or drugs causes an increase in the number of bacteria in the stomach and upper small bowel and an increase in the risk of enteric infections, particularly with *Salmonella* species. *Small intestinal motility* provides an effi-

Table 6-1
Host defense mechanisms

Type	Site	Mechanism
Acid secretion	Stomach	Destroys ingested microorganisms
Motility	Small intestine	Prevents bacterial colonization
Secretory IgA	Small intestine	Prevents colonization and bacterial attachment to enterocyte
Mucus secretion	Small and large intestine	Prevents bacterial attachment and epithelial invasion
Endogenous flora	Large intestine	Prevents colonization by pathogens

cient mechanism for clearing bacteria from the proximal gastrointestinal tract, and preventing their attachment to the mucosal surface. Alterations in motility secondary to diseases such as scleroderma and diabetes mellitus are frequently associated with overgrowth of bacteria in the small intestine, which may cause malabsorption. The secretion of *mucus* by surface enterocytes and the secretion of *IgA* also prevent adhesion and attachment of microorganisms to the mucosal surface. Recent studies have identified a unique class of immunocyte, the *M cell,* in the lamina propria of the gastrointestinal tract, which is the initial recognition site for detection and processing of foreign antigens that penetrate the mucosa. Although current understanding of the intestinal immune system remains incomplete, recent clinical experience in patients with acquired immunodeficiency syndrome (AIDS) has indicated how essential the intestinal immune system is in preventing enteric infections.

Pathophysiologic Mechanisms of Enteric Infections

The clinical hallmark of enteric infections is diarrhea, which may result from two major mechanisms: (1) release of toxins, and (2) mucosal invasion (see Table 6-1). Bacterial toxins are generally classified as being either *cytotonic,* meaning they cause fluid and electrolyte secretion by activation of the adenylate cyclase system, or *cytotoxic,* meaning they injure the mucosal cell and cause fluid secretion by mechanisms other than adenylate cyclase activation. Toxin-mediated diarrhea occurs predominantly in the proximal small bowel and is characterized by large volume, watery diarrhea. Diarrhea can be caused by ingestion of preformed bacterial toxins (*Staphylococcus aureus*), by toxins produced by sporulating organisms within the lumen of the gastrointestinal tract (*Clostridium perfringens*), or by toxins elaborated by bacteria adherent to the surface of enterocytes in the proximal gastrointestinal tract (*Vibrio cholera, Escherichia coli*). Toxin production and mucosal invasion are not mutually exclusive. Bacteria such as *Shigella dysenteriae* produce enterotoxins as well as invade the intestinal mucosa; they may cause an illness that is biphasic with toxin-mediated large-volume watery diarrhea followed by a dysenteric illness with bloody diarrhea.

The enterotoxin of *V. cholerae* has been the prototype for investigating the pathophysiology of toxin-mediated diarrhea. Cholera toxin, a protein with a molecular weight of 84,000 daltons, contains five B (binding) subunits, which surround a single A (catalytic) subunit. The B subunit complex is responsible for toxin binding to the surface of the enterocyte. Following binding of the B subunit to the cell surface, the A subunit penetrates the plasma membrane and irreversibly activates the enzyme adenylate cyclase, which, in turn, produces cyclic AMP (see Chap. 5). The end result is secretion of salt and water by the enterocyte in amounts that produce watery diarrhea. Similar mechanisms have been described for other diarrheal pathogens such as *E. coli, C. perfringens, C. difficile,* and *S. dysenteriae.*

Infections mediated by bacterial invasion usually occur in the distal ileum or large bowel and are associated with frequent passage of small volumes of mucopurulent, bloody diarrhea. Invasion of the intestinal wall is usually limited to the mucosa, although the inflammatory response to bacterial invasion commonly extends to the lamina propria. Bacteremia is unusual but does occur in the immunocompromised or splenectomized host. The mechanism by which bacteria invade the mucosa is poorly understood. Morphologic studies, however, have demonstrated bacterial replication within enterocytes, and cell to cell infection is believed to occur. The pathophysiologic mechanism responsible for diarrhea in invasive infections is controversial. Diarrhea may be secondary to concomitant release of toxins by the invasive bacteria as has been demonstrated for *Shigella* or may be secondary to release of inflammatory mediators (e.g., prostaglandins and leukotrienes). In addition, inhibition of normal fluid absorption by the damaged colonic epithelium may play a role in net fluid loss seen with invasive infections. The clinical features of toxin-mediated and invasive diarrheas are compared in Table 6-2.

Syndromes of Enteric Infections

Acute Bacterial Dysentery

Acute bacterial dysentery is characterized clinically by the frequent passage of diarrhea that is commonly mucopurulent and bloody with variable degrees of abdominal pain, fever, tenes-

Table 6-2
Toxigenic vs. invasive diarrhea

	Toxigenic	Invasive
Typical pathogens	Clostridium perfringens Staphylococcus aureus	Salmonella enteritidis Shigella flexneri
Bacterial pathogenesis	Colonization of small intestine Production of enterotoxin	Colonization of large bowel Invasion and multiplication in wall of bowel
Host response	Secretion of NaCl and water by enterocyte	Mucosal inflammation and ul- ceration
Clinical features	Large-volume, watery diarrhea	Small-volume, bloody, and mucopurulent diarrhea
Incubation period	Short (hours)	Long (days)
Fecal leukocytes	Absent	Present
Sigmoidoscopy	Normal	Acute colitis
Diagnosis	Based on clinical features; vomiting common; culture of pathogen from contaminated food	Identify pathogen in stool cul- ture

mus, and dehydration. The clinical spectrum of disease is quite variable, with an indolent diarrhea on one extreme and fulminating colitis on the other. Recent advances in bacteriologic techniques have significantly increased the number of cases in which a bacterial pathogen can be identified. Currently, a specific bacterial pathogen can be identified in more than 50 percent of diarrheal illnesses caused by ingestion of contaminated food. A recent large series identified enteric pathogens with these frequencies: Salmonella, 26 percent; S. aureus, 15.6 percent; C. perfringens, 7.1 percent; Shigella, 6.3 percent; Bacillus cereus, 0.8 percent; and V. parahaemolyticus, 0.8 percent. These figures represent outbreaks that could be traced to a common food source and may not reflect the incidence of specific pathogens in sporadic cases. The common bacterial pathogens and the food sources with which they are commonly associated are shown in Table 6-3.

Clinical diagnosis of acute bacterial dysentery relies predominantly on identification of the specific enteropathogen by stool culture. Examination of the stool will show the presence of blood and leukocytes when epithelial invasion has occurred. This simple test is extremely reliable for distinguishing diarrhea resulting from invasive pathogens in which leukocytes and erythrocytes are common from diarrhea owing to bacterial toxins in which they are absent.

Table 6-3
Bacterial pathogens and food sources

Pathophysiology	Bacteria	Common food source
Ingestion of preformed toxin	Staphylococcus aureus	Egg products, cream, mayonnaise
	Bacillus cereus	Rice
Toxin production after colonization of small bowel	Clostridium perfringes	Beef, turkey
	Escherichia coli (toxigenic)	Water, salads
	Vibrio cholera	Water
Bacterial invasion of epithelium	Salmonella enteritidis	Eggs, poultry
	Shigella species	Various
	Campylobacter fetus	Unpasteurized milk, water
	Yersinia enterocolitica	Milk, meat
	Escherichia coli (invasive)	Unknown
	Vibrio parahaemolyticus	Shrimp, crabs

Salmonella

The genus Salmonella contains three species: *Salmonella typhi,* which has a single serotype; *S. enteritidis,* which has approximately 1700 serotypes; and *S. choleraesuis,* which, as its name implies, is largely restricted to porcine hosts. *S. enteritidis* is responsible for the common dysenteric illness encountered in humans, and the single serotype *S. typhimurium* is alone responsible for 25 to 35 percent of human infections caused by Salmonella. Salmonella causes two clinically distinct syndromes in humans: *enteric fever* and *gastroenteritis*. Enteric fever caused by *S. typhi* is called *typhoid fever*; when caused by *S. enteritidis,* it is called *paratyphoid fever.*

The incidence of enteric fever has decreased in industrialized countries with improvements in sanitation and water purity but is sometimes encountered in individuals returning from underdeveloped countries. The pathophysiology of enteric fever involves two sequential bacteremic phases. The first phase is an asymptomatic bacteremia that follows invasion of the small bowel epithelium by the organism. This transient primary bacteremia occurs 24 to 72 hours following the ingestion of bacteria, which are then phagocytosed. They then multiply within cells of the reticuloendothelial system. Clinical symptoms occur approximately 10 days following the primary bacteremia and correspond to the onset of the second continuous bacteremia, which persists until intracellular organisms are eradicated by the development of delayed hypersensitivity. During the persistent bacteremia, metastatic abscess formation can occur and the biliary tract is seeded with bacteria. Bacteria multiply within the gallbladder, and stool cultures become positive secondary to passage of bacteria from the biliary tree into the gastrointestinal tract. The distinguishing clinical features of the second stage of the illness are severe generalized headache, rose spot skin eruption, abdominal pain, distention, and, often, constipation. Initially, the fever has a remittent pattern but becomes persistent with the classic relative bradycardia, with the pulse rate slower than expected for the degree of pyrexia during the second and third weeks. During this time, constipation gives way to diarrhea, and the complications of intestinal hemorrhage or perforation or both occur. Both these phenomena are secondary to ulceration of ileal mucosa overlying the inflamed Peyer's patches. The incidence of these potentially fatal complications has decreased markedly since the introduction of specific antimicrobial therapy. Salmonella can persist in the gallbladder despite antibiotic therapy, thus giving rise to the chronic carrier state and secondary spread of the disease.

Salmonella gastroenteritis is acquired by ingestion of contaminated food, most commonly poultry products, and is caused almost exclusively by serotypes of *S. enteritidis*. The peak incidence of this disease is in the months of July to November. Onset of symptoms is generally within 12 to 48 hours after ingestion of adequate bacterial inoculum, which reflects the time required for bacteria to multiply in the lumen and to invade the mucosa. The initial symptoms of nausea and vomiting give way rapidly to the development of colicky abdominal pain and diarrhea. The diarrheal phase lasts 3 to 5 days and gradually resolves in most untreated patients. Antibiotic therapy does not significantly ameliorate the disease but may prolong fecal shedding of Salmonella.

Shigella

The genus Shigella contains four subgroups (A–D), with the most common pathogens in each subgroup being *S. dysenteriae*, *S. flexneri*, *S. boydii*, and *S. sonnei*, respectively. The original Shigella bacillus, *S. dysenteriae*, is primarily isolated from travelers returning from abroad, whereas *S. sonnei* and *S. flexneri* are responsible for the majority of infections in this country. Shigellosis occurs predominantly as sporadic cases, although common source epidemics have been reported. Humans are the main reservoir for this pathogen, and infection is spread by the fecal-oral route. A distinguishing feature of this organism is the relatively small inoculum required to produce clinical disease and the resulting high attack rate in exposed individuals.

After ingestion of a sufficient inoculum, symptoms begin in 24 to 48 hours. Some strains of Shigella have a plasmid for an enterotoxin that can cause a profuse watery diarrhea in the early stages of illness. The primary pathology is due, however, to invasion and multiplication of organisms within the colonic mucosa. This causes profound inflammation and ulceration, which result in the characteristic bloody diarrhea and can be indistinguishable from acute ulcerative colitis on sigmoidoscopy. Shigellosis is usually self-limited, with fever abating in 4 days, and diarrhea and abdominal pain resolving in 7 to 10 days. In general, antibiotic therapy should be reserved for individuals with fulminant infection, for debilitated patients, and for those with evidence of metastatic foci of infection.

Campylobacter fetus

Campylobacter fetus contains two subspecies, *fetus* and *intestinalis,* which are animal pathogens; and the subspecies *jejuni,* which is becoming increasingly recognized as an important human pathogen. Campylobacter enteritis occurs most frequently during the warm months of the year and tends to be sporadic, although outbreaks traced to unpasteurized milk and contaminated water have been reported. In several recent series, Campylobacter has been isolated more frequently than Salmonella and Shigella. The pathophysiology of Campylobacter enteritis is not well understood at the present time. Invasion of jejunal and ileal mucosa by ingested organisms has been documented, with clinical symptoms beginning 3 to 5 days after ingestion of the organism. The clinical features include headache, myalgias, and severe abdominal pain, which can mimic acute appendicitis or other surgical illnesses. Diarrhea begins within a day of the initial symptoms and is watery and foul smelling. Blood and leukocytes are present in the stool, and, when the colon is involved, the clinical picture resembles acute ulcerative colitis. The illness usually lasts approximately 1 week, although protracted illnesses of several weeks are not uncommon. Erythromycin treatment may shorten the clinical illness, although, in most cases, antibiotic therapy is not required.

Yersinia enterocolitica

Yersinia has been increasingly identified as an important human pathogen as bacteriologic techniques have improved. Thirty-four serotypes have been identified, with specific serotypes being responsible for clinical disease in different countries. The pathogenic mechanism includes both the ability to invade large and small bowel mucosa and the production of a heat-stable enterotoxin. Yersinia infections cause several clinical syndromes that appear to depend on the age of the infected host. *Yersinia enterocolitis* occurs most frequently in children younger than 5 years of age and is characterized by abdominal pain, fever, cramps, and diarrhea. The illness can last from one to several weeks and, when prolonged, can mimic inflammatory bowel disease. In older children and adolescents, a syndrome of ileal infection and mesenteric adenitis is the most common presentation. The clinical symptoms in this age group often result in exploratory laparotomy to rule out acute appendicitis.

In adults, Yersinia can cause an acute dysenteric illness that resembles shigellosis. Of note is the occasional occurrence of acute arthritis with erythema nodosum several weeks after the acute diarrheal illness has abated. This occurs most commonly in individuals who are positive for the HLA B27 histocompatibility antigen and closely resembles Reiter's syndrome. Rarely, a bacteremic or typhoidal form of disease occurs in persons who are immunocompromised; this can lead to metastatic abscess formation. Although the use of antibiotics is recommended in severely ill persons, their efficacy has yet to be clearly demonstrated.

Escherichia coli

Whereas in the past, invasive forms of E. coli have been reported to cause only sporadic cases of acute bacterial dysentery, recent outbreaks associated with the hemolytic-uremic syndrome (HUS) have focused greater attention on this entity. The HUS has the clinical hallmarks of a microangiopathic hemolytic anemia in association with acute renal failure. E. coli serotype 0157:H7 has been identified as the pathogen in several outbreaks of hemorrhagic colitis in the United States and Canada. In these cases, bloody diarrhea and abdominal pain were universally present, but the development of fever was unusual. Nausea and vomiting were present in approximately half the cases. Clinical isolates of E. coli 0157:H7 produced an apparently unique cytotoxin that is toxic to Vero cells in culture (Vero toxin) and was associated with the development of the HUS in some cases. At the present time, the pathophysiologic relationship of E. coli 0157:H7, Vero toxin production, hemorrhagic colitis, and HUS is unclear but has become a focal point of investigation of the pathophysiologic mechanisms by which bacterial toxins cause human disease.

Toxin-Mediated
Diarrhea

There is significant clinical and bacteriologic overlap between the syndromes of acute bacterial dysentery and toxin-mediated diarrhea. Both infections are acquired by the fecal-oral route and are usually associated with ingestion of contaminated food. The clinical hallmarks of toxin-mediated food poisoning are the relatively short incubation period, the prominence of nausea and vomiting, and the brief duration of illness. These clinical features reflect the activity of cytotonic enterotoxins on the gastrointestinal epithelium to increase net fluid secretion in the absence of cellular injury or epithelial invasion.

Staphylococcus aureus

The pathophysiologic mechanism of food poisoning caused by *S. aureus* is the ingestion of a preformed toxin in food contaminated with the organism. In the typical outbreak, food containing egg products or cream is not adequately refrigerated after preparation, allowing *S. aureus* to grow and produce an enterotoxin. Following ingestion of the contaminated food, clinical symptoms occur 4 to 8 hours later. This short incubation period reflects the effect of the preformed toxin, which is independent of bacterial multiplication in the gastrointestinal tract.

Staphylococcal food poisoning is characterized by severe nausea and vomiting, which is followed in a matter of hours by voluminous, watery diarrhea. The disease usually lasts less than 24 hours and resolves spontaneously. The clinical diagnosis is based on the short incubation period, the presence of symptoms in other persons who ate the same food, and the presence of vomiting followed by diarrhea. Antibiotic therapy is not indicated, and therapy is largely restricted to fluid and electrolyte replacement.

Clostridium perfringens

Clostridium perfringens is an anaerobic, spore-forming organism that is nearly ubiquitous in the environment. It is present in the normal human flora of the gastrointestinal tract, in soil, and in many meats. Typical human food poisoning is caused by *C. perfringens* Type A and is frequently associated with dishes of beef, turkey, or chicken that have undergone an initial cooking in large quantities. The spores of *C. perfringens* are able to withstand the heat of the initial cooking, particularly when the internal temperatures achieved by cooking have been limited by the large volumes of meat being cooked. If the meat is then allowed to cool slowly or is simmered at inadequate temperature for long periods of time, the organisms will then begin to grow and may achieve large numbers in the previously cooked meat. If the meal is then served cold, or after minimal rewarming, the organisms will survive and provide a large infectious inoculum. The enterotoxin of *C. perfringens* Type A is a 34,000 dalton protein that is part of the spore coat and is released as the organisms sporulate within the intestinal tract.

Food poisoning caused by *C. perfringens* Type A is characterized clinically by an incubation period of 8 to 24 hours, with this time interval reflecting the growth and subsequent sporulation of the organisms within the lumen of the small intestine. Typical outbreaks occur in institutions or are associated with a social event at which large quantities of meat are cooked a considerable period of time prior to serving. Attack rates tend to be high, with as many as 50 percent of exposed individuals commonly affected. Nausea is common, but vomiting is unusual; this difference is useful in distinguishing *C. perfringens* from *S. aureus*. Diarrhea is watery and voluminous and lasts for 12 to 24 hours. Symptoms resolve spontaneously, and antibiotic therapy is not indicated. Identification of *C. perfringens* in the stool does *not* establish the diagnosis, since this organism is part of the normal colonic flora.

Bacillus cereus

Bacillus cereus has increasingly been implicated as a cause of food poisoning and appears responsible for two distinct clinical syndromes. *Bacillus cereus* is an aerobic, spore-forming organism that is often present in dried or processed foods. As its name implies, this bacteria is commonly associated with grains, particularly rice. As with *C. perfringens,* the spores of *B. cereus* are resistant to heat, and, when food is allowed to cool slowly after cooking or is maintained at a temperature from 30° to 50°C, the organism may germinate and produce the enterotoxins.

The two clinical syndromes caused by *B. cereus* are mediated by the production of different toxins. One toxin has enterotoxigenic activity similar to cholera toxin and activates adenylate cyclase within the enterocyte, causing (1) a net secretion of fluid by the gastrointestinal tract, and (2) diarrhea. The incubation period for the diarrheal illness is from 8 to 12 hours; the diarrhea lasts an average of 24 hours. As with other toxin-mediated diarrheal illnesses, the disease is self-limited and does not require specific therapy.

The other syndrome caused by *B. cereus* is characterized primarily by vomiting, although some persons also develop diarrhea. The incubation period for this illness is 2 hours, suggesting that ingestion of preformed toxin is responsible. The vomiting is often mild and persists for 6 to 12 hours and resolves spontaneously. This syndrome has strongly been associated with rice that has been cooked and then kept warm for prolonged periods of time prior to serving. The attack rate of this vomiting illness is often near 100 percent among exposed individuals.

Vibrio parahaemolyticus

Outbreaks of acute diarrheal illness have been associated with *V. parahaemolyticus,* particularly in southern coastal areas of the

United States. Contaminated shellfish, particularly shrimp, have been implicated as the source of infection. The typical illness has an incubation period of 24 to 48 hours and is characterized by a diarrheal illness that persists for approximately 24 hours. Vomiting is unusual, and the volume of diarrhea is not large, although it has a watery consistency. Severe abdominal pain, fever, and chills are common. No specific antibiotic therapy is indicated.

Traveler's Diarrhea

With international travel now an everyday occurrence, traveler's diarrhea has taken on significance far in excess of ruining an occasional overseas holiday. The volume of international travel and the common use of prophylactic antibiotics to prevent this illness have given rise to far-reaching public health concerns. The spectrum of enteric pathogens identified in traveler's diarrhea has increased enormously with improved microbiological techniques. Clinicians must commonly deal with a variety of previously exotic pathogens that return home with the international traveler. In addition, immigrants from Southeast Asia have introduced into everyday practice a variety of pathogens rarely encountered in industrialized countries.

The incidence of traveler's diarrhea varies with the country visited. In general, the attack rate in the industrialized countries of Western Europe is quite low, whereas travelers to India, Mexico, the Middle East, and Africa may experience attack rates as high as 30 to 50 percent.

The major pathogen responsible for traveler's diarrhea is enterotoxigenic strains of *E. coli,* which produce either a heat-labile or a heat-stable enterotoxin. Typically, the individual is asymptomatic for the first 2 to 3 days. The peak incidence of diarrhea is between the fourth and sixth days, and diarrhea usually persists for 2 days. Significant variation exists in the duration and severity of illness. Occasionally, the business traveler who spends a brief period of time in a foreign country develops symptoms after returning home.

Controversy exists regarding the appropriate use and indications for prophylactic antibiotics to prevent traveler's diarrhea. Recent well-designed clinical studies have indicated that trimethoprim/sulfamethoxazole and doxycycline are effective in reducing the incidence of diarrhea, but general recommendations for their widespread use are pending further review of the public health implications. Avoidance of water, ice, and salads may help to decrease the risk of acquiring traveler's diarrhea, but once symptoms have begun, therapy is restricted to supportive care with particular attention to fluid replacement. Toxigenic *E. coli* are responsible for approximately three fourths of the cases of traveler's diarrhea, but other enteric pathogens such as *Shigella, Salmonella, Entamoeba histolytica,* and *Giardia lamblia* and viruses must also be considered in the differential diagnosis. Because of the large variety of pathogens implicated in traveler's diarrhea, it is imperative to culture stool to identify bacterial pathogens a?d to examine fresh specimens for the presence of parasites and protozoa.

Antibiotic-Associated Diarrhea and Colitis

Virtually any type of antibiotic treatment, either oral or parenteral, may lead, in some patients, to colonization of the large intestine with *Clostridium difficile,* the major causative organism of antibiotic-associated pseudomembranous colitis (Fig. 6-1). This organism forms resistant spores that are frequently found in hospital wards and intensive care units. During or following antibiotic therapy, *C. difficile* is able to colonize the large bowel where it then releases several exotoxins. These, in turn, produce an inflammatory colitis manifested by watery diarrhea, crampy lower abdominal pain, and fever. Proctosigmoidoscopy may reveal rectal or colonic pseudomembranes, discrete, 2- to 4-mm whitish elevated plaques composed of inflammatory exudate, mucus, and exfoliated epithelial cells overlying a superficial ulcer. The diagnosis of *C. difficile* infection is confirmed by demonstration of the cytotoxin in stool filtrates by its cytopathic effect on cultured fibroblasts, or by anaerobic culture of the organism from stool.

For reasons not yet clear, newborns are frequently asymptomatic carriers of *C. difficile,* and the cytotoxin may be present in their feces. It has been suggested that the newborn lacks epithelial receptors for the toxins. After 6 months of age, infants are rarely colonized, and antibiotic therapy may be followed by typical features of acute *C. difficile* colitis.

Treatment of this infection requires eradication of *C. difficile* with specific antibiotics and eventual establishment of normal

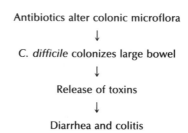

Antibiotics alter colonic microflora

↓

C. difficile colonizes large bowel

↓

Release of toxins

↓

Diarrhea and colitis

Fig. 6-1
Pathogenesis of antibiotic-associated colitis associated with *Clostridium difficile.*

flora. Apparently the normal colonic microflora provide a "natural" barrier to colonization with *C. difficile,* as infection rarely occurs in individuals not exposed to antibiotic therapy.

Parasitic and Protozoan Infections

Although relatively infrequent compared with bacterial infections, parasitic infections are an important cause of diarrhea, especially in low-income rural families, travelers, and immigrants from underdeveloped countries. Parasitic pathogens can be classified as either protozoan (single-cell) organisms (amebiasis, giardiasis), or metazoan (multicellular) organisms (roundworms and flatworms).

Amebiasis

Entamoeba histolytica infection in humans can range from the asymptomatic carrier state to fulminant colitis. Serologic evidence of prior infection is found in approximately 5 percent of U.S. citizens, most of whom have never traveled to endemic areas. Asymptomatic cyst passers serve as a source of infection and may occasionally become acutely ill by mechanisms not well understood. The most common clinical presentation is acute colitis, which presents as acute bloody diarrhea, colicky lower abdominal pain, and fever typical of acute bacterial dysentery. Toxic megacolon and perforation may occur in severe cases. The diagnosis is suggested by the finding of discrete colonic ulcers scattered on normal-appearing mucosa at sigmoidoscopy or colonoscopy. The finding in fresh stool of motile trophozoites containing ingested erythrocytes establishes the diagnosis. It is most important to distinguish amoebic colitis from acute ulcerative colitis, as systemic steroid therapy for presumed ulcerative colitis may lead to fulminant infection in patients infected with *E. histolytica.* Effective treatment is available in the form of metronidazole, alone or in combination with emetine or diiodohydroxyquin.

Giardiasis

Giardiasis is a common protozoan infection of the small intestine in travelers and can occur in local outbreaks secondary to contaminated water supplies. Recent evidence points to beavers and other wild animals as intermediate hosts for the flagellate *Giardia lamblia.* Infection with this organism can cause three distinct clinical syndromes: (1) acute diarrhea, (2) subacute diarrhea and malabsorption, and (3) asymptomatic cyst passers. The acute stage may be indistinguishable from bacterial diarrhea, with explosive watery diarrhea, mid-epigastric cramps, flatulence and distention, and nausea and vomiting. The pathogenetic mechanism by which Giardia causes diarrhea has not been established. Giardia does not appear to produce toxins, and mucosal invasion by Giardia has been suggested but not firmly documented.

The organism colonizes the upper part of the small intestine, attaching itself to the villous membrane of the enterocyte. In some individuals, persistence of the organism in this location gives rise to a syndrome of chronic diarrhea and malabsorption. Typically, the patient complains of generalized abdominal aching, passage of soft, malodorous stools, anorexia, flatulence, and weight loss. These symptoms may be intermittent, with return to normal health between attacks. The frequent occurrence of protracted giardiasis in patients with hypogammaglobulinemia suggests that altered immunity underlies chronic or subacute infection with this parasite. Some individuals become asymptomatic chronic cyst passers, with or without previous episodes of acute illness. The pathogenetic mechanisms underlying these varied manifestations of giardiasis are obscure.

Diagnosis of infection with *G. lamblia* is established by finding the trophozoite or cyst in stools. In some patients, the parasite may be present in duodenal aspirates but absent in stools. Hence, duodenal intubation and aspiration is recommended in patients suspected of having giardiasis but in whom multiple stool examinations are negative.

Treatment with quinacrine is curative in approximately 95 percent of patients. Metronidazole is a less effective but generally better tolerated alternate therapy. All forms of giardiasis, including the asymptomatic cyst passer, should be treated to eradicate the pathogen from the intestine.

Intestinal Worms

Intestinal worms are classified as roundworms (Nematoda) or tapeworms (Cestoda). Roundworms do not require a secondary host, whereas most tapeworms parasitize an intermediate host (fish, pig, or cattle). Humans become infected by eating infested fish or meat. Intestinal worms may be asymptomatic or cause mild anemia owing to blood ingestion by the worm. Eosinophilia is common with worms but rare with the protozoan parasites. Invasion of tissues outside the intestinal tract is a serious and occasionally fatal complication of these parasites.

Infestations with intestinal roundworms (nematodes) are common in rural poor persons, especially in the southern United States and among immigrant populations in urban centers. The most common parasite infection in this country is *Enterobius vermicularis*, or pinworm, which infests small children. The female worm deposits eggs on the perianal area, causing pruritis ani. Diagnosis is established by identification of eggs on adhesive tape applied to the perianal skin. *Trichuris trichiura*, or whipworm, is also common in young children, especially among those in institutions, and is generally asymptomatic. Heavy infestation may result in rectal prolapse or diarrhea. Both pinworm and whipworm infestations respond well to mebendazole therapy.

Ascaris lumbricoides, or roundworm, is a larger worm, up to 12 inches in length, which resides in the upper small intestine. Infestations are often asymptomatic, but migration of the worm into the bile duct, pancreatic duct, or appendix may produce symptoms. In heavy infestations, a mass of worms may occlude the lumen causing bowel obstruction. Mebendazole is effective in eliminating ascaris.

Hookworms (*Necator americanus* and *Ancylostoma duodenale*) attach to the mucosa of the upper small intestine where they ingest blood. In heavy infestations or in patients with borderline iron stores, severe anemia may result; abdominal pain, diarrhea, and weight loss are also occasionally seen. Passage of larvae into the lungs results in an allergic pneumonitis with a high degree of eosinophilia.

The most severe intestinal nematode infection is strongyloidiasis. *Strongyloides stercoralis* colonizes the upper small intestine, where it may cause mild abdominal pain or malabsorption. In some patients, generally those with suppressed immunity or malnutrition, dissemination or "hyperinfection" may occur. This is manifested by high fever, shock, abdominal pain and associated gram-negative septicemia. This condition is poorly responsive, even to specific therapy.

Intestinal tapeworms live in the small intestine of humans and compete with the host for nutrients. These parasites attach to the mucosa by the *scolex*, or head. The egg cases, or *proglottids*, are arranged in a tape-like series that may reach 20 feet in length. When ripe, these drop off from the tape, are shed in stools, and are then ingested by a secondary host where they ultimately form larvae in muscle tissue. The life cycle is then completed when the infected fish, pork, or beef is eaten by humans, and the larva mature to adult worms in the human intestine. The common forms of intestinal tapeworms encountered in the United States are listed in Table 6-4.

Sexually Transmitted Intestinal Infections

The lower gastrointestinal tract can become infected with several unusual pathogens during anal intercourse. These anorectal infections are often referred to as "gay bowel," although it should be noted that some of them (e.g., gonococcal proctitis and lymphogranuloma venereum) also occur in women follow-

Table 6-4
Intestinal tapeworms

Name	Intermediate host	Signs and symptoms
Diphyllobothrium latum	Freshwater fish	Anemia, vitamin B_{12} deficiency
Taenia solium	Pig	Usually asymptomatic in intestine; cysts may disseminate to all organs (cysticercosis)
Taenia saginata	Cattle	Large worms may obstruct bowel; cysticercosis may also occur
Hymenolepis nana	None, lives only in humans	Abdominal pain, pruritus ani

Table 6-5
Anorectal infections

Agent	Signs and symptoms	Diagnosis
Neisseriae gonorrhea	Creamy discharge, constipation, and pain	Culture of N. gonorrhea on selective medium
Herpes simplex	Extreme rectal pain and tenderness, bloody discharge; discrete ulcers on sigmoidoscopy	Viral isolation from stool, discharge, or rectal swab; serology of acute and convalescent sera
Treponema pallidum	Mild or no symptoms	Dark-field examination of ulcer; serologic studies
Entamoeba histolytica	Diarrhea with mucus or blood; diffuse proctitis or proctocolitis with scattered ulcers at sigmoidoscopy	Motile trophozoites or cysts in stool; serologic studies
Chlamydia trachomatis	Diarrhea, discharge; diffuse proctitis at sigmoidoscopy	Granulomata in rectal biopsy; isolation of chlamydia from tissue or stool

ing heterosexual contact. A second category of sexually transmitted intestinal infections includes those occurring in patients with AIDS. This disorder is frequently accompanied by severe intestinal infection with a variety of pathogens and parasites.

Anorectal Infection in Homosexual Males ("Gay Bowel")
Infection of the anal canal and rectum is a common venereal disease among promiscuous gay males. The most commonly encountered pathogens (Table 6-5) are *Neisseriae gonorrhea*, *Herpes simplex*, *Entamoeba histolytica*, *Chlamydia trachomatis*, and *Treponema pallidum*.

The clinical features of acute anorectal infection include anal discharge, pain on defecation or with anal intercourse, alteration in bowel habit, and fever. Since the rectal mucosa and anal canal can respond to injury in only a limited number of ways, the clinical features of these infections are similar. Multiple infections occur in approximately one third of patients with acute proctitis. It is important to distinguish between true infection and abrasion of the rectal mucosa from anal intercourse, which is usually localized to a well-defined area. Gay males presenting with these symptoms should be questioned carefully about frequency and type of recent sexual exposure. Individuals with multiple sexual partners and those engaging in receptive anal intercourse are at highest risk of developing anorectal infection. The examining physician should not hesitate to inquire about the sexual practices of any patient with symptoms of anorectal inflammation, including those suspected of having idiopathic ulcerative proctitis. Failure to obtain a history of homosexual contact is a frequent cause for misdiagnosis.

Specific diagnostic features are listed in Table 6-5. It is recommended that all patients with suspected gay bowel syndrome undergo proctosigmoidoscopy to obtain fresh material for culture and to biopsy the rectum. Careful follow-up of known contacts is mandatory, although, not infrequently, it is impossible to trace sexual partners.

In addition to anorectal infections, gay males may also be infected with the usual enteric pathogens, including Salmonella, Shigella, Campylobacter, Giardia, and various amoeba species, including E. histolytica, and the nonpathogens Endolimax nana, E. hartmanni, and E. coli. Some gay males are asymptomatic carriers of E. histolytica, whereas others may be acutely infected and present with acute colitis. A common mode of transmission of these pathogens is anilingus, with direct anal-oral spread. Diagnosis and treatment are identical to those for the nonhomosexual population.

Gastrointestinal Infections in Immunosuppressed Patients

Enteric infections are common among patients with congenital or acquired defects of the immune system. It was recognized many years ago that individuals with congenital or acquired immunoglobulin deficiency were susceptible to enteric infections such as giardiasis. Recently, the worldwide epidemic of AIDS has highlighted the importance of the cellular immune system in preventing enteric infection.

Selective IgA Deficiency
The extent of familial deficiency of secretory IgA is quite variable from patient to patient. Although most patients with IgA deficiency are asymptomatic, those who do develop infections have recurrent sinopulmonary infections and an increased incidence of giardiasis. In addition, celiac sprue and nodular lym-

phoid hyperplasia of the intestine occur more frequently, although in none of these conditions has a causal relationship with the IgA deficiency been clearly established.

Common Variable Immunodeficiencies
Common variable immunodeficiencies are characterized by low levels of serum IgG and variably abnormal levels of IgA and IgM. Chronic diarrhea may occur in up to 60 percent of such patients, owing in part to chronic giardiasis, bacterial overgrowth of the small bowel, or associated disaccharidase deficiency or villous atrophy. Treatment of these disorders is aimed at eradication of specific infections and at parenteral injections of immunoglobulins.

Enteric Infections in AIDS
The worldwide epidemic of AIDS has resulted in highlighting the important role of the intestinal immune system in preventing enteric infection. It is now well recognized that chronic opportunistic intestinal infections are common in AIDS patients; in some of these patients, the resultant diarrhea is a major source of malnutrition and death. Even though the same pathogens may be involved, enteric infections in AIDS produce different symptom complexes than are seen in anorectal infections in gay males. Enteric infections in AIDS generally involve the large and small intestine, are chronic and unremitting, and respond poorly to therapy because of the underlying derangements of host immunity. In contrast, anorectal infections in immunocompetent gay males are limited to the rectum and anal canal, are usually acute in nature, and generally respond well to specific therapy and temporary sexual abstinence.

AIDS patients with enteric infections generally present with chronic abdominal pain and diarrhea. Because the pain is often worsened by eating, anorexia and steady weight loss are common. Diarrhea may occur up to 20 times per day in severe cases; this contributes to dehydration, electrolyte disturbances, and weight loss.

Infection with *Cryptosporidium muris* is common in AIDS patients. This protozoan is sometimes identified in normal persons with transient diarrhea. AIDS patients with cryptosporidiosis generally have severe watery diarrhea and crampy diffuse abdominal pain. The oocysts are easily identified in acid-fast stains of stools or by a special isolation technique. Unfortunately, specific antibiotic therapy is not available; supportive measures to maintain hydration and caloric intake are generally required.

Cytomegalovirus (CMV) enterocolitis is another opportunistic infection in AIDS patients. This organism produces colitis that may be difficult to differentiate from idiopathic ulcerative colitis. The organism may be cultured from endoscopic biopsies or identified in histologic sections by the typical intranuclear inclusion. Therapy with experimental antiviral agents may be useful in some patients.

Herpes simplex virus may produce anorectal infection in AIDS patients similar to that described in gay males who do not have AIDS. A typical feature is widespread perianal lesions. Systemic administration of acyclovir is indicated for those in whom herpesvirus has been isolated from stool, anal swabs, or perianal exudates.

Mycobacterium avium-intracellulare (MAI) infection in AIDS patients may be manifested clinically by cholestatic hepatitis, abdominal pain, malabsorption, and severe diarrhea. The organism is cultured from blood and stool cultures. Unfortunately, conventional antituberculous therapy is ineffective for this pathogen.

In addition to these opportunistic infections, AIDS patients are susceptible to infection with conventional enteric pathogens, including Salmonella, Shigella, and Campylobacter, and to amebiasis. These are generally responsive to specific antimicrobial therapy.

Study Questions   1. Host defense mechanisms that protect against enteric infections include which of the following:
   a. Gastric acid secretion
   b. Pancreatic protease secretion
   c. Gastrointestinal motility
   d. Indigenous microflora of the gastrointestinal tract
   e. Mucus secretion by surface enterocytes
   f. Salt and water secretion by enterocytes
   g. Phagocytosis of pathogenic organisms by surface enterocytes

   Answers
   a, c, d, e

2. Answer true or false:
   a. Bacterial toxins can be divided into two general categories: (1) cytotonic, which stimulate salt and water secretion, and (2) cytotoxic, which injure epithelial cells.
   b. A bacterial pathogen can cause diarrhea by either toxin production or mucosal invasion, but not by both mechanisms.
   c. Mucosal invasion by bacterial pathogens most commonly occurs in the proximal jejunum.

    d. Typhoid fever has been effectively eradicated in underdeveloped countries and is never encountered in Western societies.

    e. The presence of nausea and vomiting preceding diarrhea indicates the presence of a viral pathogen and effectively excludes the presence of a bacterial pathogen.

Answers
a. true
b. false
c. false
d. false
e. false

3. Match the enteric pathogen in List I with the appropriate risk factor, foodstuff, or clinical feature listed in List II.

List I

1. *Staphylococcus aureus*
2. *Clostridium perfringens*
3. *E. coli* 0157:H7
4. *Giardia*
5. *Vibrio parahaemolyticus*
6. *Bacillus cereus*
7. *Clostridium difficile*
8. *Cryptosporidium muris*

List II

a. Meats
b. Shellfish, shrimp
c. Rice
d. Antibiotics
e. AIDS
f. Cream, egg products
g. IgA deficiency
h. Hemolytic-uremic syndrome

Answers
1. f
2. a
3. h
4. g
5. b
6. c
7. d
8. e

References

Andrews, H., Wyke, J., Lane, M., et al. Prevalence of sexually transmitted disease among male patients presenting with proctitis. *Gut* 29:332, 1988.

Blaser, M. J., Wells, J. G., Feldman, R. A., et al. Campylobacter enteritis in the United States. *Ann. Int. Med.* 98:360, 1983.

Dupont, H. L., Ericson, C. D., Robinson, A., et al. Current problems in antimicrobial therapy for bacterial enteric infection. *Am. J. Med.* 82(Suppl. 4A):324, 1987.

Formal, S. B., Hale, T. H., and Sansonetti, P. J. Invasive enteric pathogens. *Rev. Infect. Dis.* 5:702, 1983.

Guerrant, R. L., Shields, D. S., Thorson, S. M., et al. Evaluation and diagnosis of acute infectious diarrhea. *Am. J. Med.* 78(Suppl. 6B):91, 1985.

Laughon, B. E., Druckman, D. A., Vernon, A., et al. Prevalence of enteric pathogens in homosexual men with and without AIDS. *Gastroenterology* 94:984, 1988.

Murray, B. E. Resistance of *Shigella, Salmonella* and other selected enteric pathogens to antimicrobial agents. *Rev. Infect. Dis.* 8(Suppl. 2):172, 1986.

Siegel, D., Cohen, P. T., Neighbor, M., et al. Predictive value of stool examination in acute diarrhea. *Arch. Pathol. Lab. Med.* 111:715, 1987.

7 : Inflammatory Bowel Disease

Mark A. Peppercorn

Definition

The chronic idiopathic inflammatory bowel diseases include ulcerative colitis and Crohn's disease. Ulcerative colitis is a recurrent inflammatory process of unknown etiology, involving the mucosa and submucosa of the colon. The disease may be limited to the rectum, may involve the left colon to the splenic flexure, or may extend in a continuous fashion to the cecum. Associated changes of no clinical significance may be seen in the terminal ileum. Crohn's disease, on the other hand, is a recurrent focal inflammatory process involving any part of the gastrointestinal tract in a transmural fashion.

Epidemiology

The incidence of ulcerative colitis and Crohn's disease is highest in developed areas of the world, especially the United States, northern Europe, and Australia. About 10,000 new cases of each are diagnosed yearly in the United States. The number of new cases of ulcerative colitis diagnosed yearly has remained relatively constant over the past 30 years. In contrast, the incidence of Crohn's disease has been doubling each decade since the 1940s, such that the annual incidence of Crohn's disease is now equal to that of ulcerative colitis. In the "developing" regions, the incidence remains low, although incidence rates are beginning to increase in these areas.

Although the highest proportion of cases have their onset between the ages of 15 and 40 years, disease may occur for the first time in infancy or in old age. Males and females are affected equally. Although no ethnic, racial, or socioeconomic group is immune to inflammatory bowel disease, the incidence of ulcerative colitis and Crohn's disease is significantly higher in Jews than in non-Jews and in Caucasians than in non-Caucasians.

There is a clearly established familial tendency for inflammatory bowel disease, with 10 to 25 percent of patients having first-degree relatives with the disease. Although ulcerative colitis and Crohn's disease commonly occur in the same family, there is an 80 to 90 percent concordance for the same disease within sibships. Monozygotic twins have a much higher concordance for these disorders than do dizygotic twins. No data, including

HLA studies, have provided definite evidence for genetic versus environmental determinants of familial patterns.

Etiology

Neither the etiology nor pathogenesis of ulcerative colitis or Crohn's disease is known, although numerous theories have been proposed. Etiologies suggested include psychogenic, allergic, neuromotor, vascular, environmental, dietary, and genetic. Most recent work has focused, however, on immunologic and infectious etiologies. Abnormalities of the immune system have been detected for both disorders, but, as yet, these findings do not explain etiology or pathogenesis. There have been recent intriguing reports of the isolations of atypical mycobacterial strains from the tissue of patients with Crohn's disease. Further investigations of these findings are ongoing.

**Ulcerative
Colitis**

Pathophysiology

The major clinical features of ulcerative colitis include diarrhea with frequent, often watery stools, rectal bleeding, and abdominal pain. When severe, iron deficiency anemia and hypoalbuminemia occur. These manifestations of the disruption of the normal function can readily be explained by the pathologic changes observed in the condition.

The inflammatory process in ulcerative colitis is usually confined to the mucosa and submucosa. The major features of the process include diffuse inflammation, crypt abscesses, and chronic mucosal changes. Although the inciting factor is not known, the initial lesion in ulcerative colitis may be the crypt abscess, which occurs when polymorphonuclear leukocytes accumulate within the tip of the intestinal crypt, associated with epithelial cell degeneration. The inflammatory lesion is further characterized by crypt epithelial cell necrosis, an extension of the polyps into the crypts, along with the presence of chronic inflammatory cells. This disruption of normal colonic architecture is accompanied by diminished ability to absorb water and sodium, leading to the diarrhea, and by weeping of the protein into the gastrointestinal lumen, resulting in hypoalbuminemia.

As part of the reaction to the inflammatory process, there is engorgement of the vessels in the submucosa, and as part of the repair process, a very vascular friable granulation tissue develops in ulcerated areas. Bleeding, a common manifestation of ulcerative colitis, often leads to anemia. It results from the ulcerative process destroying the mucosa in these highly vascularized areas.

As further repair continues, granulation tissue fills in the ulcerative areas. Collagen is deposited in the lamina propria, and hypertrophy of the muscularis mucosa occurs. At times, the exuberant granulation tissue assumes a polypoid configuration and appears as a pseudopolyp on x-ray or endoscopy. Pseudopolyps have no physiologic consequence, nor any neoplastic potential. The changes in the muscularis mucosa may lead to spasm, contributing to the painful contractions felt by patients with ulcerative colitis. Moreover, the hypertrophy and spasm of muscle can appear, on x-ray, as a stricture. These "strictures" are usually reversible, since they are not caused by fibrosis.

Clinical Picture   The clinical presentation of ulcerative colitis is variable. It has been useful for therapeutic and prognostic reasons, to classify a patient's symptoms as mild, moderate, or severe. There is a correlation of extent of disease with the severity of the symptomatology. Patients with involvement limited to the rectum (proctitis) or rectosigmoid (distal colitis) often present in an insidious manner, with intermittent rectal bleeding or mild diarrhea, with fewer than four bowel movements per day. Tenesmus, mild cramping, and even periods of constipation are common in such patients, but severe pain, fever, profuse bleeding, and poor nutrition are not part of the picture of mild disease. Patients with moderate symptoms usually have involvement of more than the distal colon, with the inflammatory process extending up toward the transverse colon (left-sided colitis). Such patients may have up to 10 loose bowel movements a day, with frequent bleeding and mild anemia, but they rarely require a blood transfusion. Abdominal pain is common but not severe, and fever, if present, is of low grade. The overall nutritional status is usually adequate.

Patients with severe or even fulminant symptoms usually have extensive colonic involvement, often reaching to the cecum, although occasionally, patients with more limited disease will present with a severe picture. These patients have very frequent movements, usually greater than 10 per day, bleeding often requiring transfusion, severe abdominal pain, and fever at times as high as 103°F, with poor nutritional status. However, in some of these patients, the ulcerative process, which is usually confined to the mucosa and submucosa, extends to the muscular layers of the colon, with loss of motor tone and resulting colonic dilatation, giving the clinical picture of toxic megacolon. When the disease extends to the serosa, colonic perforation may occur.

Diagnosis   The diagnosis of ulcerative colitis rests on the historic details, coupled with findings on some form of endoscopic examination of the colon. Colonic biopsy and barium enema can be confirmatory of the findings, whereas examination of the stool for infectious agents will eliminate other diagnostic considerations.

Most patients with ulcerative colitis have a gradual onset of symptoms, sometimes heralded by a self-limited episode of rectal bleeding preceding the onset of full-blown symptoms by weeks or months. In such patients, as noted, the history is usually one of alteration of normal bowel function, with a tendency toward diarrhea, rectal bleeding, and varying degrees of crampy lower abdominal pain. Less than 10 percent of patients with ulcerative colitis will have, as an initial presentation, a fulminant picture. A family history of inflammatory bowel disease should also be sought. The findings on physical examination are nonspecific and therefore not helpful in establishing a diagnosis of ulcerative colitis; they may, however, include pallor, evidence of weight loss, abdominal tenderness, and red blood on digital examination of the rectum.

A key to the diagnosis is direct visualization of the colonic mucosa. Since ulcerative colitis always affects the rectum, the diagnosis is usually readily established by sigmoidoscopy, which can be accomplished simply with a standard rigid sigmoidoscope. A flexible sigmoidoscope is better tolerated by some patients, however, and affords the opportunity, at the outset, to establish to some degree the extent of disease. There is a spectrum of changes seen endoscopically. The earliest sign is usually a loss of the normal vascular pattern, a finely granular texture, and the appearance of microhemorrhage, when the mucosa is wiped. As the process becomes more advanced, the mucosa appears pitted, and spontaneous bleeding can be seen. In the more severe cases, macroulceration can be appreciated, bleeding may be profuse, and copious exudate is often present. Pseudopolyps, which signify some evidence of the chronicity and severity of the process, may be observed in an area of disease involvement.

It is useful to obtain a biopsy of the colonic mucosa at the time of the initial examination, as an adjunct to the endoscopic findings. A biopsy will usually confirm the presence of inflammation of the colonic mucosa, with changes ranging from mild degrees of inflammation to microscopic erosions of the epithelium and crypt abscesses (Fig. 7-1). The inflammatory process in ulcerative colitis is diffuse, involving all areas of biopsied mucosa, in contrast to the findings in Crohn's disease or infectious colitis, where the changes are usually focal, with part of the involved area appearing normal under the microscope. Moreover, patients with ulcerative colitis, unlike those with self-limited forms of colitis, will show atrophic changes in the mu-

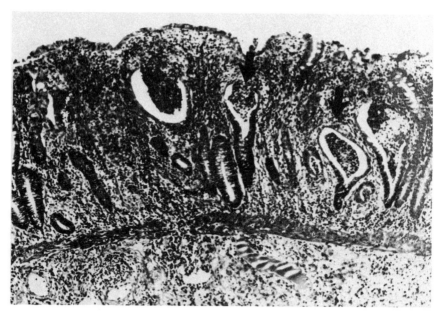

Fig. 7-1
Colonic mucosa in a patient with idiopathic ulcerative colitis. The mucosa is diffusely inflamed, and the crypts are distorted. Many crypts are dilated with epithelial destruction and intraluminal inflammation (crypt abscesses, indicated by arrow). (Courtesy of Donald Antonioli, M.D.)

cosa, with a decreased number of glands, and branching of glands, evidence of past mucosal destruction or repair. Although usually unnecessary when there is clear-cut endoscopic evidence of mucosal inflammation, the colonic biopsy is especially useful when the sigmoidoscopic findings are equivocal, since it will often detect clear abnormalities with significant inflammation in such settings.

The barium enema, like the rectal biopsy, can serve as an adjunct to the endoscopic findings and help establish extent of disease (Fig. 7-2). However, the barium enema may be normal in mild disease of limited extent. Moreover, in the sicker patients with more extensive involvement, a barium enema should be avoided, since it can contribute to morbidity and usually does not alter management. The findings on barium enema include a diffusely reticulated pattern, upon which are superimposed punctate collections of barium lodged in microulcerations. As the process advances, the colonic margins appear irregular, with spiculated collarbutton "ulcers." Pseudopolyps may also be seen. The latter stages of ulcerative colitis are characterized radiographically by shortening of the colon, loss of redundancy, disappearance of normal haustrae, and a narrowed caliber of the bowel lumen.

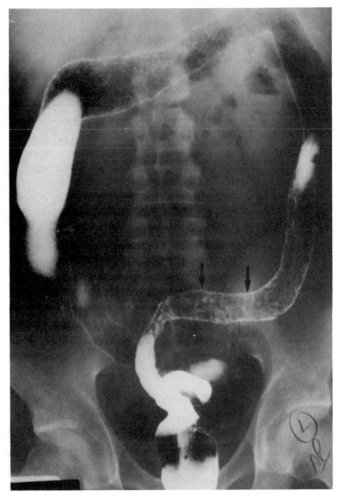

Fig. 7-2
Barium enema in a patient with idiopathic ulcerative colitis. The arrows indicate the diffusely reticulated pattern in the left colon, which represents
mucosal ulcerations. Note the pattern of continuous involvement. (Courtesy
of Norman Joffe, M.D.)

Total colonoscopy need not be done initially in patients with
ulcerative colitis, since the information gained about extent of
disease rarely contributes to the initial therapeutic approach
and, as with the barium enema in the setting of active disease,
may increase the morbidity by increasing the risk of megacolon
or perforation. Once the disease quiets down, colonoscopy
should be considered, since documentation of universal colitis
will likely influence subsequent cancer surveillance.

Differential Diagnosis	The characteristic clinical endoscopic and pathologic picture of ulcerative colitis is not pathognomonic. The other principle idiopathic form of colitis, Crohn's disease, can resemble ulcerative colitis in most ways. Features that distinguish Crohn's disease from ulcerative colitis include rectal sparing, segmental distribution, small bowel involvement, perianal disease granulomas on biopsy, focality of pathologic lesions, and fistulae development. The bacterial causes of colitis include Shigella, Salmonella, Campylobacter, invasive *Escherichia coli*, and *Aeromonas hydrophila*. These usually present with an acute self-limited picture, in contrast to the more chronic or subacute presentation of ulcerative colitis. However, stool cultures for bacterial pathogen should be obtained on any patient with an ulcerative colitis-like presentation. In the same manner, amoebic colitis can mimic ulcerative colitis in all regards. Stool for ova and parasites, amoebic serology, and even a biopsy with special stains for amoeba may be required to rule out amoebic infection. Ischemic colitis typically has its onset abruptly in elderly patients with underlying heart disease. A history of radiation therapy, often for genital or urinary tract malignancies, should direct the clinician to the possibility of radiation colitis in the patient with bloody diarrhea and evidence of colitis on endoscopy. Other disorders, such as carcinoma of the colon, irritable bowel syndrome, and even hemorrhoids, can be confused initially with ulcerative colitis. These disorders are easily distinguished from ulcerative colitis, however, by endoscopic investigation of the colon.
Complications	Complications of ulcerative colitis can be divided into local ones, involving the intestine itself, and systemic ones, involving non-colonic sites.

Local Complications

Rarely, massive hemorrhage necessitating emergency surgery may be associated with severe ulcerative colitis. More common are repeated episodes of bleeding, leading to anemia, which may require transfusions.

As discussed previously, when the ulcerative process extends into the muscle layers of the bowel, loss of motor tone may occur, with colonic ileus and distention. Patients with these complications, because of the severity of the inflammation, are often toxic with tachycardia, high fever, and leukocytosis. This clinical picture is termed *toxic megacolon* (Fig. 7-3). If the ulcerative process extends to the serosa, perforation with peritonitis may occur. It is in this group of patients with ulcerative colitis that mortalities are seen.

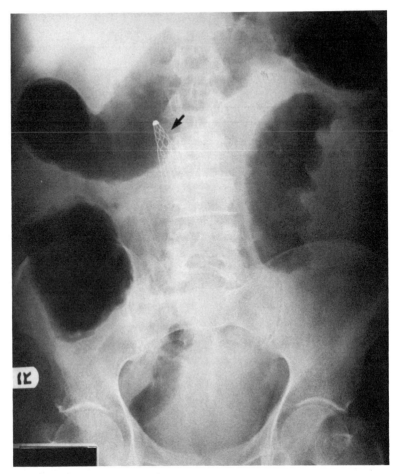

Fig. 7-3
Abdominal film in a patient with idiopathic ulcerative colitis and *toxic megacolon*. Note the dilated, gas-filled colon, whose irregular surface represents deep mucosal ulcerations. The arrow indicates an unrelated vascular filter in the inferior vena cava. (Courtesy of Julian I. Gilliam, M.D.)

Although the inflammatory process of ulcerative colitis is usually superficial, occasionally, with repeated episodes of ulceration and inflammation, enough fibrosis will occur to cause a benign stricture. Such strictures can lead to symptoms of colonic obstruction. Often troubling to the clinician is the difficulty in distinguishing benign strictures from those associated with carcinoma.

The development of carcinoma is one of the dreaded complications of ulcerative colitis. Although estimates of cancer incidence vary widely from study to study, it is indisputable that some patients with ulcerative colitis are at an increased risk for colonic cancer. That risk is highest in those with extensive involvement of the colon and those who have had disease for more than 10 years.

These cancers tend to be multiple, arise from flat mucosa, are uniformly distributed in the colon, infiltrate broadly, and tend to be anaplastic. Because of these features, early cancer detection has been difficult. Cellular atypia or dysplasia of the mucosa appears to be an early sign of impending malignant transformation. In the most severe form of dysplasia, epithelial nuclei are markedly enlarged, hyperchromatic, and tightly packed, appearing to overlap. The nuclei extend into the upper half of cells, and no mucin production is seen. Some series report at least a 50 percent association of occult malignancy with high-grade dysplasia. For this reason, there are now surveillance programs advocating periodic colonoscopy in patients at high risk, viewing dysplasia as a predictor of carcinoma. In patients in whom high-grade dysplasia is found, colectomy is strongly considered.

Systemic Complications

Erythema nodosum — painful, tender indurated subcutaneous nodules usually on extensor surfaces — and pyoderma gangrenosum — ulcerated lesions usually on the extremities associated with necrosis of the surrounding dermis — are the skin lesions most often associated with ulcerative colitis. Both lesions tend to parallel the activity of the colitis and respond to treatment of the colitis. Ocular manifestations of ulcerative colitis include episcleritis and uveitis. The former parallels colitis activity, whereas the latter occurs independent of colonic disease. Episcleritis is manifested by injection of the deep ciliary vessels. Uveitis often causes pain, distorts the interior chamber with synechiae and opacity, and can be seen in association with spondylitis and sacroiliitis.

Ankylosing spondylitis and sacroiliitis may be asymptomatic, detectible only by x-ray changes, or cause progressive symptoms of low back pain and immobility. In ankylosing spondylitis, there is obliteration of the normal disk spaces by sclerosis of the vertebral bodies. Sacroiliitis results in sclerosis and obliteration of the sacroiliac joints. These central arthritic complications do not parallel disease activity, may have their onset prior to the colitis, and can progress despite total colectomy. Both tend to occur in patients with the HLA B27 histocompatibility antigen.

In contrast, the peripheral forms of arthritis, most often involving the large joints such as the knees, ankles, and wrists, usually parallel the activity of the bowel disease. These forms of arthritis

Table 7-1
Extraintestinal manifestations of inflammatory bowel disease

Skin	Liver
Erythema nodosum	Fatty liver
Pyoderma gangrenosum	Chronic hepatitis
	Sclerosing cholangitis
Eyes	Cholangiocarcinoma
Episcleritis	Amyloid
Uveitis	
Joints	
Peripheral arthritis	
Central arthritis	
Ankylosing spondylitis	
Sacroiliitis	

differ from rheumatoid arthritis in being monoarticular, asymmetric, and not associated with positive serologies, subcutaneous nodules, or synovial destruction.

Abnormalities of the liver are common in patients with ulcerative colitis. Fatty liver is a frequent finding and may be manifested by mild elevations of transaminases. Sclerosing cholangitis can affect both the intra- and extrahepatic bile ducts. When cholangitis involves the liver itself, the portal triad is expanded with inflammatory cells, and there is ductular proliferation, erosion of the limiting plate, and periductular fibrosis. Involvement of the biliary tree causes segmental areas of stenosis and dilatation. Clinical manifestations can include abdominal pain, fever, and jaundice, and may be associated with a rising bilirubin and alkaline phosphatase. Secondary biliary cirrhosis and liver failure are dreaded consequences of these disorders. Sclerosing cholangitis occurs independently of the course of colitis and is not reversed by colectomy. Liver transplantation is a consideration in end-stage disease. Cholangiocarcinoma is difficult to distinguish radiologically from the benign strictures of sclerosing cholangitis; its incidence is increased in patients with ulcerative colitis (Table 7-1).

Therapy   Sulfasalazine has been a mainstay of therapy for patients with ulcerative colitis for more than 45 years. This drug is efficacious in approximately 80 percent of patients with mildly and moderately active disease. It also plays an important role in the prophylaxis of ulcerative colitis in patients who are in remission. About three fourths of patients maintained on sulfasalazine will stay in remission for up to at least 3 years. Similar patients on placebo, on the other hand, have a 75 percent flare-up rate in the first year alone.

Sulfasalazine consists of sulfapyridine linked to 5-aminosalicy-late (5-ASA) by an azo bond. Intestinal bacteria are responsible for cleaving the bond, with release of the two metabolites. The sulfapyridine is largely absorbed, metabolized by the liver, and excreted in the urine. The 5-ASA is largely unabsorbed, staying in contact with diseased colonic mucosa, to be excreted in the feces. Most of the drug's toxicity, including nonspecific symptoms such as headache and nausea, as well as allergic reactions, can be traced to the sulfa moiety. On the other hand, the 5-ASA appears to be clinically efficacious in its own right. Multiple studies have attested to the efficacy of 5-ASA enemas and suppositories in patients with active distal ulcerative colitis. Topical 4-ASA, an isomer of 5-ASA, appears to be as effective as 5-ASA in such patients. Even patients refractory to sulfasalazine and corticosteroids may respond to the topical 5-ASA. Moreover, sulfasalazine-sensitive patients can usually tolerate the 5-ASA and 4-ASA, which have minimal side effects.

Recent studies have established the safety and efficacy of oral 5-ASA agents in active ulcerative colitis and as prophylaxis for disease in remission. These agents include slow-release forms of the drug, a dimer of 5-ASA, which links the molecule to itself, and agents that link 5-ASA to inert molecules, via an azo bond. As of yet, only a 5-ASA enema product is commercially available in the United States.

Corticosteroids have been used successfully in patients with ulcerative colitis since their inception into clinical medicine in the mid-1940s. Topical forms of steroid, including hydrocortisone and methylprednisolone, may be administered in a retention enema form and are efficacious in about 80 percent of patients with proctitis and distal colitis. Long-term usage of these agents can result, however, in the common steroid side effects, which include changes in body habitus, alteration of glucose metabolism and bone integrity, development of cataracts, and disruption of the pituitary-adrenal axis. A new synthetic corticoid, tixocortal pivalate, appears to be as effective topically as standard formulations, but because of rapid metabolism, it does not cause the same systemic effects.

For patients with more extensive disease and more prominent symptoms, oral prednisone is very effective. Although this form of therapy is often used in conjunction with sulfasalazine, there are no data as to the adjunctive affect of one agent with the other. For patients with severe and fulminant forms of the disease, intravenous hydrocortisone, methylprednisolone, and prednisolone may alter the course and avert colectomy. Corticotropin (ACTH) appears to be even more effective than standard forms of systemic corticosteroids in patients with severe colitis who have not recently been on oral steroids.

Although they have assumed an ever increasing role in the treatment of patients with Crohn's disease, immunosuppressive drugs, such as 6-mercaptopurine and azathioprine, have a more limited role in the treatment of ulcerative colitis. They may, however, be efficacious in refractory distal colitis and are useful in allowing reduction of the steroid dosage in patients who cannot get below high or moderate doses of oral steroids without flaring.

Antibacterial agents in ulcerative colitis are reserved for patients with severe fulminant disease who either have evidence of peritoneal irritation or who, despite high-dose steroids, are doing poorly, with low-grade fever, leukocytosis, and a shift to the left in the white blood count differential.

Antidiarrheal agents, such as diphenoxylate with atropine, loperamide, and tincture of opium, must be used cautiously, since these drugs may precipitate ileus and even megacolon in patients with very active disease. However, in well-established chronic disease, the judicious use of these drugs can help to achieve a night of sleep and allay anxiety about daily functioning.

General nutrition is an important aspect of the therapeutic program in ulcerative colitis. Unfortunately, there is no evidence that specific diets are of help in this disorder. Emphasis should be placed on normalization of diet and adequate caloric intake to guard against excessive weight loss and nutritional depletion. However, in patients with diarrhea, cramps, and gas, it is reasonable to restrict certain foodstuffs, such as fresh fruit and fresh vegetables, diet gum, caffeine, and monosodium glutamate. Lactose intolerance should be sought as a possible contributor to symptoms.

For severely ill patients who require hospitalization, appropriate replacement of fluid and electrolytes is essential. For most of these patients, complete bowel rest utilizing total parenteral nutrition (TPN) will be indicated. Total parenteral nutrition can maintain and improve the nutritional status but is not efficacious as primary therapy in ulcerative colitis and does not appear to affect the course of the disease.

Surgery

There are several indications for surgery in patients with ulcerative colitis. The most common indication is that of chronic disability and recurrent symptoms despite intensive medical therapy. The toxic patient who fails medical therapy or who has an impending or actual perforation will also require colectomy. High-grade dysplasia or actual carcinoma should lead to surgery. Exsanguinating hemorrhage is an uncommon but occasionally seen cause of emergency surgery. Systemic complications rarely prompt surgery, but occasionally, colectomy will be performed for severe refractory pyoderma gangrenosum. Finally, growth retardation in children, otherwise refractory to medical therapy, may be an indication for surgery.

For many years, the only operation available to patients with ulcerative colitis was a proctocolectomy, with a permanent ileostomy. The so-called Brooke ileostomy has stood the test of time and is accepted by most patients. However, the ileostomy is incontinent and requires a permanent external appliance to be worn. In order to overcome this drawback to some extent, a continent ileostomy has been developed that creates an ileal reservoir with a nipple valve. The so-called Kock pouch requires no external appliance but does require regular catheterizations though the nipple valve for emptying (Fig. 7-4). This procedure has carried with it a high rate of complications, including "pouchitis," or mucosal inflammation in the pouch, and malfunctioning of the nipple valve, leading to further surgery. There is now a great deal of interest in sphincter-saving operations, which do not necessitate any form of permanent ileostomy. The procedure that has drawn the most recent attention is that of a mucosal proctectomy, leaving the rectal musculature in place and creating an ilealanal anastomosis, with a pouch or reservoir created out of the ileum (Fig. 7-5). Potential drawbacks include "pouchitis," anastomotic leaks, stricture formation, and partial incontinence. Nonetheless, the impressive early results with regard to a low incidence of complications and high patient satisfaction suggest that this procedure merits careful consideration as well as long-term follow-up.

Crohn's Disease

Pathophysiology

Although Crohn's disease may affect any portion of the gastrointestinal tract, there are certain areas that are more commonly involved. About one third of cases involve only the small intestine (regional enteritis), with most of these cases occurring in the distal ileum (ileitis). About 20 percent of patients with Crohn's disease have colonic involvement only (Crohn's colitis), whereas almost half of the patients have disease in the ileum and colon (ileocolitis). Although uncommon, Crohn's disease of the mouth, gastroduodenal area, and jejunum have been well described, although usually in conjunction with disease in more commonly occurring areas. In the same manner, perianal lesions are almost always associated with disease in other loca-

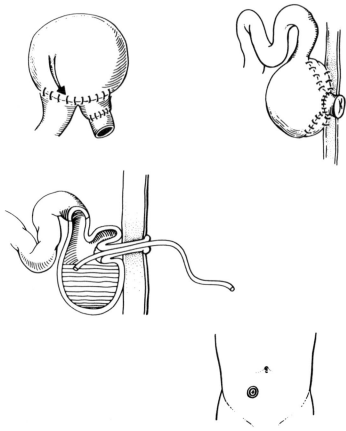

Fig. 7-4
The continent ileostomy ("Kock pouch"). The figures demonstrate how the pouch is (1) fashioned from the terminal ileum; (2) positioned with a transabdominal nipple valve, which prevents uncontrolled expulsion of the liquid contents; (3) emptied by a small catheter placed through the nipple valve; and (4) viewed by the patient, as the nipple valve does not require an external appliance. (From S. B. Hanauer and J. B. Kirsner. *Inflammatory Bowel Disease. A Guide for Patients and Their Families.* New York: Raven, 1985. P. 124.)

tions and can plague up to one third of patients with the disorder.

The anatomic distribution of disease varies so widely that it is not surprising that the clinical presentations of the disorder can be so variable. Just as the knowledge of the anatomic distribution enables one to predict the likely clinical symptoms, the recognition of the nature of the pathology of Crohn's disease leads to an understanding of the course and complications of the disorder. Crohn's disease is a transmural process. At the mucosal level, the earliest visible gross lesion, analogous to a canker sore in the mouth, is an aphthous ulcer. These discrete patchy ulcers are associated with submucosal edema and pro-

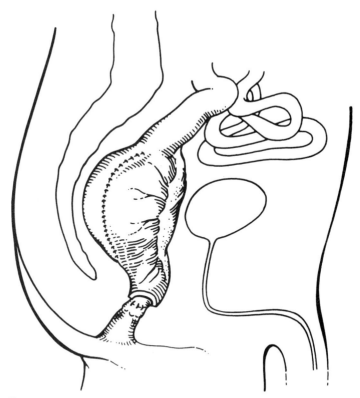

Fig. 7-5
The ileal reservoir with ileoanal anastomosis. The reservoir has been fashioned from the terminal ileum and is then joined to the anus, following a
previous mucosal proctectomy. (From S. B. Hanauer and J. G. Kirsner. *Inflammatory Bowel Disease. A Guide for Patients and Their Families.* New
York: Raven, 1985. P. 126.)

gressively enlarge, becoming confluent, destroying the surrounding normal mucosa, and giving a "cobblestone" appearance to the mucosa. The inflammatory process is not limited to
these mucosal and submucosal alterations, as in ulcerative colitis, but extends through all layers of the bowel wall, to the
serosa. On the serosal surface, mesenteric fat becomes hy-
peremic and edematous and encases the wall in a "creeping"
fashion, while the adjacent mesenteric nodes also enlarge.

The gross manifestations of ulceration are seen microscopically
initially as small mucosal defects, often overlying lymphoid follicles, with eventual extension through the bowel layer as sinus
tracts culminating in fistulae. Granulomas, inflammatory cell infiltrate, and edema are noted under the microscope in a patchy
distribution through all the layers of the bowel. Eventually, fibrosis occurs, leading to thickening of the bowel wall, luminal
narrowing, and stricturing. These mucosal uclerations, inflam-

mation, and edema of the bowel, strictures, and fistulae lead to the clinical manifestations of Crohn's disease.

The mucosal alterations and submucosal inflammation and edema cause disruption of the absorption of sodium and water and, as in ulcerative colitis, lead to diarrhea. In addition, in patients in whom the distal ileum is involved, bile acids are malabsorbed, and, in the colon, impair water absorption and promote water and sodium secretion, further adding to the diarrhea. Hemorrhage can occur when the mucosal ulceration extends to the level of the superficial blood vessels. The progressive fibrosis, which causes stricturing of the bowel and narrowing of the lumen, manifests itself as episodes of bowel obstruction. Fistulae, which penetrate the serosal surface, extend into adjacent tissues and cause pockets of extraluminal infection and drainage.

Clinical Picture   The majority of patients with Crohn's disease, regardless of distribution, have diarrhea as a major manifestation. Occasionally, a patient with disease limited to the distal ileum will have no clinical manifestations until the ileal lumen becomes very narrowed; in these instances, constipation may actually be seen. Bleeding is not as common as in ulcerative colitis. Patients with ileitis alone rarely have gross bleeding. Patients with colonic involvement can, however, bleed grossly and even massively. However, a history of prolonged diarrhea without bleeding is not unusual in patients with Crohn's colitis.

As with ulcerative colitis, crampy abdominal pain is a common manifestation of Crohn's disease, regardless of the distribution. As mentioned previously, the transmural nature of Crohn's disease leads to fibrotic strictures, which are manifested in the ileum as repeated episodes of small bowel obstruction. When these occur in the gastroduodenal area, the patients present with a picture of gastric outlet obstruction. When sinus tracts penetrate the mucosa, perforation of the bowel wall occurs. These symptoms often present as acute episodes of localized peritonitis, with fever, abdominal pain, and tenderness, with a mass sometimes noted on physical examination. Diffuse peritonitis is an unusual but reported complication of a perforation in Crohn's disease.

The clinical presentation of the fistulae that occur in Crohn's disease depends on the area of involvement adjacent to the involved bowel. Enteroenteric (bowel-bowel) fistulae often go unnoticed clinically or are evidenced by an area of localized tenderness with a palpable mass. Enterocutaneous (bowel-skin) fistulae are apparent with bowel contents draining out to the skin surface. These most often occur in areas of surgical scars or through the umbilicus by way of a persistent urachal segment. Enterovesicle (bowel-bladder) fistulae lead to a clinical history of air passage with urination and recurrent urinary tract infections. Fistulization into the retroperitoneal space can lead to ureteral obstruction and hydronephrosis.

Independent of fistulae from intraabdominal Crohn's disease are foci of disease arising from anal crypts spreading through the internal sphincter muscle. This process leads to draining anorectal fistulae, painful anal fissures, and perianal abscesses.

When Crohn's disease occurs in childhood before puberty, the only clinical manifestation of the disorder may be growth retardation. In both children and adults, Crohn's disease can present only as a fever of unknown origin.

Diagnosis

As with ulcerative colitis, the patient's history is often most suggestive of Crohn's disease. A history of prolonged diarrhea with abdominal pain with or without bleeding, along with weight loss and fever, is suggestive of Crohn's disease. A family history of inflammatory bowel disease and a history of perianal disease would add further likelihood to the diagnosis. Physical examination in itself is usually not diagnostic, although evidence of perianal disease or enterocutaneous fistulae would be suggestive. Many patients with Crohn's disease will have evidence of malnutrition or the suggestion of a tender abdominal mass on examination of the abdomen.

The diagnosis of Crohn's disease rests on endoscopic and radiographic studies of the bowel. Colonoscopy has emerged as the most effective way to diagnose Crohn's disease of the colon. Focal ulcers ranging in size from the tiny early aphthous lesions to large irregular punched-out ulcers or long latitudinal ulcers are typical of the endoscopic picture of Crohn's colitis. Pseudopolyps are also typically found in chronic Crohn's disease, as in ulcerative colitis. The segmental nature of Crohn's disease is often striking on colonoscopy, with grossly normal mucosa and well-preserved vascular markings being suddenly interrupted by focal ulcers or larger areas of obvious disease.

Although not as sensitive as colonoscopy, the air-contrast barium enema may detect the early aphthous lesion and be helpful in documenting the segmental nature of the disorder, its asymmetry, and its characteristic distribution with frequent rectal sparing and a predominance of right-sided colonic disease (Fig. 7-6).

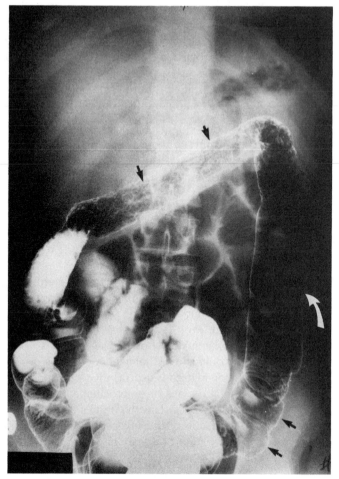

Fig. 7-6
Barium enema in a patient with Crohn's disease of the colon. The small arrows demonstrate mucosal nodularity and ulceration in the sigmoid and transverse colon. The large arrow demonstrates the uninvolved descending colon ("skip lesions"). (Courtesy of Norman Joffe, M.D.)

In contrast to colonic disease, in which colonoscopy has become a valuable tool in diagnoses, the upper gastrointestinal series and small bowel x-ray remain the mainstays of diagnosing Crohn's disease of the small intestine (Fig. 7-7). The typical radiologic features of advanced ileal Crohn's disease include nodularity, ulceration, and stricturing of the lumen, and separation of bowel loops (a reflection of bowel wall thickening), as well as evidence of fistulization. Gastroduodenal disease can be suggested on the upper gastrointestinal series by evidence of antral narrowing and segmental stricturing of the duodenum. Occasionally, the finding of small bowel Crohn's disease will be

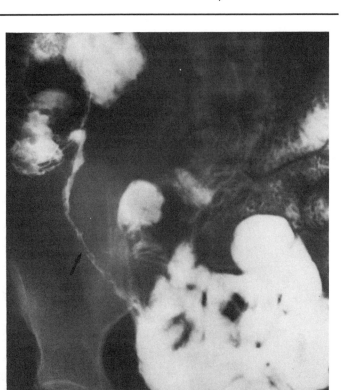

Fig. 7-7
A barium small bowel series in a patient with Crohn's disease of the small intestine. The arrow demonstrates the "string sign" produced by marked narrowing of the terminal ileum. (Courtesy of Norman Joffe, M.D.)

subtle and better appreciated on air-contrast study of the small intestine; this is known as enteroclysis.

Intestinal biopsies are usually confirmatory, rather than diagnostic, of Crohn's disease. The typical mucosal biopsy shows a focal ulcerative and inflammatory process, rather than the diffuse abnormality seen with ulcerative colitis. One finding, however, is pathognomonic for Crohn's disease in the absence of documentable infection. Epithelioid granulomas may be found in any layer of the bowel wall and may consist of giant cells and epithelioid cells surrounded by a rim of T lymphocytes (Fig. 7-8). These may be found in up to 10 percent of routine rectal biopsies in patients with Crohn's disease without gross evidence of disease in the rectum. However, the absence of granulomas does not rule out the diagnosis of Crohn's disease, since up to 50 percent of patients with Crohn's disease will not have granulomas on intestinal biopsy.

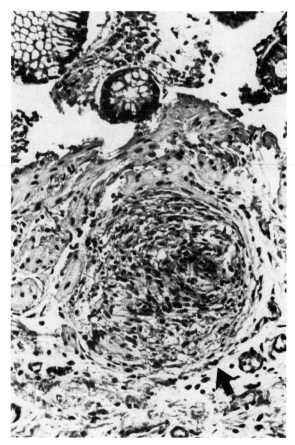

Fig. 7-8
A rectal biopsy from a patient with Crohn's disease. A non-necrotic granuloma (*arrow*) is present in the submucosa. (Courtesy of Donald Antonioli, M.D.)

Differential Diagnosis

Because of the similarities in clinical presentation, it is often difficult to distinguish Crohn's disease of the colon from ulcerative colitis. However, as noted above, reliance on clinical radiologic, pathologic, and endoscopic features will usually allow the distinction to be made. The majority of patients with Crohn's disease have small bowel involvement, and up to 50 percent will have rectal sparing — both never seen in ulcerative colitis. Up to one third of patients with Crohn's colitis will not have gross bleeding, whereas almost one third of patients will have perianal disease. The focal nature of the lesions pathologically, the presence of granulomas, the asymmetry of the disease, and the segmental distribution with skip lesions, as well as fistula formation, are all characteristic of Crohn's disease and quite atypical for ulcerative colitis.

Diverticulitis, ischemia, and colonic cancer may all be difficult to distinguish from Crohn's colitis because of their presentations, which can mimic a focal colitic process. As in patients with ulcerative colitis, it is critical to rule out bacterial and parasitic causes of colitis.

With regard to small bowel disease, Yersinia can present with an acute picture of ileitis indistinguishable from Crohn's disease except by its time course. Tuberculosis can mimic ileal Crohn's disease completely. A history of exposure to tuberculosis should be sought, and skin tests for tuberculosis should be done. Amoebiasis can be mistaken for Crohn's disease of the distal ileum and cecum. Both lymphoma and ischemia may involve the small intestine and give a clinical and radiologic picture that can be mistaken for Crohn's disease.

Finally, because the findings in early Crohn's disease can be subtle, both lactose intolerance and the irritable bowel syndrome are diagnoses frequently made in patients who subsequently show evidence of Crohn's disease of either the small or large intestine.

Complications   Local complications related to disease activity are part of the clinical picture and include intestinal obstruction, severe hemorrhage, perforation with or without abscess formation, and fistulization. These complications have been discussed previously with regard to the clinical presentation of the disease.

The systemic complications related to inflammatory activity are similar to those seen in ulcerative colitis and include erythema nodosum and pyoderma gangrenosum, uveitis, episcleritis, peripheral arthritis and central arthritis, and hepatobiliary disease. These complications tend to be more frequent in patients with colonic involvement (see Table 7-1).

There are several complications unique to Crohn's disease that occur as a result of small bowel pathophysiology. Bile acids have an enteropathic circulation with absorption in the distal ileum. With severe ileal disease, there is malabsorption of the bile acids and diminution in the size of the bile acid pool. This may lead to the development of gallstones because of the diminution in the bile acid to cholesterol ratio in bile.

Vitamin B_{12}, like bile acids, is absorbed in the distal ileum. Ileal disease can lead to malabsorption of vitamin B_{12} and the creation of a picture of pernicious anemia.

If bile acid malabsorption is severe, there will be too low a level of duodenal bile acids for effective micelle formation and, hence, the development of fat malabsorption or steatorrhea.

This can lead to all the complications of fat malabsorption, including weight loss, diarrhea, clotting abnormalities, and hypocalcemia with osteomalacia, or even tetany. Moreover, when steatorrhea is present, calcium, which normally binds dietary oxalate with excretion in the stool, preferentially binds fatty acids in the bowel lumen. This leaves oxalate free to be absorbed in the colon, leading to hyperoxaluria and the formation of oxalate kidney stones. All these abnormalities can occur with severe ileal Crohn's disease alone, but they tend to be more pronounced in patients who have had extensive ileal resections for their disease.

As with ulcerative colitis, there is an increased incidence of gastrointestinal malignancies in Crohn's disease. The incidence of small bowel cancer is much higher in patients with Crohn's disease than in the normal population, but, because of the rarity of this tumor, the numbers of patients with small bowel carcinoma is small. Many of the cancers that have been described have been found in surgically bypassed loops of the small intestine. The incidence rate of colon cancer in Crohn's disease is a topic of debate. Some studies suggest that the incidence may actually approach that of ulcerative colitis in patients with long-standing disease. To date, surveillance programs analogous to those carried out in ulcerative colitis are not routinely done in patients with Crohn's disease, but such surveillance should be considered for patients who have intact colons and long-standing disease activity.

Treatment

In many respects, the drug therapy of Crohn's disease is similar to that of ulcerative colitis (Table 7-2). Sulfasalazine is efficacious in active Crohn's colitis and ileocolitis, although it does not appear to be as effective in ileitis alone. Unlike its use in ulcerative colitis, sulfasalazine has not been shown to be effective as a prophylactic therapy for disease in remission, nor does it prevent postoperative recurrences. For patients sensitive or allergic to sulfasalazine, one of the new topical or oral 5-ASA preparations may prove effective.

Topical corticoids and parenteral steroids, as in ulcerative colitis, can be effective in limited and severe forms of Crohn's disease. For more moderate disease, oral prednisone is extremely effective in Crohn's ileitis and ileocolitis. For patients with colitis alone, there is some evidence to suggest that prednisone may not be as effective as when there is evidence of ileal disease. Nonetheless, the drug is routinely used for patients with Crohn's colitis. As with sulfasalazine, corticosteroids do not prevent flare-ups of disease in remission or prevent postoperative recurrences. It remains unclear whether sulfasalazine acts

Table 7-2
Drug therapy of inflammatory bowel disease

Drug	Ulcerative colitis	Crohn's disease
Sulfasalazine	Mild to moderate activity	Mild to moderate activity (more useful in colitis than ileitis)
Corticosteroids		
Topical	Proctitis and left-sided colitis	Proctitis and left-sided colitis
Oral	Moderate to severe activity	Moderate to severe activity
Parenteral	Severe or toxic disease	Severe or toxic disease
Immunosuppressives	Steroid sparing Refractory distal disease	Steroid sparing Fistulae Perineal disease Maintenance of remission
Metronidazole	Not useful	Perineal disease Mild to moderate activity (more useful in colitis than ileitis)

in an adjunctive way with steroids, but there is suggestive evidence that in Crohn's colitis, the combination of sulfasalazine and a corticosteroid is more effective than either agent alone.

Immunosuppressive drugs, such as 6-mercaptopurine and azathioprine, have taken on an increasing role in the therapy of Crohn's disease. When given in conjunction with other forms of therapy, these agents may be effective in improving the overall state of well-being, in fistula healing, and in allowing reduction of the dose of corticosteroids. Moreover, the immunosuppressive drugs appear to be effective as long-term maintenance therapy in patients whose disease is in remission.

Metronidazole has recently been added to the list of available agents in the treatment of Crohn's disease. The drug is as useful as sulfasalazine in Crohn's colitis, but, like sulfasalazine, is not as effective in ileitis alone. It may be especially useful in refractory perianal disease when used in high doses for prolonged periods of time.

A variety of oral antibiotics have been suggested, in uncontrolled trials, to be useful in active Crohn's disease. Broad-spectrum antibiotics, given parenterally, clearly have a major role in patients who present with signs of localized peritonitis. Most of these patients have suffered a focal perforation and will respond to bowel rest and antibiotic therapy.

As with ulcerative colitis, the judicious use of antidiarrheal agents can greatly decrease the frequency of bowel movements. Moreover, cholestyramine, a bile salt binding agent, can be especially effective in diminishing the bile salt diarrhea seen in Crohn's disease. Patients who have nonobstructing ileal Crohn's disease or who have had ileal resections can particularly benefit from this agent.

In patients with Crohn's disease who have steatorrhea related to severe ileal disease or extensive ileal resections, a low-fat diet with medium-chain triglyceride oil may diminish the diarrhea and improve the nutritional status. Such patients will often need supplements of calcium, vitamin D, and vitamin K. For patients with disease refractory to medical therapy, total parenteral nutrition may be used in an attempt to induce remission as a primary form of therapy.

Studies suggest that patients with Crohn's disease may have a higher incidence of depression than does the general population. Although, to date, no studies verify the efficacy of psychotherapy in the treatment of Crohn's disease, individual patients can clearly benefit from counseling, formal therapy, and perhaps psychoactive drugs. The same can also be said for patients with ulcerative colitis.

As with ulcerative colitis, surgery plays a major role in the management of patients with Crohn's disease. Some patients come to surgery because of intractable symptoms, despite the whole gamut of pharmacologic and nutritional treatments that are available. Another major indication for surgery in Crohn's disease is that of bowel obstruction, most often in patients who have distal ileal disease with repeated episodes of small bowel obstruction. Surgical resection should be considered in patients who have suffered a local perforation and have evidence of ongoing abscess and in those with bothersome ileocutaneous fistulae and ileovesicle fistulae. Although the latter can be managed conservatively without the threat of progressive renal damage, in most instances, medical therapy fails to heal the fistula, and surgery will be required.

Unfortunately, Crohn's disease usually recurs after resectional therapy, especially after anastomosis. There is a steady rise in the cumulative incidence of postoperative recurrence with time. Despite the high recurrence rate, most patients with Crohn's disease who undergo surgery feel improved with regard to their general psychosocial function. Surgery, therefore, should not be withheld if clearly indicated.

Study Questions 1. A 30-year-old man with known Crohn's ileitis undergoes a 30-cm ileal resection with anastomosis because of obstruction. Following surgery he develops painless, watery diarrhea not associated with abdominal pain, weight loss, or bleeding. Which of the following findings would be likely in the evaluation of the diarrhea?

a. Elevated 72-hour fecal fat
b. Early recurrent disease on x-ray or colonoscopy
c. Abnormal D-xylose absorption
d. Elevated serum gastrin
e. None of the above

Answer

e.

Watery diarrhea following a limited ileal resection is usually due to effects of poorly absorbed bile acids on colonic fluid absorption and secretion. If measured, fecal bile acids would be abnormally elevated. However, only larger resections approaching 100 cm or more result in enough depletion of the bile acid pool to cause maldigestion and steatorrhea.

2. For each of the diagnoses in List I, select the appropriate features from List II.

List I
A. Crohn's disease
B. Ulcerative colitis
C. Both of the above
D. Neither of the above

List II
1. Associated with mucosal ulceration
2. Presence of a perirectal abscess
3. No recurrence after total colectomy
4. Is frequently segmental in its involvement of the intestine
5. Continuous involvement of the entire colon (pancolitis)
6. Associated with arthritis and ankylosing spondylitis
7. Mucosal biopsy is routinely diagnostic of the disease
8. Definite high risk of carcinoma with lengthy, extensive disease

Answers
1. C
2. A
3. B
4. A
5. B
6. C
7. D
8. B

References

Driscoll, R. N., and Rosenberg, I. H. Total parenteral nutrition in inflammatory bowel disease. *Med. Clin. North Am.* 62:185, 1978.

Greenstein, A. J., Janowitz, H. D., and Sachar, D. B. Extraintestinal complications of Crohn's disease and ulcerative colitis: Study of 700 patients. *Medicine* 55:401, 1976.

Greenstein, A. J., Sachar, D. B., Smith, H., et al. Cancer in universal and left-sided ulcerative colitis: Factors determining risk. *Gastroenterology* 77:290, 1979.

Lockhart-Mummery, H. E., and Morson, B. C. Crohn's disease of the large intestine and its distinction from ulcerative colitis. *Gut* 1:89, 1960.

Mekhjian, H. S., Switz, D. M., Melnyk, C. S., et al. Clinical features and natural history of Crohn's disease. *Gastroenterology* 77:898, 1979.

Mendeloff, A. I. The epidemiology of idiopathic inflammatory bowel disease. In J. B. Kirshner and R. G. Starter (eds.), *Inflammatory Bowel Disease* (2nd ed.). Philadelphia: Lea & Febiger, 1980. Pp. 5–23.

Peppercorn, M. A. Sulfasalazine: Pharmacology, clinical use, toxicity and related new drug development. *Ann. Intern. Med.* 101:377, 1984.

Rosenstock, E., Farmer, R. G., Petrus, P., et al. Surveillance for colonic carcinoma in ulcerative colitis. *Gastroenterology* 89:1342, 1985.

Sachar, D. B., Wolfson, D. M., Greenstein, A. J., et al. Risk factors for post-operative recurrence in Crohn's disease. *Gastroenterology* 85:917, 1983.

Sack, D., and Peppercorn, M. A. Drug therapy of inflammatory bowel disease. *Pharmacotherapy* 3:158, 1983.

Sparberg, M., and Fenessy, J. Ulcerative proctitis and mild ulcerative colitis: A study of 220 patients. *Medicine* 45:391, 1966.

Taylor, B. M., Beart, R. W., Jr., Dozors, R. R., et al. The endorectal ileal pouch — anal anastomosis. *Dis. Colon Rectum* 27:347, 1984.

8 : Vascular Insufficiency of the Bowel

T. Edward Bynum

Anatomy

The intraabdominal gastrointestinal tract is supplied by the celiac axis, superior mesenteric artery, and inferior mesenteric artery. The superior mesenteric artery is the largest single branch of the aorta. The microcirculation of the bowel is composed of series-coupled (consecutive) and parallel-coupled vascular elements. The series elements consist of the arterioles, the precapillary sphincters, the capillaries, and the venules. The arterioles are the major site of resistance to blood flow; the precapillary sphincters determine capillary perfusion; the capillaries are the site of molecular and fluid exchange; and the venules act as capacitance vessels. The parallel elements consist of blood vessels in the parallel wall layers of the bowel. In the submucosa, there is an extensive arteriole network. The muscularis propria is supplied by several arterial branches.

Another way to consider the vasculature is by order of branching. The mesenteric artery branches into small mesenteric arteries. From there arises a first-order arteriole that penetrates both layers of the muscularis propria and courses along the submucosa. In the submucosa arise second- and third-order arterioles. The third-order arterioles give off branches to the muscle as well as other branches that supply the mucosa up to the tip of individual villi.

Within the villus, the main arteriole passes through the core of the villus, giving rise to smaller branches that supply the capillary network. Several capillaries drain into a small venule, and subsequently several small venules carry blood to a larger venule at the base of the villus.

The two main vessels draining blood from the bowel are the superior and inferior mesenteric veins. The splenic vein drains blood from the lower esophagus, stomach, spleen, and head of the pancreas. The juncture of the superior mesenteric and splenic veins forms the portal vein, whose blood flow constitutes one fifth of the total venous return to the heart.

Branches of the superior and inferior mesenteric arteries anastomose to form a continuous arterial pathway that courses parallel to the long axis of the colon; this anastomotic pathway is designated the "marginal artery of Drummond."

The walls of arterioles are composed chiefly of vascular smooth muscle, which reacts to changes in the biochemical environment, such as the PO_2 of the tissue and the presence of catecholamines. The rate of blood flow to the bowel is regulated by changes in the tension of the walls of these arterioles. Changes in the tension of the smooth muscle of these vascular walls can markedly alter the cross-sectional area of arterial flow. For example, norepinephrine can markedly reduce bowel blood flow by increasing smooth-muscle tension in the arteriolar walls, thereby reducing the radius of these vessels and raising the mechanical resistance to blood flow. A vasodilator agent has the opposite effects: It relaxes the muscle in the walls, increases the radius of the vessel lumen, increases the cross-sectional area, decreases mechanical resistance, and increases blood flow. Because arterioles control the mechanical impedance to blood flow, they have been termed the *resistance vessels* of the mesenteric circulation.

Nearly all the exchange of water, ions, organic solutes, gases, and heat between the cells of the body and the blood occurs across the walls of the capillaries. Thereby, the capillaries have been termed the *exchange vessels* of the mesenteric circulation. Not all the capillaries are open to the flow of blood (and therefore do not participate in exchange) at any point in time. What determines the availability of the particular capillary to blood flow is a smooth-muscle thickening at the beginning of the capillary, which is known as the precapillary sphincter. Precapillary sphincters relax in response to chemical changes in their environment that have usually occurred because of changes in the metabolic activity of nearby cells. Capillaries offer much less resistance to blood flow compared with arterioles; therefore, relaxation of precapillary sphincters is not accompanied by a major increase in blood flow. What does occur is an increase in oxygen consumption. Thus, when active transport of sodium and glucose occurs in the small intestine, there can be a 25 percent increase in oxygen consumption, accompanied by an 8 percent increase in blood flow.

The venules act as flexible reservoirs for blood (as well as acting as conduits to get "used" blood back to the heart) and have been termed the *capacitance vessels* of the mesenteric circulation.

Physiology

About half the mass of the intestinal wall is composed of the mucosa; the mucosa receives two thirds of the total blood flow.

Several factors control mesenteric blood flow. These can be organized under extrinsic and intrinsic factors. Extrinsic factors are systemic circulatory events, the autonomic nervous system, and vasoactive hormones. Intrinsic factors are changes in the metabolic environment, paracrine substances, autoregulation, and bowel distention. Systemic circulatory factors are the hemodynamic forces and physical aspects of the overall circulation, which deliver blood to the mesenteric circulation. These include systemic arterial blood pressure, total blood volume and cardiac output, and the viscosity of the blood. Any significant changes in the functional state of the heart, the blood, or the major vessels will greatly alter mesenteric blood flow. Acute hemorrhage of severe proportions will cause marked reductions in arterial blood pressure and cardiac output and increases peripheral vascular resistance; subsequently, mesenteric blood flow is reduced markedly in this circumstance.

The autonomic nervous system has direct and indirect effects on blood flow. Direct effects involve sympathetic, postganglionic vasomotor nerves, which release norepinephrine at alpha-adrenergic receptors located on the smooth muscle of resistance and capacitance vessels in the microcirculation. This leads to vasoconstriction with decreased blood flow and decreased venous capacitance. Indirect effects increase blood flow in two ways. First, parasympathetic fibers release acetylcholine adjacent to muscarinic receptors located on mucosal epithelial cells and smooth-muscle cells of the muscularis; this results in increased secretory and motor activity of the bowel, which increases local metabolism and leads to increased blood flow to support these stimulated functions. Second, if there is general activation of the sympathetic nervous system in the body, the adrenal medulla releases epinephrine, which stimulates beta-adrenergic receptors in the heart and peripheral vessels, resulting in a more forceful and more rapidly beating heart with increased cardiac output. At the same time, there is reduced resistance to blood flow in the bowel, and blood flow increases.

Intrinsic events and agents are present within the bowel itself and are important in controlling blood flow there. These include parenchymal metabolism, paracrine substances, autoregulation, and bowel distention. When secretion, active absorption, or motility are occurring, the responsible parenchymal cells consume more oxygen and release more CO_2. This changes the metabolic environment in a way that relaxes the smooth muscle of nearby resistance and exchange vessels. The increased blood flow, in turn, delivers more oxygen to the stimulated parenchymal cells and carries away waste products such as CO_2 and lactate. Paracrine substances ("hormone"-like chemicals released locally with local action) that are believed to be vasoactive in the intestinal circulation include histamine, serotonin, adenosine, certain prostaglandins, and some peptides. Autoregulation refers to the ability of certain organs to maintain a normal blood flow in the face of a decrease in mean systemic blood pressure. This occurs to a striking degree in the small intestine and somewhat less in the colon. When the bowel is severely distended, it can be accompanied by a decrease in blood flow. Such severe distention occurs only in extreme pathological conditions and is almost never seen in normal circumstances.

Pathology

In ischemic bowel disease, the gross appearance of the bowel depends on the severity and depth of injury. The external appearance of the bowel may be normal if the necrotic lesion is limited to the mucosa. When the muscularis propria of the involved portion of the bowel is ischemic but not necrotic, the muscle can contract spastically; the bowel then shows irregular shortening and sacculation. When ischemic necrosis and infarction are deep and extensive, the color of the bowel ranges from dusky gray to the frankly greenish black color that represents gangrene. Microscopically, mild mucosal ischemia exhibits a coagulative-type necrosis, often with a "ghost" appearance of the surface epithelial cells and crypts. Frequently, capillaries are distended. In the region between ischemic and normal tissue, segmented white cells are abundant and crypt abscesses are present. With more extensive ischemic necrosis, the coagulative "ghosting" and hemorrhage can extend into submucosa, muscularis propria, and even to the serosa. At times, mucosal sloughing occurs, resulting in ulcer craters of varying depth. Particularly in the colon, ischemic damage can lead to a chronic scar, often with some degree of stricture. Under the microscope, this appears as dense fibrous tissue with marked granulation tissue and thin reepithelialization over the scar.

Pathophysiology

Ischemic disease of the bowel is either occlusive or nonocclusive, with the prevalence being approximately 50 percent for each. Occlusive ischemic disease is relatively obvious and represents some type of mechanical obstruction to the flow of blood in those vessels that supply the bowel. Vascular occlusion in large and medium arteries can be caused by emboli, surgical ligation, thrombosis (often on an atheromatous plaque), or tumor. Emboli, from an artificial mitral valve or a fibrillating atrium, and surgical bypass, especially consequent to vascular surgery involving the distal aorta, are the most common. Small artery occlusion is usually due to some type of inflammatory disease of those vessels (arteritis) or to showers of small emboli. Venous occlusion is a rare cause of ischemic bowel disease. In medium and large veins, occlusion is due to thrombosis often related to hypercoagulable states such as polycythemia vera, paroxysmal nocturnal hemoglobinuria, or the use of birth control pills. Most small vein thrombosis appears to be secondary to bowel ischemia caused by nonocclusive mechanisms. Nonocclusive ischemia results from failure in blood flow. Here, there is no mechanical occlusion, or the mechanical narrowing (atherosclerosis, arteriosclerosis) does not by itself account for any reduction in blood flow to the intestine. In nonocclusive ischemic disease, the defect is a reduction in blood flow associated with either circulatory shock and hypotension or with heart failure in which there is a significant decrease in cardiac output (even without detectable hypotension). Therefore, nonocclusive ischemia is usually related to a severe derangement in the central circulation and is a consequence of such conditions as congestive heart failure, myocardial infarction, major hemorrhage, sepsis, cardiac arrhythmias, severe dehydration, severe cardiac valve disease, or administration of vasoconstrictive drugs. The intravenous administration of cardiac glycosides or digitalis toxicity have caused nonocclusive ischemia.

The pathological and clinical result is the same whether ischemic disease is due to occlusive or to nonocclusive mechanisms. Nonocclusive ischemia seems potentially more reversible, but actual reversibility may be difficult if patients are elderly and have irreversible and severe cardiac disease. Furthermore, reperfusion after nonocclusive ischemia contributes to the injury by creating toxic chemical radicals. On the other hand, the extent and severity of occlusive ischemia may be less severe than one would imagine, because of the richness of collateral blood supply to the intestine, which can play a beneficial part if central circulatory mechanisms are intact. Most ischemic bowel disease, whether occlusive or nonocclusive, is rather acute. Rarely, the intestine may suffer chronic ischemia, almost always owing to severe occlusive lesions in the vasculature. In this circumstance, the demands for increased blood supply made necessary by a functioning mucosa cannot be met by the diseased and occluded circulation. This results in a clinical syndrome that is expressed as either abdominal angina (pain while eating a meal) or malabsorption.

Clinical Considerations

Ischemic disease of the bowel varies in severity across a wide spectrum — all the way from transient hypoxia of the villus tips (perhaps accompanied by premature sloughing of a few epithelial cells at the tip of the villus) to complete transmural infarction of that segment of the bowel. Obviously, the more the situation is toward the former, the more reversible things can be. Transmural bowel infarction is not reversible. In between, a patient may develop severe ulceration, which can ultimately heal if perfusion is reestablished but may leave scarring and stricture.

Ischemic bowel disease is clinically quite different when it involves the small intestine as opposed to the colon. The mechanisms can be either occlusive or nonocclusive in either location. However, ischemia of the small bowel is a much more severe disease. It (1) is less often reversible, (2) more often goes on to complete infarction, (3) more often requires resection of bowel, and (4) far more often leads to death of the patient. For example, one collected series of patients with small bowel ischemia reported a 90 percent fatality rate. The fatality rate in ischemic disease of the colon is almost the reciprocal of that, being less than 10 percent, closer to 5 percent. Even what initially appears to be severe ischemic damage to the colon is often totally reversible with little if any ultimate residual as long as perfusion can be reestablished.

Ischemic bowel disease frequently occurs in the setting of known compromises in the general or local circulation. In other words, it is most common in elderly persons with known cardiac disease or generalized vascular disease, or in patients of any age group who have suffered significant hemorrhage or sepsis. Occasionally, there does not seem to be any background association with cardiovascular disease or other circulatory disturbance, but, often, if one looks carefully, one can identify a mitral valve source of emboli or discover that the patient is taking birth control pills.

Acute small bowel ischemia usually presents as moderate to severe abdominal pain, usually cramping in nature. Frequently, patients will have nausea and anorexia. Early in the course of the disease, the abdominal pain will be totally out of proportion to any physical finding. In other words, patients frequently have normal bowel sounds, a soft abdomen without tenderness or rebound, and a normal plain film of the abdomen. Therefore, if the patient has a background that suggests the possibility of ischemic bowel disease, one should not wait for typical physical findings to develop. Once such findings have developed, it indicates that transmural infarction has taken place, and the possibility of rescuing the patient's bowel or the patient's life is greatly diminished. Ischemic disease of the colon, also known as ischemic colitis, usually presents as bloody diarrhea, often but not always accompanied by cramping abdominal pain. If barium contrast radiographic studies are obtained (not always advisable), they may show what is known as "thumb-printing" (Figs. 8-1 and 8-2). This is due to focal areas of submucosal

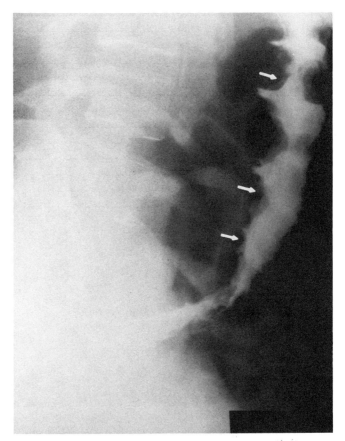

Fig. 8-1
Barium enema showing nodular impressions and irregularity ("thumb-printing") of the descending colon in a patient with ischemic colitis *(arrows)*.

hemorrhage or edema. It is believed to be quite characteristic for ischemic disease of the bowel, but it also occurs in Crohn's disease, clostridia toxin disease, and submucosal hemorrhage owing to overdose of anticoagulant medication.

Ischemic colitis has a clinical presentation that can be similar to ulcerative colitis. Its radiographic and endoscopic appearance can mimic that of ulcerative colitis, Crohn's colitis, or clostridia toxin colitis. Traditionally, it has been believed that ischemic colitis occurs characteristically at or around the splenic flexure. The explanation for this belief was that the splenic flexure is supposed to be a "water-shed" region for the colonic arterial blood supply, representing the zone between that part of the colon supplied by the superior mesenteric artery and that supplied by the inferior mesenteric artery. The "water-shed" was

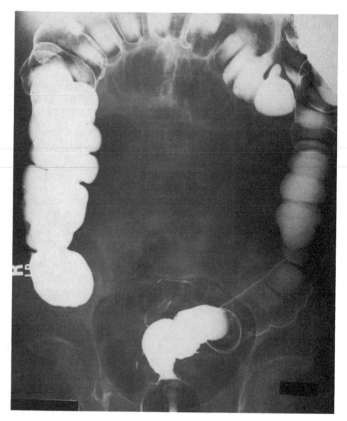

Fig. 8-2
Repeat study 4 weeks later showing complete healing of the lesion.

assumed to be relatively deprived of blood flow. However, there is no basis for this assumption; ischemic disease of the colon is not more common right at the splenic flexure.

If one suspects ischemic disease of the small bowel, everything possible should be done to improve and enhance the extrinsic factors involved in blood flow to the intestine; that is, if possible, hemorrhage should be stopped, blood volume restored, cardiac output enhanced, cardiac failure corrected, and so on. Once that has been accomplished as quickly as possible, the next step is mesenteric angiography. This will readily distinguish occlusive mesenteric vascular disease from nonocclusive disease. (One must remember that the mesenteric vasculature may appear entirely normal in patients who genuinely have nonocclusive small bowel ischemia, even with small bowel infarction.) If the patient has occlusive disease, measures must be considered to mechanically remove or bypass the occlusion. If the angiogram is compatible with nonocclusive disease, further measures must be undertaken to enhance the general circulatory situation. Additionally, one can consider the administration of vasodilator medications, often directly into the mesenteric circulation by means of the angiographic catheter. The role of angiography is very limited in ischemic colitis.

The reasons for the dramatic discrepancy in clinical severity and prognosis for ischemic disease of the small bowel compared with that for ischemic disease of the colon are not readily apparent. One might expect ischemia of the colon to have a worse outcome. The normal colon harbors an immense quantity of bacteria, including large numbers of gram-negative and anaerobic organisms. Ischemia could be expected to disrupt the barrier function of the colonic epithelium that separates the luminal contents (feces as well as large quantities of bacteria) from the systemic circulation. Disruption of this barrier ought to allow colon bacteria and bacterial products (e.g., endotoxin) access into the systemic circulation. Then, one might expect colon ischemia to lead to sepsis. Small bowel ischemia only rarely leads to bacteremia or sepsis (as one would expect), but events resulting from small bowel ischemia suggest clinical deterioration owing to some type of circulating toxin, perhaps represented by vasoactive or cardiodepressant peptides released into the circulation from ischemic small bowel mucosa.

Study Questions
1. A 60-year-old woman with diabetes experiences the subacute onset of crampy, left lower quadrant abdominal pain with watery diarrhea that becomes bloody. On admission, she is afebrile with a blood pressure of 160/90 mm Hg and a pulse of 110 per minute. Examination of the abdomen reveals it to be soft with moderate left lower quadrant tenderness but no evidence of peritoneal signs (rigidity, involuntary guarding). On sigmoidoscopy, the rectal mucosa is unremarkable, but the sigmoid mucosa is inflamed with mild bleeding. An abdominal film reveals "thumb printing" in the left colon. Answer true or false:
   a. The colonic lesion most likely resulted from a cardiac embolus to the inferior mesenteric artery.
   b. The most prudent management calls for immediate exploratory laparotomy.
   c. The lesion described will most likely resolve with conservative management.
   d. One potential sequel is a stricture of the involved segment of the colon.

   Answers
   a. False
   b. False
   c. True
   d. True

This patient has sustained an episode of ischemic colitis that is thought to result from a transient state of "low-flow" to the affected colonic segment. Spontaneous recovery is the rule although on occasion a stricture can result.

2. A 54-year-old woman is admitted to the intensive care unit with gram-negative sepsis secondary to acute pyelonephritis. On admission her systolic blood pressure is 70 mm Hg. She is treated with intravenous fluids, antibiotics, and dopamine. Six hours after admission she complains of mild abdominal pain that progresses in severity over the next 12 hours and then develops nausea. On physical examination she is noted to have mild abdominal distention with diffuse mild tenderness and hypoactive bowel sounds. A plain x-ray of the abdomen reveals dilated loops of small bowel. An abdominal angiogram is performed and demonstrates no occlusion or significant stenosis of the mesenteric arteries. Answer true or false:

a. The angiographic study has excluded mesenteric ischemia as a cause of her abdominal symptoms.
b. Progression to transmural bowel infarction is possible.
c. Optimization of systemic hemodynamics is an important step in the management of such patients.

Answers
a. False
b. True
c. True

This patient has mesenteric ischemia related to systemic hypotension with resulting splanchnic vasoconstriction (nonocclusive ischemia). If prolonged this process can lead to transmural bowel infarction. Attempts to rectify the systemic hemodynamic abnormalities can restore the splanchnic circulation with resulting resolution of the ischemia.

References

Bynum, T. E. Vascular Disease of the Intestine. In J. H. Stein (ed.), *Internal Medicine* (2nd ed.). Boston: Little, Brown, 1987.

Bynum, T. E., and Jacobson E. D. Nonocclusive intestinal ischemia. *Arch. Int. Med.* 139:281, 1987.

Bynum, T. E., and Jacobson E. D. Vascular Disorders of the Large Bowel. In J. B. Kirshner and R. G. Shorter (eds.), *Diseases of the Colon, Rectum and Anal Canal.* Baltimore: Williams & Wilkins, 1987.

Bynum, T. E., Gallavan, R. H., and Jacobson, E. D. The Pathophysiology of Nonocclusive Intestinal Ischemia. In A. P. Shepherd and D. N. Granger (eds.), *Physiology of the Intestinal Circulation.* New York: Raven, 1984.

Cooperman, M. *Intestinal Ischemia.* Mount Kisco, New York: Futura, 1983.

Tepperman, B. L., and Jacobson, E. D. Mesenteric Circulation. In L. R. Johnson (ed.), *Physiology of the Gastrointestinal Tract.* New York: Raven, 1981.

9 : Motor Disorders of the Gastrointestinal Tract

Roger J. May

The motor activity of the gastrointestinal tract is responsible for (1) transporting swallowed food into the stomach, (2) breaking solid food into small particles, (3) mixing it with digestive enzymes, (4) assisting in the absorption of digested food, and (5) transporting the undigested residue toward the rectum for eventual expulsion. In this chapter, we will discuss the normal and abnormal motor activity of the stomach, small intestine, and colon. Motor disorders of the esophagus are discussed in Chap. 1.

The motor segments of the alimentary tract consist of functionally distinct compartments that are connected to each other. Despite major differences in function and motor control, the different segments of the alimentary canal have a similar overall structural organization (Fig. 9-1). The wall of the alimentary canal consists of an outer layer of longitudinal muscle and an inner layer of circular muscle (muscularis externa). Between these two layers of smooth muscle lies the myenteric plexus, the network of intramural neurons that is essential for all coordinated and organized motor activity. The extrinsic (e.g., autonomic) nerves exert their effects on gastrointestinal motility by means of these enteric nerves. Internal to the layer of the muscular externa is the submucosa, which contains the submucosal ganglia. The physiology of the submucosal ganglia is not well understood, but this component of the enteric nervous system may regulate contractions of the muscularis mucosae and modify mucosal absorption and secretion through excitatory and inhibitory neurotransmitters. The innermost layer of the gastrointestinal tract is the mucosa, which is in contact with luminal contents and mediates absorption and secretion.

The motor activity of the gastrointestinal tract plays a major role in the physiology of this organ system. Although the stomach and segments of the small and large bowel act as a series of chambers in series, nevertheless, the motor activity of the stomach, small bowel, and large bowel are sufficiently distinct that their physiology and pathophysiology should be discussed separately.

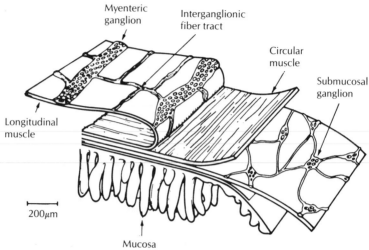

Fig. 9-1
Schematic drawing of the wall of the small intestine showing the different layers of the wall. Note the myenteric ganglion between the longitudinal muscle and the circular muscle, and the submucosal ganglion between the circular muscle and the mucosa. (From J. D. Wood. Physiology of the Enteric Nervous System. In L. R. Johnson (ed.), *Physiology of the Gastrointestinal Tract*. New York: Raven, 1981.)

Motor Functions of the Stomach

The motor activity of the stomach has at least two functions. First, the stomach acts as a reservoir to accommodate the large volume of solid and liquid contained within a meal and to deliver the ingested food into the duodenum at a rate compatible with optimal digestion. Second, the stomach acts to disperse and pulverize solids such that they are reduced to a particle size compatible with optimal digestion. The stomach achieves these functions by the contributions of two distinctly different regions of motor activity — the proximal and distal stomach.

With respect to motor activity, the proximal stomach consists of the fundus and the orad third of the gastric body. Intracellular and extracellular recordings of smooth muscle in this region have demonstrated a steady resting electrical potential with no spontaneous fluctuation in electrical activity. Intracellular recordings have suggested that the contractions of the proximal stomach result from small, slow depolarizations that are not associated with spike burst activity.

This electrical activity results in a predominant motor activity characterized by slow sustained contractions with durations of 1 to 3 minutes per contraction and amplitudes of 10 to 50 cm of water. The electrical activity, and hence the contractions, are subject to both inhibitory and excitatory effects. The vagus nerves contain neurons that indeed do have both excitatory and inhibitory effects on the motor function of the proximal

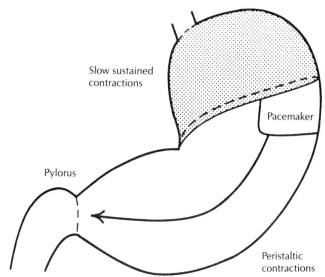

Fig. 9-2

Proximal stomach (*shaded area*) has slow sustained contractions that regulate the emptying of liquids. Distal stomal has peristaltic contractions that sweep aborally from gastric pacemaker to pylorus and control the emptying of solids. (From K. A. Kelly. Gastric motility after gastric operations. *Surg. Annu.* 6:103, 1974.)

stomach. The sympathetic innervation of this region mediates additional inhibitory effects. In addition, humoral agents influence proximal motor activity. Motilin, a gastrointestinal peptide, stimulates motor activity in this region, whereas all other gastrointestinal peptide hormones (e.g., gastrin, cholecystokinin, and secretin) inhibit proximal contractions.

The slow sustained contractions in the proximal stomach press gastric contents aborally toward the distal stomach and the duodenum. These contractions play a major role in the emptying of liquids but only a minor role in the emptying of solids. With respect to solids, these contractions hasten the movement of food into the antrum where the grinding contractions effect the fragmentation of the food necessary for normal emptying (Fig. 9-2).

The proximal stomach plays a major role in the reservoir function of the stomach. This region relaxes to accommodate the increasing volume of a meal. This phenomenon (receptive relaxation and accommodation) is important since the gastric emptying of liquids is a function of the pressure gradient between the stomach and the duodenum. With receptive relaxation, the stomach can accommodate increasing volumes without increasing gastric pressure and hence with little effect on the emptying of liquids. Receptive relaxation is mediated by inhibitory effects

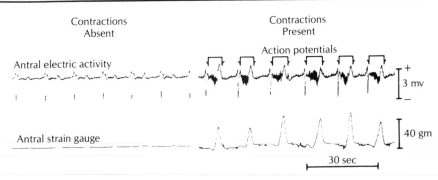

Fig. 9-3
Relationship between antral electrical activity (slow waves), action potentials (spike bursts), and muscular contractions. Note that action potentials are superimposed on the slow waves and result in contractions. (From K. A. Kelly. Gastric motility after gastric operations. *Surg. Annu.* 6:103, 1974.)

of the vagus nerve, which decrease the amplitude and frequency of the tonic contractions of the fundus. With vagotomy, this phenomenon is abolished, and, in this setting, increasing gastric volumes of solids or liquids are associated with increased gastric pressures and hence increased rates of gastric emptying. These disordered pressures and hence abnormal gastric emptying are, in part, the mechanisms of "dumping" in patients who have been subjected to a bilateral truncal vagotomy (transection of the main trunks of the vagus nerve).

The electrical activity of the distal stomach is quite distinctive and distinguishes this region from the less electrically active proximal stomach. Extracellular recordings from the smooth muscle of the distal stomach reveal slow cyclic changes in the membrane potential. These cyclic changes have been labeled *pacemaker potentials* or slow wave activity, since they do not initiate smooth muscle contraction themselves but do determine the timing and location of the action potentials (spike bursts) that produce muscle contractions. These cycles of slow waves (SW) originate in a region of the greater curvature near the junction of the proximal and middle third of the corpus. They have a regular rhythm of three cycles per minute in humans and move distally toward the pylorus at an accelerating rate (0.5 cm/second in the corpus and increasing to 4 cm/second in the distal antrum) (Fig. 9-3).

Action potentials are the electrical phenomena associated with the contractions of the gastric smooth muscles. The timing of action potentials is in phase with the SWs, but not all SWs have an associated action potential. Furthermore, when an action potential is superimposed on a SW, the resulting contraction may occur at a single location or may be propagated over a variable

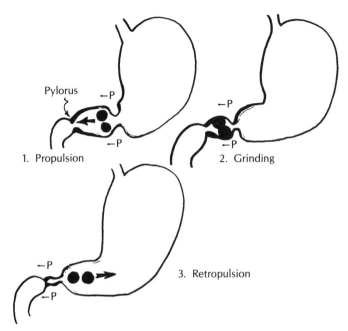

Pylorus

1. Propulsion

2. Grinding

3. Retropulsion

Fig. 9-4
The sequence of propulsion, grinding, and retropulsion by postprandial antral peristalsis (P). The process results in thorough mixing of gastric contents with gastric secretions and disperses solids into smaller pieces. (From K. A. Kelly. Motility of the Stomach and Gastroduodenal Junction. In L. R. Johnson (ed.), *Physiology of the Gastrointestinal Tract*. New York: Raven, 1981.)

distance. Some contractions arise in the pacemaker region and sweep distally to the gastroduodenal junction. In the postprandial stomach, the contractions do not usually occlude the lumen but rather propel the chyme, which is near the gastric wall, toward the pylorus and allow the contents in the more central lumen to move backward toward the proximal stomach (Fig. 9-4). In contrast, in the fasting stomach, contractions do completely occlude the lumen and propel the luminal contents distally as the affected region of the stomach empties into the duodenum.

The SW potential is an intrinsic property of the intestinal smooth muscle cells and is not affected by neural or hormonal stimulation. Stimulation by these factors, however, can affect the frequency of the action potentials and, hence, of the muscular contractions. The vagal nerves contain neurons that have both inhibitory and excitatory effects on motor functions of the distal stomach, as they do in the proximal stomach. For the most part, vagal stimulation or activity enhances contractions of the distal stomach and mediates gastric peristalsis. Indeed, following vagotomy, gastric motor activity is abolished.

Sympathetic innervation of the distal stomach mediates inhibitory effects on gastric motility. Among the hormones, gastrin, cholecystokinin, and motilin enhance gastric motor activity and peristalsis, although, to date, gastrin is the only hormone that appears to have a physiologic role in gastric motility. Secretin, gastric inhibitory polypeptide, and glucagon have inhibitory effects, but it is unclear whether these effects are physiologic.

The predominant effects of distal gastric contractions are to mix the chyme with gastric secretions and to fragment and triturate ingested solids. Peristalsis propels the solids into the antrum and toward the pylorus. However, contraction of the distal antrum results in almost complete occlusion of the pylorus, so that only liquids and extremely small particles are able to pass into the duodenum. Particles greater than 0.1 mm in size are propelled backward toward the proximal stomach (see Fig. 9-4). The shearing effect of these contractions on the to-and-fro movement of the larger particles disperses them into successively smaller particles. When the solid food has been reduced to particles of approximately 0.1 mm in size, peristalsis is able to carry this finally dispersed portion into the duodenum. Poorly digestible solids, such as dietary fiber, and indigestible solids, such as experimental markers, are retained in the postprandial stomach, since the grinding activity of the distal antrum cannot reduce them to particles of sufficiently small size. Such solids are emptied slowly or not at all during the postprandial period and are not completely emptied until the appearance of cyclic fasting motor activity, which is able to empty the stomach completely of all retained material.

The pylorus does not appear to function as a physiologic sphincter. In fasting human subjects, experimental studies using manometric (pressure-sensitive) probes have failed to demonstrate an increased resting pressure in the pyloric channel. Under basal conditions, therefore, the pylorus is patent. The narrow lumen of the pylorus at the gastroduodenal junction does not provide a barrier to the flow of liquids but does provide resistance to the emptying of solids, as described previously.

Coordination between gastric and duodenal contractions also plays a role in gastric emptying. As gastric contents are propelled through the gastroduodenal junction, the proximal duodenum relaxes and allows the chyme (dispersed food) to enter. As the contractions of the distal antrum are completed and close the pylorus, the proximal duodenum then contracts and propels luminal contents into the distal duodenum. The absence of this coordination could thus impair gastric emptying

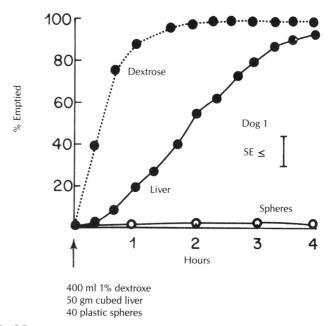

400 ml 1% dextroxe
50 gm cubed liver
40 plastic spheres

Fig. 9-5
Patterns of canine gastric emptying of a liquid (dextrose), a digestible solid (liver), and an indigestible solid (spheres) after their simultaneous ingestion. (From R. A. Hinder and K. A. Kelly. Canine gastric emptying of solids and liquids. *Am. J. Physiol.* 233:E335, 1977.)

by either increasing duodenal resistance during gastric emptying or by increasing duodenogastric reflux during periods of pyloric patency.

The stomach, therefore, has the ability to empty different constituents of a meal at different rates. Of all the constituents, liquids are emptied at the most rapid rate. For example, 50 percent of a 500-ml load of saline is emptied in 12 minutes in humans. Liquids that are hyperosmolar or of a more complex nutritional content empty at a slower rate. Digestible solids empty at a slower rate than do liquids. For example, in canine studies, 50 percent of a meal of 50 gm of cubed liver is emptied in 2 hours. Finally, as mentioned previously, indigestible solids are retained by the postprandial stomach such that particles greater than 2 mm in size are not emptied after a meal and do not leave the stomach until the reappearance of fasting motor activity (Fig. 9-5).

The composition of the meal may have additional effects on the rate of gastric emptying. For example, carbohydrate is emptied more quickly than protein, which, in turn, is emptied more quickly than fat. Furthermore, the acidity of gastric contents also slows emptying such that a meal of pH 7.0 empties more rapidly than does a more acidic meal. In addition, an inverse relationship exists between osmolarity and gastric emptying such that hyperosmolar meals empty more slowly than do isotonic ones. These "braking" effects are mediated through specific receptors in the proximal small bowel that regulate gastric emptying through feedback mechanisms that are both neural and hormonal in nature.

In summary, the motor activity of the postprandial stomach allows the stomach to (1) store the ingested meal, (2) triturate the chyme into small particles, and (3) empty the chyme into the duodenum at a rate optimal for digestion. The proximal stomach relaxes to accommodate the meal and regulates the emptying of liquids through changes in intragastric pressure. The contractions of the distal stomach fragment and disperse the chyme and regulate the emptying of solids through the sieving effects of the gastroduodenal junction. Finally, coordination between gastric and duodenal motor activity and feedback regulation through intestinal receptors enhances and optimizes the emptying with respect to efficient digestion.

Manometric studies using pressure-sensitive probes enable the characterization of gastric motor activity. Motor activity in the fasting stomach is distinctly different from that in the postprandial stomach. During the interdigestive (fasting) period, there are four periods of variable motor activity that occur in a cyclic fashion. During Phase 1, which lasts 45 to 60 minutes, few, if any, contractions occur in the stomach. During Phase 2, which lasts 30 to 45 minutes, intermittent contractions are propagated distally over short distances. This is followed by Phase 3, which lasts 5 to 15 minutes and is characterized by rhythmic (3 cycles/minute), strong (50 mm Hg) propulsive contractions. The cycle is completed by Phase 4, a brief, 5-minute period of decreasing contractions, which is then followed by Phase 1, as the cycle repeats itself. The period of an entire cycle (Phase 1 → Phase 1) is approximately 2 hours, and each phase of the cycle passes aborally through the stomach, duodenum, and small intestine. The succession of cycles has been termed the *migrating motor complex* (MMC) (Fig. 9-6A). Phase 3 originates in the proximal stomach, and, as it migrates through the distal stomach, the powerful contractions propel gastric contents through the patent pylorus. These intense propulsive contractions are the predominant mechanism by which dietary fiber and indigestible solids leave the stomach during the interdigestive period. The MMC activity is abruptly abolished by feeding and returns within 2 to 4 hours of a meal, depending on the nutritional composition of the meal. The postprandial motor pattern is

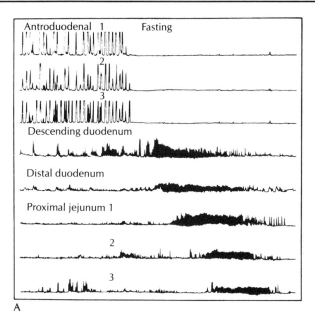

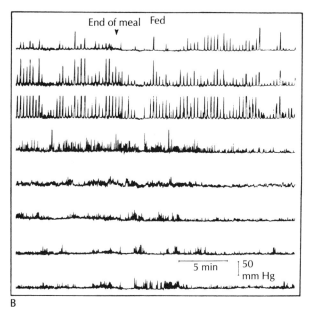

Fig. 9-6
Normal gastrointestinal motility. A. Normal migrating motor complex during the fasting period. Note the intense activity front (Phase 3) passing from the antrum into the duodenum and jejunum. B. Normal fed phase characterized by persistent antral and intestinal phasic pressure activity. (Reprinted by permission from Malagelada, J. R., et al.: *Manometric Diagnosis of Gastrointestinal Motility Disorders*, Thieme Medical Publishers, New York, 1986.)

characterized by frequent, irregular contractions of high amplitude in the distal stomach (Fig. 9-6B).

The coordination and propagation of the MMC in the distal stomach is mediated, in large part, by the vagus nerve, since truncal vagotomy abolishes MMC activity in the distal stomach and results in retention of solids. Other factors may be operative. Cyclic rises in the serum levels of motilin appear to correspond to the origination of Phase 3 in the stomach, but it is unclear whether the changes in the motilin level stimulate the MMC or modulate the cycle that has been initiated by some other mechanism. Indeed, in canine studies, surgical duodenectomy lowers serum motilin levels and abolishes gastric MMC activity, even though neural innervation of the stomach remains intact; therefore, the initiation and modulation of gastric MMC activity is probably multifactorial.

Gastric Emptying

Methods of Measurement

Radiographic techniques, such as the barium upper gastrointestinal (UGI) series, are relatively insensitive methods of measuring gastric emptying and hence of detecting gastric retention. Such studies are helpful in ruling out gastric outlet obstruction (e.g., pyloric channel ulcer, cancer) as a cause of gastric retention. Patients with disabling symptoms of gastroparesis (motility-related delay in gastric emptying), however, can have normal-appearing barium studies. This lack of sensitivity is due to the fact that: (1) the suspension of barium behaves as a liquid that empties more easily than a solid; (2) the high density of barium probably effects more rapid emptying of the suspension; and (3) these studies are performed in fasting patients and do not measure the more complex, postprandial motor activity. When barium studies do document gastric retention, subtle forms of mechanical outlet obstruction must be ruled out by gastroscopy before a firm diagnosis of gastroparesis can be made.

Radionuclide scintigraphy is a much more sensitive technique for the measurement of gastric emptying. The liquid component of the meal is labeled with the radionuclide indium (In 111). Either egg (egg salad, scrambled egg whites) or chicken liver is labeled with technetium (Tc 99^m) and can serve as a marker of the solid component of the meal. Following ingestion of radiolabeled solid and liquid meal, the patient reclines under a scintiscanner that measures the initial level of intragastric radioactivity. The scintiscanner then measures the rate of passage of radioactivity out of the stomach (i.e., gastric emptying). Differential rates of solid and liquid emptying can be detected. The rate of emptying of the solid component depends on the complexity of the test meal; for example, 50 percent of labeled egg whites is emptied in 50 minutes (T ½), whereas labeled chicken liver consumed with a balanced meal is emptied in 150 minutes.

Disorders

From the aforementioned discussion, it is apparent that gastric emptying can be impaired by any of three mechanisms: (1) pyloric obstruction, (2) dysfunction of the vagus or intrinsic gastric nerves, and (3) dysfunction of the gastric smooth muscle. Mechanical factors producing pyloric obstruction include peptic ulcer of the pyloric channel or duodenal cap (see Chap. 3), and malignancy of the distal stomach (see Chap. 4). Causes of neuromuscular dysfunction leading to delayed gastric emptying (gastroparesis) are discussed in the following paragraphs.

Vagotomy and Gastric Resection

In theory, truncal vagotomy performed in the treatment of peptic ulcer disease should greatly alter gastric emptying. Vagotomy disrupts receptive relaxation in the proximal stomach and results in a more rapid rate of emptying of ingested liquids owing to increased intragastric pressure. Furthermore, truncal vagotomy disrupts the gastric pacemaker in the corpus and thus diminishes antral motility and impairs the emptying of solids. Surgical studies in dogs have confirmed these effects. The addition of a pyloroplasty to the vagotomy improves the rate of emptying of solids. Antrectomy, by abolishing the antropyloric mechanism of dispersing and "sieving" solids, accelerates the emptying of solids.

In recent years, an alternative technique, the highy selective vagotomy (HSV), has been developed. With the HSV, vagal fibers to the proximal stomach (corpus) are selectively cut to decrease acid secretion, whereas those fibers mediating motor function remain intact. Predictably, animal and clinical studies have demonstrated a relatively normal rate of emptying of solids following HSV.

In clinical trials, truncal vagotomy with pyloroplasty or antrectomy is relatively well tolerated. Radionuclide studies demonstrate an initial postoperative slowing of emptying of solids, but emptying improves to normal or near-normal levels within 6 to 36 months of surgery. Prolonged gastric stasis resulting in serious clinical symptoms occurs in only 1 to 3 percent of patients undergoing such surgery.

It should be understood, however, that these operations do disrupt the normal physiology of gastric emptying, affect digestion, and frequently produce at least mild clinical symptoms.

Predictably, the prevalence and severity of symptoms is related to the degree with which surgery disrupts gastrointestinal physiology; for example, truncal vagotomy, antrectomy, and gastrojejunostomy (Billroth II) produce more frequent and severe symptoms than does HSV. Rapid gastric emptying of liquids can lead to symptoms of "dumping," when the accelerated passage of hypertonic liquids into the duodenum or jejunum results in mucosal fluid secretion, intestinal distention, and, at times, diarrhea. With antrectomy, solids are not dispersed into a particle size optimal for digestion, and this may mildly impair digestion. Furthermore, with the formation of a gastrojejunostomy, gastric chyme passes directly into the jejunum with resulting poor mixing of the chyme with bile and pancreatic secretions. These factors combined with the smaller capacity of the resected stomach result in weight loss in 10 to 30 percent of postoperative patients. With Billroth II anastomosis and truncal vagotomy, 35 to 50 percent of patients experience some postoperative symptoms.

Diabetic Gastroparesis

Diabetic gastroparesis is a complication usually associated with long-standing, insulin-dependent diabetes mellitus and occurs in the setting of autonomic neuropathy. Delayed gastric emptying is one of many enteric complications of diabetes. Such patients can also suffer from pseudo-obstruction of the small intestine, diarrhea, constipation, or fecal incontinence (see the following paragraph). In these conditions, pathologic studies of the gastrointestinal smooth muscle demonstrate it to be normal, suggesting that these disorders are due to diabetic neuropathy. In patients with gastroparesis, gastric manometric studies have documented disruption of MMC activity and a relative paucity of overall motor activity. Clinical studies have demonstrated at least a partial impairment of vagal innervation as the secretion of acid in response to sham feeding is decreased.

Pseudo-Obstruction

Intestinal pseudo-obstruction refers to a syndrome in which symptoms of gastrointestinal obstruction are caused by ineffective peristalsis. Although gastrointestinal involvement is usually diffuse, severe symptoms from one or more levels of the gastrointestinal tract may predominate. Occasionally, the predominant symptoms are those of gastroparesis. Those diseases that produce intestinal pseudo-obstruction will be discussed in more detail in the section on small bowel motility disorders.

Medications

Several medications have been demonstrated to delay gastric emptying. In the majority of patients, therapeutic dosages of these medications can be administered without symptoms of gastroparesis. However, in patients with underlying disorders of gastric emptying or in those receiving high doses of these medications, treatment with these drugs may lead to clinical symptoms.

Morphine and narcotic analgesics cause gastric retention and appear to exert their inhibitory influence through gastrointestinal opioid receptors and via the central nervous system.

Anticholinergic agents (e.g., atrophine, propantheline) delay gastric emptying, presumably through their inhibition of vagal and cholinergic-mediated motility. Other medications with anticholinergic properties, such as tricyclic antidepressant medications, slow gastric emptying in a similar fashion.

L-Dopa, which is used in the treatment of Parkinson's disease, has also been shown to delay gastric emptying. This effect presumably occurs through the interaction of this drug with inhibitory dopamine receptors in the stomach.

Anorexia Nervosa

Anorexia nervosa is a psychiatric disorder characterized by weight loss and disturbed body image; it is associated with gastrointestinal symptoms of anorexia, nausea, and vomiting. Scintigraphic studies have demonstrated relatively normal emptying of liquids but delayed emptying of solids. The etiology of the syndrome is unknown, and the mechanism of the delayed gastric emptying remains unclear. Although severe weight loss itself may produce a decreased rate of gastric emptying, anorectic patients who have experienced a gain in weight do not consistently correct their abnormal emptying pattern.

Idiopathic Gastroparesis

A small number of patients develop symptoms and signs of delayed gastric emptying in the absence of surgery, medication, systemic disease, or intestinal pseudo-obstruction. Antral myoelectric activity may be abnormal in some of these patients. Whereas in normal subjects, gastric slow wave activity occurs at 3 to 4 cycles/minute, patients with idiopathic gastroparesis may have regular patterns of increased frequency ("tachygastria") or irregular frequencies. Antral motility is disrupted, but the hypothesis that the gastroparesis is due to the abnormal electrical activity remains to be proved.

Symptoms and Treatment of Delayed Gastric Emptying

Since the major motility functions of the stomach are to serve as a reservoir for ingested food and to triturate food prior to digestion, one could predict the symptoms of gastroparesis: anorexia, early satiety, postprandial fullness, nausea, and vomiting. Often, patients may vomit food consumed many hours before, evidence of gastric stasis. Weight loss and malnutrition routinely occur with more severe forms of this disorder.

Dietary adjustments can reduce symptoms and improve nutritional intake. A program of frequent small feeding of liquids or soft, low-residue foods is best tolerated for the following reasons: (1) small feedings cause less gastric distention and postprandial discomfort; (2) liquids are emptied more easily by intragastric pressure than by antral peristalsis; and (3) low-fiber foods reduce the risk of gastric retention and the formation of bezoars (undigested plant residue).

Cholinergic agonists, such as bethanechol, have not been of proven benefit. Such drugs initiate gastric contraction by their action at the myoneural receptor but do not stimulate propagative contractions (peristalsis) or improve gastric emptying.

Metoclopramide, an analog of procainamide in contrast, has proved very effective. It possesses strong cholinergic properties and antagonizes the central and peripheral actions of endogenous dopamine. It increases the amplitude of antral contractions, improves coordination between gastric and duodenal contractions, and enhances gastric emptying. It has been proved effective in enhancing gastric emptying in patients with (1) diabetic gastroparesis, (2) postsurgical gastroparesis, and (3) anorexia nervosa.

Gastric surgery is not routinely effective in improving symptoms in patients with gastroparesis. In patients with diabetic gastroparesis, this may be due to coincidental motility abnormalities in the small bowel. In patients with idiopathic gastroparesis, this failure is presumably due to subsequent progression of the idiopathic motility abnormality to involve the small bowel.

Small Bowel

Motor Functions Under physiologic conditions, small intestinal peristalsis consists of coordinated contractions, which result in the effective mixing and orderly propulsion of intestinal contents. As in the stomach, the pattern of regional movement is dictated by the presence of pacesetter signals generated by the intestinal smooth muscles themselves. Whereas in the stomach the frequency of the pacesetter signals is 3 to 4 cycles/minute, in the duodenum the frequency is 10 to 12 cycles/minute; along the length of the small bowel, the frequency progressively decreases so that the ileal frequency is 8 to 9 cycles/minute. These slow waves recur continuously and impose restrictions on the timing and location of spike bursts that initiate muscular contractions. Since Phase 3 of the MMC represents the maximum coincidence of spike bursts on the slow waves, the frequency of muscular contraction in Phase 3 varies with the level of the gastrointestinal tract (e.g., 3 contractions/minute in the stomach, 10 to 12 contractions/minute in the duodenum). The autonomic nerves appear to act by means of the intramural plexuses to induce or suppress the contractile response to electrical slow waves and, in this manner, aid in coordinating contractions. The intramural plexuses also mediate intrinsic reflex contractions.

Manometric studies of the small intestine have identified and characterized a fasting pattern of intestinal motility that is analogous to that of the stomach (see Fig. 9-6A). Phase 3 of the MMC is manifested as a zone of increased motor activity that migrates caudally through the small intestine and effectively clears the gastrointestinal tract of all undigested material. During the fasting period, most but not all the MMCs originate in the stomach every 120 to 140 minutes and sweep through the small bowel to the ileum. Absorption of intestinal contents has been shown to be greatest during Phase 1, when transit is slowest and hence mucosal contact is prolonged. Predictably, absorption is least during Phase 3. In addition, the appearance of Phase 3 in the duodenum coincides with cyclic increases in biliary and pancreatic secretions.

The absence of the orderly components of the MMC has been associated with stasis of intestinal contents and abnormal intestinal functions. For example, bacterial overgrowth of the small intestine is much more likely to be present if MMC activity is absent.

As in the stomach, feeding disrupts the interdigestive cycle, and the rapidity and length of disruption depends on the nutrient properties of the meal. The contractile pattern that develops with eating is termed the *fed pattern* and resembles the pattern of Phase 2 somewhat, that is, random motor activity with occasional peristaltic and antiperistaltic complexes traveling over short distances (see Fig. 9-6B). Possibly this relatively static, phasic pattern effects luminal mixing of chyme with digestive secretions and optimizes mucosal contact time for absorption. Because specific phases of the fed pattern are not evident, further characterization has not been accomplished.

Motor Disorders   Motor disorders of the small bowel usually prolong small bowel transit and result in symptoms of "functional" small bowel obstruction. Affected patients complain of abdominal distention or bloating, crampy abdominal pain, anorexia, nausea, and vomiting. Examination of the abdomen usually reveals abdomi-

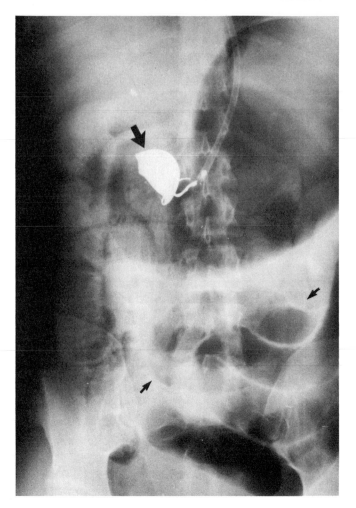

Fig. 9-7
Abdominal film in a patient with intestinal pseudo-obstruction. The large
arrow indicates the mercury bag at the tip of a Cantor tube, which has been
passed in order to decompress the gas-filled stomach and small bowel (*small
arrows*).

nal distention with decreased bowel sounds on auscultation.
Plain radiographs will demonstrate dilated, air-filled loops of the
small bowel that can usually be differentiated from that seen
with mechanical obstruction if luminal air is generally distributed throughout the gastrointestinal tract (Fig. 9-7).

Intestinal Pseudo-Obstruction
Intestinal pseudo-obstruction is a syndrome with clinical symptoms of intestinal obstruction in the absence of mechanical occlusion of the lumen. It is chronic, whereas the syndrome of

adynamic ileus is acute and self-limited. Pseudo-obstruction appears to consist of a spectrum of diseases in which disordered motility, caused by neuronal or smooth muscle dysfunction, results in functional bowel obstruction. Such syndromes can be categorized as either *primary disease,* occurring without a recognizable cause, or *secondary disease,* occurring in association with an underlying disease or drug use. Multiple causes of secondary intestinal pseudo-obstruction exist and include collagen vascular diseases, primary muscle disease (e.g., muscular dystrophy), endocrine disorders, neurologic diseases, and drug-induced dysfunction. The most frequently observed causes of secondary intestinal pseudo-obstruction include scleroderma, amyloidosis, myxedema, and diabetes mellitus.

In scleroderma, small bowel involvement always occurs in association with esophageal involvement (see Chap. 1). Pathologic findings of the small intestine consist of variable deposition of dense collagenous tissue in the submucosa, smooth muscle, and serosa, accompanied by smooth muscle atrophy.

Gastrointestinal involvement is common in systemic amyloidosis; rectal biopsy is positive for amyloid in 85 percent of patients with this disease. Although amyloid is initially deposited in the vessel walls of the submucosa, later deposition occurs in intestinal smooth muscle and seems to correlate with the degree of motor dysfunction.

Gastrointestinal symptoms, such as constipation, are quite common in hypothyroidism. Pathologic findings include mucopolysaccharide infiltration of both the smooth muscle and the myenteric plexus.

Altered small bowel motility may occur in insulin-dependent diabetics in a fashion analogous to gastroparesis and has been attributed to a visceral neuropathy in view of the frequent coexistence of symptoms of generalized autonomic dysfunction. No specific lesions have been observed in the intestinal ganglia, mucosa, smooth muscle, or microvasculature.

In patients with advanced stages of these disorders, manometric studies will usually reveal infrequent, weak muscular contractions. Barium radiographic studies will demonstrate small bowel dilatation with delayed transit of contrast material.

Primary or chronic idiopathic intestinal pseudo-obstruction (CIIP) usually presents as recurrent episodes of intestinal pseudo-obstruction without a recognizable underlying disease. It occurs in patients of all ages and both sexes. Although some kindreds with CIIP have been identified, the majority of cases are sporadic. Recurrent attacks of highly variable frequency, intensity, and duration are characterized by nausea, vomiting, cramping abdominal pain, and abdominal distention. Not infrequently, patients will have undergone one or more exploratory laparotomies in search of mechanical obstruction.

In CIIP, significant weight loss is common and physical examination may reveal evidence of wasting and malnutrition. Malnutrition is primarily caused by anorexia, nausea, and vomiting and may become so severe that it is an important contributor to the morbidity of the disease.

Diarrhea and even steatorrhea may be evident quite early in the course of the disease and are attributed to bacterial overgrowth in the poorly motile small intestine. In the healthy jejunum, bacterial counts are usually 0 to 10^4 colony-forming units per ml of gram-positive aerobic organisms. With stasis owing to either poor motility or mechanical obstruction, jejunal bacterial counts approach 10^6 to 10^8 colony-forming units per ml and consist of anaerobic and enteric gram-negative organisms. Bacterial overgrowth in the small bowel can result in mucosal injury and a severe derangement of both luminal digestion and mucosal absorption (see Chap. 5).

Radiographic and manometric studies suggest that CIIP is a heterogeneous syndrome. In some patients, such studies reveal relatively atonic bowel with infrequent, weak contractions; this pattern is suggestive of a myopathy. In other patients, high amplitude, uncoordinated contractions are demonstrated; this suggests a neuropathy. Pathologic studies have confirmed that the observed heterogeneity is due to different patterns of neuromuscular disease. In some patients, studies of surgical or autopsy specimens have demonstrated degeneration of the myenteric plexus throughout the gastrointestinal tract in the presence of normal smooth muscle. In other patients, pathologic studies have demonstrated extensive atrophy of the longitudinal or circular layer of the smooth muscle with a normal myenteric plexus.

The management of advanced primary or secondary intestinal pseudo-obstruction is difficult. No available medication, including metoclopramide, has proved effective in these syndromes. Cisapride, a prokinetic drug currently under investigation, may prove effective in improving intestinal transit and reducing symptoms. Dietary management is analogous to that used for gastroparesis: frequent small feedings of a soft solid, low-fiber diet with liquid nutritional supplements. Total parenteral nutrition may be used temporarily during acute obstructive episodes or chronically for protracted, severe disease. Trials of antibiotics directed at bacterial overgrowth may temporarily decrease diarrhea and lessen obstructive symptoms. Finally, surgery is to be avoided in small bowel patterns of CIIP since the diffuse involvement precludes any prudent bowel resection.

Adynamic Ileus

Adynamic or "paralytic" ileus refers to an acute decrease or absence of small bowel motility owing to metabolic or neurologic derangements. Severe electrolyte imbalance (hypokalemia, hypercalcemia) presumably affects intestinal smooth muscle function and results in decreased motility. Overactivity of the sympathetic nervous system is also thought to inhibit small bowel as well as gastric and colonic motility. This often occurs in the postoperative period ("postoperative ileus"), in association with peritonitis, or following spinal cord injury or pelvic fractures. Adynamic ileus is self-limited (postoperatively) or totally reversible with treatment of the underlying abnormality (peritonitis, hypokalemia).

Colon

Motor Activity

Under physiologic conditions, the colon receives approximately 1 liter of ileal effluent daily. Colonic motor activity prolongs contact between the effluent and the mucosa to optimize absorption of fluid and electrolytes and transports the waste products to the rectum for expulsion.

The patterns of myoelectric activity and muscular contraction in the colon are not as straightforward or as well understood as those of the stomach and small bowel. As in the more proximal gastrointestinal tract, the colonic smooth muscle cells are capable of generating both slow waves (pacesetter potentials) and action potentials or spike bursts (SB). However, both the myoelectric and the motor activity of the colon lack the pattern of uniform aborad propagation that characterizes these phenomena in the stomach and small bowel. Indeed, the pattern of SW propagation in the colon is not well understood, and the association among SB, colonic contractions, and movement of luminal contents is not well defined.

Slow wave frequency varies strikingly throughout the colon. Investigational studies suggest that the longitudinal and circular muscles generate separate patterns of SW frequency. In humans, the predominant SW frequency from the ascending colon to the descending colon is approximately 11 cycles/minute. Myoelectric studies suggest that a pacemaker exists in the transverse colon and that SWs arising in this region are propagated most often in an orad direction toward the cecum (Fig. 9-8). In

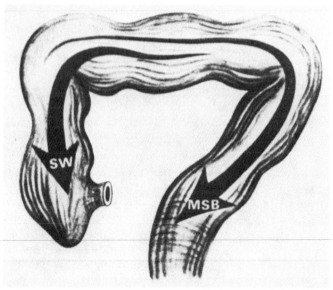

Fig. 9-8
A proposed scheme relating flow in the colon to the electrical slow waves (SW) and the migrating spike bursts (MSB). A pacemaker appears to exist at a highly variable position in the transverse colon, and slow waves appear to spread away from this site toward the cecum. Contractions paced by these slow waves should produce flow with a polarity in the same direction (arrow, SW). The migrating spike bursts began at a variable position in the proximal or transverse colon and migrate distally toward the rectum. Contractions initiated by these spike bursts should produce flow with a polarity in the same direction (arrow, MSB). (From J. Christensen, S. Anuras, and R. L. Hansen. Migrating spike bursts and electrical slow waves in the cat colon: Effect of sectioning. Gastroenterology 66:240, © by Williams & Wilkins, 1974.)

the sigmoid colon, the SW frequency decreases to approximately 6 cycles/minute, and, in the rectosigmoid, there are intermittent periods of SW frequency of 3 cycles/minute.

Two patterns of SBs exist in the colon. As in the proximal gastrointestinal tract, SBs may be superimposed on SW cycles and initiate muscular contractions. Alternatively, SBs may arise as a cluster unrelated to SW cycles. In the latter case, a complex of SBs may arise in the proximal or transverse colon and migrate distally toward the sigmoid and rectum (migrating spike bursts) (Fig. 9-8). Presumably this myoelectrical phenomenon corresponds to the periodic mass propulsion of luminal contents observed physiologically and yet the association is not precise; the rate of transit of the migrating spike bursts, measured myoelectrically, is 4 cm per second, whereas that of the mass propulsion measured radiographically is 0.25 cm per second.

Several different patterns of muscular contractions occur in the colon. The majority of contractions arising in the ascending or transverse colon are *retrograde contractions* propagated proximally toward the cecum, which corresponds to the pattern of SW propagation. Presumably this pattern of contractions slows transit through the proximal colon and enhances mucosal absorption of fluid. Periodically, *mass propulsions*, consisting of waves of contractions, originate in the proximal or transverse colon and propel varying amounts of luminal contents into the sigmoid colon. Throughout the colon, *segmented activity* combines retropulsion with propulsion and prevents rapid transit over long distances. In the sigmoid colon, relatively stationary *segmental contractions* further slow the transit of material received from the more proximal colon. Presumably these segmental contractions allow completion of mucosal absorption of fluid and electrolytes prior to expulsion of the fecal matter. Given this predominance of segmental and retrograde muscular activity in the colon, it is understandable that increased colonic motor activity is more likely to cause constipation than diarrhea.

Although the smooth muscles themselves are capable of initiating contractions, colonic peristalsis is apparently mediated by both *intrinsic* (myenteric plexus) and *extrinsic* neural control (autonomic innervation). In general, the influence of the intrinsic neural control on contractions is inhibitory. For example, the congenital absence of intramural ganglia in Hirschsprung's disease is associated with tonic contraction of the aganglionic segment. Immunohistochemical studies have demonstrated several neuropeptides in neurons of the intrinsic nervous system, and these peptides may mediate excitatory and inhibitory effects. *Substance P* is found within neurons that extend axons into the muscularis externa and appears to stimulate contraction of the circular smooth muscle. *Enkephalin*, an endogenous opioid, has also been demonstrated in these neurons, but its physiologic role is not yet understood. The administration of exogenous morphine does induce colonic SB and muscular contractions in humans and in experimental animals, and enkephalin may have a similar effect. Finally, neurons in both the submucosal and myenteric plexus contain *vasoactive intestinal peptide*, which is thought to mediate inhibitory effects on colonic motor activity.

The proximal colon receives extrinsic cholinergic fibers by way of the vagus nerve; cholinergic innervation of the left colon and rectum is by way of the pelvic sacral nerves. Although cholinergic fibers in general stimulate colonic motility, the vagus nerve does carry some inhibitory fibers. The proximal colon receives sympathetic fibers from the splanchnic nerves, which arise from the superior mesenteric ganglion. The distal colon receives adrenergic innervation from the inferior mesenteric ganglia by way of the lumbar colonic nerves. In general, adrenergic stimulation of the colon inhibits colonic motility.

With feeding, there is a prompt increase in colonic SB and muscular contractions ("gastrocolic" or postprandial reflex). The SBs are superimposed on intrinsic SW activity and produce primarily segmental contractions. The magnitude of the increased SB activity is related to the caloric content and nutritional composition of the meal. A greater increase in colonic activity occurs with a 1000-calorie meal than with a 350-calorie meal. Furthermore, fat is the major dietary stimulus to colonic motor activity and stimulates both a prompt and a late motor response. Dietary protein and carbohydrates have no effect on colonic motility. The postprandial increase in colonic motility appears to be mediated by cholinergic nerves, as it can be blocked by pretreatment with anticholinergic agents.

Anorectal Function

As the sigmoid colon extends caudad and posteriorly, it takes a more anterior course at the level of the sacral spine (rectosigmoid junction) and extends to the pelvic floor. This distal 15-cm length of the colon is termed the *rectum*. At the pelvic floor, the anal canal extends 2.5 to 5.0 cm through the muscles of the levator ani, and the sling effect of one of these muscles, the puborectalis, creates an anorectal angle of 85 to 105 degrees. The sphincter muscles that surround the anal canal play a major role in the continence of stool.

The internal anal sphincter (IAS) consists of a thickening of the rectal circular muscle that extends the length of the anal canal. It is an involuntary smooth muscle with innervation by sacral and splanchnic nerves, and its tonic contraction results in the closure of the anal canal at rest.

The external anal sphincter (EAS) consists of several bundles of striated muscle that act as a single unit and surround the IAS. It is a voluntary muscle with innervation by the pudendal nerve. The EAS demonstrates some tonic activity at rest, but its voluntary contraction is the major mechanism for continence of stool and flatus.

Rectal sensation is mediated by afferent parasympathetic fibers passing to the sacral cord and alerts one to distention produced by stool or flatus.

Under physiologic conditions, the resting closure of the anal canal provided by the IAS prevents "stress incontinence" owing to coughing and straining, and gross incontinence caused by the precipitous passage of stool into the rectum. As stool passes

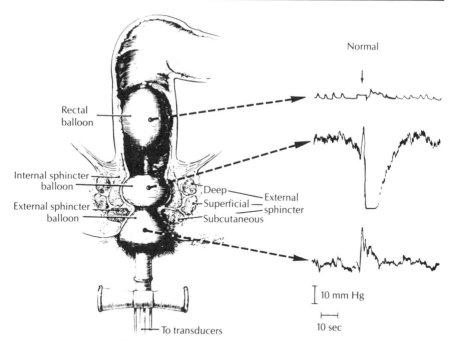

Normal

10 mm Hg

10 sec

To transducers

Rectal balloon

Internal sphincter balloon

External sphincter balloon

Deep
Superficial
Subcutaneous
External sphincter

Fig. 9-9
Schematic drawing of a balloon manometric catheter positioned in the anorectum. Note the locations of the internal sphincter and the external sphincter. The catheter has been placed with the proximal balloon in the rectum, the middle balloon in the upper anal canal (to measure the internal sphincter), and the distal balloon in the lower anal canal (to measure the external sphincter). The dotted arrows indicate that, under normal conditions, distention of the rectal balloon produces reflex-relaxation of the internal sphincter (inhibitory reflex) and reflex-contraction of the external sphincter (sphincteric reflex). (From B. T. Engel. The treatment of fecal incontinence by operant conditioning. *Automedica* 3:101, 1978. Gordon & Breach Science Publishers, Inc.)

into the rectum, distention of the rectum mediates a volume-dependent relaxation of the IAS (*anorectal inhibitory reflex*). Rectal distention also alerts one to tighten the EAS (voluntarily), thus achieving continence until defecation is appropriate. Some investigators suggest that the "flap valve" mechanism created by the anorectal angle may also contribute to the continence of solid but not liquid stool. From the aforementioned description, it should be apparent that continence is a multifactorial phenomenon involving: (1) appropriate strength in the IAS and EAS, (2) adequate rectal sensation, and (3) a normal anorectal angle. The competency of sensation and sphincter strength can be measured by anorectal manometry, using either a balloon catheter (Fig. 9-9) or a perfusion catheter.

Motor Disorders

Constipation
Constipation is not a specific disorder, but rather a symptom — the subjective sense of incomplete evacuation. No definition

of normal stool frequency exists. Some patients pass small amounts of stool several times per day but complain of a sense of incomplete evacuation and hence consider themselves "constipated." Others pass stool every 2 to 3 days but feel comfortable and hence do not consider themselves "constipated."

Simple constipation refers to brief episodes of constipation that are common and usually due to changes in diet or life-style. It usually results from ingestion of a low-fiber diet or use of a constipating drug. Colonic transit, like gastric emptying, is slowed by the ingestion of narcotic analgesics or drugs with anticholinergic activity. With more prolonged constipation, it is essential to rule out mechanical obstruction of the colon (e.g., cancer, stricture). Optimal management of simple constipation consists of increasing dietary fiber intake through a high-fiber diet (e.g., 20 to 30 gm fiber per day) or the use of bulk agents (e.g., psyllium powder). Laxative use should be discouraged, as its use leads to irregular stools and perpetuation of a sense of "constipation." In addition, chronic use of laxatives, especially those containing senna and cascara, can damage the myenteric plexus of the colon and lead to worsening constipation and increasing laxative dependency.

Severe constipation in adults may represent a *forme fruste* of intestinal pseudo-obstruction. Evidence of systemic diseases such as diabetes mellitus, hypothyroidism, scleroderma, and amyloidosis should be sought. Recent studies suggest that some cases of *severe idiopathic constipation* may result from an unexplained, acquired damage to the ganglia of the myenteric plexus. The medical and dietary management of such patients is difficult, and some have even been referred for subtotal colectomy with variable success.

Effects of Dietary Fiber
Dietary fiber refers to that part of plant material (grain, fruit, and vegetable) that can neither be digested by the gastrointestinal tract nor be fermented by colonic bacteria. Fiber is not a single dietary or chemical entity but rather a class of plant carbohydrates, including lignin, cellulose, hemicellulose, and pectin. In nutritional studies, the term *crude fiber* refers to that carbohydrate residue remaining following chemical treatment of foods with acid and alkali. This estimation of "dietary residue" does not accurately represent the results of physiologic digestion; hence, this term has been discarded from recent investigation. The term *dietary fiber* refers to the residue remaining after controlled laboratory treatments with concentrations of acid and enzymes that are more representative of physiologic digestion and is the currently preferred means of quantitating nutritional fiber (Table 9-1). As demonstrated in Table 9-2, dietary fiber has

Table 9-1
Dietary fiber in fruits, nuts, vegetables, and grains

Food*	Serving size	Dietary fiber (gm)
Fruits		
Apple	1 med	3.2
Apricots	3	2.4
Banana	1 med	5.9
Cherries	10	1.3
Cranberries	½ cup	2.3
Dates, dried	10	7.0
Figs, dried	2	18.5
Grapes, green	20	1.1
Mango	1	4.5
Cantaloupe	¼ melon	2.5
Honeydew	¼ melon	2.7
Orange	1 med	4.5
Peach	1 med	2.1
Pear	1 med	3.1
Pineapple, canned	1 cup	2.2
Pineapple, fresh	1 cup	1.9
Plums	2	2.5
Prunes, dried	4	5.2
Raisins	½ cup	5.4
Strawberries	1 cup	3.3
Nuts		
Almonds	10	3.6
Brazil nuts	10	5.4
Peanuts	½ cup	5.7
Peanut butter	2 tablespoons	2.1
Vegetables		
Asparagus	4 spears	0.9
Beans, baked	1 cup	18.6
Broccoli tops	1 cup	5.6
Brussel sprouts	1 cup	6.5
Cabbage, shredded	1 cup	1.9
Carrots	1 cup	3.2
Cauliflower	1 cup	2.5
Celery	1 stalk	0.7
Cucumber	6 slices	0.2
Green beans	1 cup	3.5
Lettuce	1 cup	0.8
Mushrooms	1 cup	1.8
Onion	1 small	1.4
Peas	1 cup	11.3
Pepper, sweet	1 cup	0.9
Potato, boiled	1 med	1.4
Spinach	1 cup	3.5
Tomato	1 med	3.0
Breads and cereals		
White bread	1 slice	0.8
Whole-wheat bread	1 slice	2.4
All-Bran	½ cup	9.9
Cornflakes	1 cup	2.8
Grape Nuts	1 cup	5.3
Rice Krispies	1 cup	1.4
Shredded Wheat	1 biscuit	3.0
Special K	1 cup	1.7

*All foods fresh unless stated otherwise.
(From J. L. Slavin and A. S. Levine. Dietary fiber and gastrointestinal disease. *Pract. Gastroenterol.* 10:56, 1986.)

Table 9-2
Effects of dietary fiber on colonic function

Increase stool weight
Increase stool water content
Accelerate colonic transit
Decrease intraluminal pressures of the colon

several effects on colonic motility and the physical properties of stool. In general, increases in dietary fiber accelerate intestinal transit, and this shortening of transit occurs almost exclusively in the colon. Whereas dietary fiber as a nutritional class produces these effects, the ability of different fiber components to produce these changes is variable. For example, wheat bran (hemicellulose) has a greater effect on intestinal transit than comparable amounts of dietary fiber obtained from cabbage, apples, or carrots (cellulose, pectin). Furthermore, the different physiologic effects of fiber do not correlate in a parallel fashion. For example, the differing abilities of fiber components to increase stool water do not correlate with their abilities to shorten intestinal transit. Dietary pectins possess the greatest ability to bind water but do not accelerate transit to the greatest degree. Indeed, pectins appear to slow gastric emptying, and this effect has been used in diabetic patients to improve glucose tolerance and in postgastrectomy patients to lessen symptoms of "dumping."

Hirschsprung's Disease
Hirschsprung's disease results from the congenital absence of the intramural ganglia of the anorectum and of variable lengths of the distal colon. Since these ganglia mediate inhibitory relaxation, their absence results in failure of relaxation of the internal sphincter and hence in persistent contraction of the aganglionic segment of the colon. The resulting obstruction to the passage of stool produces severe constipation with dilatation of the more proximal normal colon. Constipation may be apparent in neonates (e.g., meconium ileus) or may present in older children with problems of fecal impaction and megacolon.

The diagnosis is suspected by the history (e.g., neonatal onset) and the findings on barium enema and anorectal manometry. Barium enema often reveals a dilated proximal colon (which has normal ganglia) and a contracted distal colon and rectum (which are aganglionic). Anorectal manometric studies demonstrate the absence of the anorectal inhibitory reflex (relaxation of internal sphincter with balloon distention of the rectum). The diagnosis is confirmed by a full-thickness biopsy of the rectal mucosa, which documents the absence of the intramural ganglia.

Management requires surgical excision of the aganglionic rectum and colon and creation of a "neoanorectum" by pulling normal colon through the anal canal.

Irritable Bowel Syndrome

The irritable bowel syndrome (IBS) is a disturbed state of predominantly large bowel motility for which no anatomic cause can be found. It is the most common gastrointestinal disorder in the United States and the most common cause for an outpatient visit to a gastroenterologist. It ranks second to the common cold as a cause of absenteeism owing to illness. Common synonyms included *irritable colon* and *spastic colon*, but terms such as *mucous or spastic colitis* should be discouraged since IBS is not an inflammatory disorder ("colitis").

Its key features are abdominal pain and constipation with or without mucous discharge and episodic diarrhea. No pathologic changes have been identified in the colonic mucosa, smooth muscle, or myenteric plexus. Some but not all investigators have measured changes in SW patterns with an increased incidence of 3 cycles per minute and a decreased incidence of 6 cycles per minute. Manometric studies have reported increased segmental contractions in the sigmoid colon and an excessive sensitivity of the colonic contractions to emotional stress (Fig. 9-10).

Personality and behavioral profiles of these patients reveal them to be frequently rigid, methodical, and conscientious and to have obsessive-compulsive tendencies. Depression and hysteria are frequently associated with IBS. As a group, these patients have a behavior pattern characterized by increased seeking of medical care.

The most commonly accepted theory of the etiology of IBS is that the abnormal behavioral profile of these patients results in an exaggerated colonic motility response to environmental stress. The abnormal phasic motor activity in the left and sigmoid colon results in crampy, lower abdominal pain and the infrequent passage of small, hard stools.

The diagnosis is made by the positive identification of a symptom complex and natural history compatible with IBS and the thoughtful exclusion of other gastrointestinal disorders; in short, it is a diagnosis of exclusion.

Treatment consists of (1) sympathetic explanation of the disorder and reassurance, (2) a high-fiber diet, (3) anticholinergic

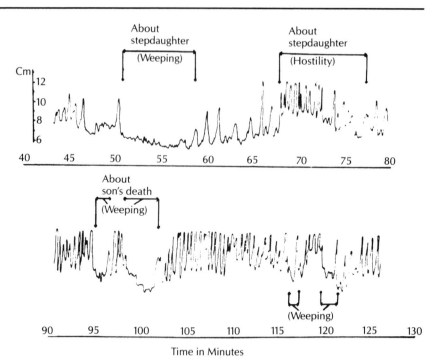

Fig. 9-10
Colonic motility recorded during stress interview in a patient with irritable bowel syndrome. Inhibition of colonic motor activity occurred with depression (weeping) and stimulation with hostility. (From T. P. Almy, F. K. Abbott, and L. E. Hiukle, Jr. Alterations in colonic function in man under stress. IV. Hypomotility of the sigmoid colon and its relationship to the mechanism of functional diarrhea. *Gastroenterology* 15:95, © by Williams & Wilkins, 1950.)

agents for increased abdominal pain, and (4) psychological support, if indicated.

Diverticulosis
It has long been recognized that diverticular disease of the colon is associated with abnormalities in colonic motility. The increased intraluminal pressures observed in this disorder are thought to be produced by increased segmenting contractions in the left colon. The pressures presumably create the diverticula by forcing the mucosa through the weaknesses in the colonic wall at the site of the penetrating vessels (see Chap. 10).

Study Questions   1. A 25-year-old woman with a 10-year history of insulin-dependent diabetes mellitus presents with complaints of anorexia, nausea, and vomiting. A barium upper gastrointestinal series demonstrates a normal gastroduodenum with no evidence of gastric outlet obstruction. A gastroscopy demonstrates no evidence of gastritis or peptic ulcer disease. Which of the following statements about the patient's complaints is/are correct?

a. The symptoms are psychogenic in origin.
b. A nuclear medicine (scintigraphic) gastric emptying study will demonstrate delayed emptying.
c. The symptoms may be reduced by treatment with metoclopramide.
d. This condition is due, in part, to autonomic neuropathy affecting the vagus nerve.
e. The treatment of choice is a hemigastrectomy with gastro-jejunostomy (Billroth II).

Answers
b, c, d
The symptoms are those of delayed gastric emptying. The patient has diabetic gastroparesis. The diminished gastric motility in this condition is felt to result, in part, from the effects of the autonomic neuropathy of diabetes on the vagus nerve. Scintigraphic studies are more sensitive than barium radiographs in the detection of disorders of gastric emptying. Metoclopramide increases the amplitude of gastric contractions and enhances gastric emptying; hence, it is likely to reduce the symptoms of gastroparesis. Since small bowel motility is often abnormal in the setting of diabetic autonomic neuropathy, gastric surgery is usually unsuccessful in relieving the symptoms of this condition.

2. A 2-year-old boy presents with a history of constipation dating from infancy. On examination his abdomen is distended, and an abdominal film confirms that he is impacted with stool. Following a satisfactory catharsis, a barium enema is performed and demonstrates a dilated colon with contraction of the distal sigmoid colon and rectum. Which of the following statements is/are correct?
a. This condition is caused by the congenital absence of sympathetic innervation of the colon.
b. Anorectal manometry will demonstrate an absence of the inhibitory reflex (relaxation of internal sphincter with distention of the rectum).
c. A full-thickness biopsy of the rectal mucosa will demonstrate an absence of intramural ganglia.
d. The segments of colon that appear dilated on barium enema are aganglionic (absence of ganglia).
e. The treatment of choice is a high-fiber diet supplemented with laxatives.

Answers
b, c
The patient has Hirschsprung's disease, a condition caused by the congenital absence of the intramural ganglia of the anorectum and variable lengths of the distal colon. Since

these ganglia mediate inhibitory relaxation, their absence results in the absence of the anorectal inhibitory reflex and in persistent contraction of the aganglionic segment of colon. A full thickness biopsy of the rectal mucosa will document the absence of the intramural ganglia. Management requires surgical excision of the aganglionic rectum and colon and creation of a "neo-anorectum" by pulling normal colon through the anal canal. The constipation caused by this condition is too severe to be treated successfully with diet and laxatives. The sympathetic innervation of the colon in this condition is normal.

References

Gastric Motor Function

Dubois, A., Gross, H. A., Ebert, M. H., et al. Altered gastric emptying and secretion in primary anorexia nervosa. *Gastroenterology* 77:319, 1979.

Feldman, M., and Schiller, L. R. Disorders of gastrointestinal motility associated with diabetes mellitus. *Ann. Intern. Med.* 98:378, 1983.

Horowitz, M., Maddox, A., Harding, P. E., et al. Effect of cisapride on gastric and esophageal emptying in insulin-dependent diabetes mellitus. *Gastroenterology* 92:1899, 1987.

Malagelada, J.-R., Camilleri, M., and Stanghellini, V. *Manometric Diagnosis of Gastrointestinal Motility Disorders.* New York: Thieme, 1986.

Meyar, J. H., Ohashi, H., Jehn, D., et al. Size of liver particles emptied from the human stomach. *Gastroenterology* 80:1489, 1981.

Minami, H., and McCallum, R. W. The physiology and pathology of gastric emptying in humans. *Gastroenterology* 86:1592, 1984.

Perkel, M. S., Moore, C., Hersh, T., et al. Metoclopramide therapy in delayed gastric emptying. *Dig. Dis. Sci.* 24:662, 1979.

Rees, W. D. W., Miller, L. J., and Malagelada, J.-R. Dyspepsia, antral motor dysfunction, and gastric stasis of solids. *Gastroenterology* 78:360, 1980.

You, C. H., Lee, K. Y., Choy, W. Y., et al. Electrogastrographic study of patients with unexplained nausea, bloating and vomiting. *Gastroenterology* 79:311, 1980.

Small Bowel Motor Function

Cohen, S. (moderator): The gastrointestinal manifestations of scleroderma: Pathogenesis and management. *Gastroenterology* 79:155, 1980.

Hohl, R. D., and Nixon, R. K. Myxedema ileus. *Arch. Int. Med.* 115:145, 1965.

Legge, D. A., Wollaeger, E. E., and Carlson, H. C. Intestinal pseudo-obstruction in systemic amyloidosis. *Gut* 11:764, 1970.

Malagelada, J.-R., Robertson, J. S., Brown, M. L., et al. Intestinal transit of solid and liquid components of a meal in health. *Gastroenterology* 87:1255, 1984.

Schuffler, M. D., Rohrmann, C. A., Chaffee, R. G., et al. Chronic intestinal pseudo-obstruction. *Medicine* 60:173, 1981.

Vantrappen, G., Janssens, J., and Peeters, T. L. The migrating motor complex. *Med. Clin. North Am.* 65:1311, 1981.

Colonic Motor Function

Christensen, J. Motility of the colon. In L. R. Johnson (ed.), *Physiology of the Gastrointestinal Tract* (2nd ed.). New York: Raven, 1987.

Haddad, H., and Devroede-Bertrand, G. Large bowel motility disorders. *Med. Clin. North Am.* 65:1377, 1981.

Read, N. W. (ed.). *Irritable Bowel Syndrome.* New York: Grune & Stratton, 1985.

Schuster, M. M. Irritable bowel syndrome. In M. H. Sleisenger and J. S. Fordtran (eds.), *Gastrointestinal Disease: Pathophysiology, Diagnoses, Management* (4th ed.). Philadelphia: Saunders, 1989.

Slavin, J. L., and Levine, A. S. Dietary fiber and gastrointestinal disease. *Pract. Gastroenterol.* 10:56, 1986.

Vahouny, G. V. Effects of dietary fiber on digestion and absorption. In L. R. Johnson (ed.), *Physiology of the Gastrointestinal Tract* (2nd ed.). New York: Raven, 1987.

Anorectal Function

Cerulli, M. A., Nikoomanesh, P., and Schuster, M. M. Progress in biofeedback conditioning for fecal incontinence. *Gastroenterology* 76:742, 1979.

Henry, M. M., and Swash, M. (eds.). *Coloproctology and the Pelvic Floor.* Boston: Butterworths, 1985.

10 : Diverticular Disease of the Colon

Marvin D. Berman

Diverticula can be present anywhere in the gastrointestinal tract. However, the site of both greatest occurrence and concentration is the sigmoid colon. Most are asymptomatic. Their origin is either on an acquired or a congenital basis.

Colonic diverticula are believed to be harbored in approximately one third of individuals over the age of 60 years and are a cause of significant morbidity and mortality in Western industrialized nations. In 1983, in the United States, diverticular disease of the colon was responsible for more than 200,000 hospitalizations and 50,000 surgical procedures with associated health care costs of more than one third of a billion dollars. Yet despite its impact on health care resources, most colonic diverticula, like those found elsewhere in the gastrointestinal tract, are asymptomatic. In order not to confuse the anatomic abnormality with that of its symptoms, it is important to accurately define *diverticulum, diverticulosis, diverticulitis,* and *diverticular disease.* A *colonic diverticulum* is a herniation of mucosa through the muscular layers of the bowel wall. *Diverticulosis* is the presence of diverticuli, whereas *diverticulitis* is the inflammatory process that develops from a perforated diverticulum. The term *diverticular disease* is any symptom or sign arising from the presence of a diverticulum.

Epidemiology

Prior to the twentieth century, diverticula of the colon were considered little more than pathologic oddities that seldom produced clinical manifestations. In Third World countries, diverticulosis is still rare, while the opposite is true in modernized societies. Despite limitations of autopsy and radiographic studies, it is apparent that the presence of diverticula increases with age and most commonly occurs after age 40. It is estimated that the prevalence of colonic diverticulosis rises from 5 percent in the fifth decade to 50 percent in the ninth decade of life. Because the true prevalence of this disease is unknown, only estimates can be made as to percentage of individuals who eventually become ill. It is speculated that only 10 to 20 percent develop signs and symptoms of disease, and 1 percent require surgical intervention. For patients younger than 40 years of age, it appears that disease manifestations are far more serious, and more than one half of these patients eventually require surgery.

Pathology

The most common site of diverticula, observed in 90 to 95 percent of all cases, is the sigmoid colon. When more proximal involvement of the colon occurs, it is usually in continuity with the sigmoid. By contrast, the occurrence of diverticular disease confined to the right colon is prominent in the Orient and Hawaii and may have a congenital origin.

On gross examination, the taeniae coli and circular muscle are thicker than normal. Because of the thickness of the circular muscle and the apparent shortening of the longitudinal axis of the colonic wall by the taeniae, an almost accordion-like semblance is created. Among the clefts of circular muscle, diverticula can usually be found between the mesenteric and antimesenteric taeniae (Fig. 10-1). The lumen of the bowel is further

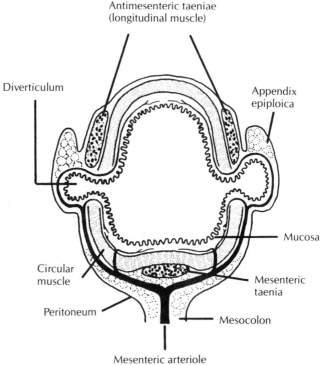

Fig. 10-1
Cross-section anatomy of a colon segment containing diverticula. The diverticula are formed by herniation of mucosa through the circular muscle on the mesenteric side of the antimesenteric taeniae. Note the relationship of a diverticulum with its mesenteric arteriole. (From P. B. Berman and J. B. Kersner. Current knowledge of diverticular disease of the colon. *Dig. Dis.* 17:741, 1972.)

narrowed by redundant folds of mucosa. When viewed either through a colonoscope or with a barium enema, diverticula appear as outpouchings whose sizes range from only a few millimeters to a centimeter or more (Fig. 10-2A, B).

Microscopically, most diverticula of the colon are pseudodiverticula because only the mucosa and submucosa herniate through the circular muscle to lie in the pericolic tissues. These pseudodiverticula occur at weak sites in the circular muscle created by penetration of the mesenteric arterioles supplying the mucosal surface (Figs. 10-1 and 10-3). This close association of diverticula with penetrating blood vessels is undoubtedly important in the pathogenesis of bleeding from diverticular disease of the colon. The thickness of the colonic wall is related in part to deposition of elastin, an important connective tissue protein, and not to hyperplasia or hypertrophy of muscle cells.

Isolated diverticula in the right colon are usually true diverticula in that the herniation involves not just the mucosa and submucosa but all layers of the bowel.

Pathogenesis

With the introduction in the 1880s of the milling of grain by steel rollers, replacing stone milling, the fiber content of wheat flour diminished by as much as 90 percent. Subsequently, epidemiologic documentation has associated diverticular disease of the colon with low dietary intake of fiber and altered colonic function. In Africans who routinely ingest a high-fiber diet and in whom diverticular disease of the colon is virtually unknown, stool weights and stool transit times (length of time from ingestion of food to excretion) are 400+ gm and 24 to 36 hours, respectively. By contrast, in individuals from industrialized nations whose diets are fiber deficient, daily fecal weights can be as low as 100 gm, stool transit times can be prolonged 72 hours or more, and diverticulosis is common.

It is hypothesized that one of the factors required for the formation of diverticula is the existence of a pressure gradient between colonic lumen and serosal surface. Based on the Law of Laplace, the tension (T) in the wall of a cylinder is directly related to the pressure (P) within and the radius (R) of the cylinder ($T = P \times R$). If one assumes that the tension of the circular muscle of the colon is constant, the intraluminal pressure will be greatest where the lumen is narrowest, that is, the sigmoid colon. Presumably, a low-residue, low-fiber diet can result in small stools, increased intraluminal pressures, and the likelihood of herniation of mucosa through areas in the circular muscle that are created vulnerable by the penetrating mesenteric arterioles. Further exacerbating the potential for diverticular dis-

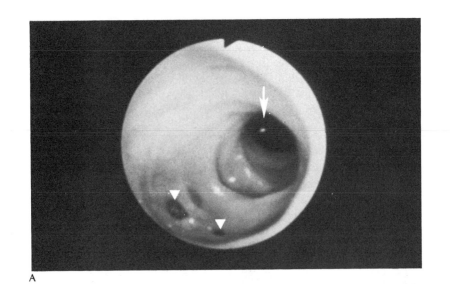

A

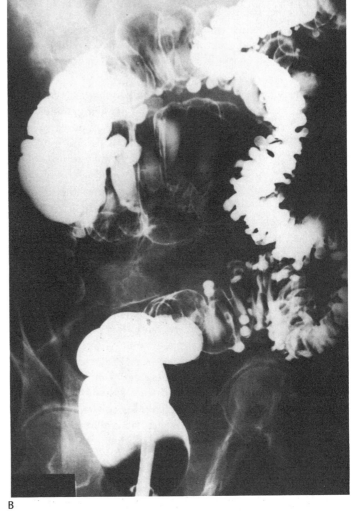

B

Colonic lumen

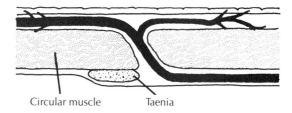

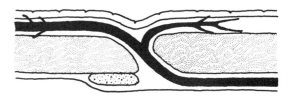

Circular muscle   Taenia

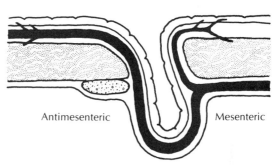

Antimesenteric   Mesenteric

Fig. 10-3
Illustration of the relationship of a developing diverticulum and a penetrating mesenteric arteriole. (From M. A. Meyers, D. R. Alonso, G. F. Gray, et al. Pathogenesis of bleeding colonic diverticulosis. *Gastroenterology* 71:577, © by Williams & Wilkins, 1976.)

Fig. 10-2
A. Colonoscopic view of lumen of the colon (*large arrow*) and several diverticular orifices (*arrowheads*). B. Numerous colonic diverticula are demonstrated by barium enema.

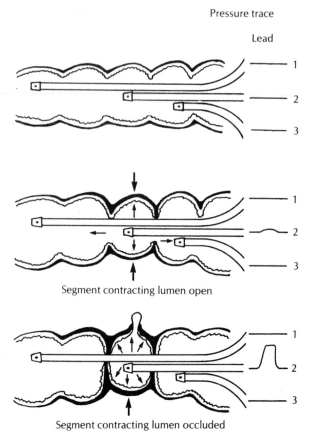

Pressure trace

Lead

Segment contracting lumen open

Segment contracting lumen occluded

Fig. 10-4
Manometric tracings from three areas of the colon. A diverticulum can be formed when the bowel lumen is sufficiently narrowed that discontinuous closed chambers are created. (From N. S. Painter. The cause of diverticular disease of the colon, its symptoms, and its complications. *J. R. Coll. Surg. Edinb.* 30:118, 1985.)

ease is the aging process, because the flexibility and tensile strength of collagen, the major connective tissue protein, diminishes with advancing age. Consequently, as an individual ages, the colonic wall has lowered resistance to distention from intraluminal pressure. It is not surprising that patients with systemic connective tissue disorders such as Marfan and Ehlers-Danlos syndromes develop diverticular disease at a young age.

The generation of intraluminal pressure is related to contraction of the colonic wall muscle. Using pressure-recording catheters and cineradiography, investigators have demonstrated that waves of high pressure coincide with bandlike contractions, which narrow and can occlude short segments of bowel into closed chambers (Fig. 10-4). These intracolonic pressures can exceed 90 mm Hg and may result in the formation of diverticula.

Measurements of intraluminal pressure have demonstrated that the intake of diets high in fiber content is associated with low intracolonic pressure suggesting that high fiber diets are protective against the development of diverticular disease.

Clinical Features

Diverticulitis

The development of diverticulitis is not the result of local inflammation within the lumen of a diverticulum; rather, it is due to the actual perforation of a diverticulum. Although the mechanism responsible for the perforation is unknown, there are at least two possibilities. In one sequence of events, inspissated stool in a diverticulum causes obstruction of its opening, which, in turn, may lead to mechanical trauma and eventual perforation at the apex of the diverticulum. In the other theory, the perforation of a diverticulum is simply an extension of the same process thought responsible for the very development of the diverticulum. High intracolonic pressure may be greater than pressure within colonic blood vessels. The mucosa may become ischemic and permit penetration of normal colonic bacterial flora through the thin diverticular wall. The coexistence of diabetes and atherosclerosis may be important co-morbid factors. Regardless of the operative mechanism, the severity of the signs and symptoms of the diverticulitis depends on the extent of the perforation. When perforation is limited to a microperforation into the pericolic tissues and mesenteric fat, the symptoms may be subclinical or mild. Less commonly, the perforation extends beyond the local pericolic tissues and even progresses to peritoneal soilage and gross peritonitis.

Despite the high prevalence of colonic diverticula, clinically apparent diverticulitis occurs in only 10 to 20 percent of patients with diverticulosis. The most common presentation is that of pain localized to the left lower abdominal quadrant, but pain can extend to the hypogastric area and even radiate to the lower back. The patient may have associated chills and fever and can be constipated because of mechanical obstruction or ileus (functional spasm of the colon). Nausea and vomiting are often present in these patients.

On physical examination, tenderness and guarding in the left lower quadrant are present. In approximately 25 percent of the cases, a mass is palpable. On rectal examination, the tender sigmoid colon may be palpable through the left wall of the rectum. The stool is rarely bloody, but occult blood can be present. Other than an elevated erythrocyte sedimentation rate and an increased concentration of polymorphonuclear leukocytes, blood values are frequently normal.

Complications of diverticulitis include abscess, fistula formation, and intestinal obstruction, but not massive hemorrhage. An intraabdominal abscess may manifest itself by persistent or spiking fevers. The abscess may occur adjacent to the involved segment of bowel or anywhere within the abdominal cavity. Rarely, extension and rupture of a diverticulum or its abscess directly into the peritoneum result in catastrophic generalized peritonitis.

The patient with peritonitis is acutely ill, has a "board-like" abdomen, and exhibits signs typical of gram-negative sepsis. In approximately 10 to 25 percent of patients hospitalized for diverticular disease of the colon, obstruction of the bowel may be observed. The mechanisms responsible for mechanical obstruction include extrinsic pressure, created by pericolic or intramural abscesses in the acute setting, and chronic fibrosis and adhesions from previous episodes of diverticulitis. Diverticular disease of the colon is second only to carcinoma as a cause of colonic obstruction in adults. Another major complication of diverticulitis is formation of fistuli. In approximately 5 percent of patients, direct perforation of the inflammatory process into another abdominal viscus can produce a fistula. Colovesical (colon to bladder) fistuli account for at least half of all fistuli associated with diverticulitis; pneumaturia (passage of gas during urination) and fecaluria (co-mingling of feces with urine passed from the urethra) are pathognomonic of colovesical fistuli. A coloenteric (colon to small bowel) fistula is usually asymptomatic but occasionally may result in symptomatic steatorrhea from bacterial overgrowth. Lastly, colocutaneous (colon to skin) fistuli may be another complication caused by acute diverticular abscesses.

The diagnosis of diverticulitis is often made on purely clinical grounds. Radiographic techniques such as plain x-rays of the abdomen, barium enema, ultrasound, and computerized tomography (CT) scan are often performed to support the diagnosis and rule out intraabdominal conditions that enter into the differential diagnosis. An example of diagnostic features on barium enema is illustrated in Fig. 10-5A and B.

A number of conditions can simulate diverticulitis; these include cancer of the colon, Crohn's disease, ischemic colitis, and appendicitis. The distinction among these conditions is based on clinical, radiologic, and laboratory findings. In the acutely ill patient, surgical exploration may be necessary for both diagnosis and treatment.

Therapy directed against acute diverticulitis depends on the severity of the clinical illness. Mild attacks are treated by placing

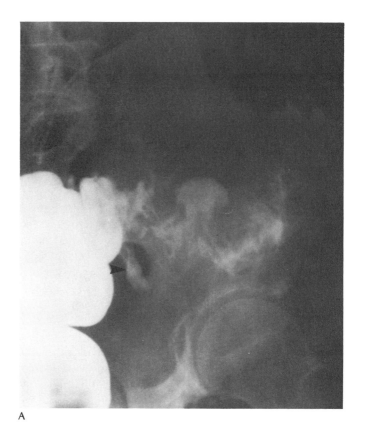

A

B

Fig. 10-5
Radiographic signs of acute diverticulitis. A. Extraluminal barium, signifying
perforation, is observed. B. Extraluminal mass narrowing the colon is demonstrated (arrowheads).

the patient on a liquid diet and an oral absorbable antibiotic such as ampicillin. For severely ill patients, treatment includes hospitalization, intravenous hydration, nasogastric suction, and broad-spectrum parenteral antibiotic coverage for gram-negative aerobes, enterococci, and anaerobic *Bacteroides fragilis*. Severe clinical illness often abates within 3 to 4 days, and the patient can begin to eat, initially with a liquid diet. Surgical intervention is required in only 30 percent of severely ill hospitalized patients. Indications for surgery include an abscess that does not respond to medical therapy, free peritoneal perforation, or intestinal obstruction. The mortality rate for surgical intervention ranges from 1.6 percent in elective cases to more than 15 percent in gravely ill patients. The type of surgical procedure is governed by the urgency and condition of the patient. Most commonly, the leaking segment is resected and a proximal colostomy is fashioned while the distal end is closed (Hartmann's procedure); at a later date, the bowel can be reanastomosed. Occasionally, it is possible to both resect the diseased bowel and perform a primary anastomosis. Following a bout of diverticulitis, either medically or surgically managed, patients should be placed on a high-fiber diet. By increasing dietary fiber to 15 to 20 gm of fiber per day, fecal weight doubles, and both stool transit times and intraluminal pressures in the left colon decrease. Although there is no evidence that the number, size, and distribution of diverticuli regress, treatment with unprocessed wheat bran and other high-fiber foods may prevent the recurrence of symptoms of diverticular disease of the colon.

Diverticular Hemorrhage

Colonic diverticulosis is the most frequent etiology of severe lower intestinal bleeding. It is believed that between 2 and 6 percent of patients with diverticulosis will suffer from an episode of severe hemorrhage.

The presumed pathogenesis of diverticular hemorrhage is related to the characteristic angioarchitecture of the mesenteric arteriole with its diverticulum. There is no evidence that diverticulitis is responsible. Instead, the mesenteric arteriole, in response to injury within the colonic or diverticular lumen, develops eccentric intimal thickening toward the luminal side. Presumably, with repeated injury, progressive weakness in the arteriole leads to vessel rupture and significant arterial bleeding (Fig. 10-6). Interestingly, the majority of bleeding from diverticula arises from those located in the right side of the colon.

Classically, patients with significant lower gastrointestinal hemorrhage experience mild lower abdominal cramps and rectal urgency. Abdominal pain is not a feature of diverticular hemorrhage. The patient passes bloody stools that range in color from

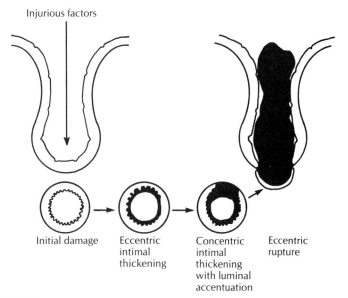

Injurious factors

| Initial damage | Eccentric intimal thickening | Concentric intimal thickening with luminal accentuation | Eccentric rupture |

Fig. 10-6
Possible pathogenesis of hemorrhage from colonic diverticulum. (From M. A. Meyers, D. R. Alonso, G. F. Gray, et al. Pathogenesis of bleeding colonic diverticulosis. *Gastroenterology* 71:577, © by Williams & Wilkins, 1976.)

bright red to maroon. Rarely, the stool may be melenic. The bleeding usually stops spontaneously, and signs and symptoms of hypotension are related to both the degree of hypovolemia and the cardiovascular reserve of the patient.

In a patient with presumed lower gastrointestinal bleeding, it is necessary to obtain a sample of stomach contents to be certain that the source of bleeding is not from a lesion above the ligament of Treitz. Sigmoidoscopy, either with a rigid or flexible instrument, should be performed to eliminate ulcerative colitis and ulcerated hemorrhoids as potential explanations for the bleeding. Because bleeding is self-limited in most patients, a barium enema or colonoscopy can be used within several days to rule out polyps, tumors, and angiodysplasia. When hemorrhage is massive, colonoscopy is often technically not feasible, and retained barium from a barium enema can obscure further testing by angiography. When blood loss is greater than 0.5 ml per minute, the site of continued hemorrhage is best visualized by either scintigraphy or angiography. Radionuclide imaging with technetium-labeled red blood cells or sulfur colloid can often localize the bleeding but is not able to identify the etiology of the hemorrhage (e.g., diverticulum, angiodysplasia, ischemia, or tumor). Angiography is capable of both localizing and controlling the hemorrhage with either selective arterial infusion of pitressin or embolization of the offending vessel. If angiography is unsuccessful, surgical resection is indicated.

Appendicitis

Epidemiology

Appendicitis is one of the most common indications for both admission to the hospital and subsequent emergency laparotomy. Like diverticular disease of the colon, appendicitis is predominantly a disease of the industrialized nations. A dramatic increase in its prominence has been identified with the beginning of the twentieth century. Appendicitis is seen less commonly in rural populations in the Third World that ingest high-fiber diets. During each of the World Wars, a fall in the incidence of appendicitis was associated with a diminished dietary intake of refined carbohydrates. A negative correlation between ingested green vegetables and tomatoes with acute appendicitis has recently been observed in England and Wales. Despite the positive association between low-fiber diets and appendicitis, for inexplicable reasons, beginning in the 1970s, there appears to be a steady decline in its incidence.

The risk of developing acute appendicitis during one's lifetime is estimated to be between 12 and 20 percent. The disease most commonly occurs in the young, with a peak incidence in the second and third decade. In the past, appendicitis affecting the elderly was considered uncommon, but recently it has risen to as many as 9% of those treated for appendicitis. There is no striking female predominance, but appendectomy for non-acute appendicitis is performed more commonly in women because of the difficulty in distinguishing the symptoms of appendicitis from gynecologic pathology.

General Considerations

In humans, the appendix has no known function and may simply be a vestige of evolution. However, because of the appendix's conspicuous amount of lymphoid tissue, which atrophies after the third decade in life, an immunologic function has been ascribed to it. Despite its possible immunologic role as the human equivalent of the avian bursa of Fabricius, there is no evidence to suggest that appendectomy predisposes to the development of neoplastic illness.

The appendix is a mobile structure whose origin from the colon is just below the ileocecal valve. Its diameter is 5 to 10 mm, and its length may vary from 2 to 20 cm, with an average of 8 cm in adults. Although the appendix has its own mesentery, it may project in one of several directions, that is, by the side of the ascending colon, in the iliac fossa, behind the cecum, or behind the ileum. The clinical signs and symptoms of appendicitis vary because of these different anatomic positions.

Acute appendicitis is an inflammatory response to obstruction of its lumen. When the disease is early, edema and vascular congestion are prominent. Initially, polymorphonuclear leukocytes appear in the mucosa and then infiltrate the entire wall. As a consequence of the inflammatory response, a fibrinous exudate grossly develops on the serosal surface. The process continues with focal and extensive necrosis of the appendiceal wall. Eventually, the gangrenous appendix perforates and results in either localized abscess or free peritonitis.

Pathogenesis
Appendicitis is precipitated by blockage of the appendiceal lumen. The rarity of acute appendicitis in neonates may be related to its wide funnel shape characteristic for this period of life. The most common cause of obstruction of the lumen is inspissated stool (fecalith). The presence of fecaliths may be related to the low-fiber Western diet, which presumably predisposes to viscous, hard feces. Uncommon causes of appendiceal obstruction include lymphoid hyperplasia, neoplasm, calculi, foreign bodies, and parasites.

With occlusion of the lumen of the appendix, continued mucosal secretion leads to increased intraluminal pressure, which limits venous blood flow. Hypoxia develops; the mucosa ulcerates; bacteria invade the tissues; the intraluminal pressure increases further; and the arterial circulation becomes thrombosed. Gangrene and perforation usually follow within 24 to 36 hours.

Clinical Features
A little more than half of the patients present with a classic history for appendicitis. The sequence of symptoms is (1) periumbilical pain, (2) anorexia/nausea/vomiting, (3) right lower quadrant tenderness, and (4) fever. When this sequence is not present, another diagnosis should be considered. The patient initially complains of vague epigastric or periumbilical discomfort, presumably associated with appendiceal peristalsis directed against the obstruction. Within the next 4 to 6 hours, the intensity of the ache increases and localizes to the right lower quadrant as the serosal surface becomes involved with the inflammatory process. In a male, testicular pain is sometimes present. A sensation of constipation is frequent, and a belief that the discomfort can be entirely relieved by a bowel motion accounts for the common administration of cathartics and enemas. Fever is usually low-grade, and the presence of high fever coincident with the start of abdominal pain argues strongly against the diagnosis of appendicitis.

Physical examination early in the course of appendicitis is usually unremarkable. The patient may often lie quietly with his right thigh flexed. As the disease progresses, the patient exhibits muscle guarding and tenderness with rebound discomfort (transient abdominal pain upon withdrawal of pressure) to the right lower quadrant. In about 50 percent of cases, hyperesthesia of the skin over the appendiceal area can be demonstrated. The obturator sign (pelvic pain precipitated by internal or external rotation of the hip) and psoas sign (pain in the pelvis caused by extension of the thigh) can sometimes be useful diagnostic maneuvers. On rectal examination, right-sided tenderness may be elicited.

The single most useful set of laboratory values is the white cell count and differential. In more than 95 percent of patients, an elevated white cell count greater than 10,000 and predominance of polymorphonuclear leukocytes (greater than 75%) or both is observed.

Like diverticulitis, the diagnosis of appendicitis is usually made on clinical grounds alone. Abdominal x-rays, ultrasound, CT scan, or barium enema should be used when the diagnosis of a surgical problem is in doubt or when appendicitis is one of many diagnostic possibilities.

The differential diagnosis of conditions that mimic appendicitis is lengthy but can be grouped into (1) intraabdominal (e.g., mesenteric adenitis, small bowel obstruction, cholecystitis, perforated peptic ulcer, diverticulitis, perforated colonic carcinoma, and infection with *Yersinia enterocolitica*); (2) retroperitoneal (renal colic and acute pyelonephritis); (3) pelvic (e.g., tubo-ovarian abscess, ectopic pregnancy, and normal ovulation [mittelschmerz]); and (4) systemic causes (e.g., pneumonia, porphyria, and diabetic ketoacidosis). The distinction among these conditions is obtained by the skillful use of clinical, radiologic, and laboratory findings.

The treatment of acute appendicitis is prompt surgical excision. Complications of appendicitis include local wound infection; abscess; sepsis; peritonitis; fistula formation between bowel, bladder, vagina or abdominal wall; and septic thrombophlebitis of the portal venous system (pylephlebitis). Because the increased morbidity and mortality associated with delays in diagnosis and treatment is so striking, finding a normal appendix in 20 to 25 percent of patients at laparotomy is considered acceptable.

In addition to delay, both on the part of the patient as well as the physician, there are groups of patients who are at particular risk for the development of perforation. In the slightly less than half of individuals who do not have classical symptoms, in the elderly and in the very young, the diagnosis of appendicitis can be extremely subtle.

When the anatomic position of the appendix is behind the cecum (retrocecal) or the ileum (retroileum), the anterior abdominal pain, localized and produced by peritoneal irritation from the inflamed appendix, may not occur. Similarly, physical signs such as right lower quadrant pain and hyperesthesia may be absent. Maximal tenderness may be present posteriorly in the right flank. Another anatomic position that poses diagnostic difficulties is the appendix that extends deep into the pelvis. In these patients, abdominal discomfort may be minimal. Instead, urinary frequency and diarrhea may be prominent. Tenderness or mass in the rectum may be appreciated. With pregnancy, the diagnosis of appendicitis may frequently be delayed. The enlarging uterus lifts the appendix out of the pelvis toward the right mid and upper abdomen. Furthermore, the symptoms of abdominal discomfort, nausea and vomiting, may be incorrectly ascribed to the pregnancy. Because of the high rate of fetal loss associated with appendiceal perforation and minimal risk of laparoscopy or laparotomy or both, prompt surgical intervention is mandatory.

Appendicitis in the very young is especially treacherous. For those younger than 2 years of age and children between 3 and 5 years of age, the rate of perforation is 93 percent and 71 percent, respectively. This extremely high rate of perforation is related in part to the nonfocality of signs and symptoms. Instead, the parent may notice only irritability, lethargy, or anorexia.

In patients older than 60 years of age, the rate of appendiceal perforation has been reported to vary from 32 to 70 percent. Furthermore, postoperative complications are high, some of which are related to pre-existing medical illnesses, and contribute to the approximately 5 percent mortality rate. There may be at least two explanations for the high rate of perforation. First, patients may delay in coming to medical attention because of mildness of the symptoms and the belief that a bowel movement would relieve the abdominal distress. The physical signs may be minimal; consequently, the surgeon may be reluctant to operate on an elderly high-risk individual without a definite diagnosis. Second, anatomic changes predispose toward early perforation. The appendiceal lumen in the elderly is often narrowed; the wall is thin, fibrotic, and devoid of lymphoid tissue; and the vascular supply may be diminished from pre-existing atherosclerosis.

Study Questions   1. A patient visits your office in Kenya complaining of lower left quadrant discomfort. He denies any fever. A barium enema demonstrates an extensive number of diverticula.
A. Which of the following would you expect to be true:
   (1) The patient is a 19-year-old Peace Corps worker from New York City.
   (2) The patient is a 60-year-old missionary from Great Britain.
   (3) The patient is a 60-year-old farmer from the Kenyan countryside.
   (4) The patient regularly eats a diet high in fiber.
   (5) The patient regularly eats a diet deficient in fiber.
B. One would expect which of the following to be true:
   (1) The diverticula are located on the mesenteric side of the antimesenteric taeniae.
   (2) The taeniae coli are thicker than normal but the circular muscle is not appreciably changed.
   (3) The circular muscle is thicker than normal but the taeniae coli are not appreciably changed.
   (4) Both the circular muscle and taeniae coli are thicker than normal.
   (5) Both the circular muscle and taeniae coli are thinner than normal.

Answers
1A. (2), (5)
The development of diverticula is associated with increasing age, Western society, and a low-fiber diet.
1B. (1), (2), (3)
Diverticula of the colon are usually acquired lesions that arise near weak areas caused by penetrating mesenteric arterioles. Both the taeniae coli and circular muscle are thicker than normal.

2. Which of the following can be complications of diverticulitis?
   (1) Urinary tract infection
   (2) Steatorrhea
   (3) Intestinal obstruction
   (4) Massive lower gastrointestinal bleeding
   (5) Development of cancer of the colon

Answer
(1), (2), (3)
Diverticulitis can perforate other organs, e.g., bladder and small bowel. A fistula between the bladder or small bowel and colon can cause urinary tract infections and bacterial overgrowth and steatorrhea.

3. A patient is being operated on for acute appendicitis. At laparotomy, the appendix is noted to be perforated. Which of the following may be associated with perforation of the appendix? (More than one may be correct.)
   (1) Age less than five years
   (2) Age greater than 60 years
   (3) Symptoms for less than 24 hours
   (4) Symptoms for greater than 36 hours

Answer
(1), (2), (4)

References

Almy, T. P., and Howell, D. A. Diverticular disease of the colon. *N. Engl. J. Med.* 302:324, 1980.

Barker, D. J. P. Acute appendicitis and dietary fibre: An alternative hypothesis. *Br. Med. J.* 290:1125, 1985.

Lau, W. Y., Fan, S.T., Yiu, T. F., Chu, K. W., et al. Acute appendicitis in the elderly. *Surg. Gynecol. Obstet.* 161:157, 1985.

Meyers, M. A., Alonso, D. R., Gray, G. F., and Baer, J. W. Pathogenesis of bleeding colonic diverticulosis. *Gastroenterology* 71:577, 1976.

Ouriel, K., and Schwartz, S. I. Diverticular disease in the young patient. *Surg. Gynecol. Obstet.* 156:1, 1983.

Painter, N. S. The cause of diverticular disease of the colon, its symptoms and complications. Review and hypothesis. *J. R. Coll. Surg. Edinb.* 30:118, 1985.

Savrin, R. A., and Clatworthy, H. W. Appendiceal rupture: A continuing problem. *Pediatrics* 63:37, 1979.

Whiteway, J., and Morson, B. C. Pathology of the aging — diverticular disease. *Clin. Gastroenterol.* 14:829, 1985.

11 : Tumors of the Small and Large Intestine

George Benes
Roger J. May

Small Intestine
Tumors of the small intestine are rare. Five percent of all gastrointestinal tumors are of small bowel origin, with malignant tumors in this viscus accounting for only 1 percent of all gastrointestinal cancers. It is striking that cancer of the small bowel is much less common than that of the large bowel. There are approximately 2,000 new cases of small bowel cancer per year in the United States versus 140,000 new cases of colorectal cancer in 1986. Several hypotheses have been put forward to explain the observed rarity of small bowel tumors, including (1) the large liquid content of the small bowel may dilute potential carcinogens; (2) the rapid transit of small bowel contents does not allow for prolonged contact time between the mucosa and possible carcinogens; (3) the small bowel has few bacteria; therefore, bile salts are not deconjugated into a potential carcinogen; (4) the small bowel has a higher concentration of detoxifying enzymes such as benzpyrene hydroxylase; and (5) increased levels of immunoglobulin IgA are present, which may be helpful in making carcinogens harmless. To date, none of these theories has been proved.

Although rare, the clinical presentation of small bowel tumors is subtle and may mimick other disease processes. A thorough understanding of the pathophysiology of small bowel tumors is therefore required to permit early detection in patients with these disorders.

Anatomy
The small bowel is approximately 600 to 700 cm in length. Three separate functional segments can be identified. The duodenum, the first segment, is easily distinguished from the more distal small intestine by the fact that its mucosa contains Brunner's glands and that the second and third duodenal portions are retroperitoneal. By convention, the boundary between the duodenum and the jejunum is the ligament of Treitz. The boundary between the jejunum proximally and the ileum distally is not so easily distinguished. By general convention, the proximal 40 percent of the small intestine is designated as jejunum and is characterized by more prominent valvulae conniventes and smaller bowel caliber than that found in the ileum.

The venous drainage of the small intestine is into the portal system, and the lymphatic drainage is into the thoracic duct by way of regional nodes.

Adenomas

Adenomas are the most common small bowel neoplasm, constituting one third of all small intestinal tumors. These tumors are discrete masses that resemble adenomas of the colon in both gross appearance and histology. They may be either *pedunculated* (attached to the intestine by a stalk) or *sessile* (arising directly from the intestine). These neoplasms occur with an increased frequency in the proximal small bowel (especially duodenum) and are composed of crowded, closely packed cells with uniform hyperchromatic nuclei. Although the entire mucosa of the adenoma is neoplastic, it is classified as benign if the mucosal architecture is preserved and no invasion of neighboring bowel is observed.

Adenomas of both the small and large bowel have been classified into two main categories: tubular and villous. Occasionally, an adenoma will have a component of both and is termed *tubulovillous*. Tubular adenomas are usually single and pedunculated with a flat top. Villous, or papillary, adenomas are usually sessile and have a cauliflower type of appearance. The histology of adenomas will be discussed in more detail in the section dealing with colonic neoplasms.

The usual presenting signs and symptoms of small bowel adenomas are occult gastrointestinal bleeding (the stool tests positive for occult blood) or melena and abdominal pain owing to either intussusception or small bowel obstruction. If the adenoma is located at the ampulla of Vater, the patient may come to medical attention rather early in the course of the tumor because of findings of biliary tract obstruction.

The diagnosis is usually made radiographically using barium studies. At times, a routine barium small bowel series may not be sensitive enough to detect a small adenoma, and more sophisticated radiographic techniques, such as an enteroclysis study (barium is instilled directly into the small bowel by a tube passed through the nose or mouth), may be required. Since most adenomas are located in the duodenum, endoscopy is often useful in making the diagnosis. If accessible to the endoscope, the adenoma can then be either biopsied or removed by snare electrocautery. Occasionally, surgery is required to remove the adenoma. Controversy exists as to the reliability of the frozen section in predicting whether simple excision is adequate, as the invasiveness of malignant cells cannot be determined accurately in all specimens.

*Adeno-
carcinomas*

Just as adenomas are the most common benign small bowel tumor, adenocarcinoma is the most common malignant tumor of the small bowel, accounting for 50 percent of all malignant tumors of this segment. Grossly, these cancers appear as annular constricting lesions or as polypoid infiltrating lesions. Microscopically, they are usually well differentiated and mucin producing. As with small bowel adenomas, adenocarcinoma occurs more commonly in the proximal small intestine. Unfortunately, this tumor may attain a size sufficient to encroach on the lumen and produce symptoms of partial small bowel obstruction before it comes to medical attention. Consequently, at the time of diagnosis, tumor has often spread beyond the bowel wall.

Treatment consists of surgical removal of the carcinoma as well as regional lymph nodes. At times, cure is impossible and only palliative surgery is performed to relieve the obstruction. Surgery is the only chance for cure, as the tumors do not respond to chemotherapy or radiation therapy. It is not surprising that the 5-year survival rate with surgery is 20 percent.

Certain diseases and syndromes are associated with an increased risk of adenocarcinoma of the small bowel. In Crohn's disease, the tumor arises in an involved segment of the intestine and may even develop in bypassed segments of intestine years after surgery for Crohn's disease. The risk is also increased in several of the inherited polyposis syndromes. In Gardner's syndrome and familial polyposis coli, small bowel adenomas may occur in addition to the classic presentation of diffuse colonic polyposis; in these diseases, duodenal adenocarcinoma and periampullary carcinoma may uncommonly occur. In addition, in the Peutz-Jeghers syndrome, which is characterized by mucocutaneous pigmentation and hamartomatous polyps of the gastrointestinal tract, duodenal and small bowel carcinoma may rarely develop, but the risk is not as high as with the other polyposis syndromes. In contrast to adenomas, hamartomas are benign growths that contain all the cellular elements of the small intestinal mucosa.

*Carcinoid
Tumors*

Carcinoid tumors are the second most common tumor of the small intestine and the most common endocrine tumor of the gastrointestinal tract. These tumors are derived from neuroendocrine cells of the gastrointestinal tract and its embryologic derivatives such as the tracheobronchial tree. Neoplasms derived from these cells demonstrate a slow rate of growth and hence their description as "carcinoma-like" or "carcinoid."

Carcinoid tumors may arise from several locations in the gastrointestinal tract as well as from extraintestinal locations such as the lungs, pancreas, and ovaries. In the gastrointestinal tract, the appendix is the most common site of origin (35 to 40%), and the ileum is the next most common site (15 to 20%). Rectal carcinoids and bronchial carcinoids are quite uncommon (12 to 14% each), and those originating at other sites (stomach, pancreas, and ovary) are rare.

Appendiceal carcinoids appear as small nodules, 1 to 2 cm in diameter. Those derived from extra-appendiceal locations present as small rounded or plaquelike tumors below the mucosa. Multiple primary tumors may be present. On histologic examination, these tumors are composed of solid nests or trabecular cords of very regular cells with variable staining with silver salts, hence, the term *argentaffin cells.*

The risk of malignant invasion and metastatic spread varies with the size and site of origin of the primary tumor. When the primary tumor is greater than 2 cm in size, the risk of malignancy is markedly increased, whereas tumors 1 cm in size or less are rarely malignant. With respect to location, carcinoid tumors of the appendix are almost exclusively benign and are usually incidental findings at appendectomy. By contrast, 20 percent of carcinoid tumors of the ileum and a smaller percentage of rectal carcinoid tumors are malignant.

Only a minority of even malignant carcinoid tumors give rise to the *carcinoid syndrome.* This syndrome consists of vasomotor disturbances, cutaneous flushing, and diarrhea, which are produced by the release of vasoactive substances from the tumor into the systemic circulation. As one might expect of such tumors of neuroendocrine origin, carcinoid tumors may produce a spectrum of bioactive substances, including 5-hydroxytryptamine (serotonin), histamine, kallikrein, bradykinin, prostaglandin E, dopamine, and norepinephrine.

Intestinal carcinoid tumors release these substances into the portal circulation, but they are then readily metabolized by the liver and do not reach the systemic circulation in concentrations sufficient to produce the carcinoid syndrome. Only when large hepatic metastases develop do enough of these bioactive factors reach the systemic circulation to produce the syndrome. However, the ability of malignant carcinoid tumors to produce the syndrome does vary with the site of the primary tumor. Only 35 percent of malignant ileal carcinoid tumors produce the clinical syndrome, and the syndrome is rare with metastatic carcinoid tumors of the rectum or colon.

By contrast, even benign carcinoid tumors of the bronchial tree can produce a dramatic syndrome of clinical symptoms. Although not all carcinoid tumors of the tracheobronchial tree synthesize and release bioactive substances, those tumors that do are able to release these factors directly into the systemic circulation without the interference of hepatic metabolism. It is not surprising, therefore, that the carcinoid syndrome associated with bronchial tumors is more extreme and prolonged in its symptomatology.

The most striking and characteristic manifestations of the carcinoid syndrome are the paroxysmal vasomotor disturbances. Affected patients develop episodic cutaneous flushing over the face and neck, which may appear deep red or cyanotic. The patient is often aware of a feeling of warmth over these areas. Episodes can occur spontaneously or may be precipitated by stress or the ingestion of alcohol. The flushing associated with ileal carcinoids is brief, but that associated with bronchial carcinoids is more prolonged and can last hours or even days. With time, telangiectasias develop over the face and neck as a result of these recurrent vasomotor disturbances. Not surprisingly, the episodes of flushing can be associated with a drop in systemic blood pressure and tachycardia. Patients with bronchial carcinoids can experience transient hypotension.

These vasomotor disturbances are believed to be caused by the release of kallikrein, bradykinin, histamine, and prostaglandins by the tumor. Gastric carcinoid tumors can release large amounts of histamine and produce a patchy pattern of flushing with serpiginous borders. The direct release of these substances into the systemic circulation by bronchial carcinoids can produce, in addition to flushing, lacrimation, rhinorrhea, and periorbital and peripheral edema.

The release of serotonin from these tumors is thought to be the major cause of gastrointestinal symptoms in these patients. Enhanced intestinal motility owing to the serotonin is associated with abdominal cramps, audible bowel sounds, rapid intestinal transit, and diarrhea. Malabsorption, if present, tends to be mild. At times, the primary carcinoid tumor itself produces symptoms of partial or total small bowel obstruction and is a cause of gastrointestinal bleeding.

The prolonged release of serotonin can also give rise to cardiac pathology. Endocardial fibrosis of the right side of the heart can develop and affect the atrium, ventricle, valves, and chordae. The clinical consequences of this process are the valvular changes of pulmonic stenosis and tricuspid regurgitation. For some patients, this can lead to the development of right-sided heart failure. Pulmonary metabolism of serotonin reduces sys-

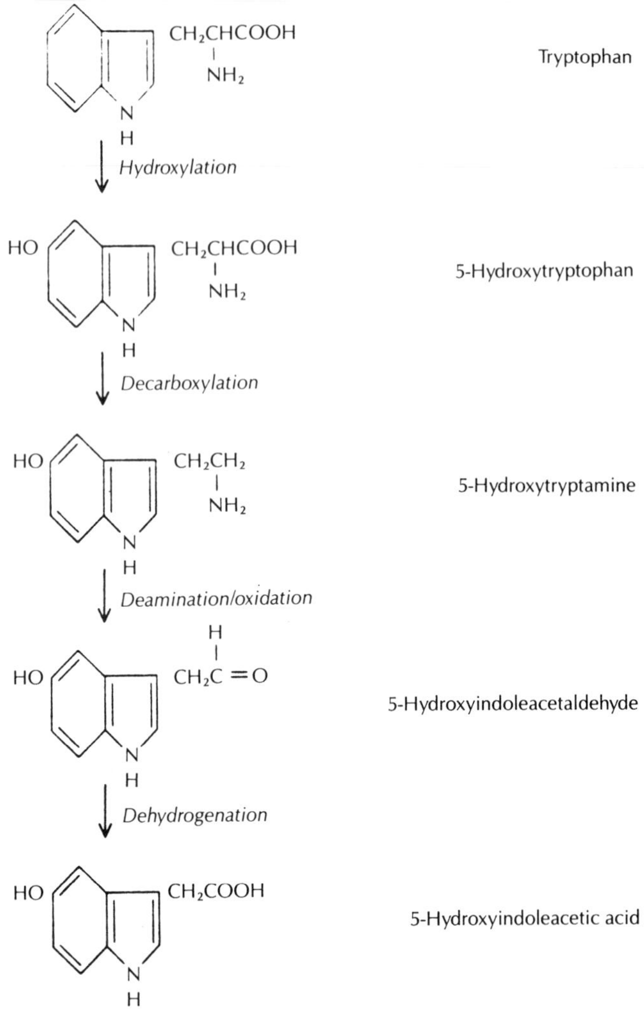

Fig. 11-1
Metabolism of tryptophan to 5-hydroxytryptamine (serotonin) by carcinoid tumor. Serotonin secreted by the tumor is then metabolized by the body to yield 5-hydroxyindoleacetic acid, which is excreted in high concentration in the urine. (From G. M. Gray. Acute Diarrhea. In E. Rubenstein and D. D. Federman (eds.), SCIENTIFIC AMERICAN *Medicine*, Section 4, Subsection III. © 1988 Scientific American, Inc. All rights reserved.)

temic levels sufficiently to prevent similar changes in the left side of the heart.

The diagnosis of the carcinoid syndrome is made by finding elevated urinary levels of 5-hydroxyindoleacetic acid (5-HIAA), a metabolite of serotonin (Fig. 11-1). Normal urinary levels of 5-HIAA are less than 9 mg per 24 hours. In the carcinoid syndrome, urinary levels are usually in the range of 30 to 500 mg per 24 hours. Lesser elevations (10–30 mg/24 hr) are not usually due to the carcinoid tumor but, rather, are caused by other gastrointestinal conditions (e.g., malabsorption) or by the ingestion of certain foods (bananas, walnuts) or drugs (glyceryl guaiacolate, phenothiazines, methenamine mandelate). Obviously, the patient must be advised to avoid these foods and drugs during the urinary collection for this analysis. Finally, it should be kept in mind that not all carcinoid tumors are associated with elevated levels of urinary 5-HIAA. As mentioned previously, if a carcinoid tumor of the gastrointestinal tract has not spread to the liver, the carcinoid syndrome will not be present and urinary screening will be unrevealing. Furthermore, if a carcinoid tumor does not produce serotonin, screening for 5-HIAA will be negative despite spread of the tumor to the liver. In this respect, gastric carcinoid tumors are noteworthy since they synthesize 5-hydroxytryptophan rather than serotonin, and hence urinary levels of 5-HIAA are normal. With gastric carcinoids, blood levels of 5-hydroxytryptophan can be measured.

Carcinoid tumors are relatively slow-growing and thus may be associated with a good prognosis despite the presence of hepatic metastases. Patients often survive beyond 5 to 10 years following diagnosis. At times, however, carcinoid tumors demonstrate undifferentiated characteristics, grow and metastasize at a rapid rate, and are associated with a poor prognosis.

For instances in which the primary tumor produces symptoms of intestinal obstruction, surgery is obviously indicated. The management of the carcinoid syndrome, however, is much more difficult. Since gastrointestinal carcinoid tumors produce the syndrome only when they are metastatic, treatment has been directed at reducing the overall tumor mass. The response of the primary or metastatic tumor to chemotherapeutic agents such as cyclophosphamide, melphalan, or streptozotocin is limited and brief. Occasionally, in a patient experiencing severe symptoms of the carcinoid syndrome, resection of large hepatic metastases may reduce the output of bioactive substances and improve the clinical status. Symptomatic management of flushing has not been very successful; where histamine appears to be the major mediator of the flushing, the combined use of antihistamines (e.g., diphenhydramine) and H_2-receptor antagonists (e.g., cimetidine) can occasionally be helpful. Since serotonin is thought to be the major mediator of diarrhea, therapy in the past has been directed at blocking the synthesis or action of serotonin. An inhibitor of serotonin synthesis, p-chlorophenylalanine can have some beneficial effect on diarrhea. The serotonin antagonist, methysergide, is also effective in reducing the diarrhea of carcinoid syndrome, but its use is limited because it produces retroperitoneal fibrosis. Most recently, somatostatin and a synthetic analog have been found to be successful in the treatment of both the diarrhea and the flushing of this syndrome. Somatostatin appears to inhibit the release of serotonin and the vasoactive factors from tumor tissue and thus reduces symptoms by reducing the circulating levels of these substances. Urinary levels of 5-HIAA often fall dramatically when patients are successfully treated in this fashion.

Leiomyomas

Leiomyomas are common benign tumors that have a uniform distribution within the small intestine. This is a tumor of smooth muscle origin arising either from the muscularis propria or externa or from the muscularis mucosa. The tumor may present as either a extraluminal, intramural mass or an intraluminal polypoid mass. Either presentation may be associated with intestinal obstruction or intussusception. The tumors vary tremendously in size, ranging from a few millimeters to 15 cm. Leiomyomas are highly vascular and can present as chronic and occult, or episodic and vigorous gastrointestinal bleeding.

Histologically, leiomyomas are composed of interlacing bundles of smooth muscle cells without a surrounding capsule. In contradistinction to leiomyomas of the stomach, leiomyomas of the small intestine are highly vascular and can therefore be diagnosed by angiography. The treatment of leiomyomas consists of surgical resection.

It is not always possible to distinguish between leiomyomas and the malignant counterpart, leiomyosarcomas. If the tumor has invaded the surrounding tissue or if metastases are noted at the time of surgery, the diagnosis of leiomyosarcoma is clear. However, in many patients, the distinction has not yet been made. Therefore, criteria have been established to better distinguish between benign and malignant tumors.

Tumors that are hypercellular, contain more than five mitoses per 10 high-power fields, demonstrate cellular atypia, and are larger than 5 cm are most likely to be malignant. Leiomyosarcomas spread by direct extension into adjacent tissues and by way of the bloodstream, with common metastatic sites being the liver, lung, and bones. Lymph node metastases are uncommon. Presenting signs and symptoms include gastrointestinal hemorrhage or abdominal pain owing to obstruction or intussusception. Barium studies and computerized tomographic (CT) scans may be helpful in diagnosing the lesion and in identifying metastases, if present. En bloc removal is curative in 65 percent of cases if wide resection margins are made and if no metastases are present. Radiation may be beneficial as adjuvant therapy. Combination chemotherapy with doxorubicin, cyclophosphamide, vincristine, and imidazole carboxamide may provide a 65 percent response rate.

Lymphomas

Primary small intestinal lymphoma (PSIL) arises from focal lymphoid tissue within the small bowel. Criteria for PSIL include (1) the absence of superficial or mediastinal adenopathy, (2) a normal peripheral white blood cell count, (3) limitation of the disease to the alimentary tract with only regional nodes, and (4) absence of hepatic and splenic involvement. Primary small intestinal lymphoma accounts for 12 to 18 percent of all small bowel tumors and 4.5 percent of lymphoid neoplasms from all sites. The peak age for childhood ileocecal lymphoma is younger than 15 years; for adult small bowel lymphoma, it is in the fifth and sixth decades. There is a 2:1 male to female ratio.

Of special interest is an unexplained association between PSIL and celiac sprue. Ten percent of patients older than 50 years with long-standing celiac sprue will develop PSIL. The diagnosis of lymphoma in these patients is difficult, because the symptoms may mimic those of the underlying sprue. Lymphoma should be suspected in patients whose sprue worsens or becomes refractory to gluten restriction. In addition, the appearance of unexplained fever or abdominal pain in a patient with sprue should raise the suspicion of a superimposed intestinal lymphoma.

Primary small intestinal lymphoma can originate anywhere in the small bowel, although it most commonly involves the ileum and the jejunum in adults. Grossly, one may see (1) diffuse infiltration over a variable length of small bowel (Fig. 11-2); (2) a focal, nodular polypoid lesion; (3) an ulcerating mass; or (4) an aneurysmal dilatation with stricturing. The tumor spreads by means of adjacent nodes or by direct extension, eventually involving distant mesenteric nodes and organs outside the abdomen.

The histologic classification of PSIL is very confusing and is constantly changing. By the fundamental Rappaport Classification, 60 to 75 percent of small bowel lymphomas are histiocytic, which are then subclassified as malignant histiocytosis and histiocytic lymphoma. Malignant histiocytosis follows a rapid course and is characterized by diffuse infiltration of the intestine. One usually sees multiple nonindurated ulcers or diffuse "hosepipe" thickening of the small bowel. These tumors stain positively for α_1-antitrypsin, lysozyme, and kappa and lambda chains with immunoperoxidase staining techniques. By contrast, histiocytic lymphoma follows a less rapid course. A discrete tumor mass is usually present, and the tumor cells are

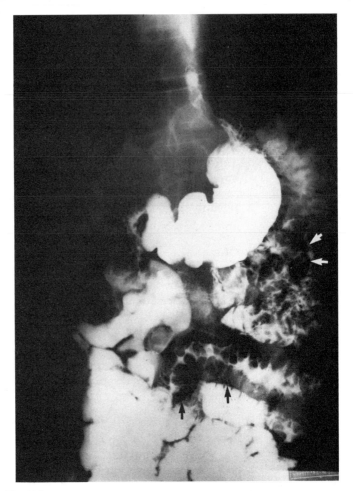

Fig. 11-2
Barium small bowel series in a patient with diffuse lymphoma involving the proximal small intestine. The arrows indicate the nodularity and diffuse thickening of the intestinal wall caused by infiltration of the tumor. (Courtesy of Norman Joffe, M.D.)

large with oval-shaped nuclei and a large amount of poorly defined cytoplasm.

Lymphocytic lymphomas, which constitute 25 percent of PSIL, are classified into poorly or well-differentiated types and are either nodular or diffuse. Monoclonal antibody production is a common feature of this type of lymphoma. Rare types of PSIL are lymphoblastic intestinal lymphoma and mixed histiocytic, lymphocytic lymphoma.

On average, 6 months have elapsed between the onset of symptoms and the establishment of the correct diagnosis. Most cases of PSIL present in an insidious manner, although, occasionally, patients present as a surgical emergency with bowel perforation or obstruction. The most common symptoms are those of partial intestinal obstruction (nausea, vomiting, anorexia, and abdominal pain) or intestinal bleeding (melena and hematochezia). An abdominal mass, fever, and occult gastrointestinal bleeding are common presenting signs. Clubbing, splenomegaly, and peripheral lymphadenopathy are rare manifestations. Laboratory examination usually reveals a mild anemia owing to either iron deficiency or chronic disease and an elevated erythrocyte sedimentation rate. Malabsorption is rare. Barium studies reveal long dilated aperistaltic segments, nodular filling defects, ulcerations, or stricture formation within the small bowel in up to 90 percent of patients. When present in the ileum, these radiographic changes can mimic those of Crohn's disease. Enteroenteric and enterocutaneous fistulae, however, are extremely uncommon.

Management consists of a combination of radiation therapy, chemotherapy, and surgery. Surgery is used primarily for making the diagnosis and for debulking large tumor masses. Radiotherapy is probably as efficacious as surgery for non-bulky early-stage tumors. Advanced stages of lymphoma require combination chemotherapy using standard protocols as first-line therapy. Chemotherapy protocols include CHOP (cytoxan, daunorubicin, Oncovin, prednisone), BACOP (bleomycin, Adriamycin, cytoxan, Oncovin, prednisone), and MOPP (methotrexate, Oncovin, prednisone, procarbazine). The stage of the tumor at the time of presentation is the most important prognostic feature. The presence of large tumors, evidence of spread to contiguous structures, malnutrition, and perforation indicate a particularly poor prognosis. Overall, the 5-year survival rate for PSIL is 40 to 45 percent.

Lymphoma of Immunoproliferative Small Intestinal Disease — Mediterranean Type

Lymphoma of immunoproliferative small intestinal disease (IPSID) is a distinct entity that affects young adults in Middle Eastern and African countries. Such patients present with an illness characterized by malabsorption and abdominal pain. The disease is usually diffuse and affects the jejunum to a greater extent than the ileum. The disease appears to arise in the lamina propria and is characterized by infiltration of the mucosa and submucosa by plasma cells, histiocytes, and abnormal lymphocytes. It may be associated with the production of an abnormal circulating IgA immunoglobulin containing only alpha chains (alpha chain disease). It has been postulated that malnutrition and repeated parasitic infections of the small bowel in susceptible individuals lead to prolonged stimulation of IgA-producing lymphocytes and can cause a "prelymphoma" state. Some investigators have observed that prolonged therapy with the antibiotic tetracycline can produce a transient regression of this "prelymphoma" state. With the actual evolution of malignant lymphoma in IPSID, the tumor becomes quite refractory to chemotherapy and radiotherapy and is associated with a poor prognosis.

Large Intestine

Neoplastic diseases of the large intestine are an important course of morbidity and mortality in the United States. Adenomatous polyps of the colon are quite common and may be found in 20 to 50 percent of autopsy subjects older than 60 years of age. In addition, colorectal cancer is second only to lung cancer as a cause of cancer-related deaths in this country. In 1986, an estimated 140,000 new cases of cancer of the colon and rectum were diagnosed, and this disease resulted in approximately 60,000 deaths. A thorough understanding of the pathophysiology of colonic tumors is therefore crucial to the detection and management of these important diseases.

Anatomy

The colon measures approximately 4.5 ft (1.5 m) from the cecum to the rectum. The most proximal portion, the cecum, has the widest lumen, and the bowel caliber progressively narrows as one proceeds distally to the sigmoid colon. The luminal diameter increases again in the most distal portion of the colon, the rectum.

Morphologically, the colon is divided into distinct layers. The mucosa, the layer in contact with the lumen, is composed of absorptive columnar cells with occasional mucus-secreting goblet cells. The muscularis mucosae separates the mucosa from the submucosa, which has no distinctive features. The muscularis externa, which contains both circular and longitudinal muscle layers, lies beneath the submucosa and is covered externally by a thin serosa.

The arterial blood supply of the colon is through the superior and inferior mesenteric arteries, whereas the portal system supplies the venous drainage by way of the superior and inferior mesenteric veins. The rectum is drained by means of the hemorrhoidal veins, which are part of the systemic circulation.

Polyps

Polyps in the colon are classified pathologically as either hyperplastic, juvenile, or adenomatous. Hyperplastic polyps are 1- to 3-mm, smooth sessile protrusions of normal mucosa that occur most often in the rectum and sigmoid colon; they are asymptomatic and have no malignant potential. Juvenile polyps are usually pedunculated hamartomas characterized by an abnormal proliferation of normal intestinal elements (mucosa, smooth muscle). Juvenile polyps may occur in both children and

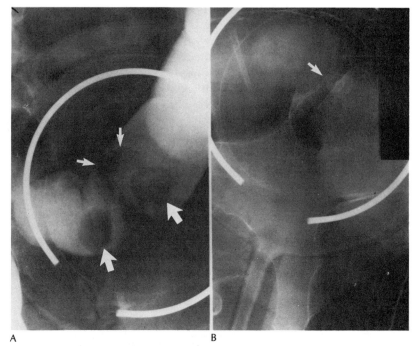

A   B

Fig. 11-3
A. Two pedunculated adenomatous polyps of the colon demonstrated on a barium enema. The large arrows indicate the adenomas. The small arrows indicate their respective stalks. B. A sessile adenomatous polyp (*arrow*) of the colon demonstrated on a barium enema. (Courtesy of Norman Joffe, M.D.)

adults and can cause modest bleeding, but they have no malignant potential. Only adenomatous polyps have the potential for malignant transformation, albeit small, and these are further subclassified as tubular, villous, or tubulovillous. As mentioned previously, approximately one third of middle-aged adults were found to have adenomatous polyps in population screening studies and autopsy surveys. As with adenomas of the small bowel, adenomatous polyps of the large bowel can be either sessile or pedunculated (Fig. 11-3). Based on the incidence of colorectal cancer, it appears that 1 to 5 percent of adenomatous polyps develop to cancer. Characteristics of adenomatous polyps that have been associated with the malignant potential of the polyps include size, histology, and the degree of atypia (change in the normal tissue architecture).

Polyps less than 1 cm in size are rarely malignant. If the polyp is between 1 and 2 cm in size, the malignant potential is as high as 10 percent and rises to as high as 46 percent in polyps greater than 2 cm in size.

Seventy-five percent of adenomas are classified as tubular adenomas, ten percent as villous adenomas, and fifteen percent as tubulovillous. The malignancy rate varies with the different architectural types and is approximately 3 to 5 percent for tubular adenomas and as high as 30 to 50 percent for villous adenomas. The rate for tubulovillous adenomas is 22 percent, suggesting that these tumors behave more like villous adenomas than tubular adenomas (as far as malignant potential is concerned). When both size and histologic types are taken into account, it appears that the size of the polyp is more important in determining malignant potential.

Benign adenomas are graded into mild, moderate, and severe degrees of epithelial atypia according to cytologic criteria (Fig. 11-4). The nuclei are enlarged and hyperchromatic with minimal loss of polarity in polyps showing minimal atypia. Severe atypia is identified by large, pleomorphic nuclei with marked stratification and loss of polarity and the presence of mitotic figures. Approximately 70 percent of adenomas show mild atypia; 20 percent are classified as showing moderate atypia; and the remaining 10 percent have features consistent with severe atypia.

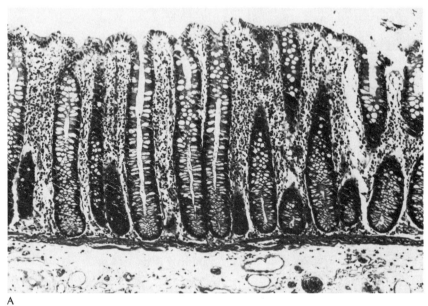

A

Fig. 11-4
A. Normal colonic mucosa. The crypts, lined by goblet and absorptive cells, are closely aligned as straight parallel tubules. The lamina propria contains a mononuclear inflammatory infiltrate. B. Portion of a colonic adenoma. The mucosa forms villous projections lined by severely dysplastic epithelium characterized by cells with enlarged hyperchromatic, stratified nuclei and diminution or loss of mucin production. C. Invasive colonic adenocarcinoma, extending into the submucosa beneath normal mucosa (present in upper right corner of photograph). The malignant glands are tightly packed, with loss of intervening mucosa, forming the so-called cribriformed growth pattern. (Courtesy of Donald Antonioli, M.D.)

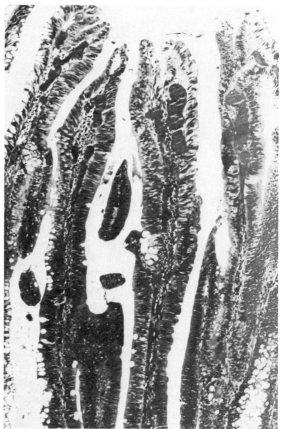

B

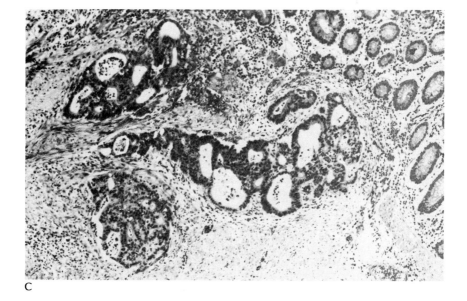

C

The malignant potential of polyps increases as the severity of the atypia increases, with mild atypia having a 6 percent potential and severe atypia having a 35 percent potential.

Occasionally, carcinoma is found within a polyp, lending credence to the theory that most adenocarcinomas of the colon arise from polyps. The depth of invasion of the carcinoma within the polyp is probably the most important prognostic feature in this setting. Polyps with the carcinoma confined to the mucosa do not pursue a biologically malignant course, and simple removal is justified. However, if carcinoma is found to be invading the submucosa, whether the polyp is sessile or pedunculated, the clinical outcome is much worse, and colonic resection and evaluation for metastatic disease is warranted. Other factors that may play a role in determining prognosis in polyps with carcinoma in situ include the location, size, and histologic type of the polyp.

Follow-up of patients in whom an adenomatous polyp was found is important, because these patients have a 30 to 50 percent chance of developing a subsequent adenoma and are at a higher risk than the general population of developing colorectal carcinoma. Current recommendations include repeat colonoscopy within one year of the original polypectomy to ensure that all original neoplasms have been removed. If no polyps are found on follow-up, repeat colonoscopic examinations are recommended at a frequency of every 3 years. These surveillance guidelines are based on the assumption that the doubling time of colonic neoplasms is sufficiently slow (300–500 days) that this schedule is appropriate for the early detection of new polyps or carcinoma.

Adenocarcinomas

Environmental factors seem to play a large role in the etiology of most colorectal cancers, with higher socioeconomic classes and people living in Western, industrialized countries having a higher incidence. Dietary patterns are generally assumed to be instrumental in the development of colorectal cancer. Epidemiologic studies in various countries have documented a direct correlation between mortality from colorectal cancer and per capita consumption of calories, dietary fat, and meat protein. For example, in Japan, where the consumption of these nutrient factors is much less than in Western countries, the incidence of colonic cancer is low. When Japanese families emigrated to the United States and adopted a Western diet, within a generation, their incidence of colonic cancer has approached that of the general American population.

At least two theories, neither of which is completely satisfactory, have been proposed to account for this relationship. First, societies that consume high amounts of fiber in their diet were found to have a lower incidence of colorectal cancer. High-fiber intake is known to increase stool bulk and may shorten colonic transit time, thereby diluting potential carcinogens and also decreasing contact time between colonic mucosa and these potential carcinogens. This theory, however, does not incorporate the myriad of other social and environmental factors that may also be playing a role.

Second, societies that ingest large amounts of animal (saturated) fats also have a higher incidence of colorectal cancer. Some researchers propose that the ingestion of saturated animal fats results in an increase in the anaerobes in the intestinal microflora, leading to the deconjugation of bile salts; this conversion may produce potential carcinogens. Indeed, several observers have found increased amounts of fecal anaerobes in the intestinal microflora of colon cancer patients; however, attempts at altering the fecal microflora profile with dietary alterations have been unsuccessful.

Another theory relating diet and colorectal cancer suggests that indole-containing vegetables, such as broccoli, turnips, cauliflower, and cabbage, may induce protective enzymes that inactivate carcinogens. In addition, diets supplemented with calcium have been shown to decrease crypt cell proliferation in the colon; this effect, in theory, may decrease the likelihood of cancer caused by promotional and initiating events. Other potentially protective dietary factors include vitamin A, C, and E and selenium.

In summary, epidemiologic evidence points to diet as the major etiologic factor in the development of colorectal cancer. No single foodstuff, however, has been found to be exclusively causative or protective. Macrobiotic diets and strict life-style modifications have not been shown to prevent colorectal carcinoma, but they may possibly reduce the risk. For now it seems prudent to advise patients to eat a diet that includes fiber and cruciferous vegetables and to limit the intake of animal fats.

As many as 25 percent of patients with colorectal cancer have a family history of the disease. Two categories exist: the uncommon polyposis syndromes, and the more common, less well-defined non-polyposis syndromes.

Familial polyposis coli, an autosomal dominant genetic disease, is characterized by the presence of thousands of adenomatous polyps within the colon. A variant, Gardner's syndrome, is characterized by extraintestinal soft tissue and bony tumors in addition to the innumerable adenomatous polyps. Turcot's syndrome consists of malignant central nervous tumors in addition to polyposis coli. Almost 100 percent of untreated patients with these syndromes of polyposis coli will develop colorectal cancer by the age of 40 years, making early and aggressive screening essential and treatment mandatory. For patients with a family history of the disease, screening should start in adolescence, because the disease is usually evident at this age; screening should include periodic colonoscopy or double contrast barium enema or both. Once the disease is confirmed, the treatment of choice is total proctocolectomy in conjunction with an ileostomy. Newer rectal-sparing surgical techniques have been developed that obviate the need for an ileostomy. If the rectal mucosa is retained, however, intense screening is necessary in such patients, because the risk for polyps and cancer remains in the retained rectum. Polyposis coli appears to result from a defect in the colonic mucosa leading to an abnormal proliferative pattern and an impaired ability for cellular repair. In normal subjects, cell proliferation is limited to the base of the colonic crypts. In persons with the syndromes of polyposis coli, the proliferation extends along the entire length of the crypts and onto the surface epithelium.

In distinction to the aforementioned syndromes are the familial colonic cancer syndromes *without* associated colonic polyposis. Patients in such families have an incidence rate as high as 50 percent of developing the disease. The trait is autosomal dominant, and the median age for the appearance of the cancer is 50 years — 10 to 15 years younger than in patients without a family history. Diffuse colonic polyposis is not a precursor state prior to the development of cancer. As in patients with polyposis coli, intense screening is mandatory and should begin by age 25 and include yearly screening of stools for occult blood and colonoscopy every third year.

There is an association between inflammatory bowel disease (IBD) and colorectal cancer. Patients with IBD have a higher incidence of colorectal cancer than does the general population; this risk is greater in patients with ulcerative colitis than in those with Crohn's disease.

The risk for colorectal cancer increases directly with the extent of the IBD as well as the length of time that the patient has had the disease. During the first 10 years after the diagnosis of IBD, the risk of colorectal cancer is small, but it then increases at a rate of approximately 1 percent per year. Screening in these patients is imperfect, because the symptoms of colorectal cancer, such as abdominal cramping or bloody diarrhea, may mimic those of the underlying colitis. Therefore, yearly colonoscopy is recommended after 10 years of disease. Mucosal biopsies are obtained every 10 cm to screen for mucosal dysplasia (alteration in size, shape, and organization of epithelial cells) or occult cancer. In patients with chronic ulcerative colitis, the finding of severe mucosal dysplasia on mucosa biopsy indicates a high risk of coexisting or future carcinoma at some other site in the colon. Consequently, many investigators recommend an elective colectomy in this setting. In patients with clinically severe or refractory disease of greater than 10- to 15-years duration, the increasing risk of colorectal cancer may become a strong factor in the decision regarding elective colectomy.

Presenting Symptoms
The anatomic location of the tumor within the colon usually determines the signs and symptoms with which the patient presents. As stool moves from the right to the left colon, it changes from a relatively liquid state to a semisolid or solid state. Owing to the liquid nature of the stool and the wide lumen in the right colon, carcinomas in this region infrequently present with obstructive symptoms and may become quite large before they are detected (Fig. 11-5). Iron deficiency anemia and symptoms of anemia (fatigue, palpitations, and new onset angina pectoris) are frequently the initial findings. Stool hemoccult tests may not be consistently positive, as the tumors often bleed intermittently.

Carcinomas located in the left colon more commonly present with obstructive symptoms, such as abdominal pain and cramping, since the lumen of the bowel is more narrow and, as mentioned previously, the stool is more solid (Fig. 11-6). Cancers developing in the rectosigmoid are associated with tenesmus (sensation of need to defecate), narrowing in the caliber of the stool, and hematochezia. Bowel perforation is a rare sign of colorectal carcinoma.

Stage and Prognosis
The prognosis for patients having adenocarcinoma of the colorectum is closely associated with the depth of tumor penetration into the bowel wall and the presence or absence of both regional lymph node involvement and distant metastases. Various staging schema, originally introduced by Dukes, have been modified over the years. Patients with superficial lesions that do not penetrate into the muscularis and do not involve regional lymph nodes have Stage A disease. Patients whose tumors pen-

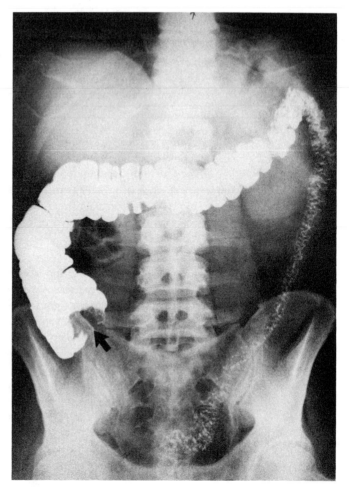

Fig. 11-5
Barium enema in a patient with adenocarcinoma of the cecum (*arrow*). Note that the tumor does not obstruct the lumen. (Courtesy of Norman Joffe, M.D.)

etrate more deeply but still have not spread to lymph nodes are designated as having Stage B_1 if the tumor is restricted within the muscularis mucosa or Stage B_2 if it penetrates through the serosa. The presence of regional node involvement defines Stage C disease; that stage is also subdivided into C_1 or C_2 by the degree of tumor penetration into the bowel wall. The appearance of metastases in the liver, lung, bone, or other anatomically distant sites classifies a patient has having Stage D disease (Fig. 11-7). In the absence of distant metastases, staging classification cannot be determined prior to surgery.

The majority of recurrences for colorectal cancer occur within the initial 3 to 4 years following resection. Therefore, the 5-year

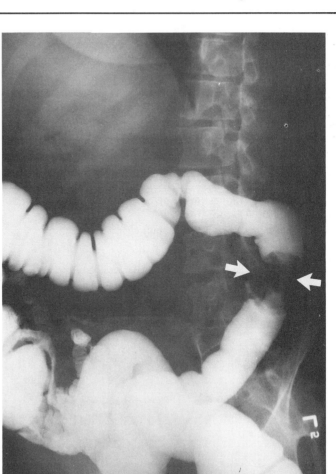

Fig. 11-6
Barium enema in a patient with adenocarcinoma of the descending colon (*arrows*). Note that the tumor constricts and partially obstructs the lumen. (Courtesy of Norman Joffe, M.D.)

survival rate is a reasonable indication of cure. The probability of cure is closely related to the stage of the disease at the time of surgery (Table 11-1).

More favorable prognosis in patients with colorectal cancer, irrespective of staging, includes the involvement of four or less regional nodes, the absence of tumor adherence to other organs, a well-differentiated histology, the absence of venous invasion, and detection and resection of the tumor prior to colonic obstruction by the tumor.

The liver is the most common visceral site of metastases, being the initial location of distant spread in one third of patients at

Table 11-1
Staging and prognosis of colorectal cancer

Stage	Description	Five-year survival (%)	
		1940s and 1950s	1960s and 1970s
A	Infiltration no deeper than submucosa	80	>90
B₁	Infiltration of muscularis; no penetration of wall; no lymph node involvement	60	85
B₂	Extension through colonic wall; no lymph node involvement	45	70–75
C₁	Infiltration of muscularis; no penetration of wall; lymph node involvement	15–30	35–65
C₂	Extension through colonic wall; lymph node involvement		
D	Distant metastases	<5	<5

Source: R. M. Mayer. Gastrointestinal Cancer. In E. Rubenstein and D. D. Federman (eds.), SCIEN-TIFIC AMERICAN *Medicine*, Section 12, Subsection VIII. © 1988 Scientific American, Inc. All rights reserved.

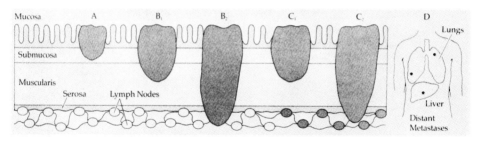

Fig. 11-7
A staging classification for colorectal cancer, which incorporates modifications of the Dukes' system. A tumor is classified according to the extent of infiltration of the bowel wall and by whether it has spread to lymph nodes or distant organs. Staging is significant for determining prognosis. (From R. M. Mayer. Gastrointestinal Cancer. In E. Rubenstein and D. D. Federman (eds.), SCIENTIFIC AMERICAN *Medicine*, Section 12, Subsection VIII. © 1988 Scientific American, Inc. All rights reserved.)

the time of initial resection and eventually becoming involved in two thirds of patients at the time of their death. The metastases spread by way of regional lymph nodes and by the portal circulation; therefore, supradiaphragmatic sites are rarely involved without concomitant involvement of the liver. Rectal cancers are a major exception, because tumor cells that are shed from these lesions may enter the paravertebral venous plexus and reach the lungs or supraclavicular lymph nodes, bypassing the liver. The median survival time following the detection of distant metastases is 6 to 9 months.

Screening

The goal of colorectal cancer screening programs is the detection of localized superficial neoplasms in asymptomatic individuals, leading to an increase in the surgical cure rate. The ideal screening program should be (1) both sensitive and specific, (2) relatively noninvasive, (3) easily and widely applicable, and (4) "cost-effective." To date, no program has met these goals.

The most widely used screening method for the early detection of colorectal cancer is assessing the stool for the presence of occult blood. The most common method involves placing a small sample of stool onto guaiac-impregnated paper and adding hydrogen peroxide (e.g., Hemoccult Kit). Hemoglobin in the stool causes oxidation of a phenolic compound in the paper, yielding a blue color. False-positive test results may occur in patients who take oral iron supplements or eat large quantities of red meat. If test subjects adhere to a high-residue diet, avoid vitamin C, and submit only fresh stool specimens, the potential for false-negative results is minimized.

Even under the best of circumstances, the test is limited as a screening technique for the following reasons: (1) colorectal cancers bleed only intermittently; therefore, between 35 and 50 percent of patients with known bowel cancer will have a negative reaction on a single stool specimen; (2) only 5 to 10 percent of patients who test positive for the presence of occult blood will be found to have colorectal cancer; (3) compliance in the general population is only approximately 75 percent; and (4) a false-positive rate of 7 to 12 percent exposes a large number of people to unnecessary barium enemas or colonoscopies or both.

The American Cancer Society recommends rigid proctosigmoidoscopy as a screening test for colorectal cancer in asymptomatic patients between the ages of 40 and 50 years every 3 to 5 years. This recommendation was based on the assumption that more than 60 percent of cancers are located within the distal 25 cm of the colon, within reach of the proctosigmoidoscope. For unexplained reasons, the incidence of cancers found proximal to this point is increasing, placing the tumor out of reach of the rigid scope. The advent of the flexible sigmoidoscope allows visualization of the colon to 60 cm but at much greater expense and is only performed by specially trained personnel.

To date, no satisfactory clinical trial of screening tests has been performed to evaluate their safety, direct and hidden costs, and efficacy in prolonging the life of patients with colorectal cancer. Until such trials are conducted, the evaluation of the stool for occult blood and periodic proctosigmoidoscopic examinations should be performed in patients older than 45 years who do not have a family history of early colorectal cancer.

Treatment

The only curative treatment for colorectal cancer is resection of the lesion with wide surgical margins and appropriate excision of neighboring mesentery and regional nodes. Tumors of the right colon are managed by a right colectomy with a subsequent primary anastomosis (ileocolostomy). In similar fashion, carcinoma of the left colon is managed by left colectomy. When carcinoma of the rectum occurs more than 6 to 8 cm above the anal verge, an appropriate low resection of the tumor is performed through an abdominal incision, and an anastomosis is fashioned between the sigmoid colon and the distal rectum (low anterior resection). When the rectal cancer occurs less than 6 to 8 cm from the anal verge, the rectum must be resected by both an abdominal and a perineal approach, and a functioning colostomy is fashioned in the distal sigmoid colon (abdominoperineal resection).

In general, colorectal cancer is only mildly sensitive to radiation therapy; hence, this modality is used primarily in a palliative role for unresectable rectal cancer and metastatic cancer (e.g., bone metastases). As a rule, adjuvant radiotherapy administered to the tumor site after apparent complete resection of the cancer has not been shown to decrease the rate of recurrence or to improve survival. The exception to this rule is the group of patients with stage B_2 or C rectal tumors. Such patients may experience a local recurrence rate of 30 to 40 percent despite apparently adequate surgery owing to early local spread of the tumor through the extensive pelvic lymphatic system. In these patients, postoperative radiotherapy seems to destroy tumor cells in the perirectal tissue and reduces the postoperative rate of recurrence.

As with radiotherapy, chemotherapy is not strikingly effective in colorectal cancer. Therapy with 5-fluorouracil (5-FU), the most widely used agent, produces only a 15 to 20 percent success rate among patients with metastatic disease. Unfortunately, the response is only limited and temporary. Predictably, adjuvant chemotherapy given after apparently complete resection of advanced staged tumors does not reduce the rate of recurrence or prolong survival. In investigational studies with patients with hepatic metastases, infusions of 5-FU by way of the hepatic artery have been performed in hopes of maximizing delivery of the drug to the tumor site while minimizing systemic toxicity. Unfortunately, controlled studies have not demonstrated an advantage of this approach over conventional systemic chemotherapy.

Study Questions

1. Which of the following factors is or are thought to be associated with the malignant potential of adenomatous colonic polyps?
   a. Size of the polyp
   b. Colonic site of the polyp (right versus left colon)
   c. Histology of the polyp (tubular versus villous)
   d. Age of the patient
   e. Degree of cellular atypia in the polyp

   Answer

   a, c, e

   The malignant potential of an adenomatous polyp increases with its size — rare in polyps less than 1 cm and 46% in polyps greater than 2 cm in size. The malignancy rate is greater with villous adenomas (30–50%) than with tubular adenomas (3–5%). The malignant potential increases as the severity of cellular atypia increases, with mild atypia having a 6% potential and severe atypia having a 35% potential. The colonic site of an adenomatous polyp and the age of the patient affected are *not* associated with the malignant potential of the polyp.

2. Which of the following statements about adenocarcinoma of the colon is or are correct?
   a. More common in developed countries than underdeveloped countries.
   b. Typically arises de novo, without prior adenomatous changes in the colon.
   c. Most common sites are rectum and sigmoid colon.
   d. Chemotherapy is preferred over surgical resection in the treatment of early colon cancer.
   e. Cancer of the right side of the colon is more likely to cause obstructive symptoms than that of the left side of the colon.

   Answer

   a, c

   Adenocarcinoma of the colon is more common in developed countries possibly because of the higher fat and lower fiber content of the diet in these countries. Although this cancer can occur at any site in the colon, it arises more commonly in the rectum and sigmoid colon. The majority of colonic adenocarcinomas are thought to develop through malignant transformation of adenomatous polyps. Surgery is the only curative treatment of colon cancer; chemotherapy plays largely a palliative role. Because of the larger lumen and the more liquid stool in the right colon, carcinomas arising here are more likely to present with signs of occult gastrointestinal bleeding than with symptoms of colonic obstruction.

References

Small Bowel Tumors

Herbsman, H., Wetstein, L., Rosen, Y., et al. Tumors of the small intestine. *Curr. Probl. Surg.* 17:121, 1980.

Laws, H. L., Han, S. Y., Aldrete, J. S. Malignant tumors of the small bowel. *South. Med. J.* 77:1087, 1984.

Perzin, K. H., and Bridge, M. F. Adenomas of the small intestine: A clinicopathologic review of 51 cases and a study of their relationship to carcinoma. *Cancer* 48:799, 1981.

Carcinoid Tumor/Syndrome

Feldman, J. M. Carcinoid tumors and syndromes. *Semin. Oncol.* 14:235, 1987.

Krols, L. K., Moertel, C. G., O'Connell, M. J., et al. Treatment of the malignant carcinoid syndrome: Evaluation of a long-acting somatostatin analogue. *N. Engl. J. Med.* 315:663, 1986.

Intestinal Lymphoma

Gray, G. M., Rosenberg, S. A., Cooper, A. D., et al. Clinical conference: Lymphomas involving the gastrointestinal tract. *Gastroenterology* 82:143, 1982.

Weingrad, D. N. Primary gastrointestinal lymphoma. A 30-year review. *Cancer* 49:1258, 1982.

Large Bowel Tumors

Simon, J. B. Occult blood screening for colorectal carcinoma: A critical review. *Gastroenterology* 88:820, 1985.

Sugarbaker, P. H., and Corlew, S. Influence of surgical techniques on survival in patients with colorectal cancer. *Dis. Colon Rectum* 25:545, 1982.

Wynder, E. L., and Reddy, B. S. Dietary fat and fiber and colon cancer. *Semin. Oncol.* 10:264, 1983.

Hereditary Syndromes of Colonic Polyposes/ Cancer

Bulow, S. Colorectal polyposes syndromes. *Scand. J. Gastroenterol.* 19:289, 1984.

Santos, M. J., Kursh, A. J., and Cameron, J. L. Three varieties of hereditary intestinal polyposes. *Johns Hopkins Med. J.* 145:196, 1979.

Winawer, S. J., and Sherlock, P. Surveillance for colorectal cancer in average risk patients, familial high risk groups, and patients with adenomas. *Cancer* 50(Suppl.):2609, 1982.

12 : Jaundice and Inherited Hyperbilirubinemic Disorders

John P. Vermeulen
Sanjiv Chopra

Bilirubin is the primary waste product of heme metabolism. A normal serum bilirubin concentration (0.3–1.0 mg/100 ml) represents a balance between the rate of heme production and the hepatic clearance of bilirubin. Hyperbilirubinemia results when bilirubin formation exceeds clearance, as in hemolytic states, or when elimination is impaired owing to a liver abnormality. This is manifested clinically in the form of jaundice (icterus) with the visible accumulation of excess bilirubin in the skin, mucous membranes, or sclera, imparting a distinct yellow discoloration to these tissues. The only other condition with which it can be confused is in the rare individual who has ingested large quantities of foods rich in the yellow pigment carotene, notably carrots, or foods rich in lycopene such as tomato juice. Additionally, chronic ingestion of certain drugs, such as Atabrine or busulfan, can occasionally impart an orange-yellow color to the skin.

Jaundice is usually observable when serum bilirubin levels reach 2.5 mg/100 ml. The accumulation of bilirubin in soft tissue (skin, sclera) lags behind the serum levels. Consequently, if the onset of hyperbilirubinemia is rapid, very high serum levels may be attained before clinical jaundice is evident. In the same manner, clinical jaundice may persist for several days after serum levels have returned to normal.

By itself, hyperbilirubinemia is generally benign except when high levels are present in neonates or in those with an inheritable defect in bilirubin metabolism (Crigler-Najjar type I disease) in whom high levels of bilirubin (generally greater than 15 mg/dl) can accumulate in the brain, leading to brain damage referred to as *kernicterus*. This form of encephalopathy is often rapidly fatal, with survivors suffering irreversible brain damage variably manifested by hearing loss, mental retardation, and cerebral palsy with athetosis. The primary significance of hyperbilirubinemia is its value as a signal to the clinician that the balance between the production and clearance of bilirubin has been disturbed. Thus, it can direct the clinician toward the underlying disease states associated with jaundice so that appropriate therapy may be initiated.

To understand these disease processes, a fundamental knowledge of heme metabolism is necessary. The first half of this chapter deals with normal bilirubin metabolism; the second half details the pathologic conditions associated with jaundice.

Bilirubin

Physical Properties

Bilirubin is a tetrapyrrole formed by the cleavage of the cyclic tetrapyrrole ferroprotoporphyrin IX (heme) at the α-methene bridge position (Fig. 12-1). The conformation of bilirubin is not planar as simplistically depicted in Fig. 12-1A, but, because of strong intramolecular hydrogen bonding, it is an involuted structure as shown in Fig. 12-1B. The intramolecular hydrogen bonding shields the hydrophilic sites of the bilirubin molecule, resulting in a hydrophobic structure (bilirubin-IXα, Z,Z configuration) virtually insoluble in water but very soluble in lipid. However, on exposure of bilirubin-IXα, Z,Z to light of wavelength 400 to 500 nm, rotation can occur around the double bonds of either of the outer pyrrole rings, resulting in the more polar Z,E; E,Z; and E,E isomers. These photoisomers are more polar because they lack the intramolecular hydrogen bonding of the bilirubin-IXα, Z,Z configuration and therefore are readily excreted in bile. Although the photoisomers are normally a very small fraction of the total bilirubin, they can be used to advantage in hyperbilirubinemic infants, in whom phototherapy-induced isomers of unconjugated bilirubin-IXα can be excreted in the bile. In this situation, neonates with high levels of unconjugated bilirubin are placed under fluorescent light that emits in the 400- to 500-nm range (blue light). Consequently, the water insoluble bilirubin-IXα, Z,Z in the dermis undergoes photoisomerization to the more polar isomers, which are then excreted in the bile.

The most polar and therefore water-soluble form of bilirubin is conjugated bilirubin-IXα Z,Z (Fig. 12-1C). This is the main excretory form of bilirubin. The liver enzymatically attaches a glucuronic acid to one or both of the propionic side chains of bilirubin-IXα Z,Z. This esterification converts the lipid-soluble bilirubin with its internal hydrogen bonding to the more polar, water-soluble carbohydrate ester, which has no intramolecular hydrogen bonding. The conjugated bilirubin can then be excreted in the bile. If the serum level of conjugated bilirubin becomes greater than 2 mg/dl, it will also be excreted in the urine. Unconjugated bilirubin cannot be excreted in the urine but readily diffuses across biological membranes such as intestinal epithelium or the blood-brain barrier. In general, the bili-

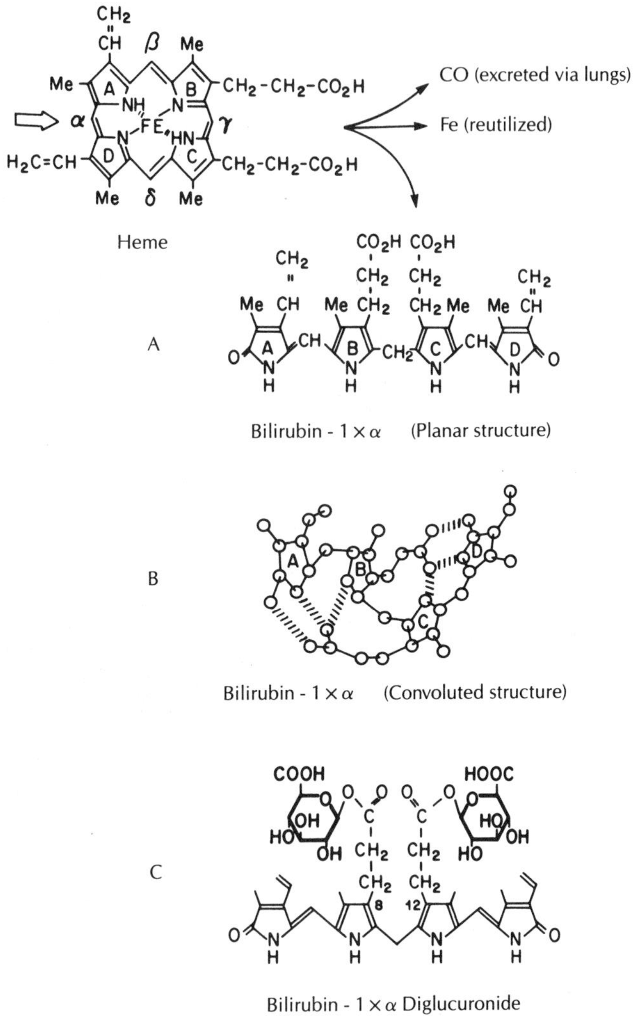

Fig. 12-1

A. Catabolism of heme to bilirubin and carbon monoxide (conventionally written structure). B. Involuted hydrogen-bonded molecular structure of bilirubin. In the presence of hydrogen-bonding (as predicted by hatched lines), bilirubin is nonpolar and therefore insoluble in water. C. The liver enzymatically attaches one or two (as depicted here) glucuronide groups to the propionic side chains of bilirubin. This prevents intramolecular hydrogen bonding. The bilirubin molecule is hence water-soluble and readily excreted in the bile.

rubin level must be greater than 20 mg/dl in full-term infants before kernicterus results. In premature, low-birth-weight infants, lower levels of bilirubin can result in kernicterus.

Sources

In adults, the daily production of bilirubin is 250 to 300 mg. About 70 percent of this is from degradation of heme from senescent red blood cells (about 1% of the total red blood cells

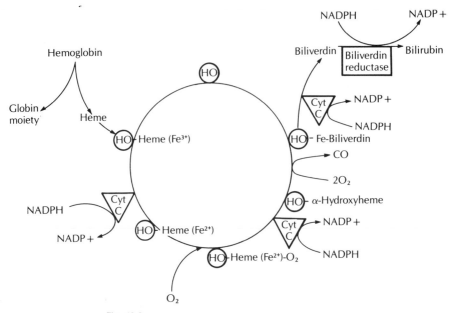

Fig. 12-2
Postulated mechanism of heme degradation to bilirubin by the microsomal heme oxygenase system and cytosolic biliverdin reductase. (Key: HO = heme oxygenase; Cyt C = NADPH-cytochrome c reductase)

per day) by the reticuloendothelial system of the spleen, bone marrow, and liver. Another 25 to 35 percent of bilirubin is from the hepatic turnover of hemoproteins such as cytochrome P-450 and catalase. Rarely, the destruction of young or developing erythroid cells can contribute significantly to the total daily bilirubin production in disease processes of ineffective erythropoiesis such as megaloblastic anemias, iron deficiency anemia, sideroblastic anemia, lead poisoning, and thalassemia minor.

Formation After senescent red blood cells are engulfed by phagocytic cells of the reticuloendothelial system, primarily in the spleen and liver, hemoglobin is catabolized and the constituents of the globin moiety are returned to the amino acid pool. The heme moiety undergoes catabolism by three separate enzyme systems as it is degraded to bilirubin (microsomal heme oxygenase, NADPH-cytochrome c reductase, and biliverdin reductase; Fig. 12-2). After dissociation from the globin, heme is transferred to microsomal heme oxygenase in the endoplasmic reticulum. The ferric-heme is reduced to the ferrous form following the donation of an electron by NADPH. This reaction is catalyzed by the NADPH-cytochrome c reductase system. Molecular oxygen binds to this reduced complex, and a second electron is donated by the NADPH-cytochrome c reductase system. This reduction of iron is accompanied by oxidation of the heme ring at the α-methene bridge with liberation of carbon monoxide (CO) and formation of the biliverdin-iron complex. This complex is hydrolyzed to biliverdin and iron, with the iron ultimately being transferred to the iron-carrying proteins (i.e., transferrin and ferritin) to be partially reutilized for heme synthesis. At this point, three moles of oxygen have been consumed per mole of heme catabolized, with 1 mole of CO released. For research purposes, the rate of formation of bilirubin can be estimated by CO production.

The third enzyme system, biliverdin reductase (located in the cytosol), completes the catabolism to bilirubin. This enzyme catalyzes the NADPH-dependent hydrolysis of biliverdin to bilirubin.

Plasma Bilirubin Transport

Unconjugated bilirubin, essentially insoluble in aqueous solutions at physiologic pH, is transported to the hepatocyte bound reversibly to albumin. There is a fraction of free or unbound bilirubin in plasma, but in an exceedingly small quantity, such that it is difficult to obtain accurate determinations of the amount of free bilirubin in plasma. However, there are numerous compounds that will compete with bilirubin for albumin binding, thereby increasing free bilirubin. In the jaundiced neonate, this can lead to increased transfer of bilirubin into the brain with subsequent development of kernicterus. Some of the compounds that compete with the albumin binding site include antibiotics (sulphisoxasole and penicillin derivatives), analgesics and non-steroidal anti-inflammatory agents (aspirin and indomethacin), food additives (parabens), x-ray contrast media for cholangiography, and diuretics (furosemide). The physician must be cautious in the use of these compounds in the jaundiced neonate at risk for the development of kernicterus.

There is an additional form of albumin-bound bilirubin variously termed *delta bilirubin, BIL-ALB,* or *bili-protein.* This is a nondissociable form of albumin-bound bilirubin that reacts directly with the commonly used diazo reagent (indicative of conjugated bilirubin). Only recently has it been recognized by the use of reverse phase high-performance liquid chromatography that delta bilirubin is distinct from conjugated bilirubin. Delta bilirubin is not detectable in normal serum or in patients with unconjugated hyperbilirubinemia (hemolysis, physiologic neonatal jaundice, Gilbert's syndrome), but it can be a significant component (up to 90%) of the total plasma bilirubin in hepatobiliary conditions such as acute and chronic hepatitis, biliary obstruction or Dubin-Johnson syndrome. This fraction increases with the duration of the disease. Because the bilirubin is so tightly

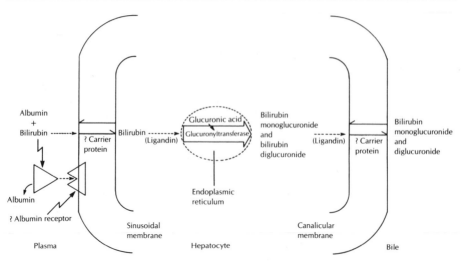

Fig. 12-3
Bilirubin uptake, intracellular transport, glucuronidation, and excretion into the bile.

bound to albumin in this form, it is not available for hepatic uptake and excretion, nor is it excreted in the urine. Consequently, it has a long plasma half-life (roughly equivalent to the half-life of albumin, i.e., 12–14 days) and can persist long after the disease process that contributed to the hyperbilirubinemia has subsided. This can lead to unnecessary evaluation and concern as the physician searches for the cause of the persistent hyperbilirubinemia.

Hepatic Uptake and Transport

Once the albumin-bound bilirubin reaches the space of Disse by passing through the fenestrations in the hepatic sinusoids, the complex comes in contact with the hepatocyte membrane. At this point, it is unclear how bilirubin separates from albumin and passes into the cell, although evidence does exist for a specific albumin receptor or binding site (Fig. 12-3). This hypothesized binding site does not appear to be specific for the albumin-bilirubin complex but is shared by a variety of other organic anions (e.g., sulfobromophthalein [BSP] and indocyanine green). Once the albumin-bilirubin complex is attached to the binding site, there is rapid transfer of bilirubin to the hepatocyte membrane, with albumin detaching and returning to the circulation. The bilirubin then appears to be transported through the hepatocyte membrane to the cytosol by means of a high-capacity, carrier-mediated transport system. It is estimated that about 30 percent of unconjugated bilirubin initially taken up by the hepatocyte refluxes back into the plasma by way of this bi-directional carrier system.

Once in the cytosol, bilirubin appears to be transported by another carrier-mediated transport system to the endoplasmic reticulum. This system is composed of two proteins, ligandin (glutathione S-transferase) and Z-protein (fatty acid–binding protein), which also bind conjugated bilirubin and other organic anions (e.g., BSP, indocyanine green). Ligandin may also serve to decrease efflux of bilirubin out of the hepatocyte and act as a storage system in conditions of unconjugated or conjugated bilirubin excess. Recently, there has been evidence of an additional means of intracellular bilirubin transport by membrane-to-membrane transfer.

Conjugation

Once the bilirubin arrives at the hepatocyte endoplasmic reticulum, either attached to ligandin or by direct membrane-to-membrane transport, it undergoes conjugation through an ester linkage to the sugar, UDP-glucuronic acid. This esterification with glucuronic acid converts the water-insoluble bilirubin to the water-soluble form needed for excretion in the bile. As mentioned previously, glucuronic acid is attached to one of the carboxyl groups of either of the two propionic acid side chains of bilirubin to form either the C8 or C12 isomers of bilirubin monoglucuronide, or to both propionic side chains, forming bilirubin diglucuronide (see Fig. 12-1C).

Conjugation of bilirubin is catalyzed by the membrane-associated enzyme bilirubin UDP-glucuronyltransferase (bilirubin-GT), which is located primarily in the smooth and rough endoplasmic reticulum of the hepatocyte. Both monoglucuronide and diglucuronide formation are catalyzed by this enzyme. Under normal circumstances, bilirubin diglucuronide represents the major pigment fraction in human bile (almost 80%), whereas the monoglucuronide represents only a minor fraction. The monoglucuronide can become a larger portion of the conjugated bilirubin in conditions of decreased bilirubin-GT activity, such as in Gilbert's syndrome and Crigler-Najjar type II disease. This is because in conditions of relative bilirubin excess, bilirubin-GT favors the formation of bilirubin monoglucuronide. UDP-glucuronyltransferase is actually a family of at least four different isoenzymes, each with specificity for different types of substrates. The many lipophilic substrates other than bilirubin that are glucuronidated by UDP-glucuronyltransferase include drugs such as morphine, propranolol, and chloramphenicol; endogenous compounds such as estrone, testosterone, and thyroxine; and certain bile acids (e.g., chenodeoxycholate). A specific isoform for the glucuronidation of bilirubin is not detectable in Crigler-Najjar type I disease (or in the Gunn rat animal model), whereas glucuronidation of other substrates remains unimpaired or minimally reduced.

Excretion

Once the bilirubin has been conjugated, it must be transported to the canalicular membrane for excretion in the bile. The manner in which conjugated bilirubin arrives at the canalicular membrane is unclear but may involve binding to ligandin or transport in the form of intracellular vesicles. When conjugated bilirubin arrives at the canalicular membrane, it is thought to undergo carrier-mediated transport into the bile. This process appears to be the rate-limiting step for the overall transhepatic transport of bilirubin, and it is the interference with this step that is presumed to be primarily responsible for the hyperbilirubinemia associated with hepatocellular disorders. Competition for this membrane carrier occurs with various organic anions, including BSP, indocyanine green, and iodinated contrast agents, but not with bile acids, which appear to have a distinct membrane carrier system of their own.

Bilirubin diglucuronide is the major pigment in human bile, and, once excreted into the small intestine, it is not significantly absorbed. Unconjugated bilirubin, which under normal circumstances constitutes less than 1 percent of excreted pigment, can be reabsorbed. In the rat model, approximately 25 percent of unconjugated bilirubin introduced experimentally into the intestine is absorbed and re-excreted in the bile, primarily in the conjugated form. In the healthy adult, conjugated bilirubin passes through the small bowel largely intact. However, in the terminal ileum and colon, bacterial β-glucuronidase hydrolyzes a portion of conjugated bilirubin to the unconjugated form (Fig. 12-4). Further reduction by bacteria to a complex series of colorless tetrapyrroles, collectively called *urobilinogen,* occurs in the colon. Approximately 20 percent of urobilinogen undergoes enterohepatic circulation with reabsorption in the colon and re-excretion into the bile. A small fraction (about 2%) of the daily production of urobilinogen is excreted in the urine. This fraction is increased in hemolytic disorders and hepatocellular disease and in the presence of portosystemic shunts.

Clinical Disorders of Hyperbilirubinemia

There are four general pathologic mechanisms by which hyperbilirubinemia can result: (1) increased bilirubin production from breakdown of red blood cells, (2) decreased bilirubin uptake or transport by the hepatocyte, (3) a defect in hepatic conjugation of bilirubin, and (4) a defect in the excretion of bilirubin either from the hepatocyte into the bile or from the bile collecting system into the small intestine. Hyperbilirubinemia can be classified into the following three subgroups: *Prehepatic* (i.e., increased bilirubin production such as from hemolysis); *in-*

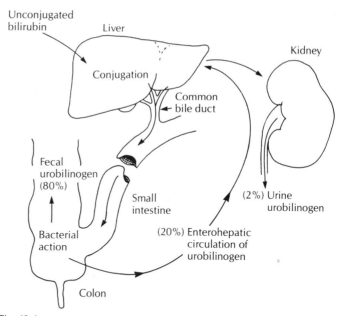

Fig. 12-4
Schematic diagram illustrating the major steps in the metabolism and excretion of bilirubin.

trahepatic (i.e., a defect in uptake, transport, or conjugation of bilirubin by the hepatocyte); and *posthepatic* (i.e., a defect in biliary excretion as would occur in obstructive jaundice; Table 12-1).

Prehepatic Hyperbili- rubinemia

Prehepatic hyperbilirubinemia (increased bilirubin production) can result from one of four mechanisms: (1) increased destruction of circulating red blood cells (i.e., hemolysis), as occurs in autoimmune hemolysis or transfusion of stored blood; (2) the destruction of abnormal erythrocytes in the bone marrow (dyserythropoiesis), as might occur in pernicious anemia; (3) increased breakdown of heme-containing cytochrome enzymes in the liver; and (4) phagocytic destruction of extravasated erythrocytes, such as in resorption of a hematoma or pulmonary infarction.

The hyperbilirubinemia resulting from hemolysis is generally mild (rarely greater than 4 mg/100 ml). This is because the normal liver has a high capacity for processing and excreting bilirubin. In fact, the bilirubin level may still be near normal in patients with a 50 percent reduction in red cell survival. Only in cases of severe hemolysis, as might occur in acute sickle cell crisis or paroxysmal nocturnal hemoglobinuria, does the serum bilirubin rise transiently above 4 mg/100 ml.

Table 12-1
Causes of jaundice

Prehepatic (pigment overload)	Intrahepatic (hepatocellular or cholestasis)		Posthepatic (obstructive)
Hemolysis (drugs, auto-immune, hemoglo-binopathies)	Congenital	Acquired	Common bile duct stone
	Gilbert's syn-drome	Viral hepatitis	Benign common bile duct strictures
Dyserythropoiesis	Crigler-Najjar syn-drome (types I and II)	Alcohol-related	
Multiple transfusions		Drugs	Pancreatic cancer
Hematoma resorption		Sepsis	Pancreatitis
	Dubin-Johnson syndrome	Congestive heart failure	Bile duct cancer
	Rotor's syndrome	Total parenteral nutrition	Ampullary cancer
			Choledochal cyst
		Postoperative status	Sclerosing cholangitis
		Malignancy	
		Primary biliary cirrhosis	

In the absence of liver disease, hemolysis results in a pure un-conjugated hyperbilirubinemia. The liver conjugates the in-creased load of bilirubin presented to it and excretes it into the bile. As mentioned previously, this results in increased produc-tion and absorption of urobilinogen. Unconjugated bilirubin cannot be excreted in the urine. Thus, the hallmark of hemolytic jaundice is a mild unconjugated hyperbilirubinemia and in-creased urinary excretion of urobilinogen in the absence of bili-rubinuria. However, occasionally in severe hemolytic crises, the biliary excretory mechanism for the excretion of conjugated bili-rubin is overwhelmed. In this situation, conjugated bilirubin refluxes back into the serum, resulting in a mild degree of con-jugated hyperbilirubinemia along with the predominantly un-conjugated hyperbilirubinemia.

The conjugated hyperbilirubinemia resulting from hemolysis is, in itself, a benign condition. Only in the newborn does the unconjugated hyperbilirubinemia pose the risk of kernicterus. With long-standing hemolysis, as is seen in hereditary spherocy-tosis and sickle cell anemia, the risk of cholelithiasis is increased because of the precipitation of bilirubin in the bile in the form of pigment gallstones.

Dyserythropoiesis, or ineffective erythropoiesis, results in a very mild hyperbilirubinemia associated with the premature de-struction of defective immature red cells in the bone marrow or spleen. The reticulocyte count is often normal or only slightly increased. Disorders associated with dyserythropoiesis include megaloblastic anemia, thalassemia, sideroblastic anemia, lead poisoning, and erythroleukemia. A rare cause of ineffective erythropoiesis is "primary shunt hyperbilirubinemia" or "idiopathic dyserythropoietic jaundice." This disorder results in asymptomatic jaundice starting in the second or third decade of life. The underlying defect in this disorder is unknown, and other than predisposing to cholelithiasis, this condition is generally considered benign.

Hyperbilirubinemia from increased breakdown of heme-containing cytochrome enzymes in the liver has been observed in experimental animals but has never been documented to occur in humans. Jaundice resulting from the breakdown of extravasated red blood cells, as from a hematoma, is unusual unless there is coexistent liver disease.

Intrahepatic Hyperbilirubinemia

Intrahepatic causes of hyperbilirubinemia can be divided into hereditary defects and acquired disturbances. Hereditary defects can be further subdivided into those resulting in an unconjugated hyperbilirubinemia (Table 12-2), and those manifesting

Table 12-2
Hereditary nonhemolytic unconjugated hyperbilirubinemia

	Crigler-Najjar disease type I	Crigler-Najjar disease type II	Gilbert's syndrome
Incidence	Rare	Uncommon	3–7% of adult population
Inheritance	Autosomal recessive	? autosomal dominant with variable penetrance	? autosomal dominant; more common in males
Bilirubin UDP-glucuronyltransferase activity	Undetectable	Markedly decreased (<10%)	⅓ normal
Clinical features	Severe jaundice (>20 mg/dl) beginning 3–4 days after birth Kernicterus usually in infants; occasionally in early adulthood Death in infancy/early adulthood	Jaundice noted in 1st year of life (usually <20 mg/dl, average 14 mg/dl) Usually asymptomatic; kernicterus is rare	Mild jaundice (bilirubin <6 mg/dl, usually <3 mg/dl) asymptomatic
Routine liver function tests (SGOT, SGPT, alkaline phosphatase, albumin, prothrombin time), liver histology	Normal	Normal	Normal
Therapy	Liver transplantation	Phenobarbital for cosmetic reasons	None needed

Table 12-3
Hereditary conjugated hyperbilirubinemia

	Dubin-Johnson syndrome	Rotor's syndrome
Incidence	Uncommon	Rare
Inheritance	Autosomal recessive	Autosomal recessive
Clinical features	Bilirubin 2–5 mg/dl (rarely up to 20 mg/dl)	Bilirubin 2–5 mg/dl (rarely up to 20 mg/dl)
	Usually recognized in early adulthood	Usually recognized in early adulthood
	Asymptomatic/normal life expectancy	Asymptomatic/normal life expectancy
Routine liver function tests	Normal	Normal
Liver histology	Black-brown pigment granules in hepatocytes; otherwise normal	Normal
Therapy	None needed	None needed

predominantly as a conjugated hyperbilirubinemia (Table 12-3). The hereditary disorders resulting in an unconjugated hyperbilirubinemia include Crigler-Najjar disease (types I and II) and Gilbert's syndrome, whereas those resulting in predominantly a conjugated hyperbilirubinemia include Dubin-Johnson syndrome and Rotor's syndrome. The acquired disturbances leading to hyperbilirubinemia are numerous (from viral hepatitis to toxic-metabolic defects; see Table 12-1). In spite of severe hepatocellular damage, the liver is still able to conjugate bilirubin. Therefore, the hyperbilirubinemia associated with acquired hepatocellular diseases is primarily conjugated. The approach to the evaluation of these acquired disorders is discussed at the end of this chapter.

Hereditary Unconjugated Hyperbilirubinemia
Crigler-Najjar Type I Disease
First described in 1952, Crigler-Najjar type I disease is a rare autosomal recessive disease characterized by the complete absence of bilirubin glucuronyl-transferase activity. Consequently, those genetically afflicted with this disease present in the first few days of life with a severe unconjugated hyperbilirubinemia. Most patients die within the first 18 months of life with bilirubin encephalopathy; however, rarely, individuals have survived into young adulthood before the onset of kernicterus and subsequent death.

Except for occasional bile thrombi, liver histology on light and electron microscopy is normal. Other than the isolated unconjugated hyperbilirubinemia (usually greater than 20 mg/dl), all other laboratory tests are normal, including hepatic clearance of BSP. The treatment of Crigler-Najjar type I disease has included exchange transfusions, phototherapy, and plasmapheresis. None of these modalities has consistently proved effective in reducing serum bilirubin and improving survival. However, liver transplantation has recently been used and appears promising.

Crigler-Najjar Type II Disease

Crigler-Najjar type II disease is also characterized by a defect in bilirubin conjugation; however, unlike Crigler-Najjar type I disease, this defect is only partial, albeit severe (bilirubin UDP-glucuronyltransferase activity is less than 10% of normal). Consequently, the serum unconjugated bilirubin level is almost always less than 20 mg/dl (usually about 14 mg/dl). The onset of hyperbilirubinemia is most often recognized in the first year of life but occasionally is not manifest until young adulthood. The prognosis appears to be good with neurologic damage occurring only rarely. Phenobarbital treatment, an inducer of glucuronyltransferase activity, will decrease serum bilirubin levels considerably in type II disease, but not in type I disease. As in type I disease, liver histology and other routine laboratory tests are normal. The mode of inheritance appears to be autosomal dominant with variable penetrance.

In type II disease, phenobarbital therapy is very helpful in maintaining a reduced serum bilirubin level for cosmetic reasons and to decrease the remote potential for the development of kernicterus.

Gilbert's Syndrome

Gilbert's syndrome is a genetically inherited condition characterized by a mild elevation in serum unconjugated bilirubin (1–3 mg/dl) in the absence of other laboratory abnormalities of liver dysfunction (i.e., serum glutamic oxalotransferase, alkaline phosphatase, albumin, prothrombin time are all normal) or of overt hemolysis (although a mildly shortened red blood cell [RBC] survival can be detected in 60% of patients by use of 51Cr-tagged RBCs). A percutaneous liver biopsy (which is seldom necessary to make the diagnosis) shows normal histology. The condition is considered totally benign except for the cosmetic effect of mild jaundice: There is no hepatosplenomegaly; kernicterus never develops; and there appears to be no predisposition to pigment gallstones. This condition is probably inherited as an autosomal dominant trait with incomplete penetrance, affecting a large proportion of the population (3–7%). It is most commonly diagnosed in the second to third decade, and males predominate over females in a ratio of between 2:1 and 7:1.

The primary defect responsible for the elevated serum unconjugated bilirubin is thought to be depressed hepatic bilirubin clearance owing to a decrease in the activity of bilirubin UDP-glucuronyltransferase (usually one third of normal activity). Enzyme inducers, such as phenobarbital, will decrease the serum level of bilirubin, which supports decreased enzyme conjugating activity as the major cause of hyperbilirubinemia. However, in approximately one third of patients, there are abnormalities in the hepatic clearance of the organic ion, BSP, either in uptake or excretion. Furthermore, tolbutamide, an organic ion that does not undergo glucuronidation, has a prolonged half-life in patients with Gilbert's syndrome, probably as a result of impaired hepatic uptake; thus, Gilbert's syndrome may represent a heterogeneous group of disorders.

There have been several tests devised to confirm the diagnosis. The simplest one consists of decreasing the caloric content of the diet to less than 400 calories per day for 1 to 2 days. This usually results in a doubling of the serum bilirubin with a subsequent return to baseline values within 6 hours of refeeding. The mechanism of this phenomenon is unclear but may be secondary to an increased load of bilirubin presented to the liver from breakdown of fat-stored bilirubin during the dieting. This is coupled with an increased reflux of unconjugated bilirubin from the hepatocyte back into the serum resulting from a decrease in hepatic ligandin concentration attributable to fasting. The administration of nicotinic acid is another provocative test. This test also exacerbates the hyperbilirubinemia; however, it does so by increasing the osmotic fragility of erythrocytes, thereby resulting in a mildly increased load of bilirubin presented to the hepatocyte. Neither of these tests is particularly sensitive or specific.

Because of its benign nature, no specific therapy for Gilbert's syndrome is necessary. However, on rare occasions, phenobarbital is sometimes prescribed to decrease the jaundice for cosmetic reasons. Although the clearance of certain drugs (e.g., tolbutamide, acetaminophen) is prolonged in Gilbert's syndrome, no important clinical consequences have been reported. It is important that the physician recognize this benign condition and thus avoid performing unnecessary and potentially harmful tests.

Hereditary Conjugated Hyperbilirubinemia
Dubin-Johnson Syndrome
Dubin-Johnson syndrome is an uncommon benign disorder characterized by chronic or intermittent jaundice (predominantly conjugated bilirubin) in the absence of demonstrable

liver disease. Inherited as an autosomal recessive trait, it is found most commonly among Iranian Jews (1 in 1300). The serum bilirubin is usually between 2 and 5 mg/dl but, occasionally, may be as high as 20 mg/dl. The diagnosis is usually made after puberty — at a time when the degree of jaundice may be enhanced by a concurrent illness, various drugs (e.g., oral contraceptives), or pregnancy. It is an asymptomatic condition, although, on rare occasions, hepatosplenomegaly is noted, and, in Iranian Jews, a clotting factor VII deficiency has been reported. On gross inspection, the liver is pigmented with a dark brown or black color. The liver histology is normal except for the presence of dark pigment granules predominantly in the centrilobular zones. This dense pigment appears to be contained within lysosomes; chemical analysis suggests that it is probably composed of polymers of epinephrine, although its exact chemical nature remains unclear. Interestingly, the pigment granules will transiently disappear during coincident disease, such as acute viral hepatitis.

Dubin-Johnson syndrome is thought to be the result of a defect in the canalicular transport of anions. This is suggested by BSP administration, which results in a slow to normal uptake by the liver, normal to mild retention at 45 minutes, but a characteristic rise in serum BSP at 90 minutes owing to a reflux of conjugated BSP from the liver back into the circulation. Oral cholecystography will not usually visualize the gallbladder in patients with this disorder, because the liver is unable to excrete this radiographic contrast material. Unique to this syndrome is an abnormal pattern of urinary excretion of coproporphyrins. Coproporphyrins exist in two isomeric forms, I and III. Coproporphyrin III is a precursor of heme; coproporphyrin I is a metabolic by-product of no known function. Both are excreted in the bile and urine. Normally, in the urine, 75 percent of total coproporphyrin is isomer III. However, in Dubin-Johnson syndrome (and in no other known condition), 80 percent of urine coproporphyrin is isomer I, whereas the total urine coproporphyrin level remains normal. It is not known why the ratio of isomer I to isomer III in urine is essentially reversed in this syndrome, but the uniqueness of this abnormal excretion has made it possible to diagnose Dubin-Johnson syndrome even in neonates.

Rotor's Syndrome

Rotor's syndrome is similar to Dubin-Johnson syndrome in that it is a rare, benign syndrome characterized by a predominantly conjugated hyperbilirubinemia (with other liver function tests being normal) and is inherited as an autosomal recessive trait. However, unlike Dubin-Johnson syndrome, liver histology is completely normal in that there is no pigment accumulation in the hepatocyte. Furthermore, the gallbladder is usually visualized on oral cholecystogram, and the urinary excretion of total coproporphyrins is markedly increased (200–500% of control values), with coproporphyrin I the predominant fraction. This pattern of increased coproporphyrin excretion is not unique to Rotor's syndrome — it is seen in many other hepatobiliary diseases. As in Dubin-Johnson syndrome, this is an asymptomatic syndrome with serum bilirubin levels in the range of 2 to 5 mg/dl and, rarely, up to 20 mg/dl. The diagnosis is usually not made until young adulthood, and no treatment is necessary. The pattern of BSP plasma disappearance is different than in Dubin-Johnson syndrome in that there is no secondary rise in plasma BSP at 90 minutes, and there is very slow initial disappearance. The nature of the organic anion transport defect in the liver is unknown.

Posthepatic Hyperbili-rubinemia

Posthepatic hyperbilirubinemia refers to conditions that interfere with the passage of conjugated bilirubin from the canalicular membrane to the intrahepatic bile ducts or the extrahepatic ducts or into the small intestine. Disorders affecting this step include extrahepatic obstruction secondary to stone, stricture, sclerosing cholangitis, or cancer (ampullary carcinoma, cholangiocarcinoma, pancreatic cancer, or metastatic cancer). Conjugated bilirubin that cannot be excreted secondary to a bile duct obstruction refluxes back into the plasma, producing primarily a conjugated hyperbilirubinemia.

Clinical Approach to Patients with Jaundice

The first step in evaluating a jaundiced patient is to take a thorough history from which important clues can be obtained to help direct further evaluation. For example, if the patient is a young intravenous (IV) drug abuser or an active homosexual or has recently received a blood transfusion, one would suspect a viral hepatitis as the most likely cause of jaundice. However, in an elderly male presenting with painless jaundice, pruritis, and weight loss, one would place extrahepatic obstruction secondary to pancreatic carcinoma high in the differential diagnosis.

After a thorough history has been taken, a complete physical examination is performed — again looking for clues that will aid in the differential diagnosis. Thus, if a palpable gallbladder is discovered, a diagnosis of extrahepatic obstruction would be supported. On the other hand, the findings of a tender enlarged liver, splenomegaly, ascites, spider angiomata, palmar erythema, Dupuytren's contractures, and gynecomastia in a patient with a long history of alcohol abuse would support the diagnosis of acute alcoholic hepatitis in the background of chronic alcoholic liver disease.

The initial laboratory assessment of the jaundiced patient generally includes a complete blood count, urinalysis, liver function tests (SGOT, SGPT, alkaline phosphatase, total and direct reacting serum bilirubin, albumin, and prothrombin time) and stool examination for occult blood. If the patient is anemic and the urine is negative for bilirubin, one would suspect an unconjugated hyperbilirubinemia, with hemolysis as the most likely etiology. This theory would be supported by the findings of primarily an indirect-reacting hyperbilirubinemia, a high reticulocyte count, and fragmented RBCs on peripheral smear examination of the blood.

If a conjugated (direct-reacting) hyperbilirubinemia is discovered, one must then decide whether the disorder is primarily hepatocellular or cholestatic in origin. If the SGOT and SGPT are greater than 500 IU and the alkaline phosphatase is less than three times normal, an hepatocellular disorder would be suspected (i.e., viral hepatitis, drug-related hepatitis, or ischemic hepatitis). If the SGOT and SGPT are less than 500 IU and the alkaline phosphatase is greater than three times normal, a cholestatic cause of jaundice would be more likely. In this case, it becomes very important to distinguish intrahepatic cholestasis (sometimes called *medical jaundice*) from extrahepatic cholestasis (i.e., obstructive juandice, sometimes called *surgical jaundice*). Consequently, if features of a patient's illness are highly suggestive of hepatocellular disease, one would observe the patient while awaiting the return of viral serologies or while observing the response to withdrawal of a potentially hepatotoxic drug. If, after a period of observation, the diagnosis is still unclear, a liver biopsy may be indicated. On the other hand, if obstruction is suspected, additional studies should be performed. This work-up generally includes an abdominal ultrasound as the first imaging technique obtained. The sonographic finding of dilated bile ducts is highly predictive of extrahepatic obstruction, with false-positive findings generally being less than 5 percent. A computerized tomography (CT) scan is also useful in this situation but is more expensive and exposes the patient to radiation. However, if obstruction exists, a CT scan can provide more information as to the location and etiology of the obstruction.

Finally, in evaluating obstructive jaundice, it often becomes necessary to more clearly visualize or outline the biliary ductal system. Hepatobiliary scintigraphy with ^{99m}Tc-labeled diethyl acetanilid iminodiacetic acid or related compounds is helpful in establishing the diagnosis of acute cholecystitis or evaluating biliary duct leaks. However, this technique is not sensitive or specific enough to differentiate between intrahepatic and extrahepatic cholestasis. In general, direct cholangiography by percutaneous transhepatic cholangiography (PTC) or endoscopic retrograde cholangiopancreatography (ERCP) is better for visualizing the intrahepatic and extrahepatic bile ducts. There are many reasons why one would favor ERCP over PTC or vice versa in a particular clinical situation. In general, PTC is useful when the bile ducts are dilated and one suspects a proximal bile duct obstruction amenable to transhepatic stenting to relieve the obstruction. However, ERCP is preferred in most situations, because, with this procedure, the success rate for visualization of the biliary tree does not depend on whether the ducts are dilated; the pancreatic duct can also be visualized; and if needed, a sphincterotomy with bile duct stone removal or placement of a biliary stent can be performed at the same time. ERCP would also be preferred in conditions that would increase the risk of PTC, such as marked ascites or a severe coagulopathy. Obviously, both of these procedures depend on the availability of skilled personnel.

Study Questions

1. A 62-year-old female presents to her physician with a two-week history of nausea, anorexia, and fatigue. She had also noted progressively darker-colored urine, lighter-colored stools, and mild jaundice. Two months ago, an abdominal aortic aneurysm repair had been performed, at which time she received several blood transfusions. Physical examination revealed a mildly jaundiced ill-appearing woman. Her liver was enlarged and tender. The spleen was not palpable. Laboratory examination revealed a normal complete blood count, an SGOT that was 15 times normal, a normal alkaline phosphatase, and an elevated total bilirubin of 4.5 mg/dl and direct-reacting bilirubin of 3.5 mg/dl. Which of the following are likely to be true in this patient:

a. A urine test for urobilinogin will be strongly positive.

b. A urine test for bilirubin will be strongly positive.

c. Because the stools are lighter in color, this patient must have a component of obstructive jaundice.

Answer

b

This patient most likely has acute viral hepatitis from a blood transfusion. (Ninety percent of all transfusion-associated viral hepatitis is non-A, non-B.) There will be very little urobilinogen in the urine because in acute viral hepatitis, there is less bilirubin excreted into the bile and therefore less urobilinogen made by colonic bacteria for enterohepatic circulation and urinary excretion. Stool color becomes lighter with decreased hepatic excretion of bilirubin, but this does not differentiate hepatocellular jaundice from obstructive jaundice. Direct-reading (conjugated) bilirubin is water soluble and will be excreted in the urine.

2. A 69-year-old male presents to his physician with a three-month history of weight loss. In the last week he has noted light-colored stools, dark-colored urine, jaundice, and pruritis. Physical examination revealed a jaundiced, cachetic man with a nontender palpable mass in the right upper quadrant of the abdomen. Rectal examination revealed heme positive stool. Total serum bilirubin was 18 mg/dl with a direct-reacting component of 14 mg/dl, alkaline phosphatase was 5 times normal, and the SGOT was twice normal. An abdominal ultrasound demonstrated dilated common and intrahepatic bile ducts. The gall bladder was also markedly dilated, and no stones were seen. The pancreas appeared normal and no masses were detected. Which of the following statements is or are true:

   a. In obstructive jaundice, unconjugated bilirubin cannot be taken up by the liver.
   b. An ERCP would be useful in delineating the cause of the obstructive jaundice.
   c. Some component of this patient's direct-reacting bilirubin may represent delta bilirubin, which should be detectable in the urine.

Answer

b

This patient clearly has obstructive jaundice. The finding of heme positive stool with an abdominal ultrasound demonstrating a dilated common bile duct makes ampullary carcinoma a likely diagnosis. In this situation, an ERCP is very helpful as it would allow direct visualization of the ampulla at which time biopsies could be taken. In obstructive jaundice, unconjugated bilirubin can be taken up by the liver and conjugated but cannot be excreted into the bile. With long-standing obstructive jaundice (or jaundice of hepatocellular origin that results in primarily conjugated hyperbilirubinemia), delta bilirubin (bilirubin that is covalently bound to albumin) can become a significant part (up to 90%) of the total serum bilirubin. Delta bilirubin gives a direct reaction with the commonly used diazo reagent. Because it is irreversibly bound to albumin it cannot be excreted in the urine.

3. A 24-year-old obese medical student presented to the University Clinic with a one-day history of jaundice. He felt well in spite of having been on a very strict diet in the last three days in an attempt to lose weight. A thorough history revealed no risk factors for viral hepatitis or toxin exposure. Physical examination revealed an obese, mildly jaundiced, but otherwise healthy-appearing male. Laboratory examination revealed a total serum bilirubin of 3.5 mg/dl and a direct-reacting bilirubin of 0.5 mg/dl. All other routine laboratories — including SGOT, SGPT, alkaline phosphatase, albumin, and hematocrit — were normal.

a. Which of the following diagnoses should be considered?
   (1) Acute viral hepatitis
   (2) Gilbert's syndrome
   (3) Common bile duct obstruction

Answer

a. (2)

This patient almost certainly has the benign "intrahepatic" disorder Gilbert's syndrome. In this disorder, indirect hyperbilirubinemia is often first detected during a period of decreased caloric intake, which characteristically increases the serum bilirubin in these patients. The mechanism for the caloric restriction-induced increase in bilirubin is unclear but may be partially related to release of bilirubin from fat stores during the dieting. With other laboratory tests being normal, one need only rule out hemolysis as a potential cause for the indirect hyperbilirubinemia. Hemolysis is unlikely in view of the normal hematocrit; however, the blood smear should be examined and a reticulocyte count checked to rule out this possibility. Acute viral hepatitis can be excluded since the patient feels well and has normal serum SGOT and SGPT levels. The hyperbilirubinemia seen in patients with common duct stones is conjugated, and characteristically the serum alkaline phosphatase is elevated

b. Which of the following are true:
   (1) Liver histology would show dark pigment in the hepatocyte
   (2) A test for bilirubin in the urine would be positive
   (3) Phenobarbital would decrease the serum bilirubin

Answer

b. (3)

Liver histology in Gilbert's syndrome is normal. (Black pigment is seen in Dubin-Johnson syndrome.) Indirect (unconjugated) bilirubin is not water soluble and therefore cannot be excreted in the urine. Phenobarbital induces the activity of bilirubin uridine diphosphate-glucuronyl-transferase in the liver and thereby decreases the serum bilirubin in Gilbert's syndrome.

4. A four-week-old male infant has been markedly jaundiced since birth. His serum bilirubin is 25 mg/dl and is all unconjugated. The serum SGOT, SGPT, alkaline phosphatase, prothrombin time, albumin, and complete blood count are normal. Except for his profound jaundice, the physical examination is unremarkable.

 a. Which of the following are diagnostic considerations?
    (1) Gilbert's syndrome
    (2) Physiologic jaundice of the newborn
    (3) Dubin-Johnson syndrome
    (4) Crigler-Najjar syndrome, type I

Answer

a. (4)

This patient has the rare entity Crigler-Najjar type I syndrome. The onset of jaundice is within the first three days of life and the hyperbilirubinemia is all unconjugated. Kernicterus usually develops in the first few weeks of life followed by death in infancy. Gilbert's syndrome and Dubin-Johnson syndrome manifest as a mild hyperbilirubinemia in the second to third decade of life and Dubin-Johnson syndrome produces a conjugated hyperbilirubinemia. Physiologic jaundice of the newborn is associated with a mild unconjugated hyperbilirubinemia (mean of 6–8 mg/dl) and usually has resolved by the second to third week of life.

 b. Which mode of therapy should be considered?
    (1) Liver transplantation
    (2) Phenobarbital administration

Answer

b. (1)

Liver transplantation, which has only recently been performed in these patients, holds great promise for long-term survival. Since there is a complete absence of bilirubin uridine diphosphate-glucuronyl-transferase activity, phenobarbitol is of no value in these patients.

References

Blanckaert, N., and Schmid, R. Physiology and pathophysiology of bilirubin metabolism. In D. Zakim and T. D. Boyer (eds.), *Hepatology: A Textbook of Liver Disease*. Philadelphia: Saunders, 1983. Pp. 246–296.

Chan, K., Scott, M. G., Wu, T., et al. Inaccurate values for direct bilirubin with some commonly used direct bilirubin procedures. *Clin. Chem.* 31:1650, 1985.

Chopra, S., and Griffin, P. H. Laboratory tests and diagnostic procedures in evaluation of liver disease. *Am. J. Med.* 79:221, 1985.

Chowdhury, J. R., and Chowdhury, N. R. Conjugation and excretion of bilirubin. *Sem. Liver Dis.* 3:11, 1983.

Gollan, J. L., and Knapp, A. B. Bilirubin metabolism and congenital jaundice. *Hosp. Pract.* 20:83, 1985.

Gollan, J., and Schmid, R. Bilirubin Metabolism and Hyperbilirubinemia Disorders. In R. Wright et al. (eds.), *Liver and Biliary Disease* (2nd ed.). London: Saunders, 1985. Pp. 301–357.

Hauser, S., and Gollan, J. Recent Developments in Hyperbilirubinemia and Bilirubin Metabolism. In G. L. Gitnick (ed.), *Current Hepatology*, Vol. 4. New York: Wiley, 1984. Pp. 453–477.

Okolicsanyi, L., Fevery, J., Billing, B., et al. How should mild, isolated unconjugated hyperbilirubinemia be investigated? *Sem. Liver Dis.* 3:36, 1983.

Reichen, J. Familial unconjugated hyperbilirubinemia syndromes. *Sem. Liver Dis.* 3:24, 1983.

Richter, J. M., Silverstein, M. D., and Schapiro, R. Suspected obstructive jaundice: A decision analysis of diagnostic strategies. *Ann. Intern. Med.* 99:46, 1983.

Scharschmidt, B. F., Goldberg, H. I., and Schmid, R. Approach to the patient with cholestatic jaundice. *N. Engl. J. Med.* 308:1515, 1983.

Stremmel, W., Travoloni, N., and Berk, P. D. Uptake of bilirubin by the liver. *Sem. Liver Dis.* 3:1, 1983.

Weiss, J. S., Gautam, A., Lauff, J. J., Sundberg, M. W., et al. The clinical importance of a protein-bound fraction of serum bilirubin in patients with hyperbilirubinemia. *N. Engl. J. Med.* 309:147, 1983.

Wolkoff, A. W. Inheritable disorders manifested by conjugated hyperbilirubinemia. *Sem. Liver Dis.* 3:65, 1983.

13 : Viral Hepatitis

Alexandra L. Gibas
Jules L. Dienstag

Overview of Viral Hepatitis

Major advances have been made in identifying the agents responsible for viral hepatitis. With the identification of specific viruses and the discovery of serologic markers has come, in turn, a broadening of our knowledge of the pathophysiology of viral hepatitis. Descending from this progress, advances have followed in the application of this information to the prevention of hepatitis B with vaccines, to cultivation of hepatitis A virus in tissue culture, and to antiviral therapy.

In addition to the three major types of viral hepatitis, type A, type B, and "non-A, non-B," the delta agent, now referred to as hepatitis D, has recently been identified and characterized (Table 13-1). Although non-A, non-B has not been characterized, epidemiologic and experimental data are consistent with the existence of non-A, non-B agents, including a distinct enterically transmitted non-A, non-B agent. Cytomegalovirus and Epstein-Barr virus, both associated with mononucleosis, can also cause hepatitis in humans. However, because the hepatitis associated with these other infections is not their primary manifestation, their discussion is beyond the scope of this chapter.

Hepatitis B
Molecular Structure

Hepatitis B virus (HBV) is a double-stranded DNA virus belonging to, and the only known representative in humans of, the hepadnavirus group (hepatotropic DNA viruses). Originally labeled "serum hepatitis" because of its transmission by inoculation with serum, HBV and HBV antigens circulate in abundance in the blood of infected patients. Three particulate (intact virion, hepatitis B surface antigen, and hepatitis B core antigen) and one soluble (hepatitis B e antigen) components of hepatitis B are commonly recognized, but other complexities of this virus and its structure have been elucidated.

The intact hepatitis B virion is a double-shelled 42-nm structure, the outer shell of which consists of hepatitis B surface antigen, HBsAg. Discovered originally in the serum of an Australian aborigine, this antigen had been called Australia antigen, one of several labels abandoned after its association with HBV was es-

Table 13-1
Abbreviations used in viral hepatitis

anti-HAV	antibody to hepatitis A virus
anti-HBc	antibody to hepatitis B core antigen
anti-HBe	antibody to hepatitis B e antigen
anti-HBs	antibody to hepatitis B surface antigen
anti-HD	antibody to hepatitis D antigen
HAV	hepatitis A virus
HBcAg	hepatitis B core antigen
HBeAg	hepatitis B e antigen
HBV	hepatitis B virus
HBsAg	hepatitis B surface antigen
HDV	hepatitis D virus (delta agent)
NANB	non-A, non-B

tablished. Excess HBsAg, indistinguishable from that in intact virions, also circulates as 22-nm-diameter spherical particles and tubular structures (Fig. 13-1). It is composed of two major polypeptides, a nonglycosylated one with a molecular weight of 24,000 daltons and its glycosylated counterpart with a molecular weight of 29,000 daltons. This HBV protein can be detected in all body fluids and in hepatocyte cytoplasm. Several HBsAg subdeterminants have been identified that allow distinction of subtypes of HBV. All HBsAg isolates share a common group determinant, *a*, as well as one of the allelic pairs *d* or *y* and *w* or *r*; therefore, the major subtypes of HBV are *adw, adr, ayw,* and *ayr*. Actually, more extensive analysis has revealed the marked subtype diversity of HBV, and we now recognize many more than the original four HBV subtypes. These subtypes can be used for epidemiologic analysis to establish the source of infection; they have no impact on clinical outcome.

The inner shell of HBV is the nucleocapsid core, measuring 27 nm in diameter and expressing on its outer surface hepatitis B core antigen (HBcAg), an antigen that cannot be detected in the circulation but that can be found primarily in hepatocyte nuclei and, to a lesser degree, in peripheral cytoplasm and the cell membrane. The nucleocapsid contains HBV DNA, DNA polymerase, and protein kinase, as well as a nonparticulate circulating antigen with a molecular weight of 34,000 daltons, hepatitis B e antigen (HBeAg). The 3200 base pair genome of HBV has an unusual structure; it is composed of circular DNA in which one strand is complete with a nicked end, while the other is incomplete. As a result, the genome is only partially double stranded, containing a single-stranded region. Four open reading frames

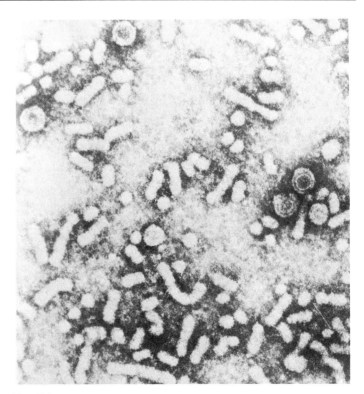

Fig. 13-1
Electron micrograph of the three morphological forms of hepatitis B virus in the serum of a patient with this condition. Note 22-nm spheres and tubules and intact virions.

have been recognized, comprising the now recognized four HBV genes: S, which codes for HBsAg; C, which codes for HBcAg and HBeAg; P, which codes for DNA polymerase; and X, which codes for a protein of limited characterization and unknown role. Additional complexity of the S gene has also been recognized. There is, in addition to the S region, which directs the replication of HBsAg, a pre-S region that contains pre-S1 and pre-S2, which code for larger HBsAg proteins, including HBV surface receptors for polymerized human serum albumin and for hepatocytes. These receptors have been postulated, but never proved, to account for the hepatotropism of HBV, and evidence suggests that HBsAg containing pre-S may be more immunogenic than HBsAg lacking pre-S products. Study of recently discovered hepadnaviruses in other animal species, for example, woodchuck hepatitis B virus, ground squirrel hepatitis virus, and duck hepatitis B virus, has illuminated much about the structure and replication of such viruses. These other viruses share the HBV structural and pathophysiologic features.

They all contain surface, external nucleocapsid (core), an internal nucleocapsid (e) antigen; the same three morphologic particulate structures; the partially single-stranded, partially double-stranded genome with its four genes; and an association with acute and chronic hepatitis and hepatocellular carcinoma. From the study of these animal "models" has emerged the recognition that all hepadnaviruses, including HBV, rely on a retroviral replicative strategy, requiring reverse transcriptase to replicate new DNA from an RNA intermediate.

Virologic and Serologic Events

Hepatitis B antigens and antibodies to them can be detected in serum and provide valuable diagnostic information.

After infection with HBV, the first viral marker to appear in the blood is HBsAg, present 4 to 12 weeks (but occasionally as early as 1 week) after viral exposure and prior to the onset of clinical hepatitis (Fig. 13-2). It persists through the clinical illness and remains present for a variable period of time. Although patients with acute hepatitis may clear HBsAg from their systems within 6 to 8 weeks after symptoms begin, persistence for 4 to 6 months is not uncommon, and, by definition, chronic infection exists if HBsAg is present beyond 6 months. The presence of HBsAg indicates active infection. In most cases of HBV infection, anti-HBs appears only after HBsAg has been cleared, as clinical symptoms are resolving. Occasionally, the appearance of anti-HBs lags several weeks. Anti-HBs is the protective antibody, and, after acute infection, the appearance of anti-HBs correlates with subsequent immunity to reinfection. In 10 to 20 percent of patients with chronic HBV infection, however, low-titer, low-affinity anti-HBs can also be detected. It does not represent protective antibody; it is not a prediction of imminent clearance of HBsAg; it is directed at a different subtype from that of the circulating HBsAg; and it is of no clinical or prognostic significance.

Hepatitis B core antigen does not circulate freely in the blood; therefore, it is not a useful clinical marker. However, antibody to HBcAg (anti-HBc) appears in virtually every case of HBV infection and can be detected within 1 to 2 weeks after HBsAg, long before anti-HBs becomes demonstrable. After acute HBV infection, whether infection resolves or remains chronic, anti-HBc persists indefinitely. A simple distinction between recent and remote HBV infection can be made by determining the antibody class of anti-HBc. High-titer IgM anti-HBc predominates during approximately the first 6 months after acute infection, whereas IgG anti-HBc is predominant thereafter. Therefore, testing for IgM anti-HBc provides a reasonable reliable clinical marker to determine the relative vintage of HBV infection in patients pre-

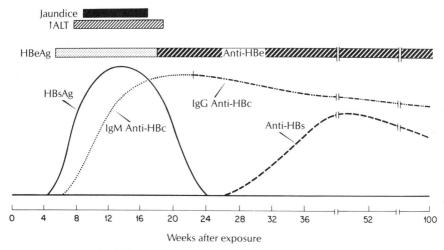

Fig. 13-2
Serologic and clinical events in hepatitis B virus.

senting for the first time with HBsAg. Occasionally, anti-HBc is the only detectable marker of HBV infection. This can occur in the small proportion of patients (1–5%) with acute HBV infection in whom HBsAg never reaches the threshold for detection with conventional assays (anti-HBc will be of the IgM class); in patients with chronic HBV infection whose HBsAg level is below the detection threshold, that is, a "low-level carrier" (IgG anti-HBc); in persons who have recovered from hepatitis B and whose infection occurred in the very remote past (IgG anti-HBc); and, rarely, in persons who are in the "window" between disappearance of HBsAg and appearance of anti-HBs (IgM anti-HBc if occurring during resolution of acute infection, IgG anti-HBc if occurring during resolution of chronic infection).

Routine commercial assays are available to detect HBeAg and antibody, anti-HBe. HBeAg appears concurrently with or shortly after HBsAg in all persons with acute HBV infection and correlates with ongoing viral synthesis, a high-titer of HBsAg, the presence of circulating virions, DNA polymerase, and HBV DNA. Because neither virions, DNA polymerase, nor HBV DNA are measurable with routinely available assays, HBeAg serves as a useful clinical tool to identify high infectivity. In acute HBV infection, HBeAg appears transiently, to be replaced early by circulating anti-HBe. In chronic HBV infection, the duration of HBeAg is variable, and a conversion from HBeAg to anti-HBe may coincide with improvement in liver disease. The study of markers of HBV replication has led to the distinction in cases of HBV infection between replicative and nonreplicative stages. The replicative stage is characterized by high levels of circulating virions, DNA polymerase, and HBV DNA; detectable HBeAg; free, episomal HBV DNA in hepatocyte nuclei; a tendency toward more severe hepatocellular injury; and high infectivity for contacts. The nonreplicative stage, which tends to occur late in the life cycle of infection, is characterized by a paucity or absence of circulating virions (only 22-nm spheres and tubules can be seen); absence of circulating DNA polymerase and HBV DNA; presence of circulating anti-HBe; relatively low infectivity; limited hepatocellular injury; and integrated HBV DNA in hepatocytes. Although the general rule is that replicative HBV infection gives way in time to nonreplicative infection, occasionally nonreplicative infection can be interrupted by spontaneous reactivation and re-expression of replicative infection.

Tissue culture to identify the presence of HBV plays no role in the diagnosis of infection with this virus. HBV cannot be cultivated in vitro in the classical sense; however, several cell lines have been transfected with HBV DNA, and they support replication of the intact virion and its associated viral proteins.

Epidemiology

Approximately 25,000 cases of new acute hepatitis B in the United States are reported to the Centers for Disease Control each year; however, a high frequency of subclinical infection and marked underreporting of clinical cases render the reported incidence a low estimate indeed. Seroepidemiologic surveys show that in the United States, 0.1 percent of adults harbor circulating HBsAg, and the frequency of previous exposure to HBV, reflected by the frequency of anti-HBs, is approximately 5 to 10 percent in adults. Thus, there are approximately 1 million HBsAg carriers in the United States. This figure is dwarfed, however, by the much higher frequency of HBV on a global scale. In certain parts of the world, especially the Far East and sub-Saharan Africa, HBV is endemic; 5 to 20 percent of the population are HBsAg-positive, and, among those who are HBsAg-negative, up to 90 percent have circulating HBV antibodies, indicative of infection in the past. Worldwide, therefore, the estimated number of HBsAg carriers reaches 200 million, or 5 percent of the Earth's population. This well-entrenched viral infection relies for its perpetuation on the maintenance of a carrier state in humans and on three primary modes of transmission. These are percutaneous inoculation or transmucous-membrane penetration, perinatal spread from mother to offspring, and intimate — primarily sexual — contact. The type of transmission and the onset of infection vary as a function of the endemicity of HBV infection. In low-prevalence areas, such as North America and northwestern Europe, most infections occur during adolescence and early adulthood. This is the age when sexual activity commences, when intravenous drug use begins, and when careers that pose occupational exposures, such as those in the health professions, begin. Therefore, in the United States, for example, most cases of HBV are transmitted by intimate contact and percutaneous inoculation/mucous-membrane penetration, and most cases do not occur until early adulthood. In contrast, in high-prevalence areas, such as Southeast Asia, most infections occur shortly after birth in offspring of HBsAg carrier mothers and result from perinatal transmission.

Certain population subgroups are at increased risk for HBV infection because of behaviors that foster one or more of the modes of HBV transmission or because of substantial exposure to blood or blood products. These include hemodialysis patients, health care workers exposed to blood, intravenous drug users, sexually promiscuous persons — especially noted in homosexual men and prostitutes — institutionalized mentally retarded/developmentally handicapped persons, and persons requiring multiple transfusions or repeated infusions of blood products (e.g., hemophiliacs). Ironically, HBV, which was once called *serum hepatitis,* is now rarely acquired as a result of blood transfusion. Since the early 1970s, all donated blood has been screened for HBsAg, eliminating almost all units containing HBV. The only exceptions, and the cause of the rare residual cases of transfusion-associated hepatitis B, are those donor units containing HBsAg levels below the sensitivity threshold of current-generation screening tests.

Because of the high frequency of HBV infection in certain parts of the world, and because of the large contribution of perinatal transmission in these countries, perinatal spread is perhaps the most important mode of HBV transmission on a global scale. Such infection occurs in babies born to HBsAg carrier mothers or to babies whose mothers are infected acutely primarily during the third trimester of pregnancy and in the immediate postpartum period. Although as many as 10 percent of such infections may occur in utero through breaks in the integrity of the barrier between the maternal and fetal circulation, almost all cases are thought to occur at the time of birth. Breast feeding has not been shown to have an impact on the likelihood of transmission. In contrast, HBeAg status is crucial. In the absence of preventive measures, babies born to HBsAg-positive mothers with HBeAg have a 90 percent likelihood of becoming HBsAg carriers, whereas babies born to HBsAg-positive mothers with anti-HBe have no greater than a 10 to 15 percent chance of becoming HBsAg carriers. Fortunately, measures are currently available that may limit the spread of HBV both in exposed newborns and in other exposed populations.

Although oral inoculation is occasionally successful, it is an inefficient mode of HBV transmission, and fecal-oral transmission plays no role in the spread of HBV. Arthropod-borne infection, although theoretically a potential mode of HBV transmission, has never been shown to play a role in the natural spread of HBV. It is worth emphasizing that not only blood, but all other body fluids as well, are potentially infectious, although less so than blood. In addition, HBV is a very stable agent that will retain its infectivity even after prolonged exposure on environmental surfaces.

Clinical Features The incubation period of hepatitis B averages about 2 months but can range from 1 to 6 months. In 5 to 20 percent of patients with acute hepatitis B, a serum sickness-like illness may occur within approximately 1 to 2 weeks prior to the icteric phase; it may consist of fever, arthralgias, arthritis, rash, or angioedema and is the result of tissue deposition of circulating HBsAg-anti-HBs immune complexes.

Other constitutional symptoms precede the icteric phase in most patients by 2 days to 3 weeks. Anorexia, altered olfactory/gustatory sense, nausea, right upper quadrant pain, malaise, and fatigue are common symptoms. Vomiting, weight loss, headache, photophobia, and upper respiratory symptoms can occur. In this early phase, physical findings are rare; slight hepatomegaly and abdominal tenderness may be present. Often, the most noticeable feature is the development of dark urine, usually just preceding the onset of clinically recognized jaundice.

During the icteric phase, which usually lasts from 2 to 10 weeks, many of the constitutional symptoms tend to subside, but anorexia and malaise may persist. Clinically, the sclerae and skin are icteric, there is right upper quadrant or epigastric tenderness, and adenopathy and splenomegaly can be detected in a small proportion of patients.

The diagnosis of hepatitis can be made based on elevations of the levels of the serum aminotransferase enzymes alanine aminotransferase (ALT, formerly called serum glutamate pyruvate transaminase [SGPT]) and aspartate aminotransferase (AST, formerly called serum glutamate oxaloacetic transaminase [SGOT]). The levels tend to rise to levels in the high hundreds to low thousands, and the ALT tends to be higher than the AST. Although alkaline phosphatase levels are often elevated as well, their elevations are not as striking as those of the aminotransferases. Bilirubin levels vary considerably, occasionally surpassing a level of 20 mg/100 ml. In typical cases, slight changes in white blood cell counts may occur; there is a relative lymphocytosis, and atypical lymphocytes are not uncommon. In very severe cases, the serum prothrombin time may lengthen, and blood sugar may be low. In protracted severe acute cases, albumin levels may also fall.

Establishing a diagnosis of hepatitis B is accomplished in almost all cases by finding HBsAg in serum. In the rare case in which levels of HBsAg are too low to be detected, the presence of IgM anti-HBc is sufficient to establish the diagnosis. Occasionally, other types of viral hepatitis, for example, type A, D, or non-A, non-B, occur in HBsAg carriers; in such cases, additional serologic data or clinical/epidemiologic findings will identify evidence for infection with more than one agent.

In 90 percent of patients with acute HBV infection, there is complete recovery, with resolution of hepatocellular injury, clearance of HBV from the liver and circulation, the development of anti-HBs and anti-HBc, and immunity from reinfection. In a small percentage of patients (0.1%) with acute HBV infection, fulminant hepatitis develops; such severe massive liver injury is associated with a very high (80%) mortality rate. By definition, the term *fulminant hepatic failure* is reserved for those patients who develop massive liver cell death within 2 months of the development of acute hepatitis. Clinically, these patients are confused, somnolent, or comatose, and they usually have ascites, edema, coagulopathy, and a shrinking liver. The bilirubin rises rapidly, and a significant prolongation of the prothrombin time is apparent; hypoglycemia is common, especially in the pre-terminal period. Death occurs as a result of gastrointestinal bleeding, sepsis, brainstem compression from cerebral edema, or multisystem failure. In the 20 percent of patients who survive fulminant hepatitis, recovery is the rule, and chronic liver disease does not follow.

Approximately 10 percent of patients with acute icteric hepatitis B will continue to be HBsAg-positive 6 months after acute illness. Approximately one half of these patients will clear their HBV infections more slowly over the next 1 to 2 years. Therefore, approximately 5 percent will remain infected chronically. In several recent studies of the natural history, estimates of chronic infection after acute infection were substantially lower, yielding a chronicity rate of approximately only 2 percent. On the other hand, many patients with chronic hepatitis B have not had a clinically recognizable acute illness. Thus, the frequency of chronic hepatitis B cannot be calculated accurately on the basis of documented acute cases. Among persons with chronic HBV infection are asymptomatic carriers and those with a spectrum of chronic hepatitis. Chronic hepatitis ranges from (1) the relatively mild and nonprogressive chronic persistent hepatitis (primarily portal and periportal inflammation, with maintenance of the integrity of the limiting plate of hepatocytes bordering portal tracts, and with minimal lobular activity), to (2) chronic lobular hepatitis, a more pronounced inflammatory process that resembles protracted acute hepatitis (in addition to portal/periportal inflammation, increased lobular activity, without erosion of the limiting plate) and that does not progress, to (3) chronic active hepatitis (more severe portal and lobular inflammation and necrosis, erosion of the limiting plate of periportal hepatocytes ["piecemeal necrosis"]; some cases of chronic active hepatitis are even more severe, with necrosis that spans lobules ["bridging necrosis"] or even multilobular collapse), a progressive process that tends to lead to fibrosis, scar formation, and architectural reorganization (i.e., cirrhosis).

Few clinical features are predictive of the likelihood for progression to chronic infection and chronic hepatitis. Infection during early childhood, natural or pharmacologic immunosuppression, and male gender are factors that increase the chances for chronicity. Although a confident distinction between progressive and nonprogressive forms of chronic hepatitis B requires histologic verification, clinical and virologic indicators may provide clues. Disabling systemic symptoms, very elevated aminotransferase levels, elevation of the prothrombin time, and depression of the albumin level are more common in chronic active hepatitis. In addition, patients with replicative chronic HBV infection (detectable serum HBeAg and HBV DNA) tend to have more severe histologic activity and are more likely to have chronic active hepatitis, whereas those with nonreplicative infection (detectable anti-HBe and undetectable HBV DNA) tend to have more quiescent necroinflammatory processes, such as chronic persistent hepatitis and the "healthy" carrier state. It is worth noting that the stage of replication in chronic HBV infection is not static; approximately 15 percent of patients with replicative chronic HBV infection convert to the nonreplicative stage each year; this tends to be associated with an improvement in liver injury. Recent observations have shown that occasionally, nonreplicative HBV infection may revert spontaneously back to the replicative stage. Such an event is accompanied by the reexpression of serologic markers of replication (HBeAg, HBV DNA) and by a resumption of liver injury. Reappearance of IgM anti-HBc is an inconstant finding and is therefore not a reliable marker of reactivation. The seroconversion rate for chronically

HBsAg-positive persons is substantially lower; only 1 percent per year clear their HBsAg and convert to anti-HBs positivity.

Cirrhosis and its associated portal hypertension lead to the development of variceal bleeding, ascites and edema, and hypersplenism; coagulopathy, cachexia, and hepatic encephalopathy may also follow. Eventually patients succumb. The other fatal complication of chronic HBV infection is hepatocellular carcinoma, which may occur in patients with chronic hepatitis and cirrhosis and in "healthy" carriers. This occurs rarely in persons who become chronically infected during adulthood but is a frequent outcome in those who acquire their infections during infancy, recognized especially in the Far East and Africa. In these areas of the world with the highest prevalence of HBsAg positivity, the annual incidence of hepatocellular carcinoma is also the highest in the world. The relative risk of dying from liver cancer in HBsAg-positive persons in the Far East, for example, has been documented to be more than 200 times higher than that in those persons who are HBsAg-negative; the estimated lifetime risk of hepatocellular carcinoma in HBsAg positive Asians has been estimated to be 40 to 50 percent! Although the exact molecular mechanism and events required for the oncogenicity of HBV are not known, the epidemiologic link between chronic HBV infection and hepatocellular carcinoma is established with high confidence (see Chap. 18). In addition, in these liver tumors, HBV DNA is integrated into the host genome, and cell lines derived from these primary liver tumors contain several copies of the HBV genome and express HBV proteins. The discovery that other hepadnaviruses, such as woodchuck hepatitis virus, are also associated with hepatocellular carcinoma in their respective animal species adds even further to the mounting evidence that HBV is an oncogenic virus.

Because of the characteristic clinical and virologic features of viral hepatitis in general and hepatitis B in particular, confusion with other clinical entities is infrequent. Still, the differential diagnosis includes infections with other hepatitis viruses, other viral diseases in which the liver becomes affected as part of a systemic illness (e.g., cytomegalovirus and Epstein-Barr virus infections, yellow fever), parasitic (toxoplasmosis, malaria) and rickettsial (Q fever) infections, drug-induced hepatitis, alcoholic hepatitis, biliary tract disease, and passive congestion of the liver secondary to right heart failure. In addition, the initial presentation of chronic liver diseases such as chronic active hepatitis may mimic acute hepatitis. Chronic active hepatitis is an important category of chronic liver disease; in the absence of a viral (hepatitis B, D, or NANB) or metabolic (e.g., copper overload in Wilson's disease) cause, autoimmune mechanisms are believed to be involved in the pathogenesis of this type of liver disease. A proportion of cases are associated with autoimmune features, for example, the presence in the circulation of antinuclear antibodies (ANA) and LE cells ("lupoid hepatitis"), and, histologically, the features are the same as those previously described for chronic active hepatitis B. Some authorities believe that autoimmune chronic active hepatitis is a distinct clinicopathologic entity, whereas others maintain that chronic active hepatitis is a single disease and that some, but not all, patients have autoimmune features. In this category of chronic active hepatitis ("autoimmune" or of unknown cause), characteristic features include symptoms and clinical signs similar to those described for acute and chronic hepatitis B. In addition to autoantibodies, elevated globulin levels are characteristic. The onset may be insidious or characterized by episodic illnesses resembling acute hepatitis. The mildest form of chronic active hepatitis is characterized histologically by features of lobular necrosis and inflammation with piecemeal necrosis (erosion of the limiting plate of periportal hepatocytes). Fibrosis and bridging necrosis are less common in this subset, clinical features are less severe, and progression to cirrhosis is not invariable. The more severe forms of chronic active hepatitis are characterized by aminotransferase levels 10 times the upper limit of normal, very high globulin elevations, aggressive-appearing morphologic changes on liver biopsy (bridging necrosis, multilobular collapse, coexistent cirrhosis), and a 1-year mortality rate approaching 40 percent. This severe form of chronic active hepatitis can lead to rapid clinical deterioration on the one hand but is very responsive to anti-inflammatory/immunosuppressive therapy, on the other hand. In marked contrast, chronic active hepatitis resulting from viral hepatitis is rarely responsive to anti-inflammatory/immunosuppressive therapy, which tends to provide a permissive environment for an increase in the level of virus replication.

Diagnostic confusion is also common when patients with acute and chronic hepatitis B present with extrahepatic manifestations. During the late incubation period of acute hepatitis B, the prodromal arthritis/dermatitis or serum-sickness-like syndrome can be mistaken for allergic cutaneous reactions and rheumatologic disorders. In chronic hepatitis B, chronic arthritis and dermatitis may occur as well as glomerulonephritis and generalized vasculitis (polyarteritis nodosa). These extrahepatic syndromes result from deposition in tissue vessel walls of HBsAg/anti-HBs immune complexes.

Although the pathogenesis of extrahepatic manifestations is well understood, an adequate explanation for liver injury and variable outcomes in patients infected with HBV is lacking. Substantial evidence suggests that HBV is not cytopathic for hepatocytes and that liver cell injury depends on the host's immune response to virus antigen(s) expressed on virus-infected hepatocytes. This hypothesis is supported by the occurrence of asymptomatic "healthy" HBsAg carriers, which harbor large numbers of virus-laden hepatocytes but have minimal or no liver cell injury. Cellular, rather than humoral, immunity appears to be the important immunologic component in the pathogenesis of liver cell injury in hepatitis B. For example, both acute and chronic hepatitis B can occur in patients with agammaglobulinemia. Similarly, there is an increased prevalence of chronic HBsAg carriage (i.e., without substantial liver injury) in patients with cellular immune defects, such as Down syndrome, chronic renal failure, organ transplants, and leukemia.

The currently favored hypothesis is that cytotoxic T cells are directed against a viral antigen target, HBcAg rather than HBsAg, on the hepatocyte surface membrane. This concept accommodates the observation that more severe liver injury tends to be associated with the replicative phase of HBV infection. During the replicative phase, increased virus replication is reflected not only by higher circulating levels of HBV and HBV antigens but also by increased expression in hepatocyte nuclei and on cytoplasmic membranes of HBcAg. Therefore, during the replicative stage, the target antigen for cytolytic T cells is expressed more abundantly and can provide the necessary ingredient for increased virus-antigen–initiated but host immune-response–effected hepatocyte injury. Although factors that favor the perpetuation of HBV infection are elusive, differences in outcome may be related to competition between cytolytic T cells and circulating anti-HBc for HBcAg on hepatocyte surface membranes. Other modulating factors, such as immunoregulatory influences, may also be involved.

Prevention and Management

There is no specific therapy for acute hepatitis B. Supportive measures such as maintenance of hydration and caloric intake are advised. Medications (especially those metabolized by the liver) should be used sparingly, and alcohol should be avoided. No other restrictions in diet or activity are necessary. For chronic active hepatitis B, the use of corticosteroids and other immunosuppressive agents has fallen out of favor. Although such therapy is effective for nonviral forms of chronic active hepatitis, it has not been shown to be effective in controlled trials. Treated patients actually tend to do less well than untreated controls, and virus replication is enhanced by such therapy. Current attention has shifted to experimental application of specific antiviral chemotherapy.

Because therapy for hepatitis HBV is lacking, prevention of infection has been emphasized. Simple commonsense precautions and methods to interrupt the spread of infection mechanically can be quite effective. For example, screening blood donors for HBsAg has led to the near-elimination of hepatitis B as a transfusion-transmitted disease, and segregating HBsAg-positive from HBsAg-negative hemodialysis patients and introducing surveillance and teaching programs in hemodialysis units have reduced dramatically the incidence of new HBV infections in these units. For optimal prevention, vaccination is the preferred approach; both passive immunization with globulin containing high-titer anti-HBs and active immunization with vaccine composed of HBsAg are available. Passive immunization provides immediate but short-lived protection, whereas active immunization involves a delay before the immune response to HBsAg develops but provides long-lasting immunity. Between the two approaches, passive immunization with hepatitis B immune globulin tends to be less effective. Evidence has accumulated to show that hyperimmune globulin tends to lengthen the incubation period of hepatitis B and to attenuate clinical illness rather than to prevent infection. As a rule, hyperimmune globulin is administered too late after exposure; it is an example of "too little, too late."

Emphasis has shifted, therefore, to active immunization with vaccine. Two forms of vaccine are available. The first consists of 22-nm spherical HBsAg particles purified from the plasma of HBsAg carriers. It is inactivated with pepsin, urea, and formalin, a process that destroys the infectivity of every virus, without exception, including human immunodeficiency virus. It has been shown to be immunogenic, effective in preventing HBV infection, and extraordinarily safe and free of serious adverse effects. Administered in three deltoid intramuscular injections at time 0, 1, and 6 months, this vaccine induces protective anti-HBs in greater than 95 percent of immunocompetent adults and children. Protection appears to last at least 5 years, if not longer. The other vaccine is made by genetic engineering. A recombinant yeast into which the gene for HBsAg has been inserted produces nonglycosylated HBsAg spherical particles. This vaccine appears to be comparable to the plasma-derived vaccine in immunogenicity, protective efficacy, and safety. Because hepatitis B vaccines contain only HBsAg and not other viral components, successful vaccines can be distinguished by the absence of anti-HBc from persons infected in the past with HBV.

Hepatitis B vaccine is recommended prior to exposure for groups with an increased risk of HBV infection (see section entitled Epidemiology). For persons who are not vaccinated but who sustain an accidental or unavoidable exposure to HBV (e.g., needle-stick inoculation, sexual exposure, or birth to a HBsAg-positive mother), a combination of passive immunization with hyperimmune globulin immediately after exposure and active immunization with vaccine is recommended.

Delta Hepatitis (Hepatitis D)
Virology

The delta agent is a defective RNA virus that measures approximately 35 to 37 nm and requires the helper function of HBV (or other hepadnaviruses) for successful infection. Hepatitis delta virus (HDV) has an unusual hybrid structure; its nucleocapsid core expresses an antigen unique to the delta agent, delta antigen (HDAg), and contains a very small circular single-stranded RNA genome similar in structure to that found in plant satellite viruses and viroids. Its outer shell consists of HBsAg (Fig. 13-3).

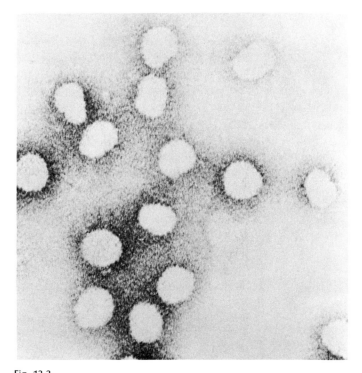

Fig. 13-3
Electron micrograph of delta particles purified from the serum of a chimpanzee.

Relying on HBV for its replication and for its outer component, HDV infection can occur only in the presence of HBV infection; therefore, acute HDV and HBV infections can occur simultaneously (coinfection), or delta infection can be superimposed on an already existing chronic HBV infection (superinfection). The delta agent acquires the HBsAg subtype of its host. If, for example, HDV infection is transmitted from one HBsAg carrier to another, and if the two HBsAg carriers have different subtypes, the HDV in the recipient will assume his, not the donor's, HBsAg subtype. In addition, because HDV and HBV rely on the same replicative processes and apparatus, often HDV superinfection of a host with HBV infection will be associated with a reduction in levels of the markers of HBV replication.

During HDV infection, delta antigen can be detected readily in the nuclei of hepatocytes; however, because the level of detectable virus antigenemia is low, delta antigen can be detected only rarely in serum. The humoral immune response to HDV consists of IgM and IgG antibody to HDAg (anti-HD). During acute HDV infection, high-titer, primarily IgM anti-HD predominates, and once such acute infection resolves, the level of anti-HD falls rapidly, rarely remaining detectable. In chronic HDV infection, both IgM and IgG anti-HD persist in high titer. In acute and chronic HDV infection, delta RNA can be detected with an experimental complementary DNA probe; the presence of delta RNA correlates well with the intranuclear expression of HDAg and is an excellent marker of HDV replication.

Epidemiology   Two patterns of delta infection have been recognized. In endemic areas, which include Mediterranean countries (southern Italy, northern Africa, the Middle East), a substantial proportion of those with chronic hepatitis B have delta markers, and transmission of HDV infection appears to occur via nonpercutaneous routes, primarily intimate contact. In nonendemic areas, such as North America and northern Europe, HDV markers are uncommon in those with HBsAg, except in population groups with frequent percutaneous exposures, that is, intravenous drug addicts and hemophiliacs. These broad distinctions are becoming blurred by population migrations from endemic to nonendemic areas and, in nonendemic areas, by the amplification of HDV infection within and outside of such populations as drug addicts, whose behavior facilitates spread of blood-borne infections. With increasing frequency, large, sustained outbreaks of simultaneous acute HDV plus HBV infections as well as of superimposed HDV infection in HBsAg carriers are being recognized, even in supposedly nonendemic areas.

Clinical Features   The duration of HBV infection determines the duration of HDV infection; clearance of HBV imposes an absolute limit on the perpetuation of HDV infection. Therefore, HDV coinfection does not increase the likelihood of chronicity of the simultaneous HBV infection. On the other hand, HDV infection is unlikely to resolve in the presence of chronic HBV infection. As long as its helper virus continues to persist, HDV can continue to replicate.

When coinfection with both HBV and HDV occurs, the clinical features are often indistinguishable from those of acute hepatitis B alone; however, occasionally, two sequential peaks of amino-transferase elevation occur, representing first acute hepatitis B, then acute hepatitis D. Superinfection with HDV of a patient with chronic hepatitis B often presents as an acute hepatitis–like exacerbation superimposed on an otherwise clinically stable HBV infection. The diagnosis of delta coinfection or superinfection can be made in most cases by demonstrating the presence of anti-HD in serum (see above); intrahepatic HDAg and circulating HDV RNA, when these markers are available, can also be helpful (Fig. 13-4). Clinical and biochemical features are similar to those of acute and chronic hepatitis B, except that hepatitis D tends to be more severe.

This increased severity is the basis for the clinical importance of delta hepatitis. Delta hepatitis accounts for approximately 30 percent of all cases of fulminant hepatitis in patients with acute hepatitis B and 70 percent of fulminant hepatitis cases in patients with chronic hepatitis B. In addition, histologic evaluation in patients with chronic delta hepatitis almost always shows the presence of chronic active hepatitis or cirrhosis or both. In general, HDV tends to increase the virulence and severity of HBV infection. The delta agent can transform acute or chronic hepatitis B into fulminant hepatitis, asymptomatic HBsAg carriage or chronic persistent hepatitis B into chronic active hepatitis, or mild chronic active hepatitis into severe and rapidly progressive chronic active hepatitis. The only serious outcome of HBV infection that has not been linked to HDV is hepatocellular carcinoma, presumably because patients with delta infection succumb to the more immediate severe complications previously described.

Prevention and Management   For those who are susceptible to HBV infection, successful vaccination with hepatitis B vaccine will prevent not only hepatitis B but also hepatitis D. For those with chronic hepatitis B, the only preventive, albeit often impractical, measure available is to avoid close personal contact with persons known to have delta

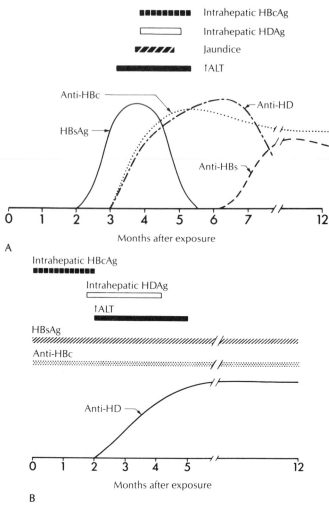

Fig. 13-4
A. Virologic and serologic events during acute hepatitis D virus (HDV) and hepatitis B virus (HBV) coinfection. B. Virologic and serologic events during acute HDV superinfection of a chronic HBV carrier.

hepatitis. Corticosteroid/immunosuppressive therapy has been shown to be unsatisfactory in severe chronic active hepatitis associated with HDV. The only promising therapeutic approach in chronic hepatitis D has been the use of alpha-interferon, which has had a beneficial effect in approximately 50 percent of treated patients.

Hepatitis A

Molecular Structure

Hepatitis A virus (HAV) is a 27-nm nonenveloped single-stranded RNA virus (Fig. 13-5) with properties of the enterovirus genus of the picornavirus family; it has been classified as en-

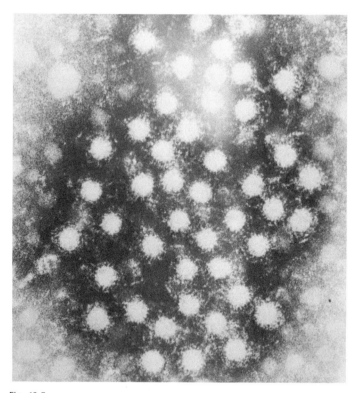

Fig. 13-5
Electron micrograph of hepatitis A virus (HAV) particles in the stool of a patient with acute hepatitis A virus.

terovirus type 72. Like other similar picornaviruses (small RNA viruses), it has four capsid polypeptides, virus protein (VP) 1 to 4. It has a 7800 nucleotide RNA genome that is similar in structure to those of other picornaviruses. In nature, only a single serotype of HAV has been identified; however, the genome of HAV has been cloned and characterized, and a number of minor differences have been identified among isolates from different parts of the world. In the three strains identified by such genomic analysis, 90 percent of nucleotides and 98 percent of predicted amino acids are identical. Hepatitis A virus is the only hepatitis virus that has been cultivated in vitro; it is noncytopathic and grows in a variety of epithelial cell lines.

Virologic Events and Serology   Humans are the primary host for HAV, but the virus can be transmitted experimentally to chimpanzees and marmosets, though less well to other species of monkeys. In the liver and in tissue culture, HAV antigen is localized to the cytoplasm. In infected persons and experimental animals, the virus can be detected in hepatocytes, blood, bile, and feces. Because viremia

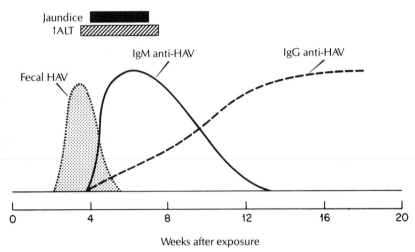

Fig. 13-6
The virologic events in hepatitis A virus.

is limited quantitatively and very transient, and because bile and liver tissue are rarely available in patients with acute hepatitis A, for practical purposes, HAV is not readily identified in blood, bile, or liver. The virus can be detected in feces, where it is shed in abundance during the late incubation period and first few days of clinical (or subclinical) illness, as early as 1 to 2 weeks after the host's exposure to the virus (Fig. 13-6). Still, detection of HAV in feces is impractical for routine diagnostic purposes. Fecal excretion of HAV peaks before the onset of clinically recognized hepatitis; therefore, by the time that a patient comes to medical attention, little, if any, fecal excretion of HAV is present. More convenient for clinical diagnostic purposes is reliance on serum markers of HAV infection. Because viremia is so transient, detection of virus in serum is too difficult; however, the humoral immune response to HAV provides a simple, convenient, and reliable diagnostic handle. As fecal virus excretion is waning, just as infection is becoming expressed clinically (biochemical indicators of hepatocellular inflammation and necrosis, i.e., ALT and AST elevations, with or without clinical symptoms), antibody to HAV (anti-HAV) becomes detectable.

During the early period of infection, anti-HAV is primarily of the IgM class, typical for primary immune responses. Although IgG anti-HAV is also produced relatively early, IgM anti-HAV is the predominant antibody for at least 3 months after the onset of acute hepatitis A; sometimes, lower levels of IgM anti-HAV can be detected for up to 6 months, rarely for up to a year. Detection of IgM in high titer, however, is a reliable marker of current or very recent HAV infection (Fig. 13-6). During convalescence,

IgG becomes the predominant class of anti-HAV, which persists indefinitely. If a patient with acute hepatitis has IgG anti-HAV in the absence of IgM anti-HAV, a diagnosis of acute HAV infection can be ruled out with confidence; the IgG anti-HAV in this case would have derived from HAV infection in the remote past.

Epidemiology

The distribution of hepatitis A, like that of hepatitis B, is worldwide. Because hepatitis A is spread almost exclusively by the fecal-oral route, contaminated food and water play a major role in its transmission, and conditions of overcrowding, poor hygiene, and poor sanitation favor the likelihood of infection. Groups at particular risk include institutionalized persons, promiscuous homosexual males, children in day-care facilities, the military, and persons who work with imported primates.

Both sporadic and epidemic cases of HAV infection occur. Among adults, HAV accounts for 20 to 30 percent of cases of sporadic hepatitis. Almost one half of urban American adults have anti-HAV, but only 5 percent of these persons recall having had clinical hepatitis. Exposure to HAV increases with age and decreasing socioeconomic status. In developing countries, inadequacy of personal and environmental hygiene leads to almost universal HAV infection during early childhood. Because viremia is transient, and because there are no chronic HAV carriers, HAV is almost never transmitted percutaneously; therefore, intravenous drug users, health workers, hemodialysis patients, and transfusion recipients are not at increased risk of infection.

Clinical Course

Most HAV infections, especially those acquired during childhood, are subclinical. In adults, however, HAV infections are much more likely to be associated with jaundice and other disabling symptoms. The post–World War II generation is much less likely to have been infected in early childhood because of improvements in personal/environmental hygiene; however, clinically apparent and often severe cases of hepatitis A are being recognized with increasing frequency in young adults.

The incubation period for HAV is approximately 25 days. Symptoms generally begin to occur 4 weeks after exposure, with the usual prodrome of low-grade fever, fatigue, nausea, anorexia, myalgias, and malaise. Coryza, cough, and pharyngitis are occasionally present. The early, nonspecific symptoms are followed by dark urine, light stools, and right upper quadrant discomfort. Jaundice then becomes clinically apparent, coinciding with a marked decrease in viral shedding and infectivity. Except for their relative mildness and transience, the symptoms of hepatitis A are indistinguishable from those of other types of viral hepatitis. Symptoms generally last a few weeks.

Physical findings include jaundice, tender hepatomegaly, and, rarely, splenomegaly. Immune-complex disease is uncommon.

As with hepatitis B, aminotransferase levels begin to rise prior to the onset of jaundice, and ALT levels tend to exceed AST levels. Peak levels vary from several hundred to several thousand units and are reached at the time of clinical jaundice, with diminishing values occurring during the recovery period and reaching normal levels within several weeks. Elevations in bilirubin and alkaline phosphatase can also occur, as in other types of viral hepatitis. Occasionally, severe cholestasis accompanies hepatitis A. In such cases, elevations of bilirubin and alkaline phosphatase are pronounced. As noted previously, the diagnosis of acute hepatitis A is made by demonstrating the presence in serum during acute illness of IgM anti-HAV.

Most patients with hepatitis A infection recover from the acute attack with no complications and with lifelong immunity. Rarely, however, hepatitis A is a cause of fulminant hepatic necrosis and death. In series of cases of fulminant hepatitis, hepatitis A accounts for only 1 to 2 percent.

Hepatitis A does not progress to chronic liver disease, and there is no chronic carrier state. Occasionally, patients can have a protracted course with clinical, virologic, and biochemical relapses that last for several months; however, relapsing hepatitis A is followed by complete recovery. During relapse, fecal excretion of HAV recurs.

The rarest clinical variant of hepatitis A is the cholestatic form. This is characterized by often protracted jaundice, pruritus, and acholic stools, with higher than usual levels of bilirubin and alkaline phosphatase. Histologically, prominent cholestasis is present. Although cholestatic hepatitis A can last for several months, it is followed by complete recovery.

Prevention and Management

In the absence of effective antiviral therapy for HAV infection, management is supportive, and attention is focused on prevention. Because peak infectivity precedes clinical illness, however, recognition of infection often comes too late to allow timely precautions in and prophylaxis of contact. Although HAV has been cultivated in vitro, currently, hepatitis A vaccines are not available. Work is underway to develop killed, live-attenuated, and recombinant hepatitis A vaccines, and preliminary trials in high-risk groups are already underway.

In the absence of active immunization, we rely instead on commonsense hygienic precautions to minimize fecal-oral spread and on the timely administration of immune globulin, that is, standard gamma globulin prepared by cold-alcohol fractionation of globulin from pooled plasma. Postexposure prophylaxis is recommended for household and institutional contacts of index cases. If globulin is administered within 2 weeks after exposure, it is 80 to 90 percent effective in preventing infection entirely; in the proportion of cases in which prevention is not accomplished, attenuation of clinical severity may result. Ironically, in those patients who are protected completely, long-lasting immunity does not result. In contrast, among those whose prophylaxis is not as successful and in whom attenuated clinical illness occurs, subclinical HAV infection results in lasting immunity.

Preexposure prophylaxis is recommended for those who travel to HAV-endemic areas, especially when outside of normal tourist routes, and for handlers of nonhuman primates. If such exposures are likely to last longer than 3 months, higher doses of globulin and repeat injections are suggested.

Non-A, Non-B Hepatitis

Virology

Cases of hepatitis are recognized with clinical and epidemiologic features of viral hepatitis but in which markers of HAV and HBV infection are absent. Identified initially in patients with transfusion-associated hepatitis, these cases have been classified as "non-A, non-B" (NANB) hepatitis. Despite numerous descriptions of putative NANB agents and serologic markers notwithstanding, no agent or marker has been identified that fulfills accepted criteria for a causative agent of NANB hepatitis; therefore, the diagnosis remains one of exclusion. Although NANB hepatitis agent(s) have not been identified, successful transmission in experimental animals, most reproducibly chimpanzees, suggests that there are at least two blood-borne NANB hepatitis agents. One was isolated from a clotting factor VIII concentrate, is inactivated by chloroform, and induces ultrastructural tubular changes in the cytoplasm of hepatocytes of experimentally infected chimpanzees. The other was isolated from a clotting factor IX concentrate, is not inactivated by chloroform, and does not induce tubular ultrastructural changes in hepatocytes. In chimpanzee cross-challenge experiments, the two appear to be immunologically distinct; infection with one does not confer immunity from infection with the other.

In addition to the agent(s) of blood-borne NANB hepatitis familiar in North America and in Europe, another form of NANB hepatitis transmitted by contaminated water has been identified in Asia and the Indian subcontinent. Whereas the blood-borne type of NANB hepatitis resembles hepatitis B epidemiologically and clinically, the so-called epidemic form of NANB hepatitis is more similar in epidemiologic and clinical features to hepatitis A. Recently, a 27-nm virus particle similar in appearance to (but distinct immunologically from) HAV has been detected in the feces of patients with epidemic NANB hepatitis. This type of hepatitis has been transmitted successfully to chimpanzees, and serologic responses to the 27-nm virus agent have been described and the initial reports confirmed. Detailed studies of serologic patterns have yet to be done, however, and routine tests to identify serologic responses in epidemic NANB hepatitis are not yet available.

Epidemiology   The absence of serologic markers for NANB hepatitis limits the extent of our understanding of the distribution and modes of transmission of these agents. In general, the blood-borne type of NANB hepatitis recognized primarily in transfusion recipients appears to resemble hepatitis B epidemiologically. Hepatitis occurs in approximately 5 to 10 percent of transfusion recipients, and NANB hepatitis accounts for more than 95 percent of these transfusion-related cases. In addition, NANB hepatitis is a major contributor to all categories of percutaneously transmitted hepatitis (e.g., in intravenous drug users, in hemodialysis and organ-transplant patients, and in hemophiliacs). In urban adults, 15 to 30 percent of sporadic hepatitis cases and about 25 percent of fulminant hepatitis cases have been attributed by serologic exclusion to NANB hepatitis. Although sexual and maternal-neonatal transmission of NANB hepatitis are not well documented, the observed parallelism in epidemiology between hepatitis B and NANB hepatitis suggests that, like hepatitis B, NANB hepatitis can be transmitted by these routes. On the other hand, secondary cases of NANB hepatitis in spouses of patients with transfusion-associated NANB hepatitis are rare.

The epidemic form of NANB hepatitis is distinct epidemiologically from the blood-borne variety. It is transmitted by the fecal-oral route and tends to be recognized in large outbreaks among those exposed to contaminated water. Recognized primarily in India and Asia, several cases imported from these parts of the world have been observed in North America. The contribution of epidemic NANB hepatitis to sporadic NANB hepatitis cases in both Asian and non-Asian countries remains to be determined.

Table 13-2
Comparative features of viral hepatitis

	Hepatitis A	Hepatitis B	Non-A, Non-B	Hepatitis D
Incubation period	25 days	75 days	50 days	?
Principal mode of spread	Fecal-oral	Nonpercutaneous and percutaneous	Nonpercutaneous and percutaneous	Nonpercutaneous and percutaneous
Chronicity	None	5–10%	10–50%	Occurs
Contribution to posttransfusion hepatitis	Almost never	5%	95%	Rare
Contribution to fulminant hepatitis	1–2%	60%	<30%	30–60% of fulminant hepatitis B cases
Contribution to sporadic hepatitis	30%	50%	20%	?
Virus characteristics	RNA	DNA	Unknown	Defective RNA

Clinical Features   Symptoms, signs, biochemical changes, and histologic pertur-
bations are similar in NANB hepatitis to those that occur in the
other viral hepatitides; therefore, clinical features cannot be
relied on to distinguish NANB from the other types of viral
hepatitis. Yet, certain generalizations have emerged from the
study of NANB hepatitis. Clinically, the blood-borne type of
NANB hepatitis resembles hepatitis B. In typical transfusion-
associated cases, the mean incubation period is approximately 7
weeks, longer than the 4 weeks for hepatitis A, and shorter than
the 12 weeks for transfusion-associated hepatitis B (Table 13-2).
In cases following infusion of clotting factor VIII concentrates
(in hemophiliacs), shorter incubation periods ranging from 1 to
4 weeks are more characteristic. Transfusion-associated NANB
hepatitis tends to be less severe than type B hepatitis during
acute illness. Only approximately 25 percent of such NANB
cases are icteric, mean aminotransferase elevations are only approximately 300 units, and many patients do not experience
characteristic or typical symptoms. A clinical feature that occurs
in up to one half of patients is a fluctuating pattern of aminotransferase elevation.

Despite its relative acute clinical benignity, however, transfusion-associated acute NANB hepatitis progresses to chronic

hepatitis in approximately 50 percent of cases, independent of whether the acute illness was mild or severe. Liver histology in the majority of these chronic cases is consistent with chronic active hepatitis (piecemeal necrosis), but clinical progression is relatively slow and insidious. Despite the fact that in some patients with chronic active posttransfusion NANB hepatitis, follow-up biopsies may show milder lesions (chronic persistent hepatitis), and despite the fact that biochemical abnormalities may be negligible and symptoms absent, over the course of 10 years, the frequency of progression to cirrhosis reaches 20 percent among those with chronic NANB hepatitis. Therefore, if NANB hepatitis develops in 10 percent of transfusion recipients, if chronic hepatitis occurs in 50 percent of these 10 percent, and if cirrhosis follows in 20 percent of the 5 percent with chronic hepatitis, these figures translate to a 1 percent incidence of cirrhosis within 10 years in recipients of blood and blood products.

Moreover, the fact that volunteer blood donors with normal aminotransferase levels can transmit NANB hepatitis to recipients suggests that, as is true for hepatitis B, there is an asymptomatic NANB hepatitis carrier state. Based on observations in recipients of single-unit' transfusions, the estimate has been made that the NANB carrier state is substantially higher, perhaps as high as 3 to 7 percent, than the hepatitis B carrier state.

In series of patients with fulminant hepatitis, NANB hepatitis has been blamed by exclusion for one fourth to one third of cases. Inevitably, some of these cases are not viral, and although fulminant transfusion-associated NANB hepatitis is extraordinarily rare, NANB hepatitis can be a cause of fulminant hepatitis.

The likelihood of chronic hepatitis after acute sporadic NANB hepatitis is reported to be substantially lower, but a definitive estimate is lacking. The epidemic form of NANB hepatitis can be quite severe. In Asian and Indian outbreaks, the mortality rate has been as high as 10 percent, primarily in pregnant women. The mean incubation period of 40 days tends to be slightly longer than that for hepatitis A, and epidemic NANB hepatitis cases are frequently cholestatic. Chronicity, however, has not been observed.

Prevention and Management

Preliminary results of a trial of alpha-interferon in a small group of patients with chronic NANB hepatitis are promising and being pursued in a large, controlled trial. At the present time, however, little more than supportive measures are available for the management of acute and chronic NANB hepatitis.

As is true for the other hepatitides, emphasis tends to be placed on prevention. For the prevention of transfusion-associated NANB hepatitis, virus-specific blood-donor screening tests have yet to be identified. Currently, limiting the occurrence of transfusion-associated NANB hepatitis relies on avoiding commercial blood donors, avoiding pooled blood products, and limiting to an absolute minimum the number of blood products transfused. In addition, the use of nonvirus-specific "surrogate" tests to "weed out" donors with an increased likelihood of exposure to and infection with NANB hepatitis agents has been adopted. Despite their limited sensitivity, specificity, and predictive value, both ALT and anti-HBc are such surrogate markers. It has been predicted that their introduction into blood-donor screening has the potential to reduce the frequency of transfusion-associated hepatitis by 30 percent.

The efficacy of immune globulin in preventing transfusion-associated NANB hepatitis, especially when volunteer blood donors are the only donor source, has not been demonstrated consistently; therefore, immune globulin is not recommended for prophylaxis in transfusion recipients. Because needlesticks, sexual exposures, and neonatal exposures represent much smaller inocula than that represented in a transfused blood unit, and because immune globulin is safe and inexpensive, many authorities recommend immune globulin for such exposures to NANB hepatitis. Studies of efficacy in these settings have not been done.

Study Questions

1. Which of the following statements about delta hepatitis is or are correct?
   a. Persons who respond to hepatitis B vaccine are immune to delta infection.
   b. The delta agent is a defective DNA-containing virus.
   c. Delta hepatitis cannot occur in the absence of HBV infection.
   d. Delta hepatitis can be associated with both acute and chronic hepatitis B infection.
   e. The fecal-oral route is the primary mode of HDV transmission.

Answer

a, c, d

The delta agent depends on hepatitis B for its replication and cannot occur in the absence of HBV infection. Therefore, persons who are immune to HBV infection will also be immune to delta hepatitis. Delta hepatitis can occur simultaneously (as a coinfection) with acute hepatitis B or can be superimposed on chronic HBV infection; HDV remains active only as long as there is ongoing HBV infection.

2. Which serologic patterns are compatible with the associated clinical situations?

a. HBsAg$^+$, HBeAg$^+$,   chronic persistent hepatitis
   IgG anti-HBc$^+$ B

b. HBsAg$^+$, IgG anti-HBc$^+$,   acute coinfection with
   anti-HD$^+$ hepatitis B and D

c. IgG anti-HAV$^+$ acute hepatitis A

d. IgM anti-HAV$^+$,   acute hepatitis A in a
   HBsAg$^+$, IgG anti-HBc$^+$ hepatitis B carrier

e. anti-HBc$^+$, anti-HBs$^+$,   immunity to hepatitis B
   anti-HBe$^+$

Answer

a, d, e

The HBsAg$^+$, HBeAg$^+$, IgG anti-HBc$^+$ serologic pattern represents chronic HBV infection. Histologically normal hepatocytes, chronic persistent hepatitis, chronic active hepatitis, chronic lobular hepatitis, or cirrhosis may exist. The presence of IgM anti-HBc$^+$, not IgG anti-HBc$^+$ with HBsAg$^+$ and anti-HD$^+$ serology, would represent simultaneous acute infection with hepatitis B and D; likewise, IgM anti-HAV$^+$, not IgG anti-HAV$^+$, would be serologic evidence of acute infection with HAV. The presence of anti-HBs correlates with immunity to hepatitis B.

3. Which of the following types of hepatitis can progress to chronic liver disease?
a. Hepatitis A
b. Hepatitis B
c. Blood-borne non-A, non-B hepatitis
d. Epidemic non-A, non-B hepatitis
e. Hepatitis D

Answer

b, c, e

Hepatitis A is always a self-limited infection and never progresses to chronic liver disease or cirrhosis. Epidemic non-A, non-B hepatitis can be quite severe, but chronicity has not been observed. In contrast, the blood-borne type of non-A, non-B hepatitis is very likely to progress; chronic hepatitis follows in up to 50 percent of acute cases. Hepatitis B becomes chronic in 5 to 10 percent of those with acute infection, and delta superinfection can occur in these cases and persist along with HBV infection.

4. Which of the following are true for hepatitis B?
   a. HBsAg can be detected prior to the appearance of jaundice and usually remains detectable after jaundice subsides.
   b. The appearance of anti-HBc precedes the appearance of anti-HBs and anti-HBe.
   c. Anti-HBe confers immunity to HBV infection.
   d. Detection of anti-HBc in the blood is useful clinically to detect acute HBV infection.
   e. Persistence of HBsAg longer than six months is followed inevitably by chronic liver disease and cirrhosis.

Answer

a, b

Circulating HBsAg can occur in the prodromal phase, prior to the onset of jaundice, and usually persists beyond the resolution of clinical symptoms. Patients are therefore infectious often before hepatitis is recognized. Beyond six months, patients can still clear HBsAg; those who remain HBsAg-positive may be "healthy" asymptomatic carriers or progress to chronic liver disease and cirrhosis. Anti-HBs is associated with immunity to HBV infection; anti-HBe is not a protective antibody. Acute HBV infection can be detected by the presence of IgM anti-HBc in the blood. The presence of anti-HBc (i.e., antibody class not specified) does not distinguish among acute infection, chronic infection, or resolved infection.

5. Which of the following are true for hepatitis A?
   a. The fecal-oral mode of transmission is the most common route.
   b. Immune globulin provides protection against hepatitis A.
   c. Infectivity begins after jaundice appears and persists for two to four weeks.
   d. A chronic carrier state occurs occasionally.
   e. Multiple serotypes have been found.

Answer

a, b

Hepatitis A is usually transmitted through contaminated food and water when a breakdown in sanitation occurs. The infectious period begins prior to clinical symptoms, when virions are being excreted in the stool. By the time jaundice appears, infectivity has subsided. Standard immune globulin, when given early enough, prevents HAV infection. This passive protection lasts only several months and therefore repeated dosing may be necessary to prevent HAV infection in those at risk (i.e., travelers to endemic areas). Viremia occurs only transiently, and no carrier state exists. Only one HAV sero-type has been identified.

References

Bonino, F., and Smedile, A. Delta agent (Type D) hepatitis. *Semin. Liver Dis.* 6:28, 1986.

Centers for Disease Control. Recommendations for protection against viral hepatitis. (Recommendations of the Immunization Practices Advisory Committee.) *Ann. Intern. Med.* 103:391, 1985.

Dienstag, J. L. Viral hepatitis type A: Virology and course. *Clin. Gastroenterol.* 9:135, 1980.

Dienstag, J. L. Non-A, non-B hepatitis. I. Recognition, epidemiology, and clinical features. *Gastroenterology* 85:439, 1983.

Dienstag, J. L., and Alter, H. J. Non-A, non-B hepatitis: Evolving epidemiologic and clinical perspective. *Semin. Liver Dis.* 6:67, 1986.

Hoofnagle, J. H., and Schafer, D. F. Serologic markers of hepatitis B virus infection. *Semin. Liver Dis.* 6:1, 1986.

Hoofnagle, J. H., Shafritz, D. A., and Popper, H. Chronic type B hepatitis and the "healthy" HBsAg carrier state. *Hepatology* 7:758, 1987.

Jacobson, I. M., and Dienstag, J. L. Viral hepatitis vaccines. *Ann. Rev. Med.* 36:241, 1985.

Lemon, S. M. Type A viral hepatitis: New developments in an old disease. *N. Engl. J. Med.* 313:1059, 1985.

Popper, H., Shafritz, D. A., and Hoofnagle, J. H. Relation of the hepatitis B virus carrier state to hepatocellular carcinoma. *Hepatology* 7:764, 1987.

Rizzetto, M. The Delta agent. *Hepatology* 3:729, 1983.

Seeff, L. B., and Koff, R. S. Evolving concepts of the clinical and serologic consequences of hepatitis B virus infection. *Semin. Liver Dis.* 6:11, 1986.

Seeger, C., Ganem, D., and Varmus, H. E. Biochemical and genetic evidence for the hepatitis B virus replication strategy. *Science* 232:447, 1986.

Tilloais, P., Pourcel, C., and Dejean, A. The hepatitis B virus. *Nature* 317:489, 1985.

Update on hepatitis B prevention. *M.M.W.R.* 36:353, 1987.

14 : Alcoholic Liver Disease

David E. Johnston
Marshall M. Kaplan

Alcoholism as a Health Problem

Alcoholism is a major cause of disease and trauma worldwide. It is equally important as a cause of personal and social disruption. Perhaps 10 to 20 million Americans are alcoholics, and many more may be problem drinkers. Alcohol is a factor in two thirds of homicides and one third of suicides. It plays a role in about half of vehicular deaths, including not only cars but also boats, private planes, snowmobiles, and other vehicles. It also plays a major role in other types of trauma. Few organ systems escape alcohol-related diseases. In addition, alcoholic cirrhosis is the leading cause of death related to alcoholism, the eighth leading cause of death in the United States, and the fourth leading cause of death among men in urban areas. Alcoholism possibly does even more damage to personal and family life, but this is more difficult to measure.

Although alcoholism is a form of drug abuse, it has no universally accepted definition. Some pundits say an alcoholic is someone who drinks more than his or her doctor; others say that an alcoholic is someone who takes a first drink before lunchtime. Alcoholism is not defined by a particular level or pattern of intake, and it does not necessarily imply drunkenness. It does imply loss of self-control over one's intake, and the presence of problems in health, job, personal or family life, or trouble with the law. An alcoholic may drink daily or drink only on weekends. He or she may live as a derelict on the streets, or hold a high, responsible position in business or the professions. Alcoholism can remain hidden from co-workers, since individuals can develop a high degree of tolerance to the intoxicating effects of alcohol. The ability to appear sober in the presence of a high blood alcohol level is itself evidence of an alcoholic drinking pattern.

The abuse of alcohol is poorly understood. The prevalence of alcoholism varies greatly from one society to another, apparently related to varying attitudes toward alcohol consumption. It is striking that per capita alcohol consumption in a community or country is proportional to the alcoholic cirrhosis death rate. Studies show that communities with a high per capita alcohol consumption have a higher percentage of individuals with very high alcohol consumptions; thus, consumption statistics are determined mainly by the heavy drinkers. Countries with higher rates of alcohol consumption have a higher male:female ratio of cirrhosis.

The availability of alcohol influences the prevalence of alcoholism and cirrhosis. Rationing of wine in France during World War II correlated with a steep decline in cirrhosis deaths, and cirrhosis returned to its former prevalence after the end of rationing. Falling alcohol prices in Canada correlated to increased cirrhosis. Various studies show a link between increased income, increased alcohol consumption, and increased deaths from cirrhosis. The relationship between social class and alcoholism is complex, because whereas income influences the availability of alcohol, peer group attitudes influence drinking habits. In some societies, alcohol is used by the whole family on a daily basis, but drunkenness is socially unaccepted. In societies where drunkenness is viewed with more tolerance, alcoholism is more prevalent. Furthermore, certain occupational groups that involve close proximity to alcohol, such as workers in taverns and restaurants, have a high prevalence of alcoholism. Heavy drinking is common in some industrial and sales jobs. The low prevalence of alcoholism among Orientals is attributed to the high frequency of a deficiency in ethanol metabolism (decreased aldehyde dehydrogenase) that causes uncomfortable flushing reactions. Otherwise, ethnic differences in the frequency of alcoholism have no apparent relationship to differences in alcohol metabolism.

There is no evidence that a specific personality type predisposes to alcoholism, although some persons with anxiety or depression may use alcohol as a sedative. Family studies do suggest a familial or genetic tendency toward alcoholism. A first-degree relative of an alcoholic has about a 15 percent chance of becoming an alcoholic. Studies of adopted infants show that the individual's risk of alcoholism is related more to the presence or absence of alcoholism in the natural parents than in the adoptive parents. Furthermore, multiple studies have examined alcoholism in identical versus fraternal twins. When one identical twin becomes an alcoholic, the other has three or four times the likelihood than would be expected for fraternal twins. Thus, multiple studies suggest a genetic factor in susceptibility to alcoholism, but little progress has been made in understanding the nature of this factor. It would seem most likely to have a neurologic basis but is not simply a difference in ethanol metabolism.

Alcoholism is maintained by the psychological defenses of denial and distortion. Alcoholics believe that they do not drink excessively, and, to support this belief, they gravitate toward friends with similar drinking habits. Alcoholics apparently misperceive the extent of their alcohol consumption and its implications. "I never touch the hard stuff" is frequently heard from the case-a-day beer drinker, and "I only drink on weekends" from the individual who binges uncontrollably. The alcoholic distorts events. The alcoholic may conclude that his employer makes unreasonable demands, when, in fact, job performance and punctuality are very poor due to alcoholism. The alcoholic may conclude that her family picks fights with her, when, in fact, she acts aggressively while under the influence. Alcoholics are adept at concealing evidence of their addiction and frequently see physicians for vague, shifting complaints and numerous "accidents." This wall of denial and distortion can lead to frustration on the part of physicians and others in dealing with the alcoholic.

Among heavy drinkers, no more than 15 to 30 percent ever get significant alcoholic liver disease, no matter what the level or duration of their consumption. In the United States, several autopsy series totaling 2,045 chronic alcoholics showed a prevalence of cirrhosis between 1.2 and 19.1 percent, with an average of 8.7 percent. Series from other parts of the world give similar results, with figures ranging up to 30 percent. The reason cirrhosis affects only a fraction of long-term alcoholics is unknown. However, the risk of alcoholic liver disease is clearly related to consumption. Pequignot and associates found the risk of cirrhosis linear with the logarithm of alcohol intake. To summarize a number of studies, the average male alcoholic has consumed 150 to 200 gm of ethanol a day for 15 to 20 years by the time he is found to have alcoholic hepatitis or cirrhosis.

Alcoholic women seem more susceptible than men to alcoholic liver disease and may present with alcoholic hepatitis after a shorter period of alcoholism than do men. The prevalence of cirrhosis in alcoholics seems to be greater in women, especially among the elderly. Alcoholic women begin their heavy alcohol consumption later in life than do men, so they tend to present with alcoholic liver disease at about the same age as men, that is, in the late 40s on average. The average woman with alcoholic liver disease has consumed about 120 to 160 gm of ethanol a day for 12 to 15 years by the time of diagnosis. On average, women have a lower body mass and greater percentage of fat than do men; thus, their volume of distribution of ethanol is lower. This may explain why women get liver disease at lower ethanol con-

Table 14-1
Ethanol content of alcoholic beverages

Beverage	Serving	% Ethanol (ml/100 ml)	Ethanol/serving (gm)
Beer	12 oz	5	14.2
Table wine	5 oz	12	14.2
Whiskey (80 proof)	1½ oz	40	14.2

Key: 1 oz = 30 ml; 1 ml = 0.789 gm ethanol; 1 gm = 7 kilocalories

sumptions than do men, although there may also be a difference in the female liver's innate susceptibility to alcohol. There are clearly differences in liver physiology between males and females, perhaps based on differences in sex hormone metabolism.

An absolutely safe level of daily alcohol consumption is difficult to define, with estimates ranging from 20 to 80 gm. The cirrhosis risk is probably small — below 80 gm of ethanol per day — but some persons seem to get liver disease at consumptions that seem modest. There is no evidence that one form of alcoholic beverage is any more likely to cause liver disease than another, given equal amounts of ethanol. That is, alcohol in the form of beer can cause the same problems as an equivalent amount of liquor. There is no evidence that fusel oil (branched chain aliphatic alcohols) or other constituents of alcoholic beverages have any bearing on liver disease.

It is simple to translate grams of ethanol into everyday terms (Table 14-1). One should remember that one proof means one half percent ethanol by volume. The specific gravity of ethanol is 0.789 gm/ml. Thus, one can see that a 1.5-oz shot of 80 proof whiskey is 45 ml of 40 percent ethanol, or 19.35 ml of pure ethanol. This comes to 14.2 gm of ethanol. The ethanol in a 1.5-oz shot of whiskey, a 5-oz glass of table wine, and a 12-oz glass of beer is roughly equivalent. To imbibe 150 gm per day of ethanol, a person would need about 10 drinks, or approximately one pint of whiskey. This translates into 1,050 calories in the form of ethanol, a major fraction of total nutritional intake.

The Metabolism of Alcohol and Its Consequences

Absorption

Ethanol is absorbed by passive diffusion, starting at first contact with mucous membranes. A small amount is absorbed in the stomach, with the remainder in the small intestine. Simultaneous intake of food delays gastric emptying and slows absorption of ethanol, so that peak blood levels are decreased. Depending on body weight and other factors, the ingestion of three to six drinks would give a peak blood alcohol level of over 100 mg per dl (100 mg/100 ml, or 0.1%), which is considered intoxicated for purposes of driving in most states.

Primary Organ *of Elimination:* *The Liver*

At lower blood alcohol levels, 80 to 90 percent of absorbed ethanol is oxidized in the liver. Many tissues can oxidize ethanol to a limited extent. The lungs and kidneys can excrete up to 15 percent of ethanol when the blood level is very high. The kinetics of elimination are difficult to describe because of the multiple pathways involved, but at moderate blood levels, the alcohol elimination rate can appear nearly independent of the blood alcohol level. The estimated maximal rate of ethanol metabolism is 200 to 240 gm/day for a 70-kg male casual drinker, and up to 370 gm/day for an alcoholic. Thus, a nondrinker could metabolize about one and a half pints of whiskey in 24 hours. A few hours after ethanol ingestion, the rate of ethanol oxidation and oxygen uptake by the liver temporarily increases by 50 percent or more, the so-called swift increase in ethanol metabolism. This is mediated by catecholamine secretion. On the other hand, chronic alcohol ingestion causes a prolonged increased rate of ethanol metabolism that may persist for weeks after the cessation of drinking.

Three liver enzymes in three different subcellular compartments play a role in ethanol oxidation (Fig. 14-1). These are (1) alcohol dehydrogenase (ADH) in the cytoplasm, (2) the microsomal ethanol oxidizing system (MEOS) in the smooth endoplasmic reticulum, and (3) catalase, in the peroxisomes. ADH catalyzes the transfer of hydrogen from ethanol to NAD to yield acetaldehyde and NADH. Such an enzyme probably exists to dispose of small amounts of ethanol and other short-chain alcohols that are generated in the gastrointestinal tract and elsewhere. ADH is found in very high activity in the liver cytosol and has an apparent Km of about 1 mM (about 5 mg/dl). This means that at typical blood alcohol levels after even one drink, the ADH pathway is working at near maximal activity. Experimentally, ADH can be inhibited by 4-methylpyrazole. At moderate ethanol levels (<100 mg/dl), 4-methylpyrazole inhibits ethanol metabolism by 90 percent. This and other evidence shows that the ADH pathway is by far the major route of ethanol metabolism in the occasional drinker who takes one or two drinks. However, at high blood levels (200–300 mg/dl), especially in the chronic heavy drinker, 4-methylpyrazole may inhibit ethanol oxidation by as little as 50 percent. These studies pointed to a non-ADH pathway of etha-

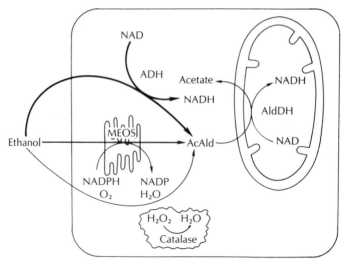

Fig. 14-1
Metabolism of ethanol in the hepatocyte by the three major pathways, ADH (alcohol dehydrogenase) in the cytoplasm, MEOS (microsomal ethanol oxidizing system) in the smooth endoplasmic reticulum, and a small amount oxidized by catalase in the peroxisomes. (AcAld = acetaldehyde; AldDH = aldehyde dehydrogenase.)

nol oxidation. Early studies showed that chronic alcohol feeding induced proliferation of the smooth endoplasmic reticulum and suggested a role for the microsomes in ethanol metabolism.

The liver microsomal fraction oxidizes a significant amount of ethanol. This MEOS uses NADPH and molecular oxygen to hydroxylate ethanol and thus oxidizes it to acetaldehyde. It has a relatively high Km of about 10 mM (roughly 50 mg/dl), but it can increase its activity significantly over weeks of alcohol exposure. The hydroxylating enzymes of the microsomes generally contain various types of P-450 heme-containing proteins. Recently, a specific species of P-450 that is induced by ethanol was isolated and characterized. This should permit better analysis of the interactions between alcohol and metabolism of other drugs. The significance of the MEOS is demonstrated by a strain of deermouse that lacks ADH. In these mice, the MEOS maintains ethanol oxidation at nearly normal levels. Catalase, the third pathway of ethanol oxidation, accounts for only a few percent, at most, of ethanol metabolism. Catalase normally detoxifies hydrogen peroxide in peroxisomes by catalyzing the transformation of two molecules of hydrogen peroxide into water and molecular oxygen. However, it can also use hydrogen peroxide to oxidize ethanol to acetaldehyde. The rate of this reaction is believed to be limited in vivo by the concentration of hydrogen peroxide in peroxisomes.

An individual's tolerance for ethanol increases with chronic alcohol intake. Most of this tolerance occurs at the level of the central nervous system, by unknown mechanisms. In addition, the metabolism of ethanol can increase by 50 percent or more after chronic use. Levels of ADH remain unchanged or even decrease in alcoholism. As will be discussed, ADH typically outruns the ability of the cell to reoxidize NADH back to NAD, and NAD becomes rate-limiting. An increase in the oxidation of NADH back to NAD can increase the rate of the NAD pathway, and this probably occurs to some extent in both the swift increase and in chronic adaptation to alcohol. The MEOS increases substantially after exposure to high alcohol concentrations, and the MEOS can increase more than the ADH pathway. The MEOS has a tenfold higher Km than ADH, so that adaptive increases in ethanol oxidation are more striking at high blood alcohol levels, as seen in the heavy drinker.

Acetaldehyde from these reactions is a very reactive, toxic metabolite. An aldehyde dehydrogenase present in the mitochondrion oxidizes acetaldehyde to acetic acid and NADH. The low Km and high total activity of this enzyme are such that blood acetaldehyde concentrations are about 1,000-fold lower than ethanol concentrations. Chronic alcoholics have higher blood acetaldehyde levels for a given alcohol level than do casual drinkers, and chronic alcoholic rats clear an acetaldehyde load more slowly than do nonalcoholics. The higher blood acetaldehyde levels in alcoholics result from both increased production and decreased clearance of acetaldehyde. Abstinence seems to permit recovery of aldehyde dehydrogenase activity in alcoholics, so that the defect is caused by alcohol and not by a preexisting defect. Chronic alcohol ingestion causes morphologic changes in liver mitochondria, so this decreased acetaldehyde oxidation may relate to the other observed mitochondrial abnormalities.

Acetate produced from acetaldehyde has three possible fates in the liver: (1) terminal oxidation by way of the Krebs cycle, (2) metabolism into lipids or ketone bodies, or (3) exit into the bloodstream. As will be discussed subsequently, the NADH produced from ethanol oxidation inhibits operation of the Krebs cycle, so acetate oxidation is inhibited. Whereas the abundance of acetate and hydrogen equivalents (as NADH and NADPH) encourages lipid synthesis, nevertheless, a significant amount of acetate enters the bloodstream. Blood acetate not only stimulates cardiac contractility but also inhibits the release of free fatty acids from adipose tissue. This latter phenomenon probably accounts for the fall in free fatty acids observed with alcohol consumption.

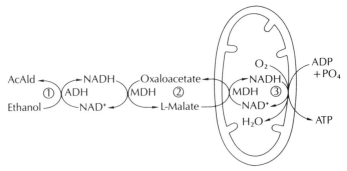

Fig. 14-2
The alcohol dehydrogenase pathway and the malate/oxaloacetate shuttle. The transfer of hydrogen equivalents from ethanol into the mitochondrion is illustrated. Under various conditions, the slow step can be determined by (1) alcohol dehydrogenase (ADH), (2) malate dehydrogenase (MDH) or availability of oxaloacetate, or (3) the oxidation of NADH in the mitochondrion.

Ethanol Increases the Hepatocyte NADH/NAD Ratio

The rate of ethanol oxidation through the ADH pathway is often less than expected based on ADH activity measured in the test tube. In other words, the level of ADH is not the rate-determining step in the ADH pathway. As mentioned previously, it is the availability of NAD that determines the rate of the pathway. Ethanol oxidation proceeds so rapidly that it often outruns the ability of the cell to oxidize the NADH produced back to NAD, and the NADH/NAD ratio becomes greatly increased. Consequently, even at modest blood levels, alcohol metabolism largely takes over energy metabolism in the liver and supplants other energy sources.

NADH is normally reoxidized as it supplies hydrogen equivalents to the mitochondrial electron transport chain, resulting in coupled oxidative phosphorylation and the oxidation of hydrogen to water. However, NADH must enter the mitochondrion to be oxidized, and the mitochondrion is not permeable to NADH or NAD. Several "shuttle" cycles are believed to transfer hydrogen equivalents from NADH in the cytoplasm to NAD inside the mitochondrion.

The most important of these is thought to be the malate/oxaloacetate shuttle (Fig. 14-2). Malate dehydrogenase transfers hydrogen from NADH to oxaloacetate to give L-malate. The malate enters the mitochondrion, where it is oxidized back to oxaloacetate and generates NADH inside the mitochondrion. This shuttle may often represent the slow step in the total ADH pathway. Increases in malate dehydrogenase or in oxaloacetate may account for the swift increase in alcohol metabolism and for a part of the more chronic increases. Under some circumstances, especially in the relatively hypoxic area of the liver lobule near the central vein, the mitochondrial oxidation of NADH may become rate-limiting. In this circumstance, modest ethanol concentrations may result in large increases in the cellular redox potential.

Hepatocytes near the portal areas and those near the central veins live in very different environments in terms of the hormones and metabolites to which they are exposed. Blood in sinusoids around portal areas has a PO_2 of about 65 mm Hg, but this drops to about 30 mm Hg near the central veins. ADH is spread fairly evenly throughout the lobule. Since oxygen is more limited near the central veins, the NADH/NAD ratio would be expected to be higher there. In fact, it is possible to measure the NADH/NAD ratio over small parts of the lobule with a microscopic fluorescence light probe that can detect the fluorescence of NADH. These experiments have confirmed that ethanol induces an increase in the redox potential primarily around the central vein. The intracellular redox potential can also be assessed by the ratio of lactate/pyruvate in blood entering and leaving the liver. The lactate/pyruvate ratio should reflect the NADH/NAD ratio of hepatocytes near the terminal hepatic venules, and this ratio dramatically increases after ethanol intake.

This major increase in intracellular redox potential has major implications for metabolism, since all enzymatic reactions coupled with NAD are affected (Table 14-2). For example, the ratio of malate/oxaloacetate is shifted to malate; lactate/pyruvate is shifted to lactate; and beta-hydroxybutyrate/acetoacetate is shifted to beta-hydroxybutyrate. As long as ethanol is present, the synthesis of glucose from amino acids (gluconeogenesis) is inhibited by the lack of available pyruvate and oxaloacetate, key intermediates in production of glucose. If glycogen stores are depleted and there is no dietary intake of carbohydrate, severe

Table 14-2
Some metabolic consequences of the increased NADH/NAD ratio

Metabolic effect	Clinical correlate
Decreased gluconeogenesis	Hypoglycemia
Increased lactate	Elevated blood lactate Possible gout
Possible increased ketoacids	Ketoacidosis
Decreased Krebs (TCA) cycle	
Inhibition of most oxidations that use liver NAD	Inhibition of some drug and hormone metabolism
Decreased fatty acid oxidation and increased fatty acid synthesis	Fatty liver Elevated blood lipids

low blood sugar can result. This is the biochemical mechanism for alcohol-induced hypoglycemia. Gluconeogenesis is restored as soon as alcohol disappears from the system.

The combination of starvation and alcoholism can also result in a metabolic acidosis from the accumulation of lactate and ketoacids, mainly beta-hydroxybutyrate and acetoacetate. The degree of acidosis is mild to moderate, and the routine urine test for ketones is negative or trace, because it does not detect beta-hydroxybutyrate. The situation begins with starvation, which causes mobilization of fat stores as free fatty acids. Given the scarcity of glucose, insulin levels fall, and levels of glucagon, cortisol, and growth hormone rise to promote gluconeogenesis and ketogenesis. However, alcohol inhibits ketogenesis. The biochemical nature of this inhibition is not known for certain but can be explained in terms of the increased NADH/NAD ratio in the mitochondrion. Acetoacetyl CoA is a necessary intermediate in ketogenesis, and it can be interconverted with beta-hydroxybutyryl CoA, which cannot be used for ketogenesis. At some point in the binge, the individual is forced to stop drinking because of illness or lack of alcohol, and the blood alcohol level falls. The blockade of ketogenesis is removed, and ketone synthesis increases. Low insulin levels decrease the peripheral utilization of ketone bodies. The "ketones" exist mostly in the form of beta-hydroxybutyrate because of the high NADH/NAD ratio.

Elevated serum uric acid levels are common in alcoholics, and ethanol has long been considered a precipitant of gout attacks. The mild chronic acidosis seen in the chronic alcoholic, with accumulation of lactate and other organic acids, inhibits the renal secretion of uric acid. Ethanol also appears to stimulate production of uric acid.

Alcoholic Fatty Liver

The ingestion of alcohol, even on a casual basis for a short period of time, results in accumulation of fat droplets in hepatocytes, especially near the central vein (or terminal hepatic venule). This is usually a harmless, fully reversible change. It is easy to understand how it occurs (Fig. 14-3). Ethanol oxidation causes a major increase in the NADH/NAD ratio; this is most prominent near the central vein. The high NADH/NAD ratio inhibits the Krebs cycle by depriving it of oxaloacetate and NAD. This means that acetate cannot be oxidized. The accumulated acetate and hydrogen equivalents stimulate the synthesis of fatty acid. The high redox potential also promotes the reduction of dihydroxyacetone phosphate (DHAP) to alpha-glycerol phosphate, an important substrate in triglyceride synthesis. These metabolic changes tend to increase triglyceride production, especially in central areas of the liver lobule. On the other hand,

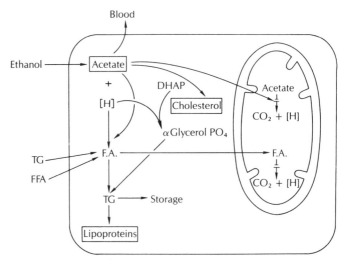

Fig. 14-3
Effect of ethanol on fat metabolism in the hepatocyte. Ethanol is oxidized to
acetate and hydrogen equivalents (H). The oxidation of acetate in the mitochondrion is inhibited by the high NADH/NAD ratio, so acetate is either
turned into fatty acid or other lipids, such as cholesterol. The high NADH/
NAD ratio increases the production of alpha-glycerol phosphate, which increases the esterification of fatty acids into triglyceride. This is either stored
or is secreted as lipoproteins. Fatty acid absorbed from extrahepatic sources
such as adipose tissue and the gastrointestinal tract cannot be oxidized,
again partly because of the high NADH/NAD ratio in the mitochondrion.
Fatty liver results.

the oxidation of fatty acids is less rapid in central than in portal
areas of the lobule, even in the absence of ethanol. Furthermore, the ethanol-induced increase in acetate and NADH suppresses fatty acid oxidation even further. Chronic alcoholism
also causes abnormal mitochondrial forms, with decreased
levels of the enzymes of fatty acid oxidation. Finally, alcohol also
inhibits secretion of lipoproteins and glycoproteins and causes
an accumulation of protein in the Golgi complex. Of the excess
liver mass seen in alcoholic fatty liver, more than half consists of
protein, water, and electrolytes. The inhibition of protein secretion may result from the toxic effect of acetaldehyde on microtubules, which participate in many secretory processes.

Under most circumstances, decreased fatty acid oxidation and
decreased lipoprotein secretion are the dominant factors in fatty
liver. Depending on the circumstances, increased lipid synthesis, decreased lipid oxidation, decreased lipoprotein secretion,
or mobilization of peripheral fat stores may all play a dominant
role in the origin of fatty liver. The amount of fat accumulated
can be increased or decreased by altering the fat content of the
diet. At some point, the fatty liver reaches a steady state from
which it no longer increases in mass. One would expect that the

NADH/NAD ratio effect of alcohol must be attenuated; otherwise, the fat content might continue to increase. In fact, the lactate/pyruvate ratio induced in the liver in response to ethanol declines after establishment of fatty liver. This is good evidence that the NADH/NAD ratio induced by ethanol declines after a steady state of fat accumulation is reached. Long-term alcohol abuse is associated with elevated blood triglycerides. Little imagination is needed to see how alcohol could promote this.

The Spectrum of Alcoholic Liver Disease

Overview

Alcohol can cause fatty liver (steatosis), hepatitis (steatonecrosis), cirrhosis, and a form of fibrosis around the terminal hepatic venules. For many years, the serious forms of alcoholic liver disease were believed to result from malnutrition rather than from alcohol itself. The typical alcoholic with liver disease consumes 150 to 200 gm of ethanol per day, or 1,050 to 1,400 calories as ethanol. Ethanol often suppresses appetite, so the alcoholic could easily consume more than half his or her diet in the form of ethanol. Even if a diet is nutritionally complete, alcohol can cause numerous vitamin and mineral deficiencies. Some forms of protein-calorie malnutrition have been associated with cirrhosis. For many years, it was impossible to produce alcoholic liver disease in animals.

Finally, experiments by Lieber and co-workers in the 1970s demonstrated that ethanol ingestion could produce liver disease in baboons on an adequate or supplemented diet. In these experiments, each alcoholic baboon had a control with the same nutrient intake except that alcohol was replaced by carbohydrate. After several years of heavy alcohol intake, liver biopsies showed varying degrees of liver disease, some of which simulated human cirrhosis. As in the human, the majority of baboons did not get significant liver disease. Today, the role of nutritional factors in causing alcoholic liver disease is questionable.

Our current understanding of alcoholic liver disease places alcoholic hepatitis on the pathway to cirrhosis, whereas fatty liver is merely a frequent co-existing lesion not directly related to cirrhosis (Fig. 14-4). Probably most individuals with alcoholic hepatitis will progress to cirrhosis if they continue drinking. Current controversy centers on whether alcoholic cirrhosis is always preceded by alcoholic hepatitis. The alcoholic baboon model of cirrhosis does not generally involve a stage of hepatitis similar to the human disease.

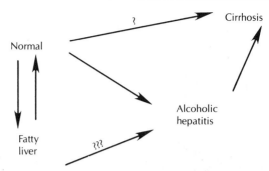

Fig. 14-4
This diagram represents current thinking on the relationship of alcoholic liver lesions. Fatty liver is probably not an important precursor to the serious lesions. Alcoholic hepatitis lies on the pathway to cirrhosis, but cirrhosis may sometimes occur without preceding inflammation.

Several generalizations are in order regarding the pathology of alcoholic liver disease. Much of the pathology is centered around the central vein, probably reflecting the great metabolic differences between the portal and central zones. However, lesions are found in all parts of the lobule. The current emphasis on the central lesions is ironic considering that only 15 or 20 years ago alcoholic liver disease was termed *portal cirrhosis*, and most authorities denied the importance of the centrilobular lesions. None of the histologic features of alcoholic liver disease is entirely specific for alcohol. It is a combination of features that makes the diagnosis more certain. Several drugs can produce a picture essentially identical to alcoholism, and the features that point to an alcoholic lesion tend to fade after months of abstinence. Cirrhosis in an alcoholic who has abstained for a year is often histologically indistinguishable from cirrhosis from other causes. Consequently, it is difficult to interpret all the histologic and functional changes in the liver that result from alcohol. Many of these changes are expected physiologic responses to alcohol metabolism, whereas others may represent cell damage.

Fatty Liver

As mentioned previously, fat droplets accumulate in hepatocytes centered around the central vein, even after rather casual alcohol intake, and this can disappear after days or weeks. On a liver biopsy routinely stained with hematoxylin and eosin, these droplets appear as empty spaces, sometimes displacing the nucleus to the side of the cell (Fig. 14-5A). Similar fatty changes in the liver (macrovesicular fat) can also be seen in diabetes, obesity, protein malnutrition, and several other conditions. Such changes may be seen in apparently normal individuals. Although in rare cases of massive fatty liver this condition may lead to elevated portal pressure and liver dysfunction, it usually

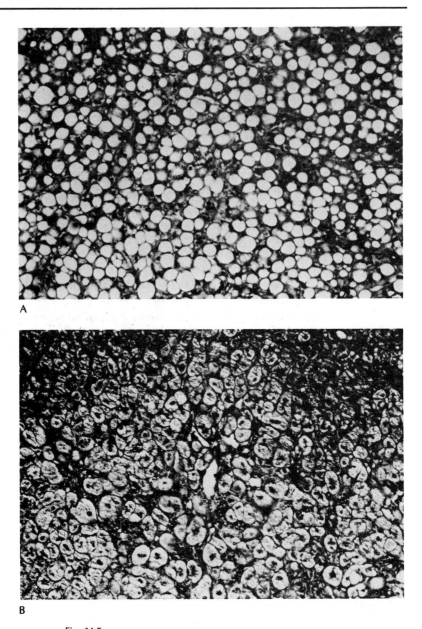

Fig. 14-5
A. The "macrovesicular" fatty liver seen in alcoholism is shown. On a routinely fixed and stained liver biopsy, the fat droplets appear as holes that often displace the nucleus to the side of the cell. B. "Microvesicular" fatty liver for comparison. This type of fatty infiltration is seen in conditions such as Reye's syndrome and acute fatty liver of pregnancy. Tiny fat droplets give the cytoplasm a vaguely "foamy" appearance that cannot be distinguished from glycogen or other substances without special fat stains done on a fresh specimen. The nucleus is not displaced to the side of the hepatocyte.

causes little problem. Alcoholic fatty liver is thought to have little to do with the progression to more serious forms of liver disease.

This type of fatty liver should be distinguished from the microvesicular fatty liver that occurs in acute fatty liver of pregnancy and Reye's syndrome. In these serious conditions, the nuclei are usually centered in cells, and the cytoplasm appears pale and vaguely foamy (Fig. 14-5B). This can be recognized as fat only with special fat stains performed on a frozen specimen.

Alcoholic
Hepatitis

A small percentage of alcoholics develop alcoholic hepatitis (Fig. 14-6). This may produce the same symptoms as in other forms of hepatitis, such as fatigue, anorexia, fever, an enlarged, tender liver, and jaundice with dark urine. The pathology of alcoholic hepatitis is centered around the central vein. Fatty change is usually present. Megamitochondria, similar in size and staining to red blood cells, are sometimes seen. They can be seen in low numbers in nonalcoholic liver disease, often as needle or cigar-shaped megamitochondria. Round megamitochondria in central areas are more specific for alcohol. Abnormal mitochondrial forms can be seen on electron microscopy of livers of many heavy drinkers, even with normal-appearing histology by light microscopy. These abnormal mitochondrial forms are caused by alcohol per se and are not due to malnutrition. One must think of the mitochondrion as a major target of alcohol, a target with implications that go far beyond energy metabolism (Table 14-3). Experimentally, chronic alcoholism leads to decreased mitochondrial oxidation of acetaldehyde, fatty acids, and succinate, with decreased cytochrome levels and total respiratory capacity.

Hepatocyte swelling or "ballooning" often occurs, especially in pericentral hepatocytes. Hepatocytes may appear three times the diameter of normal cells. These swollen cells often contain clumps of fine eosinophilic granules or a fine web-like pattern. Such swelling is thought to involve damage to the cytoskeleton, with disruption of the transport of proteins and ions. Hepatocyte ballooning probably contributes to liver enlargement and to portal hypertension in alcoholic hepatitis; it is a prelude to cell necrosis.

Many cells contain irregular clumps of eosinophilic material in the cytoplasm called Mallory's alcoholic hyaline. This often occurs in central areas and adjacent to areas of fibrosis, especially in ballooned hepatocytes. "Alcoholic" hyaline is not completely specific for alcoholic liver disease; however, in non-alcoholic disease, it tends to occur more frequently in portal areas. By electron microscopy, alcoholic hyaline has the appearance of

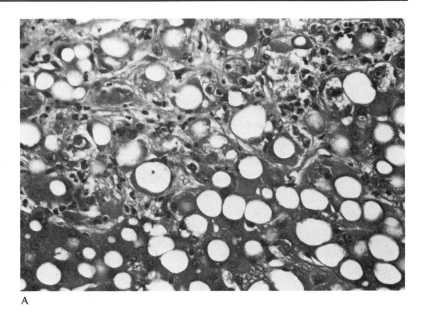

A

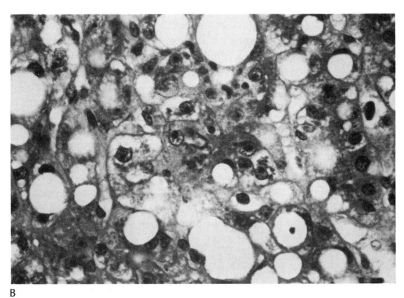

B

Fig. 14-6
Alcoholic hepatitis. A. A liver biopsy from a patient with alcoholic hepatitis, with a prominent infiltrate of polymorphonuclear leukocytes. These are not always present in abundance, but, when they are, there are few explanations except alcohol. B. Several cells with alcoholic hyaline, especially the two just to the right and left of center. Alcoholic hyaline often forms clumps that ring the nucleus. Alcoholic hyaline stands out well on a routine H&E–stained section.

Table 14-3
Metabolic activities of mitochondria

Electron transport and oxidative phosphorylation
Krebs (tricarboxylic acid) cycle
   Oxidation of acetate
   Synthesis of alpha-ketoglutarate (and thus glutamate)
Special oxidations
   Fatty acids
   Acetaldehyde
   Alpha-ketoacids of amino acids
   Amine oxidases, e.g., monoamines
Ketogenesis
Urea synthesis
Pyrimidine synthesis (dihydroorotase dehydrogenase)
Porphyrin synthesis
Calcium uptake, with a possible role in controlling intracellular calcium levels

fibrils with a diameter of 12 to 20 nm. Given this filamentous appearance, there has been suspicion that alcoholic hyaline might be composed of one of the three types of filaments in the cytoskeleton, namely microfilaments, intermediate filaments, or microtubules. Studies suggest that alcoholic hyaline represents aggregates of proteins found in intermediate filaments, although this issue is unsettled. Conceivably, acetaldehyde damages the cytoskeleton by covalently binding to cytoskeletal proteins.

Areas of alcoholic hyaline are often surrounded by polymorphonuclear leukocytes (PMNs) and some lymphocytes. The presence of PMNs is considered a very important criterion in the diagnosis of alcoholic hepatitis by some authorities, although alcoholic hepatitis can be diagnosed without PMNs. Appreciable numbers of PMNs are reliable evidence of alcoholic hepatitis, since liver infiltration with PMNs occurs in few other types of hepatitis. Some reports suggest that alcoholic hyaline is chemotactic for PMNs and that it can also activate lymphocytes from these patients. This picture is often completed by fibrosis extending out from the central vein. Initially, strands of fibrous tissue surround individual hepatocytes. In more advanced stages, hepatocytes disappear to leave bands of connective tissue radiating from the central vein. The central vein, which normally possesses a thin layer of connective tissue, is often surrounded by marked fibrosis.

This picture of alcoholic hepatitis identifies a subset of alcoholics who are susceptible to serious liver disease. It is considered a step in the pathway to cirrhosis, although not an inevitable one. With abstinence, further damage may be arrested. Even some individuals who continue to drink may have a continued form of hepatitis on biopsy without progression to cirrhosis. However, in general, alcoholic hepatitis is an indicator of serious trouble in years to come, if not the immediate future.

Alcoholic Fibrosis and Cirrhosis

With progressive damage, hepatocytes disappear around the central vein and are replaced by extensive fibrous tissue. This lesion, termed *central hyaline sclerosis*, can massively increase the connective tissue of the liver and lead to blockage of blood flow out of the sinusoids, without causing cirrhosis (Fig. 14-7A). Grossly, the cut surface of the liver is studded by white, hard connective tissue, but without the nodular appearance of cirrhosis. This type of alcoholic fibrosis is recognized more commonly in Europe than in the United States. Cirrhosis means more than just fibrous tissue in the liver. It means destruction of the normal architecture by fibrous tissue bridging from one lobule to another, and the formation of regenerative nodules that replace the lost cells (Fig. 14-7B). The result is a disturbed microcirculation with an altered quality and quantity of blood flow to the hepatocytes, shunting of blood flow through fibrous tissue, and usually an increase in total resistance to blood flow through the liver (portal hypertension). If the problem were merely destruction of hepatocytes, this would be easy for the liver to solve, since hepatocytes have a remarkable capacity to regenerate. Alcoholic cirrhosis is usually micronodular; that is, the regenerative nodules are less than 1 cm in diameter. The most viable hepatocytes are usually nearer the portal area than the central vein. Regenerative nodules grow from the most viable cells, so that the central veins tend to be pushed to the sides of the nodules. Likewise, alcoholic hyaline tends to be absent from the nodule and most prominent at its periphery. The liver may show both cirrhosis and active hepatitis. After a period of abstinence, alcoholic cirrhosis may look like any other cirrhosis. It may even be difficult to diagnose cirrhosis by liver biopsy because of sampling error. If the needle goes through a large regenerative nodule, it may yield an uncharacteristic biopsy and show little fibrous tissue. Suspicion may be aroused only because of the lack of central veins in the biopsy.

Alcoholic cirrhosis is often accompanied by iron overload, which can cause some confusion between cirrhosis and familial hemochromatosis. Heavy alcohol ingestion causes increased liver iron stores, even in the absence of liver disease. The mechanism is not clear but may relate to stimulation of iron absorption by alcohol. Nevertheless, by iron stains of the biopsy, the hepatic iron concentration is usually unimpressive and less than that seen with hemochromatosis. Quantitative measurements of

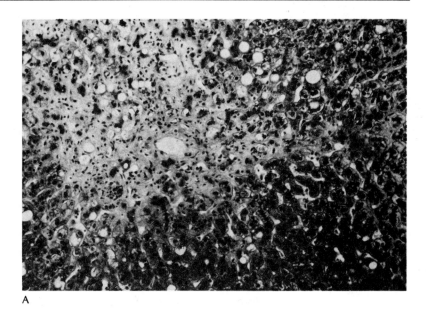

A

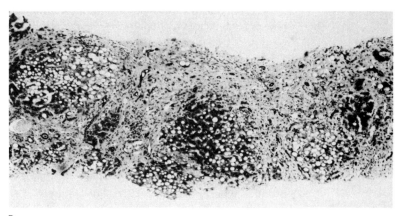

B

Fig. 14-7
Fibrosis and cirrhosis. A. Alcoholic cirrhosis with bands of fibrous tissue extending from one lobule to another, and nodules of hepatocytes remaining. B. Alcoholic fibrosis, so-called sclerosing hyaline necrosis, extending out from the central vein shown just off center. Both of these lesions would be easier to see in color with a connective tissue stain such as Masson's trichrome.

iron in the biopsy can clearly differentiate the mild overload of alcoholism from the vast excess seen in hemochromatosis.

Connective tissue in the normal liver contains mainly collagen types I and III and a variety of other components. Collagen type I predominates around the portal and central areas. Type III collagen is found in the same locations as type I, but also in sinusoids, where it stains as "reticulin." Normal sinusoids lack a true basement membrane, but sinusoids do contain a loose network of types III, IV, and V collagen lining the Disse's space. Other proteins such as fibronectin, and possibly laminin, are associated with collagen. Sulfated glycosaminoglycans such as heparin also form part of the "matrix" that helps hepatocytes adhere to each other and to sinusoidal cells. Recent work suggests that matrix components such as heparin are quite important in maintaining differentiative function in hepatocytes in culture and probably in vivo.

In cirrhosis, the increased collagen is initially type III but in later stages is also type I. Glycosaminoglycans are also greatly increased. In the sinusoids, the thin meshwork of collagen thickens into a virtual basement membrane as fibrogenesis advances. Hepatic endothelial cells normally are loosely knit and contain large pores, but, with advancing cirrhosis, they resemble a true "tight" endothelium. Even without cirrhosis, alcohol can cause the endothelial cell pores to close. These phenomena have been termed *capillarization* of the sinusoids. This process could isolate hepatocytes from factors in the serum, decrease the uptake of such factors by hepatocytes, and interfere with secretion of hepatic products into the bloodstream.

The cellular source of the collagen in cirrhosis has been a debatable issue. Liver contains few fibroblasts, and they do not increase in number during fibrogenesis. Hepatocytes in culture can secrete collagen and glycosaminoglycans. However, the major collagen-secreting cells may be the lipocyte (Ito cell or fat-storing cell) and the fibromyoblast. Lipocytes are found mainly in Disse's spaces throughout the sinusoid. They are the major storage site of vitamin A in the liver. In culture, these cells produce type I collagen and smaller amounts of type III collagen, laminin, and proteoglycans. Lipocytes have some properties of both fibroblasts and smooth muscle cells and are often seen in areas of active fibrosis. Alcoholism causes an apparent transformation of lipocytes into transitional cells, which have properties intermediate between lipocytes and fibroblasts. Increased connective tissue deposition occurs near these cells even in the absence of overt fibrosis. Myofibroblasts are related cells found in the sinusoids, especially around the central vein. They also produce collagens in culture and represent the most abundant collagen-producing cells near the central veins. Myofibroblasts and transitional cells may both be derived from lipocytes, but this is uncertain. In human cirrhosis and in animal models, these cells increase in number, change morphology, and appear directly contiguous to areas of fibrogenesis. Thus, they are probably the source of fibrous tissue in cirrhosis.

The accumulation of fibrous tissue is also probably related to a decrease in the degradation of connective tissue. Although some investigators have reported subnormal levels of collagenase in cirrhosis, this remains an uncertain observation because of the technical difficulties of collagenase assays.

Physiologic Consequences of Alcoholic Liver Disease

Alcoholic liver disease causes clinical problems similar to those seen in other forms of liver disease, except that alcohol adds many toxic effects of its own. (The complications of severe liver disease are discussed in Chap. 17.) Cirrhosis can cause a high resistance to blood flow through the liver, resulting in a high portal vein pressure and enlarged veins in the lower esophagus (esophageal varices) that can bleed profusely. High outflow pressure in the splenic vein can cause a large spleen with anemia and low leukocyte and platelet counts. Low serum albumin and high pressure in hepatic sinusoids can lead to fluid accumulation in the peritoneal cavity (ascites). Failure of hepatocytes to function can cause blood clotting disorders and a form of confusion or coma (hepatic encephalopathy; see Chap. 17).

The combination of alcoholism and liver disease often causes signs of feminization and testicular failure in male alcoholics. A variety of defects is involved, including decreased androgen production, defective clearance of estrogens, and increased conversion of weak androgens into weak estrogens in the skin and other estrogen-sensitive sites. Alcohol decreases testosterone synthesis by suppression of the hypothalamic-pituitary-gonadal axis, and by a direct and immediate inhibitory effect on the testis. Testicular atrophy occurs in vitamin A deficiency. Ethanol in vitro inhibits the oxidation of vitamin A alcohol to its active aldehyde form in the testis, so testicular atrophy may be caused by end-organ vitamin A deficiency. (Of interest, a similar phenomenon occurs in the retina.) Partial portal vein ligation in young male rats causes major portal-systemic shunting of blood, and this alone can cause testicular atrophy without intrinsic liver damage. Many authors cite the liver's failure to clear estrogens as the cause of feminization in liver disease; however, estradiol levels differ little between feminized patients and controls. Although in feminized patients, estrone levels are about twice those found in normal persons, estrone is a weak estrogen. Ethanol increases levels of the enzyme aromatase, which can metabolize weak androgens (e.g, androstanedione) to weak estrogens (e.g., estrone) at the site of action in the skin, breast, and other estrogen-sensitive tissues. It may be the combination of decreased androgens and increased estrogens that results in clinical evidence of feminization. This phenomenon is seen more often in alcoholic cirrhosis than in other forms of liver disease.

Pathogenesis of Alcoholic Hepatitis and Cirrhosis

Overview

Multiple mechanisms have been proposed to explain how alcohol causes hepatitis and cirrhosis, but the exact mechanism is unknown. This uncertainty is not unusual, since there are few hepatotoxic drugs or other chemicals for which we can give more than a general description of the mechanism. In most cases, the drug is metabolized to a highly reactive intermediate that reacts with membranes, proteins, or nucleic acids and either damages vital cellular structures or provokes an autoimmune response against the cell. The specific cellular sites of action of greatest importance are not generally known. Ethanol itself dissolves well in both the aqueous and lipid phases of the cell. It can alter the fluidity of membranes, but whether this has any pathologic significance is unknown. More likely theories include toxicity from acetaldehyde, lipid peroxidation related to depletion of glutathione, hypoxic damage owing to increased oxygen consumption, autoimmunity related to altered cell constituents, and direct stimulation of connective tissue deposition caused by metabolic effects of ethanol metabolism. These ideas are not mutually exclusive. An important requirement for any theory is the explanation of why only a minority of heavy drinkers get serious liver disease.

Acetaldehyde as a Toxin

Acetaldehyde is highly reactive with amines and other nucleophiles. Blood levels are low after alcohol ingestion in casual drinkers (about 50 micromolar) but are significantly greater than this in alcoholics. Acetaldehyde can react with amines, such as the side chains of lysine groups in proteins, and these Schiff bases can then react with other amine groups to cross-link proteins. In chronic alcoholic animals, acetaldehyde is known to bond covalently with some hepatocyte proteins whose exact identity is not known. The fact that acetaldehyde reacts with proteins is totally expected, does not prove that this plays a role in pathogenesis, and does not identify the specific targets that may be important. If cytoskeletal proteins are a major target, this could explain the accumulation of aggregated intermediate filament protein as alcoholic hyaline and might also explain why alcohol interferes with secretion of proteins by the liver. Otherwise, acetaldehyde could attack key enzymes or damage key membrane proteins, perhaps in mitochondria. If the critical point of attack by acetaldehyde were known, specific therapeutic steps might be taken.

*Lipid
Peroxidation*

Alcohol causes peroxidation of hepatic lipids and may cause hepatocyte damage by means of this mechanism. For example, acetaldehyde promotes formation of peroxides that can attack unsaturated fatty acids and thus could attack the integrity and function of membranes. Alcohol also promotes oxidative damage through depletion of reduced glutathione, a cysteine-containing tripeptide that is effective in neutralizing peroxides and other potent oxidizing agents. Alcohol oxidation by the MEOS also produces peroxides and other reactive species as a by-product. Large doses of methionine can protect rats from lipid peroxidation by ethanol, apparently by increasing the synthesis of glutathione or other protective thiols. Alcohol thus causes production of metabolites that can oxidatively damage cell membranes, and it reduces cellular defenses against lipid peroxidation.

*Increased
Susceptibility
to Other Toxins*

Chronic moderate intake of alcohol can increase the toxicity of other chemicals by increasing the activity of microsomal P-450 enzymes, which metabolize chemicals to toxic species. An example is the increase in chloroform hepatotoxicity seen in alcoholic animals. In addition, alcoholics have an increased risk of cancer, even in many sites that are not directly exposed to high concentrations of ethanol. Studies in animals suggest that this phenomenon may be due to the ability of alcohol to activate carcinogens. On the other hand, alcohol can enhance toxicity of a chemical by interfering with its metabolism and elimination. Ethanol inhibits the metabolism of xylene (dimethyl benzene) and leads to elevated blood and tissue levels in workers exposed to this common industrial solvent.

Alcoholism can increase the liver's susceptibility to damage from acetaminophen, the commonly used analgesic. At therapeutic doses, a small fraction of this drug is metabolized to a highly reactive, harmful intermediate, which is quickly detoxified by reaction with glutathione. In the alcoholic, microsomal metabolism of acetaminophen to the toxic metabolite is increased, and levels of glutathione are decreased. It is not surprising, therefore, that clinical reports suggest that even conventional therapeutic doses of acetaminophen can cause liver injury in alcoholic humans.

Ethanol alters the metabolism of a variety of vitamins and hormones that can undergo microsomal metabolism. As discussed previously, alcoholic liver disease may produce systemic signs of feminization by altering sex hormone metabolism. Ethanol can also alter vitamin D metabolism; hence, alcoholism is a major risk factor for osteoporosis. Clinical and experimental observations suggest that vitamin A levels are decreased in the alcoholic liver. This appears to result from increased degradation of vitamin A. It is unclear, however, whether this deficiency contributes in any way to liver injury or dysfunction.

The Hypermetabolic State and Hypoxia

As previously discussed, ethanol can increase metabolic oxygen consumption, and this increase may be more marked in the chronic alcoholic patient than in the casual drinker. As mentioned, alcoholic liver damage is usually most severe around the central vein and indeed may resemble that seen in hypoxia or hyperthyroidism. These observations suggest that alcohol induces a hypermetabolic state that harms the liver by inducing focal hypoxia. A number of theories have been proposed to explain this hypermetabolism and focal hepatic hypoxia, but the exact mechanism remains unknown.

It is also not known whether this increased oxygen consumption could cause liver damage. In a basically healthy animal or human given large amounts of alcohol, increased liver oxygen consumption is matched by increased blood flow. Perhaps there are circumstances in which blood flow fails to keep up with oxygen consumption. It is not known whether anemia or hypoxia in humans exacerbates alcoholic liver disease. Clinical trials have evaluated the use of antithyroid drugs to decrease oxygen consumption in patients with alcoholic hepatitis. They have met mixed success, however, and the concept is quite controversial.

Immunologic Abnormalities

In view of the importance of polymorphonuclear leukocytes and lymphocytes in alcoholic hepatitis, the immune system has been a focus of attention. Much thought centers on the notion that "neoantigens" formed from normal cell constituents by alcohol metabolites may provoke an immune response against the liver. Although various defects of cellular immunity have been described, the role of these immunologic abnormalities in causing liver injury is still unknown. For example, Mallory bodies and intermediate filaments are chemotactic for PMNs. Lymphocytes from patients with alcoholic liver disease are activated on exposure to alcoholic hyaline. In addition, the incidence of autoantibodies such as antinuclear antibody is increased in patients with alcoholic liver disease. Finally, some reports suggest the presence of antibodies directed against liver membrane constituents.

Direct Stimulation of Fibrous Tissue Production

Alcoholic hepatitis is often a precursor to cirrhosis, but in some parts of the world where alcoholic cirrhosis is common, florid alcoholic hepatitis is uncommon. Interest has focused on alcohol metabolism as a direct stimulus to the production of fibrous tissue, independent of inflammation.

In cell culture, myofibroblasts can be stimulated to produce collagen by exposure to lactate or acetaldehyde, but not ethanol. Stimulated Kupffer's cells and other inflammatory cells may produce mediators that stimulate production of fibrous tissue. These observations can integrate ideas regarding acetaldehyde toxicity, hypermetabolism, hypoxia, and the elevated NADH/NAD ratio with elevated lactate concentrations.

Nutrition and Cirrhosis

Remarkably little evidence now exists to support a role for dietary deficiencies as a cause of alcoholic cirrhosis, even though many vitamins and minerals may be inadequate in the alcoholic's diet, and alcohol interferes with many aspects of the metabolism of these substances. Alcohol can increase the degradation of choline and cause choline deficiency, which produces hepatic fibrosis in some species. Abnormalities of vitamin A metabolism have been discussed previously. Despite the controversial role of nutrition in the pathogenesis of alcoholic liver damage, nutritional support clearly speeds recovery from alcoholic hepatitis.

The Diagnosis of Alcoholic Liver Disease

Modes of Presentation

Persons with alcoholic liver disease come to the physician with varied symptoms and signs. Alcoholic hepatitis may smolder indefinitely without producing symptoms. Symptoms of alcoholic hepatitis usually start insidiously with mild fatigue and loss of appetite, although more severe symptoms such as nausea, an enlarged, tender liver, jaundice, and fever may be the initial manifestations. Right upper quadrant pain and jaundice can be mistaken for cholecystitis, with disastrous consequences. Severe alcoholic hepatitis can produce encephalopathy, ascites, or bleeding esophageal varices. Esophageal varices may even regress as the hepatocellular inflammation and swelling subside. Patients with cirrhosis may be discovered because of an enlarged liver on physical examination, although this could represent only fatty liver. Cirrhosis without acute hepatitis does not produce many symptoms until it is far advanced, when it may come to attention because of the development of ascites, encephalopathy, or bleeding varices. Any one of these clinical problems can predominate. These problems can occur, however, with any form of cirrhosis.

Alcoholism is often strenuously denied by the patient, and sometimes by his or her family. Alcoholics are skilled at concealing their alcoholism, often seeing doctors for vague and shifting complaints. A blood test or other biological indicator of alcoholism would be welcome, but a sensitive screening test does not yet exist. Only in alcoholic hepatitis is there a distinctive laboratory test abnormality. The AST (aspartate aminotransferase, formerly SGOT) is usually higher than the ALT (alanine aminotransferase, formerly SGPT) by about 2:1, and the AST is rarely greater than 300. These typical AST and ALT findings reflect a decrease in levels of these enzymes in the liver. Levels of pyridoxal phosphate, a cofactor for transaminases, are low in alcoholics, and the deficiency affects ALT more than AST. Serum ALT levels in alcoholic hepatitis may rise as the liver recovers and pyridoxal phosphate is repleted. It should be remembered that in cirrhosis without active inflammation, the liver enzymes are often completely normal, and they may be nearly normal even with serious ongoing damage.

The definitive diagnostic test for alcoholic hepatitis or cirrhosis is a liver biopsy. This can be done at the bedside with a local anesthetic but may be unsafe if the patient has massive ascites or a severe clotting disorder. Ideally, the liver biopsy will demonstrate a combination of suggestive histologic features, but the changes characteristic of alcohol may fade with months of abstinence. The biopsy helps to confirm or rule out alternative diagnoses, since 10 to 20 percent of heavy drinkers with liver disease may have a non-alcoholic cause for their liver disease.

Prognosis

Many individuals with mild alcoholic hepatitis probably stop drinking and recover without medical attention. Of patients sick enough to be admitted to a hospital, perhaps 10 to 20 percent die. When tests that reflect liver function (bilirubin, albumin, prothrombin time) are markedly abnormal, the prognosis is predictably poor. For patients with hepatic encephalopathy not related to drugs or reversible electrolyte abnormalities, the mortality may be higher than 50 percent. For the patient who continues drinking despite an encounter with alcoholic hepatitis, the likelihood of progression to cirrhosis is very great. The abstinent patient with hepatitis may improve slowly over a year or so. Many patients with cirrhosis go undetected indefinitely, so long as they do not develop variceal bleeding, encephalopathy, or ascites. In the authors' opinion, the best study of the natural history of alcoholic cirrhosis is that of Powell and Klatskin (Figs. 14-8 and 14-9). Of their cirrhotic patients without

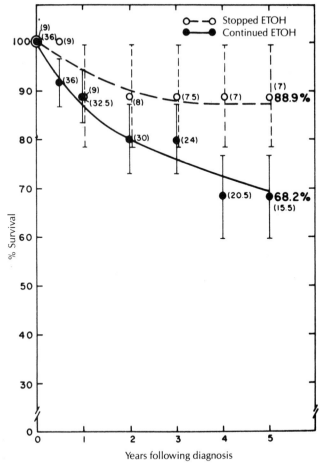

Fig. 14-8
Survival after diagnosis of alcoholic cirrhosis without ascites, jaundice, or upper gastrointestinal bleeding in 45 patients. Patients who gave up alcohol (*dashed line*) are compared to those who continued to drink (*solid line*). The differences shown are not statistically significant. (From W. J. Powell and G. Klatskin. Duration of survival in patients with Laennec's cirrhosis. *Am. J. Med.* 44:406, 1968.)

ascites, jaundice, or bleeding, the 5-year survival rate was 89.9 percent for patients who abstained, and 68.2 percent for those who continued drinking. As expected, patients who had these complications on entry to the study did much worse (Fig. 14-9), yet patients who ceased drinking still had a 60 percent 5-year survival rate. Thus, survival is quite varied, and the outlook is good and comparable to the general population for the asymptomatic cirrhotic patient who stops drinking.

Treatment

There is no established treatment for alcoholic liver disease other than abstinence and the treatment of alcoholism. A nutri-

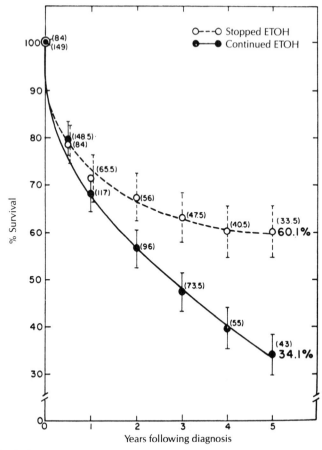

Fig. 14-9
Survival after onset of ascites, jaundice, or upper gastrointestinal bleeding in
233 patients with alcoholic cirrhosis. Patients who gave up drinking (*dashed
line*) are compared to those who continued to drink (*solid line*). The differences between the two groups are statistically significant at the third, fourth,
and fifth years. (From W. J. Powell and G. Klatskin. Duration of survival in
patients with Laennec's cirrhosis. *Am. J. Med.* 44:406, 1968.)

tious diet is prudent, given the many types of nutritional depletion caused by alcoholism, but there is no firm evidence that it
affects the outcome of the liver disease. Despite the inflammatory nature of alcoholic hepatitis, anti-inflammatory drugs such
as prednisone have shown no consistent benefit for most of
these patients. Therapies of potential benefit include propylthiouracil (PTU), given in hopes of reducing the hypermetabolic
state of alcoholism, and colchicine, given in hopes of preventing hepatic fibrosis.

Study Question   1. A 54-year-old man comes for a routine insurance physical
examination. He has had no significant illnesses in his life,

and he feels well now. He says he drinks a six-pack of beer almost every day but he doesn't "touch the hard stuff." On physical exam you feel a firm liver edge 4 cm below the right costal margin. Liver function tests show a very slightly elevated AST (SGOT) and ALT (SGPT) but are otherwise normal. Do you consider the following statements true for false?

a. He almost certainly has marked centrilobular fatty change on his liver biopsy.

b. He almost certainly has cirrhosis, given his alcohol intake and enlarged liver.

c. Half or more of the increase in his liver mass is made up of protein, water, and electrolytes.

d. This man almost certainly does not have alcoholic cirrhosis since he has never had a symptomatic episode of alcoholic hepatitis.

e. This man is more likely to get cirrhosis than his wife, who drinks the same amount.

f. This man cannot have any severe liver disease since his liver function tests are nearly normal.

Answers

a. True, given his alcohol intake and enlarged liver.

b. False. He is at some increased risk for cirrhosis but at most 15 to 30 percent of heavy alcohol users get cirrhosis.

c. True. In fatty liver about half of the increase in liver mass is protein and water. If this man has cirrhosis, then an even larger part of the increase in liver mass is protein and water.

d. False. Many patients get alcoholic cirrhosis without any history of overt alcoholic hepatitis.

e. False. Women are considered more susceptible to alcoholic cirrhosis than men.

f. False. "Liver function tests" such as ALT and AST measure ongoing destruction of liver cells. The bilirubin and prothrombin time measure the liver's function, but a large part of the liver must be destroyed before these are abnormal. Thus this patient could still have quite marked cirrhosis despite his blood tests.

References

Alcohol and disease. Proceedings of the first Acta Medica Scandinavica International Symposium. Nov. 22–23, 1984. *Acta Med. Scand.* (Suppl.) 703:1, 1985.

Fleming, K. A., and McGee, J. O'D. Alcohol-induced liver disease. *J. Clin. Pathol.* 37:721, 1984.

Galambos, J. T. Alcoholic Liver Disease: Fatty Liver, Hepatitis, and Cirrhosis. In J. E. Berk (ed.), *Bockus Gastroenterology* (4th ed.). Philadelphia: Saunders, 1985.

Galambos, J. T. *Cirrhosis.* Philadephia: Saunders, 1979.

Geokas, M. C. (ed.) Symposium on ethyl alcohol and disease. *Med. Clin. North Am.* 68:1, 1984.

Geokas, M. C., moderator, Lieber, C. S., French, S., and Halsted, C. H. Ethanol, the liver, and the gastrointestinal tract. *Ann. Intern. Med.* 95:198, 1981.

Johnson, R. D., and Williams, R. Genetic and environmental factors in the individual susceptibility to the development of alcoholic liver disease. *Alcohol Alcoholism* 20:137, 1985.

Kershenobich, D., et al. Colchicine in the treatment of cirrhosis of the liver. *N. Engl. J. Med.* 318:1709, 1988.

Lieber, C. S. Metabolism of Alcohol and Associated Hepatic Effects. In J. E. Berk (ed.), *Bockus Gastroenterology* (4th ed.), vol. 5. Philadelphia: Saunders, 1985.

Lieber, C. S. Alcohol and the liver: 1984 update. *Hepatology* 4:1243, 1984.

Orrego, H., et al. Long-term treatment of alcoholic liver disease with propylthiouracil. *N. Engl. J. Med.* 317:1421, 1987.

Powell, W. J., and Klatskin, G. Duration of survival in patients with Laennec's cirrhosis. *Am. J. Med.* 44:406, 1968.

Savolainen, E.-R., Leo, M. A., Timpl, R., and Lieber, C. S. Acetaldehyde and lactate stimulate collagen synthesis of cultured baboon liver myofibroblasts. *Gastroenterology* 87:777, 1984.

West, L. J., moderator, Maxwell, D. S., Noble, E. P. and Solomon, D. H. Alcoholism. *Ann. Intern. Med.* 100:405, 1984.

15 : Drug-Induced and Circulatory Disorders of the Liver

Roger J. May

The liver is a highly active metabolic organ. In addition to synthesizing numerous substances, it is also crucial to the modification and excretion of many endogenous compounds. Furthermore, the liver is a major site for the metabolism of exogenous substances such as medications and environmental toxins. To support this prominent metabolic activity, it receives approximately 25 percent of the cardiac output, both directly by the hepatic artery and indirectly by the portal venous system. It is not surprising, therefore, that the liver is susceptible to injury from both toxic metabolites of exogenous compounds and circulatory changes that compromise hepatic oxygen delivery.

The understanding of hepatic architecture and microcirculation is important to the recognition of the mechanisms by which toxic and ischemic injury occur. As shown in Fig. 15-1, the conventional concept of the hepatic acinus (lobule) is that it occupies adjacent sectors of neighboring hexagonal fields. Blood flow into the acinus occurs by the hepatic artery and portal vein in the portal space. Terminal afferent vascular branches extend from there into the hepatic lobule and empty into the sinusoids. Subsequent venous drainage of the sinusoids occurs by the terminal hepatic veins ("central veins"). The parenchymal regions of the lobule have arbitrarily been divided into zones 1, 2, and 3, respectively, which represent areas supplied with blood of first, second, and third quality with regard to substrate, oxygen, and nutrients. As will be discussed, the distribution over the lobule of enzymes that mediate drug and toxin metabolism often determines the resulting pattern of liver injury. In addition, the pattern of diffusion of oxygen from zone 1 to zone 3 determines the pattern of hepatic injury that occurs with circulatory failure.

Toxic Hepatic Injury

Toxic hepatic injury refers to damage to hepatocytes or interference with bile flow produced by the direct or indirect action of medications or environmental toxins. In the past, toxic hepatic injury was uncommon and was primarily caused by environmental toxins. Predictably, with the development of an increasing number of new drugs, deleterious effects of medication have become more common and represent a significant component

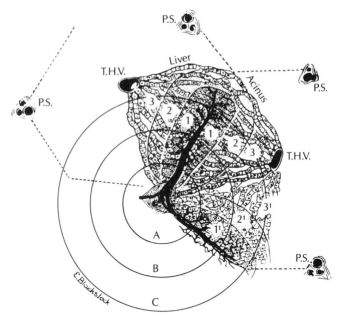

Fig. 15-1
Blood supply of the hepatic acinus and the zonal arrangement of cells. The acinus occupies adjacent sectors of neighboring hexagonal fields (*dotted lines*). Zones 1, 2, and 3, respectively, represent areas supplied with blood of the first, second, and third quality with regard to substrate, oxygen, and nutrients. The zones center around the terminal afferent vascular branches and extend into the triangular portal field. Zones 1′, 2′, and 3′ designate corresponding areas in a portion of an adjacent acinar unit. In zones 1 and 1′, the afferent vascular twigs empty into the sinusoids. Circles B and C indicate peripheral circulatory areas as commonly described around a "periportal" area, A. (Key: P.S. = portal space; T.H.V. = terminal hepatic venules ["central vein"].) (From A. M. Rappaport. Physioanatomic Considerations. In L. Schiff and E. R. Schiff (eds.), *Diseases of the Liver* (6th ed.). Philadelphia: Lippincott, 1987.)

of toxic injury. Hepatic injury by these mechanisms is a relatively minor cause of acute liver disease and represents less than 5 percent of all causes of jaundice. Despite this low frequency, however, the clinical importance of this disorder is obvious from the fact that, in the United States, approximately 25 percent of all cases of fulminant hepatic failure are due to toxic injury.

An understanding of drug metabolism is essential to understanding the mechanisms of toxic injury. Pharmacologic agents are either water-soluble or lipid-soluble. Water-soluble drugs are quickly excreted unchanged in either the urine or bile. Lipid-soluble agents are retained in the body for a longer period of time and must be converted to either less active compounds or more soluble metabolites, which are more easily excreted. The conversion of nonpolar substances to more polar compounds takes place primarily in the liver through metabolizing enzymes present in the mitochondria and microsomes.

There are two major routes involved in drug metabolism — phase I reactions and phase II reactions. Phase I reactions consist of the oxidation, reduction, and hydrolysis reactions whereby the initial compound acquires polar chemical groups (e.g., −OH or −COOH groups). These enzymatic modifications occur by means of the mixed function oxidase (MFO) system, which is located in the smooth endoplasmic reticulum. The chief enzyme of the MFO system, cytochrome P-450, consists of a number of isoenzymes that differ in their specific capacity to catalyze the metabolism of various compounds. In general, the activity of these enzymes decreases significantly with increasing age. Within the hepatic lobule, the concentration of the MFO enzyme increases as one moves from zone 1 to zone 3, and this variation in enzyme concentration is the presumed mechanism for the pattern of liver injury seen with some compounds; that is, compounds that produce injury through the action of toxic metabolites produced by the MFO are characterized by a predominant pattern of centrizonal injury resulting from the higher concentration of MFO enzymes in this region.

Phase II reactions consist of conjugation or synthetic reactions that couple the initial compound with an endogenous substance, such as sulfate or glucuronic acid, to form polar metabolites that are more readily excreted. Reactions such as glucuronidation occur in the microsomes, whereas other reactions, such as acetylation or sulfation, occur in other regions of the hepatocytes. Not uncommonly, both phase I and phase II reactions are involved in the metabolism and excretion of a compound. In such cases, phase I reactions usually precede phase II reactions as the initial compound undergoes modification before conjugation. In general, phase II reactions do not play an etiologic step in the formation of toxic metabolites in the same fashion as do phase I reactions.

The medications and environmental factors capable of producing hepatic injury are too numerous to review in detail in this chapter. The goal of this chapter is to discuss the mechanisms by which hepatotoxic reactions occur and the histologic patterns of injury that most commonly result.

In general, hepatotoxins produce injury by either an *intrinsic* or an *idiosyncratic* mechanism. *Intrinsic hepatotoxins* produce predictable injury unaffected by host sensitivity. Therefore , there is a very high, if not universal, incidence of injury, and an analogous lesion can often be produced in experimental animals. The injury is usually dose-dependent and appears in a rather short period of time after exposure to the toxin.

Idiosyncratic toxins, by contrast, produce unpredictable injury as a result of an unusual host susceptibility or metabolism. Therefore, the incidence of idiosyncratic toxicity is low. In general, a similar lesion cannot be induced in animals. The toxicity is not dose-dependent and can occur within a quite variable period of time (days to months) after the initiation of exposure.

Intrinsic Hepatotoxins

Intrinsic hepatotoxins can produce liver injury by either a *direct* or an *indirect* pathway. Quite often, intrinsic hepatotoxins act by way of both direct and indirect pathways to produce toxicity. With *direct toxicity,* the offending agent or its metabolite *directly* injures the structure or membrane of the hepatocyte or injures one of the hepatocellular organelles with resulting cellular dysfunction or death. The injury is by direct physical or chemical injury, such as the peroxidation of membrane lipids. A well-studied example of intrinsic hepatotoxicity is carbon tetrachloride (CCl_4). This compound produces direct injury to the hepatocellular membrane with associated damage to the cell's calcium pump. These effects result in a sharp rise in calcium levels in the cytosol. Carbon tetrachloride is metabolized by the MFO system, and the resulting metabolite appears to be a highly reactive free radical (CCl_3). This toxic metabolite results in peroxidation of membrane lipids and produces covalent binding with cellular macromolecules. The combined effect of these directly toxic actions is hepatocellular necrosis (Fig. 15-2). Because of the action of the MFO system in the production of the toxic metabolite, the predominant pattern of injury is centrizonal (zone 3) necrosis.

Indirect hepatotoxins act *indirectly* to produce cell dysfunction or death. Either the agent itself or its metabolite produces injury by selective interference with specific metabolic pathways or organelle structure. The injury itself can result in hepatocellular necrosis (cytotoxic) or can interfere with bile flow (cholestatic). The antibiotic tetracycline represents an example of *indirect cytotoxic* injury. As with other intrinsic agents, the toxicity is dose-related and is reproducible in animals. The major result of tetracycline hepatotoxicity is the inhibition of hepatic excretion of lipid. This presumably results from the known interference of tetracycline with protein synthesis. Tetracycline appears to inhibit protein synthesis through binding of transport RNA. In the liver, this presumably prevents the synthesis of the apoprotein necessary for the synthesis of very low density lipoprotein (VLDL) or interferes with the assembly of the components of VLDL prior to excretion. The cellular injury results in a histologic

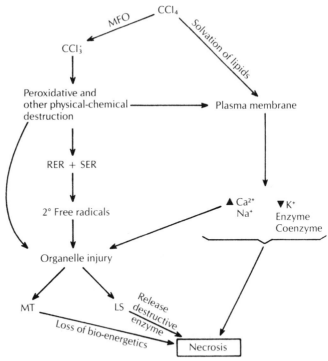

Fig. 15-2

Hypothetical scheme for overall mechanism of CCl_4-induced hepatic necrosis. Increased cytosol levels of Ca^{2+} reflect leakage from organelles and entry from extracellular fluid secondary to early changes in membranes. (Key: RER = rough endoplasmic reticulum; SER = smooth endoplasmic reticulum; MT = mitochondria; LS = lysosome.) See text for details. (From H. J. Zimmerman and W. C. Maddrey. Toxic and Drug-Induced Hepatitis. In L. Schiff and E. R. Schiff (eds.), *Diseases of the Liver* (6th ed.). Philadelphia: Lippincott, 1987.)

pattern of microvesicular fat deposition similar to that seen in Reye's syndrome or in the acute fatty liver of pregnancy.

Hepatotoxicity owing to the C-17 alkylated anabolic steroids and the ethinylated contraceptive steroids represents an example of *indirect cholestatic injury*. The exact mechanism of injury is unknown but is presumably related to the structure of the compounds. There is a specific structural requirement for the toxicity in that only those steroid compounds with alkylation at the C-17 site produce this effect. For example, testosterone does not produce this effect, but methyltestosterone does. Presumably, this class of compounds produces a rather mild interference in bile flow in a large number of subjects but produces clinically significant disease in only a minority of patients. It is probable that genetic factors play an additional role in the susceptibility to the injury or the severity of the injury. Women who experience the genetically determined condition *benign choles-*

tatic jaundice of pregnancy are very likely to experience jaundice with the ingestion of these steroid compounds. Studies suggest that the mechanism of toxicity may be related to induced alterations in the plasma membrane of the hepatocytes. The anabolic steroids may act at the canalicular membrane, whereas the contraceptive steroids act on the basolateral membrane, reducing membrane fluidity and decreasing Na^+, K^+-ATPase activity. These effects on the basolateral membrane could result in decreased uptake of bile salts and hence decreased bile flow.

Idiosyncratic Hepatotoxins

Whereas hepatic injury caused by intrinsic hepatotoxins is due to the "intrinsic toxicity" of the drug, liver injury resulting from *idiosyncratic* reactions is due to the "host *idiosyncrasy*." These reactions occur in individuals in an unpredictable fashion that is not dose-related. Although the term *idiosyncratic* is often used interchangeably with the term *hypersensitivity*, the two are not synonymous, and a distinction should be made between the two in the description of mechanisms of hepatotoxicity. *Idiosyncratic reactions* can occur by means of either a *hypersensitivity* or a *metabolic* mechanism. In a given patient, the unpredictable metabolism of a drug by the liver could lead to the accumulation of a metabolite that could act either as a haptene (producing a *hypersensitivity* reaction) or as a cytotoxin (producing *metabolic* injury).

Idiosyncratic hypersensitivity reactions tend to occur soon after initiation of drug therapy (within weeks) and are associated with clinical signs of a strong immune response. Evidence of hepatic injury is associated with fever, rash, and often eosinophilia. When the drug is stopped, the hypersensitivity reaction resolves. If the patient is then rechallenged with the offending drug, a prompt toxic response ensues. *Phenytoin* hepatoxicity is an example of this mechanism of injury. Liver injury caused by this drug is uncommon and occurs almost exclusively in adults. The onset occurs within the first several weeks of treatment and is associated with fever, lymphadenopathy, and a skin rash that may evolve into an exfoliative dermatitis. The liver shows diffuse degeneration and multifocal necrosis. The inflammatory infiltrate may include eosinophils and lymphocytes, and granulomas have been described. The hepatic injury may be severe, and the mortality rate may approach 40 to 50 percent. Patents with phenytoin-induced liver injury have been documented to have an altered metabolism of this drug. Furthermore, some relatives of these patients also exhibit similar abnormalities of phenytoin metabolism. These individuals produce highly reactive arene oxides that accumulate in the liver rather than being converted to the inactive compound dihydriol. These arene oxides may then bind covalently to tissue macromolecules, and this may result in either an antigen to stimulate the hypersensitivity reaction or a metabolic toxin to produce tissue injury.

Idiosyncratic metabolic reactions occur when, for unclear reasons, metabolism of the drug yields compounds that are injurious. In contrast to the hypersensitivity reaction, the metabolic reactions occur at a variable time after initiation of drug therapy; the onset may be as late as weeks to months after starting therapy. Liver injury occurs in the absence of systemic signs of a strong immune response. When the drug is stopped, the liver injury will resolve. If the patient is rechallenged with the offending drug, the hepatic response is delayed days or even weeks. Liver injury owing to *isoniazide* (INH) is an example of this mechanism of hepatotoxicity.

Clinically significant liver injury owing to INH is uncommon. Jaundice occurs in only 1 percent of patients. The toxicity is age-related and is rare in patients younger than 20 years of age but increases to an incidence of more than 2 percent for those older than 50 years. A transient period of hepatic dysfunction may occur in 10 to 20 percent of patients receiving INH, but this resolves despite continuation of therapy and is unrelated to the more severe hepatic injury. Signs and symptoms of disease appear within the first year of treatment, and 50 percent of affected patients will become ill within 2 months of initiation of therapy. Histologic features on liver biopsy resemble those of viral hepatitis with portal inflammation and diffuse hepatocellular degeneration and necrosis. In some patients, the histologic features may resemble those of chronic active hepatitis with extension of the inflammatory infiltrate into the lobule. The clinical course can be severe, and the mortality rate can be as high as 10 percent. The mechanism of cellular injury is thought to be secondary to the production of toxic metabolites that bind covalently to macromolecules, leading to cell necrosis. Earlier studies that suggested that patients who acetylated INH rapidly were at greater risk of hepatic injury have not been confirmed. Combined treatment of INH with rifampin, another antituberculous drug, appears to increase the risk of INH hepatotoxicity, presumably by stimulating increased production of the toxic metabolite.

Histologic Patterns of Injury

Acute Injury

All histologic patterns of liver injury, both acute and chronic, have been described with toxic hepatic injury. Although the serum biochemical abnormalities (liver function test) and pathologic patterns are usually nonspecific, certain findings may be identified that allow characterization of the disease process (Table 15-1).

1. *Cytotoxic pattern.* In this pattern, injury occurs primarily to the hepatocytes and can result in either a *zonal* or a *diffuse* pattern of injury. Zonal necrosis is most characteristic of *intrinsic hepatotoxins* and predominantly involves one of the zones of the hepatic lobule. Centrizonal (zone 3) necrosis is typically found in toxicity owing to carbon tetrachloride and acetaminophen. Hepatic injury owing to intrinsic toxins is usually associated with either a scant inflammatory infiltrate or one consisting of predominantly neutrophils.

Diffuse hepatocellular injury that resembles the pattern seen in viral hepatitis is more typical of *idiosyncratic* reactions (e.g., isoniazid, methyldopa, halothane). The inflammatory infiltrate consists of eosinophils and lymphocytes. The cellular infiltrate may be less prominent than that associated with a comparable degree of necrosis owing to viral hepatitis.

Hepatic steatosis can also result from intrinsic toxins. The deposition may be *microvesicular* as the hepatocyte is filled with many tiny droplets of fat, which do not displace the nucleus (tetracycline). Alternatively, the deposition may be *macrovesicular* as the hepatocyte is filled with a single large droplet that does displace the nucleus (ethanol, methotrexate).

2. *Cholestatic pattern.* Some *intrinsic* hepatotoxins are capable of producing injury that arrests bile flow with little evidence of parenchymal damage. The morphologic pattern is one of predominant injury to bile secretion with bilirubin casts in the canaliculi and relative sparing of the parenchyma (Fig. 15-3). Cholestasis may be associated with a prominent portal inflammatory infiltrate (with pericholangitis), such as with chlorpromazine. Alternatively, the cholestasis may be entirely bland without inflammation (without pericholangitis), such as with anabolic and contraceptive steroids.

3. *Mixed pattern.* In some forms of hepatotoxicity, there may be morphologic elements of cytotoxicity and cholestasis (phenylbutazone).

4. *Granulomatous pattern.* Hypersensitivity reactions can produce liver injury associated with granulomatous inflammation (allopurinol, quinidine). The mechanism prompting the formation of granulomas rather than a diffuse inflammatory infiltrate is unknown.

Table 15-1
Histologic types of acute toxic hepatic injury and associated biochemical and clinical aspects

Histologic lesion	Biochemical abnormalities in serum*			Clinical aspects	Examples
	SGOT and SGPT	Alkaline phosphatase	Cholesterol		
Cytotoxic					
Zonal necrosis	10–500×	1–2×	N or ↓	Hepatic and renal failure	Carbon tetrachloride, MSH, ACM, HALO
Diffuse necrosis	10–200×	1–2×	N or ↓	Severe hepatitis-like disease	INH, methyldopa, HALO
Steatosis	5–20×	1–2×	N or ↓	Resembles fatty liver of pregnancy and Reye's syndrome	Tetracycline
Cholestatic					
With pericholangitis (hepatocanalicular)	1–10×	1–10×	↑	Resembles obstructive jaundice	CPZ, EE
Without pericholangitis (canalicular)	1–5×	1–3×	N or ↑	Resembles obstructive jaundice	Anabolic and contraceptive steroids
Mixed (mixtures of cytotoxic and cholestatic)	10–100×	1–10×	N or ↑	May resemble hepatitis or obstructive jaundice	PBZ, PAS, sulfonamides

*Degree of abnormality indicated as fold increases: N, normal; ↓ = reduced; ↑ = increased.
(Key: PAS = p-aminosalicylic acid; MSH = poisonous mushrooms; ACM = acetaminophen; HALO = halothane; INH = isoniazid; CPZ = chlorpromazine; EE = erythromycin estolate; PBZ = phenylbutazone)
SOURCE: From H. J. Zimmerman and W. C. Maddrey. Toxic and Drug-Induced Hepatitis. In L. Schiff and E. R. Schiff (eds.), Diseases of the Liver (6th ed.). Philadelphia: Lippincott, 1987.

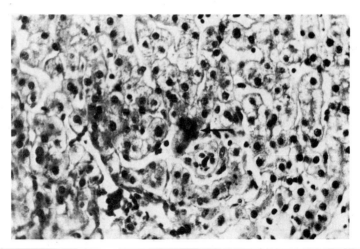

Fig. 15-3
Liver biopsy demonstrating focally prominent canalicular bile stasis (*arrow*) in a patient with estrogen-induced cholestasis. Note the absence of an inflammatory infiltrate in the hepatic parenchyma. (Courtesy of Donald Antonioli, M.D.)

Chronic Injury

Chronic hepatotoxicity can result from continued or repeated injury. The ongoing findings can be so subtle as to escape clinical detection until a more advanced morphologic lesion results. The sequellae may be *parenchymal, vascular,* or *neoplastic.*

1. *Chronic active hepatitis.* This lesion may resemble that chronic active hepatitis seen in autoimmune ("lupoid") hepatitis. Histologically, there may be a striking portal inflammation with extension of the inflammatory infiltrate into the periportal parenchyma (piecemeal necrosis"). This pattern has been seen with several drugs, including dantrolene and methyldopa. In a given patient, if cirrhosis has not evolved, the pathology will resolve with discontinuation of the drug.

2. *Vascular pattern.* Long-term treatment with some medications has led to vascular lesions of the liver. *Hepatic vein thrombosis* has been observed in women taking oral contraceptives and has been attributed to the thrombogenic effect of these drugs. *Veno-occlusive disease* is characterized as injury to and occlusion of the central hepatic venules. It differs from hepatic vein thrombosis in that the caliber of the vessels involved is much smaller than the hepatic vein. The morphologic pattern is one of hepatic congestion and centrizonal necrosis caused by the obstruction of venous outflow from the hepatic lobule. This lesion has been associated with the intake of pyrrolizidine alkaloids ("bush tea") and with certain chemotherapeutic agents (thioguanine, mitomycin C). *Peliosis hepatis* refers to the large,

blood-filled cavities that can occur in the hepatic parenchyma and are often associated with marked sinusoidal dilatation even in sites remote from the actual lesion. This lesion is seen most commonly in patients receiving long-term therapy with anabolic steroids.

3. *Neoplastic pattern.* Several neoplasms have been associated with the chronic use or exposure to medications or toxins. There is general agreement that *hepatic adenomas* are more common in women receiving oral contraceptives; indeed, some cases of adenomas have shown marked regression or even disappearance of the tumors after contraceptives have been discontinued. The chronic ingestion of foods contaminated with mycotoxins have long been suspected to be the cause of *hepatocellular carcinoma.* In addition, there is an association between this cancer and the long-term use of anabolic steroids. Rare cases of *cholangiocarcinoma* have been associated with the past use of Thorotrast, an obsolete contrast agent that was formerly used for radiographic studies. *Angiosarcoma* (hemangioendothelial sarcoma) has been associated with prolonged exposure to vinyl chloride (see Chap. 18).

Acetaminophen Hepatotoxicity

Acetaminophen (ACM) is an effective, mild analgesic that is used frequently. In therapeutic doses, it is well tolerated with few side effects. In large doses, however, it is a potent *intrinsic* hepatotoxin, which produces centrizonal necrosis by *direct* organelle injury. Since the mechanism of its toxicity and the rationale for its treatment have been well studied, a discussion of ACM hepatotoxicity is helpful in understanding general concepts of toxic hepatic injury. In addition, hepatotoxicity owing to ACM is not rare. In the United Kingdom, overdosage with ACM is a popular means of attempted suicide and is one of the most prominent causes of severe hepatic necrosis in that country.

Under normal conditions, therapeutic doses of ACM are metabolized by hepatic phase II reactions and are excreted following conjugation with either glucuronic acid or sulfate. With increasing doses, increasing amounts of ACM are metabolized by the MFO system, yielding an electrophilic metabolite, which is highly reactive. When generated in small amounts, this metabolite is immediately bound by cellular stores of glutathione, forming a stable non-toxic compound. If the concentration of the electrophilic metabolite exceeds the capacity of glutathione to neutralize it, however, the toxic metabolite binds covalently with cellular macromolecules and produces cytotoxicity (Fig. 15-4). The risk and severity of hepatic injury, therefore, depends on (1) the dose of ACM ingested, (2) the

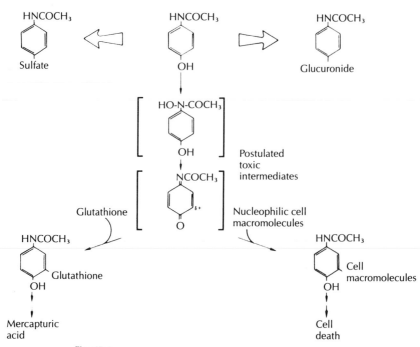

Fig. 15-4
Scheme for the physiologic and pathologic metabolism of acetaminophen. Acetaminophen (*structure in upper center*), ingested in therapeutic dosages, undergoes hepatic metabolism by conjugation with either sulfate or glucuronide (*large arrows*). When ingested in excessive dosages, the drug undergoes an alternative metabolism (*small arrows*), which results in the formation of toxic intermediates. These metabolites may then combine with glutathione, forming a stable product or with cellular macromolecules, leading to cell death. (From H. J. Zimmerman. *Hepatotoxicity*. Norwalk, Connecticut: Appleton-Century-Crofts, 1978.)

activity of the MFO system, and (3) the cellular stores of glutathione. Since the activity of the MFO system is greatest in zone 3, the highest concentration of the toxic metabolite accumulates in hepatocytes in this region, and centrizonal necrosis results.

In general, toxicity with ACM occurs with doses greater than 10 gm, and 80 percent of all severe cases have occurred with doses greater than 15 gm. Owing to the multiple factors affecting toxicity, however, an exact relationship between dose and severity of injury does not exist. This uncertainty may also result from inaccurate reporting by patients of the dose ingested plus the vomiting of the drug that occurs after large overdoses. Measurement of blood levels of ACM between 4 and 10 hours after ingestion offers a more reliable prediction of toxicity. Patients with blood levels greater than 300 µg/ml at 4 hours are likely to develop toxicity, whereas all those with levels less than 100 to

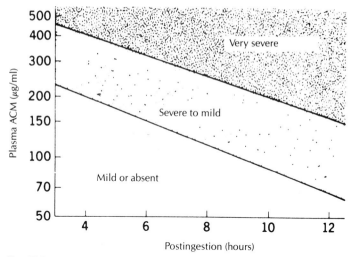

Fig. 15-5
Nomogram demonstrating the relationship between the plasma level of acetaminophen (ACM) at different times postingestion and the degree of hepatotoxicity. (From H. J. Zimmerman. *Hepatotoxicity*. Norwalk, Connecticut: Appleton-Century-Crofts, 1978.)

150 μg/ml at this time are not. A nomogram has been developed based on these observations; it is used in the clinical management of acute ACM overdoses (Fig. 15-5).

Since the activity of the MFO system affects the cellular concentration of the toxic metabolite, changes of MFO activity should alter the degree of injury caused by a given dose. Indeed, in experimental studies, pretreatment of animals with phenobarbital, a stimulant of MFO activity, increases the toxicity of a given dose of ACM. Alternatively, pretreatment with pipernyl butoxide, an inhibitor of MFO activity, decreases toxicity.

In clinical practice, chronic alcohol ingestion is the most common factor increasing MFO activity. It is not surprising, therefore, that chronic alcoholic patients are at increased risk for ACM toxicity. Indeed, mild to severe hepatotoxicity may occur in these patients at levels of ACM intake less than 10 gm. There are well-documented cases of chronic alcoholic patients developing ACM hepatotoxicity with the chronic ingestion of the drug in doses of 5 to 8 gm/day.

Studies in experimental animals have also confirmed that cellular stores of glutathione do affect the severity of ACM hepatotoxicity. Injury is more severe if glutathione stores are depleted by fasting or by pretreatment with diethyl maleate; injury is less severe if glutathione stores are replenished and maintained with the administration of sulfhydryl-containing compounds. In clinical practice, this effect is also significant in chronic alcoholic patients, in whom poor dietary intake and alcohol-mediated inhibition of glutathione regeneration combine to reduce cellular stores of this factor.

With ACM overdose, the first phase of symptoms, lasting for several hours after ingestion, is characterized by anorexia, nausea, and vomiting. Thereafter, the patient may feel relatively well for 24 to 48 hours, but laboratory testing will demonstrate early signs of evolving hepatotoxicity. If treatment is delayed or is inadequate, clinical signs of liver injury appear 3 to 5 days after ingestion and can progressively worsen. At its worst, ACM-induced hepatotoxicity can result in fulminant hepatic failure with jaundice, coagulopathy, encephalopathy, and renal failure. In such patients, the mortality may be greater than 30 percent, even with aggressive supportive therapy.

Treatment with acetylcysteine during the first 16 hours following ingestion of the overdose can reduce the hepatotoxicity of ACM. The mechanism of action of acetylcysteine appears to be the repletion and maintenance of hepatocellular stores of glutathione during the metabolism of the ACM overdose. Early administration of this drug appears to lessen the severity of cellular injury caused by the production of the toxic metabolite of ACM. Administration of acetylcysteine more than 16 hours after the overdose seems to be of no benefit. Although an intravenous form of the drug is available in the United Kingdom, acetylcysteine is administered orally in the United States. Treatment is then carried on over the initial days following the overdosage. Therefore, the recommended clinical management of ACM overdose consists of drawing blood levels during the first 4 to 12 hours following ingestion and initiating treatment immediately with acetylcysteine pending the results of these levels. If the initial blood levels subsequently indicate no risk of hepatotoxicity, treatment can be discontinued. If the initial blood levels are in the toxic range, treatment is continued and the patient is monitored for signs of liver injury.

Ischemic Injury to the Liver

Oxygen is delivered to hepatocytes by means of erythrocytes passing through the sinusoids. As demonstrated in Fig. 15-1, blood enters the lobule throughout the terminal vascular branches of the hepatic artery and portal vein. It then passes from the portal sinusoids to the centrizonal sinusoid and then leaves the lobule by way of the central vein. Oxygen delivery to the hepatocytes, therefore, occurs along a gradient between the portal (zone 1) sinusoids and the centrizonal (zone 3) sinusoids. The partial oxygen tension (PO_2) of blood falls from 65 mm of

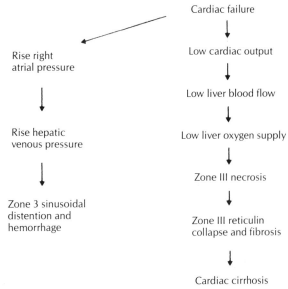

Fig. 15-6
Scheme of the mechanisms by which cardiac failure leads to hepatic injury and cirrhosis. (From S. Sherlock. The Liver in Circulatory Failure. In L. Schiff and E. R. Schiff (eds.), *Diseases of the Liver* (6th ed.). Philadelphia: Lippincott, 1987.)

mercury in the portal sinusoids to 30 mm of mercury in the centrizonal sinusoids.

From the aforementioned description of the hepatic microcirculation, it is apparent that oxygen delivery to the lobule can be comprised by either decreased vascular pressure in the portal tract (owing to decreased cardiac output or shock) or increased venous pressure in the hepatic and central veins (owing to increased right atrial pressure). Given the pattern of oxygen delivery, with circulatory failure, ischemic cellular injury and necrosis will be greatest in the centrizonal region owing to its lower PO_2. The severity of the ischemic hepatic injury should correlate with the severity and duration of the circulatory disturbance (Fig. 15-6). Systemic blood pressure measurements, however, may not accurately reflect the status of hepatic blood flow, since constriction of both the splanchnic vasculature and the hepatic artery occur with decreased cardiac output and shock.

Several syndromes of circulatory injury to the liver have been identified. In each of the syndromes, hepatic injury occurs by the mechanisms just described.

1. *Chronic hepatic congestion.* With chronic elevation of right atrial pressure, pressures are elevated in the inferior vena cava and the hepatic veins. This results in congestion of the centri-

zonal sinusoids with hemorrhage into the lobule. If the congestion is prolonged, the resulting ischemia produces centrizonal necrosis, fibrosis, and, eventually, cirrhosis ("cardiac cirrhosis"). The syndrome can be seen with any disorder resulting in chronic elevation of right atrial pressure (e.g., cardiomyopathy, tricuspid regurgitation, constrictive pericarditis). On clinical examination, the liver is enlarged and can be pulsatile owing to the transmission of cardiac impulses to the liver by an incompetent tricuspid valve. Ascites is often present.

2. *Acute hepatic congestion.* The acute elevation of right atrial pressure (pericardial tamponade) produces an acute increase in hepatic venous pressure with resulting centrizonal necrosis. If prolonged, the increased hepatic venous pressure can result in hepatomegaly, which may be painful and tender to palpation owing to acute stretching of the hepatic capsule.

3. *Ischemic hepatitis.* In patients with cardiac disease, an apparent mild decrease in cardiac output (arrhythmia, worsening ventricular function), even in the absence of overt congestive heart failure, can result in symptoms (anorexia, fatigue) and serum biochemical abnormalities (elevated transaminases) suggestive of viral hepatitis. The histologic pattern is that of centrizonal necrosis without inflammation (Fig. 15-7). The ischemic injury is thought to be due to decreased oxygen delivery by way of the portal tracts.

4. *Hepatic injury in shock.* In any patient, prolonged systemic hypotension (owing to trauma, hemorrhage, or sepsis) can result in hepatic centrizonal necrosis of varying severity as a result of decreased oxygen delivery. In patients with cardiac disease, prolonged shock can produce extensive hepatocellular necrosis culminating in hepatic failure with jaundice, coagulopathy, and encephalopathy.

With acute circulatory injury to the liver, such as with shock, the serum biochemical abnormalities reflect the resulting hepatocellular injury. Serum transaminase levels are elevated and often exceed 1000 IU/ml, mimicking changes seen in acute viral hepatitis. With chronic injury, as with chronic congestive heart failure, the transaminase levels are not as strikingly elevated, and the serum bilirubin is modestly elevated (2–5 mg/100 ml). The mechanism of the abnormal bilirubin levels is not well understood but is thought to result from ischemic liver dysfunction and increased bilirubin production, possibly owing to small infarct in the lungs and other organs.

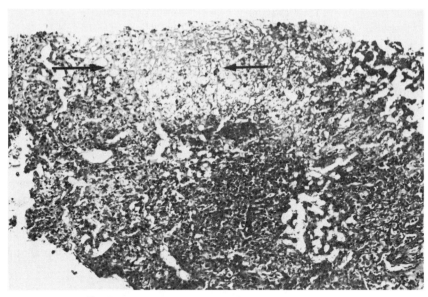

Fig. 15-7
Liver biopsy demonstrating prominent centrilobular necrosis (*arrows*) in a patient with ischemic liver injury. In the necrotic zone, the hepatocytes have disappeared, leaving the reticulin framework intact. (Courtesy of Donald Antonioli, M.D.)

Budd-Chiari Syndrome

The Budd-Chiari syndrome is an uncommon disorder caused by the obstruction of the hepatic veins. Although not strictly a circulatory disorder, this syndrome does produce clinical and pathologic findings typical of acute and chronic hepatic congestion. Despite its rarity, several different causes have been associated with the Budd-Chiari syndrome (Table 15-2). Occlusion of the hepatic veins can occur by (1) thrombosis, (2) tumor, (3) venal caval web, and (4) idiopathic mechanisms. Of these potential causes, detection of the venal caval web is most important since disruption of the web can lead to resolution of the hepatic congestion. This fibrous web, considered by some to be congenital, occurs at or above the level where the hepatic veins enter the inferior vena cava. Although this condition appears to be more common in South Africa and the Orient, well-documented cases have occurred in the United States.

With acute occlusion of the hepatic vein, the liver becomes swollen. Pathologic studies demonstrate engorgement of the centrizonal sinusoids with erythrocytes and associated ischemic atrophy of hepatocytes in this region. With prolonged obstruction, the centrizonal congestion continues, and the increasing loss of hepatocytes results in a centrilobular network of stroma

Table 15-2
Causes of the Budd-Chiari syndrome

Thrombosis
  Myeloproliferative disease (e.g., polycythemia vera)
  Paroxysmal nocturnal hemoglobinuria

Tumor
  Hepatocellular carcinoma
  Hypernephroma
  Adrenal carcinoma

Venal caval web

Idiopathic

that fills the collapsing central vein. In the advanced stages of the Budd-Chiari syndrome, hepatic necrosis progresses with resulting increased fibrosis and the eventual development of cirrhosis.

The most important clinical signs of this syndrome are hepatomegaly and ascites. Acutely, abdominal pain can be present because of the intense distention of the hepatic capsule. More often, the onset of this syndrome is subacute, and with chronicity, the condition mimics cirrhosis and portal hypertension of other etiologies. Patients often develop severe ascites. If the vena cava is also obstructed, there can be marked edema of the lower extremities and a pronounced pattern of venous collaterals on the abdominal wall.

The definitive diagnosis of this condition is provided by radiographic contrast studies (hepatic venogram) that document obstruction of the hepatic vein. On occasion the demonstration on percutaneous liver biopsy of centrizonal loss of hepatocytes with the characteristic collapse of the central vein can yield a clue to the diagnosis prior to venography.

The prognosis is variable. Patients suffering acute total occlusion of the hepatic vein experience rapid, progressive deterioration with death within weeks to months. Those with a subacute, less extensive occlusion may have a more prolonged clinical course over several years with increasing morbidity from ascites, encephalopathy, and bleeding esophageal varices.

The ascites and complications of portal hypertension in this syndrome are managed by conventional techniques (see Chap. 17). The ascites can be reduced either by chronic diuretic therapy or the use of a peritoneovenous (LeVeen) shunt. Some evidence exists that the side-to-side portacaval shunt can lead to striking clinical improvement by decreasing the hepatic congestion and central necrosis. It remains to be seen whether the frequent use of this surgery improves the survival of patients with this syndrome.

Study Questions   1. In general, hepatotoxins produce injury via either an intrinsic or an idiosyncratic mechanism. Match the most appropriate choice in List I with the statements in List II.

List I

A. Intrinsic hepatotoxins
B. Idiosyncratic hepatotoxin
C. Both
D. Neither

List II

a. Toxicity arises as a function of hepatic phase II reactions (e.g., glucuronidation).
b. Analogous lesions can be produced in experimental animals.
c. May be associated with fever, rash, and eosinophilia.
d. Can produce fatal hepatic failure.
e. Very high incidence of hepatic injury.
f. Toxicity can occur 1 to 2 months after initiation of drug.
g. Mechanism of carbon tetrachloride-induced injury.
h. Mechanism of isoniazid-induced injury.

Answers

a. D (toxicity usually arises as a result of phase I [mixed function oxidase] reactions).
b. A
c. B
d. C
e. A
f. B
g. A
h. B

2. Which of the following statements regarding acetaminophen (ACM)-induced liver injury is or are correct?
a. Toxicity occurs via an idiosyncratic mechanism.
b. Hepatotoxicity of ACM is dose-dependent (severity of injury increases with the dose ingested).
c. Hepatic injury with a given dose of ACM is enhanced in chronic alcoholic patients.
d. Clinical signs of ACM-induced liver injury occur within hours of ingestion of a toxic dose.
e. Treatment with acetylcysteine during the first 16 hours following ingestion of an overdose can reduce the hepatotoxicity of ACM.

Answer

b, c, e

If ingested in large doses (10 gm), ACM is a potent intrinsic hepatotoxin whose toxicity is dose-dependent. Since liver injury occurs via toxic metabolites produced by mixed function oxidase (MFO) activity, chronic alcohol ingestion enhances toxicity by increasing MFO activity. Early administration of acetylcysteine reduces hepatotoxicity by maintaining adequate hepatocellular stores of glutathione, which safely bind the toxic metabolites. Because liver injury occurs via toxic metabolites, clinical signs of liver injury usually appear 3 to 5 days after ingestion.

3. A 60-year-old woman with chronic congestive heart failure due to aortic stenosis and mitral stenosis suffers a cardiac arrest. Following resuscitation, there is a several hour-period of hypotension and pulmonary edema before her circulatory status can be stabilized. Forty-eight hours after the cardiac arrest, her cardiovascular status is stable, but she is noted to be mildly jaundiced. Which of the following statements is or are correct?

a. The serum transaminase levels will be strikingly elevated.
b. The severity of the hepatic injury will correlate with the severity and duration of the circulatory disturbance.
c. A percutaneous liver biopsy will demonstrate periportal inflammation with focal necrosis of hepatocytes.
d. Management should consist of optimizing cardiac output and reducing peripheral venous congestion, if possible.

Answer

a, b, d

The patient has sustained ischemic injury to the liver due to a combination of decreased vascular pressure in the portal tract (shock) and increased venous pressure in the central vein (increased right atrial pressure). The severity of the hepatic injury will correlate with the severity of the circulatory disturbance. The serum transaminase levels are usually strikingly elevated and mimic those seen in viral hepatitis. Liver histology is characterized by centrizonal congestion and necrosis *without inflammation*. Management consists of improving oxygen delivery to the liver by optimizing cardiac function.

References

Toxic and Drug-Induced Disorders of the Liver

Barker, J. D., et al. Chronic excessive acetaminophen use and liver damage. *Ann. Intern. Med.* 87:299, 1977.

Benjamin, S. B., et al. The morphologic spectrum of halothane-induced hepatic injury: Analysis of 77 cases. *Hepatology* 5:1163, 1985.

Black, M. Acetaminophen hepatotoxicity. *Ann. Rev. Med.* 35:577, 1984.

Fisher, M. D. Mechanisms of drug-induced cholestasis. *Semin. Liver Dis.* 1:151, 1981

Ishak, K. G., et al. Hepatic lesions caused by anabolic and contraceptive steroids. *Semin. Liver Dis.* 1:116, 1981.

Kaplowitz, N., et al. Drug-induced hepatotoxicity. *Ann. Intern. Med.* 104:826, 1986.

Maddrey, W. C. Isoniazid-induced liver disease. *Semin. Liver Dis.* 1:129, 1981.

Maddrey, W. C., and Boitnott, J. K. Drug-induced chronic liver disease. *Gastroenterology* 72:1348, 1977.

Spielberg, S. P., et al. Predisposition to phenytoin hepatotoxicity assessed in vitro. *N. Engl. J. Med.* 305:722, 1981.

Zimmerman, H. J. *Hepatotoxicity: The Adverse Effects of Drugs and Other Chemicals on the Liver.* Norwalk, Connecticut: Appleton-Century-Crofts, 1978.

Zimmerman, H. J. and Maddrey, W. C. Toxic and Drug-Induced Hepatitis. In L. Schiff and E. R. Schiff (eds.), *Diseases of the Liver* (6th ed.). Philadelphia: Lippincott, 1987.

Circulatory Disorders of the Liver

Cohen, J. A., and Kaplan, M. M. Left-sided heart failure presenting as hepatitis. *Gastroenterology* 74:583, 1978.

Dunn, G. D., Hayes, P., Breen, K. J., et al. The liver in congestive heart failure. *Ann. J. Med. Sci.* 265:174, 1973.

Lamont, J. T., and Isselbacher, K. J. Current concepts: Postoperative jaundice. *N. Engl. J. Med.* 288:305, 1973.

Novel, O., Henrion, J., Bernuau, J., et al. Fulminant hepatic failure due to transient circulatory failure in patients with chronic heart disease. *Dig. Dis. Sci.* 25:49, 1980.

Sherlock, S. The liver in heart failure: Relation of anatomical, functional and circulatory changes. *Br. Heart J.* 13:273, 1951.

Budd-Chiari Syndrome

Mitchell, M. C., et al. Budd-Chiari syndrome: Etiology, diagnosis, and management. *Medicine* 61:199, 1982.

Orloff, M. J., and Johansen, K. H. Treatment of Budd-Chiari syndrome by side-to-side portacaval shunt: Experimental and clinical results. *Ann. Surg.* 188:494, 1978.

Reynolds, T. B. Budd-Chiari Syndrome. In L. Schiff and E. R. Schiff (eds.), *Diseases of the Liver* (6th ed.). Philadelphia: Lippincott, 1987.

16 : Metabolic Liver Diseases (Hemochromatosis, Wilson's Disease, and Alpha$_1$-Antitrypsin Deficiency) and Primary Biliary Cirrhosis

Stephen Crane Hauser
John L. Gollan

Hemochromatosis

Iron Metabolism

Iron deficiency is extremely common, affecting more than 500 million persons worldwide, whereas iron overload is a much less common disorder. About 1 to 2 mg/day of iron is lost from the body by desquamation of epithelial cells from the skin and gastrointestinal tract, and by red blood cell losses from the gastrointestinal and genitourinary tracts (Fig. 16-1). To replace these obligatory iron losses, the small bowel absorbs iron from dietary sources. Although the average daily North American diet contains 10 to 15 mg of iron, the small intestine absorbs only 1 to 2 mg, an amount sufficient for balancing the daily iron losses (Fig. 16-1). Iron absorption is exquisitely regulated by the intestinal mucosal cell. Increased absorption occurs in the presence of decreased iron stores, hypoxia, or an increased rate of erythropoiesis. In contrast, abnormally elevated total body iron stores result in a decrease in the rate of intestinal iron absorption. The duodenum and proximal jejunum constitute the primary sites of iron absorption; hence, diseases of the small bowel, such as celiac sprue, are often characterized by decreased iron absorption and iron deficiency.

The exact mechanism by which iron is transported across the intestinal mucosal cell and into plasma is unknown, but, once in the circulation, it is bound principally to transferrin. This beta$_1$-globulin, which possesses two binding sites for iron, consists of a single polypeptide chain with a molecular weight of 80,000 daltons. The synthesis of transferrin in the liver is increased in the presence of a low hepatic iron concentration and is decreased by a high hepatic iron content. Normally, only about 30 percent of plasma transferrin is saturated with iron. The so-called plasma iron-binding capacity or the maximal amount of iron that can be bound by transferrin ranges from 250 to 400 mg/dl. Most of the dietary iron absorbed and bound to transferrin in plasma is transported to reticuloendothelial cells in the bone marrow for incorporation into newly synthesized hemoglobin, and a small amount is delivered to the liver for storage. Cellular uptake of transferrin-iron complexes is mediated by cell surface

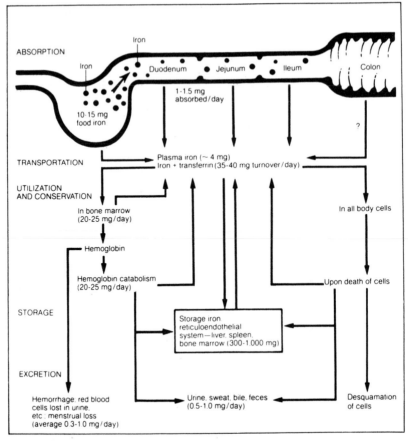

Fig. 16-1
Schematic diagram depicting pathways of normal iron metabolism in adults.

transferrin receptors, which initiate endocytosis of the complex, with subsequent transport of iron into the cell, and return of the transferrin receptor to the plasma membrane and of transferrin itself into plasma.

The majority of body iron is contained in functional proteins such as hemoglobin and myoglobin. Most non-heme iron is stored in the reticuloendothelial cells of the liver, spleen, and bone marrow and to a lesser extent, in hepatocytes as ferritin. Ferritin consists of 24 polypeptide subunits arranged in a hollow spherical form. There are two distinct subunits, L and H, which combine in different proportions to account for organ-specific isoferritins. The cavity of each apoferritin molecule may contain up to 4500 iron atoms. Degradation of cellular ferritin results in a readily available intracellular iron pool. Partial degradation of ferritin results in formation of the iron storage pigment hemosiderin, and in the normal liver, iron is stored in nearly equal amounts as ferritin and hemosiderin. Ferritin is also found in serum and in general reflects total body iron stores (1 μg/liter equals 8–10 mg storage iron). Circulating serum ferritin, which is mostly apoferritin without iron in its core, is of obscure origin and function.

Internal iron exchange is poorly understood. The majority of daily iron exchange appears to take place between macrophages and the bone marrow cells that synthesize hemoglobin or the erythron. The parenchymal cells of the liver (hepatocytes, heart (myocardial cells), and other tissues appear to act as a "sink" for excessive amounts of iron, although normally, little iron is deposited in these tissues.

Definitions

Hemochromatosis or iron storage disease is attributable to excess quantities of total body iron. Iron overload may be primary, as in the genetic disorder hereditary idiopathic hemochromatosis, or it may be secondary to other processes. Three defects appear to contribute to iron overload in patients with hereditary idiopathic hemochromatosis. First and foremost, there is increased intestinal absorption of iron relative to total body iron stores. Even in the presence of gross body iron overload, the intestine continues to absorb inappropriate amounts of iron. Second, there appears to be a defect in the ability of the reticuloendothelial cells to retain iron, resulting in a shift of iron transport to parenchymal cells, such as hepatocytes, and pancreatic and myocardial cells. Third, there may be an increased pool of non-transferrin bound iron in serum, which is preferentially taken up by parenchymal cells.

Secondary iron overload may complicate a number of disorders; dietary-induced iron overload is rare because of the limited capacity and close regulation of iron absorption by the intestine, whereas transfusion-related iron overload is not unusual. In the presence of various anemias, including thalassemia, sideroblastic anemia, and hypoproliferative anemias, repeated transfusions will result in iron overload. Each unit of transfused blood contains about 200 mg iron, so that a patient requiring four units of blood per month over a 2-year period will receive about 20 gm of iron. Because of the limited ability of the body to excrete and store iron in reticuloendothelial cells, the increased load of iron is ultimately stored in parenchymal cells of the liver, heart, pancreas, and other organs.

Incidence and Genetics

The true incidence of hereditary idiopathic hemochromatosis is uncertain but is probably between 1 : 1,000 and 1 : 20,000. There is an association between hereditary hemochromatosis and certain HLA haplotypes, such as HLA-A3 (73–78% vs. 29–36% in control populations), HLA-B14 (27–31% vs. 3–8%), and in some studies, HLA-B7. This is believed to be consistent with two homologous alleles on chromosome 6, inherited in an autosomal recessive manner. In the state of Utah, it is estimated that up to 6 percent of the population may be heterozygous for idiopathic hemochromatosis.

Pathogenesis
The mechanism of end-organ damage in both primary and secondary hemochromatosis is unknown. There is some experimental evidence suggesting that iron may induce lipid peroxidation, possibly as a consequence of free radical formation, and thus lead to membrane damage (e.g., lysosomal membranes) and cell death. Because iron is a cofactor for proline and lysine hydroxylase — two critical enzymes involved in the synthesis of collagen — it has been postulated that elevated tissue iron levels may also result in disordered collagen metabolism. An animal model of iron storage disease, the common starling, has been identified recently and may shed further light on the pathogenesis of iron overload itself and the process of cellular injury.

Clinical Manifestations
Hereditary idiopathic hemochromatosis is usually characterized by the insidious onset of symptoms, usually between the ages of 30 and 60 years. The male to female ratio is between 5 : 1 and 10 : 1, with females presenting some 10 years later than males, most likely because of the increased iron losses incurred by most women (e.g., menstruation and childbirth). Secondary hemochromatosis presents with similar clinical manifestations, but the age of onset is often much younger. Nonspecific symptoms such as weakness, weight loss, arthralgia, abdominal pain, and impotence, infertility, and loss of libido are common in the early stages. On physical examination, hyperpigmentation, hepatomegaly, and testicular atrophy may be found. However, the majority of patients remain asymptomatic for many years despite ever-increasing iron deposition in parenchymal organs.

Hepatic iron deposition may progress to cirrhosis. However, liver failure and variceal bleeding are uncommon except in symptomatic patients in whom treatment is deferred. Between 10 and 30 percent of patients (in different series) with cirrhosis will develop hepatocellular carcinoma, but this does not appear to occur in hemochromatotic patients without cirrhosis. Iron deposition in the heart frequently results in dysrythmias and congestive cardiomyopathy. Pancreatic involvement commonly presents as diabetes mellitus. A deforming arthritis similar to degenerative joint disease or rheumatoid arthritis may be seen. Characteristic involvement of the second and third metacarpophalangeal joints, as well as chondrocalcinosis, may also be

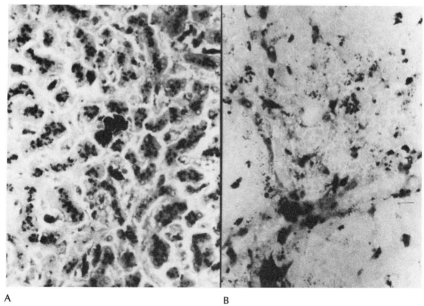

Fig. 16-2
A. Prussian blue–stained liver biopsy from a patient with idiopathic hemo-chromatosis. Iron is deposited primarily in the parenchymal cells (hepato-cytes). B. Prussian blue–stained liver biopsy from a patient with secondary iron overload. Iron is deposited mainly in reticuloendothelial (Kupffer's) cells.

found in patients. Skin involvement may be manifest by bronze or slate gray color, as well as by soft skin and scant body hair. The hyperpigmentation is particularly prominent around the face, neck, distal extremities, oral mucosa, and scars. Hy-pogonadism is common in men and is manifest by testicular atrophy, impotence, and decreased libido. Iron deposition in the pituitary gland or testicles accounts for the hypogonadism. Of interest is the recent observation that hemochromatotic pa-tients are at increased risk of developing severe infection with bacteria, such as *Yersinia enterocolitica* and *Vibrio vulnificus*. Sepsis, enterocolitis, peritonitis, and hepatosplenic abscesses have all been reported. The ingestion of raw seafood appears to contribute to the risk of these infections. It is hypothesized that because most bacteria require iron, increased availability of iron may make hemochromatotic patients more susceptible to infec-tion. Moreover, the iron-chelator desferrioxamine (vide infra) may contribute to the risk of infection by functioning as a siderophore, thereby promoting the delivery of iron to bacteria.

Pathology

In the early phase of idiopathic hemochromatosis (Fig. 16-2), iron is stored primarily in hepatocytes, especially in the peripor-tal region, with an intracellular pericanalicular distribution. In contrast, the pattern of hepatic iron loading in early, secondary hemochromatosis (Fig. 16-2) is characterized by primary deposition in reticuloendothelial cells (e.g., Kupffer's cells). With more advanced degrees of iron loading owing to either primary or secondary hemochromatosis, the patterns may become indistinguishable, with iron deposited in both parenchymal and reticuloendothelial cells, as well as in bile duct epithelium. Pathologically, iron deposition can be demonstrated both in myocardial cells and in the conducting tissue of the heart. The pancreas, pituitary gland, small blood vessels in the testicles, basal cells of the epidermis, and eccrine sweat glands are all frequently involved by iron deposition in hemochromatosis. The deposition of iron in the skin accounts for the slate gray color of some patients, whereas the bronze color in other patients is due to increased melanin deposition. A variety of pathological processes may involve the joints, including chondrocalcinosis, bony sclerosis, joint-space narrowing, subchondrial cysts, loss of articular cartilage, osteopenia, and osteophyte formation.

Diagnosis

Patients with hemochromatosis are frequently asymptomatic at diagnosis (i.e., with or without abnormal liver function tests). Nonspecific symptoms or physical findings (i.e., weakness, impotence, hepatomegaly, diabetes mellitus, or arthritis) may occur. Abnormal liver function tests, such as mildly elevated serum transaminases, may be the only clue to the diagnosis. Fortunately, sensitive blood tests exist to screen suspected patients for hemochromatosis. Virtually all hemochromatotic patients have an elevated (greater than 50%) transferrin saturation owing to a combination of an increased serum iron concentration and a decreased serum transferrin level (i.e., decreased plasma total iron binding capacity). In addition, serum ferritin is usually greater than 500 ng/ml, and often exceeds 1000 ng/ml. Except in very young patients or in unusual cases, a normal ferritin and transferrin saturation rule out iron overload. However, serum ferritin concentration may be elevated in other conditions, such as acute and chronic liver disease, inflammatory diseases such as rheumatoid arthritis, leukemia and other malignancies, and hyperthyroidism. The definitive diagnosis of hemochromatosis requires a liver biopsy with quantitative determination of the hepatic iron content. Qualitative grading by histochemical staining (i.e., Prussian blue) can be misleading, since liver biopsies from patients with alcoholic liver disease may demonstrate increased iron staining, yet quantitative determination may reveal insignificant hepatic iron stores. Normal hepatic iron concentration is 7 to 100 µg/100 mg dry weight, whereas adult hemochromatosis patients exhibit values in excess of 1000 μg/100 mg (or 1% dry weight). It is believed that alcoholic patients with hepatic iron stores similar to those found in hemochromatosis patients most likely are genetic hemochromatotics who also drink.

Computed tomographic (CT) scanning has recently been demonstrated to be of value in the diagnosis of hemochromatosis. Increased levels of iron in the liver are associated with an increased CT density or attenuation coefficient. Only the cardiac drug amiodarone or the presence of abnormal amounts of glycogen in the liver (i.e., glycogen storage diseases) also increase the attenuation coefficient. Thus, if the CT number is elevated, it is quite specific, but because fat lowers the CT number, a normal attenuation coefficient does not rule out the diagnosis of hemochromatosis. SQUID (superconducting quantum interference device susceptometer) involves the use of a magnetic field to determine hepatic iron concentrations noninvasively. Although still investigational, SQUID appears to be extremely sensitive, specific, and accurate.

Once a person is identified as having idiopathic hemochromatosis, it is crucial to screen other family members by regular measurement of serum ferritin and transferrin saturation. If these parameters are normal or only mildly abnormal, HLA typing is useful in the diagnosis of siblings of patients. Siblings having both HLA haplotypes (A3 and B14 or B7) in common with the proband are at high risk of developing hemochromatosis, whereas those with one identical haplotype are at some risk, and those with neither haplotype are at no risk. Heterozygotes may exhibit some increase in intestinal iron absorption, a serum ferritin up to 800 ng/ml, or a transferrin saturation as high as 90 percent. However, in these patients, quantitative hepatic iron concentrations are only slightly above normal, and clinical evidence of iron overload does not develop. Screening of family members should commence at age 10.

Treatment and Prognosis

Patients with idiopathic primary hemochromatosis require removal of iron by phlebotomy for life. The removal of 1 unit of blood per week (200–250 mg iron/unit) results in a gradual decline in serum ferritin followed by a fall in serum iron and an increase in plasma total iron binding capacity (i.e., decreased transferrin saturation). In time, the hematocrit will fall as iron stores are depleted, and periodic phlebotomies (every 3 months) are then required for life to prevent reaccumulation of excess iron. Approximately 20 gm of iron can be mobilized from the average symptomatic patient. Survival, general well-being, liver function tests, and, in most patients, diabetes mellitus, cardiac disease, and skin discoloration are all improved. Endocrine dysfunction and arthritis, if present, do not usually respond to the removal of iron. The risk of hepatocellular carcinoma in cirrhotic patients remains unchanged, despite the removal of iron.

Hemochromatosis secondary to chronic anemia (such as thalassemia major), requiring multiple transfusions, presents at a young age. The typical thalassemia patient, having received more than 100 blood transfusions, suffers from failure of normal growth and sexual development in adolescence, and hepatic fibrosis and death owing to cardiac disease by young adulthood. Phlebotomy cannot be performed because of the anemia. However, before end-organ damage develops, iron may be removed by chelation therapy with subcutaneous nightly infusions of desferrioxamine (a polyhydroxamic acid derivative of Streptomyces), which results in excretion of chelatable iron into urine and stool. There are reports of sudden cardiac death in these patients after vitamin C administration, possibly as a result of sudden shifts of iron from reticuloendothelial to parenchymal (i.e., myocardial) cells; hence, vitamin C supplementation should be avoided. Hypersensitivity reactions to desferrioxamine as well as ocular and otologic complications have also been reported. Although still under active scrutiny, desferrioxamine chelation therapy appears to protect these patients from cardiac disease and to improve their prognosis.

Wilson's Disease

Copper Metabolism

Copper is an essential component of a variety of metalloenzymes and, as such, is critical to a variety of mammalian functions. Because of the ubiquitous presence of copper and its relative excess in most diets, acquired copper deficiency in humans is unusual. Similarly, owing to the efficiency of physiologic mechanisms controlling copper balance, toxic accumulation is rare.

Total body copper in normal adults ranges between 50 and 150 mg, with the highest concentrations found in the liver, followed in decreasing order by the brain, heart, and kidneys. The concentration of copper in fetal liver is considerably higher than that in adults, but it rapidly falls during early infancy, owing to its redistribution to other organs, the postnatal growth spurt, and the relatively low copper content of human milk. By 3 months of age, hepatic copper concentration is comparable with that of adults.

The estimated daily copper requirement for adults is 1.3 to 1.7 mg. The daily average North American diet contains 2 to 5 mg copper, with oysters, other shellfish, liver, nuts, chocolate, mushrooms, legumes, and cereals containing the highest concentrations of copper. Metabolic studies using radiocopper indicate that 40 to 60 percent of dietary copper is absorbed, principally in the upper gastrointestinal tract.

The regularity mechanisms governing mucosal transport of copper are poorly understood. It has been postulated that two distinct cytosolic copper-binding proteins, the enzyme superoxide dismutase and the sulfhydryl-rich protein metallothioneine, may mediate the absorption of copper, with the metal being complexed by amino acids for transport across the serosal surface and released into the portal circulation. However, unlike iron, there is no evidence that copper homeostasis is regulated significantly at the level of the intestine.

Copper absorbed from the intestine is bound in plasma to albumin. This copper is cleared rapidly by the liver, and, over time, a portion of it is incorporated into the blue copper-binding glycoprotein, ceruloplasmin, an $alpha_2$-globulin, which is synthesized in the liver prior to its appearance in blood. Copper incorporated into the ceruloplasmin molecule appears to be released only in the course of hepatic degradation of the protein; thus, ceruloplasmin does not appear to function as a copper transport protein. Serum ceruloplasmin concentration is low in human newborns but increases to near adult levels during the first 2 years of life, coincidental with the postnatal decrease in hepatic copper concentration. The mean serum concentration of ceruloplasmin in adults is about 30 mg/dl, and ceruloplasmin-bound copper constitutes 95 percent of the total serum copper content. Copper bound to amino acids (e.g., histidine) constitutes a small, highly labile and functionally important ultrafilterable plasma fraction of non–ceruloplasmin-bound copper, which most likely is responsible for copper transport across cell membranes.

In the liver, as in other tissues, copper is found both in association with binding proteins, particularly metallothioneine, and as a specific component of metalloenzymes, such as superoxide dismutase. Copper-binding proteins may be critical in the temporary storage and detoxification of copper or as donors for the synthesis of ceruloplasmin or excretion of copper into bile.

Since very little copper is excreted in urine — less than 70 µg daily — the maintenance of copper balance depends primarily on biliary excretion. In healthy adults, mean biliary copper output ranges between 1.2 and 1.7 mg/day. The immediate hepatic precursor pools of biliary copper have not been defined, although cytosolic copper bound to metallothioneine or copper in hepatic lysosomes has been postulated to represent the pre-biliary copper compartments.

Genetics and Pathogenesis

Wilson's disease is a familial syndrome manifest by progressive lenticular degeneration (degeneration of the basal ganglia in the brain) associated with cirrhosis. The disease exhibits an auto-somal recessive mode of inheritance and has been reported in virtually all races. The overall gene frequency or heterozygote carrier rate has been estimated to be $1:200$ to $1:400$, which corresponds to an incidence of the disease of about five persons per million. The clinical manifestations of Wilson's disease are the result of excessive accumulation of tissue copper. Copper absorption in both homozygotes and heterozygotes with Wilson's disease does not differ from that in either normal subjects or cirrhotic patients. The reversal of abnormal copper metabo-lism in patients who have undergone orthotopic liver transplan-tation strongly supports the concept that the primary defect is located in the liver.

It is apparent that patients with Wilson's disease have dimin-ished fecal excretion of copper, owing to impaired biliary excre-tion of the metal. Although the primary defect has yet to be defined, there is evidence to suggest that a hepatic lysosomal abnormality may account for the diminished biliary excretion of copper. The Bedlington terrier appears to be an animal model of Wilson's disease, but, unlike humans, the Bedlington terrier does not develop neurologic disease or exhibit Kayser-Fleischer rings or a low serum ceruloplasmin.

Clinical Manifestations

The age of symptomatic onset and the clinical pattern of disease vary considerably among patients. The manifestations of hepatic involvement tend to occur at a younger age (rarely before 6 years of age) than those of the central nervous system; they are often nonspecific and quite similar to those of a variety of acute and chronic liver diseases. Asymptomatic patients may have minor histologic findings on biopsy or an inactive cirrhosis, with or without mildly abnormal liver function tests. Most com-monly, the hepatic disease begins insidiously and, if untreated, pursues a chronic course characterized progressively by the de-velopment of fatigue, jaundice, spider angiomas, and spleno-megaly, attributable to cirrhosis and portal hypertension. Many patients will present with a complication of advanced and previ-ously unrecognized liver disease, such as bleeding esophageal varices or hepatic encephalopathy. Between 10 and 30 percent of patients with Wilson's disease may present with clinical, biochemical, and histologic features similar to those of chronic active hepatitis. Thus, it is essential to seek the diagnosis of

Wilson's disease in all patients younger than 40 years of age with clinical, biochemical, or pathological findings compatible with chronic active hepatitis.

Occasionally Wilson's disease may present as fulminant hepatic failure, which may be clinically indistinguishable from massive hepatic necrosis secondary to a viral etiology. Concomitant hemolytic anemia owing to copper-induced hemolysis strongly suggests the diagnosis of fulminant liver failure secondary to Wilson's disease. Finally, cirrhosis and hemolysis, both of which are frequent manifestations of Wilson's disease, predispose to the development of cholelithiasis.

Patients may also present with neurologic or psychiatric manifestations, often between the ages of 12 and 30 years. Invariably, these patients also manifest Kayser-Fleischer rings. Early, subtle neurologic findings include deteriorating performance in school, incoordination, particularly involving fine movements, resting and intention tremors, dysarthria, dysphagia, and drooling. Dystonia, spasticity, and rigidity with flexion contractures are late manifestations of undiagnosed and untreated disease. Psychiatric manifestations may be prominent but are generally nonspecific and include a broad range of behavioral changes, neuroses, and even frank psychoses.

The Kayser-Fleischer ring is a golden-brown or greenish discoloration in the limbic region of the cornea, which represents copper deposition in Descemet's membrane. This bilateral discoloration appears initially at the superior pole, then the inferior pole, followed by circumferential deposition. With treatment, the rings disappear in reverse order, so that the superior pole is the last to be cleared. These pigmented rings also may be seen in any long-standing cholestatic disorder, such as primary biliary cirrhosis or partial biliary atresia.

Other less common manifestations of Wilson's disease include acute intravascular hemolysis, which usually is transient and, at times, may present in association with acute hepatic failure owing to release of copper from the liver. Proximal tubular copper deposition may lead to Fanconi's syndrome, renal tubular acidosis, and renal stones. Bone demineralization and other nonspecific osteoarticular lesions (i.e., osteopenia, spontaneous fractures, subarticular cysts, osteochondritis desiccans and chondrocalcinosis), sunflower cataracts, and blue lunulae of the fingernails may also be seen.

Natural History   The natural history of Wilson's disease can be considered in four interrelated stages (Fig. 16-3). In Stage I, patients remain asymptomatic while copper accumulates in the cytosol of hepa-

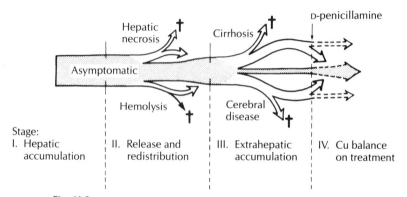

Fig. 16-3
Stages of the natural history of Wilson's disease.

tocytes. Once copper accumulation reaches a critical level, it is redistributed from the cytosol to the lysosomes, and a proportion is released into the blood (Stage II). This process of hepatic redistribution and release of copper occurs gradually in most patients (about 60%), and the disease remains clinically inapparent. However, when the hepatic release of copper is rapid, there may be an abrupt rise in blood levels sufficient to cause hemolysis, and, similarly, if the redistribution of hepatocyte copper from cytosol to lysosomes is rapid, hepatic necrosis of chronic active hepatitis may ensue. These patients may succumb as a result of hepatic failure or again become asymptomatic.

During Stage III, copper continues to accumulate in hepatic lysosomes with the development of hepatic fibrosis and cirrhosis, as well as in extrahepatic tissues (i.e., brain, cornea, and kidneys). If the cirrhosis is inactive and cerebral accumulation is slow, patients may remain asymptomatic for many years. Alternatively, patients may present with hepatic or neurologic manifestations. Finally, if diagnosed in time, patients will achieve a stage of copper balance after prolonged therapy (Stage IV) and most become asymptomatic, although some will exhibit residual evidence of portal hypertension or irreversible brain injury.

Pathology

In asymptomatic patients, even during the first decade of life, histologic changes are usually evident in the liver. The earliest light microscopic changes are nonspecific and include glycogen in the nuclei of periportal hepatocytes and moderate fatty infiltration. Coexistent or even preceding these changes, mitochondrial abnormalities (i.e., heterogeneity in size and shape, increased matrix density, separation of inner and outer mitochondrial membranes, and various vacuolated and crystalline inclusions) may be present. All these nonspecific abnormalities may regress as fibrosis and cirrhosis ultimately develop.

Some patients develop a histologic picture indistinguishable from chronic active hepatitis; this lesion may evolve into macronodular cirrhosis or progress rapidly to fulminant hepatic necrosis. Mallory's hyaline may be identified in the cytosol of hepatocytes. In contrast to idiopathic hemochromatosis with cirrhosis, hepatocellular carcinoma rarely complicates the course of Wilson's disease. Special histochemical stains for copper or copper-associated proteins lack sensitivity as well as specificity and therefore are of little value.

Diagnosis

The diagnosis of Wilson's disease relies on clinical or biochemical data or both. The presence of Kayser-Fleischer rings, some of which are apparent only on slit-lamp examination, strongly suggests Wilson's disease in the absence of other cirrhotic cholestatic disorders. Virtually all Wilson's disease patients with neurologic findings will have Kayser-Fleischer rings. In contrast, in many patients presenting with hepatic manifestations, Kayser-Fleischer rings will be absent.

Most patients with Wilson's disease have a serum ceruloplasmin concentration of less than 20 mg/dl. This finding does not appear to be directly related to the pathogenesis of the disease. Indeed, 10 percent of heterozygous carriers of the Wilson's disease gene (in whom clinical features never develop) display low serum ceruloplasmin levels (i.e., 1 in 2000 persons). Occasionally, patients with non-Wilsonian fulminant hepatitis may have low ceruloplasmin levels, owing to diminished synthetic function of the liver, as may patients with severe intestinal or renal protein losing states. Prior to 6 months of age, serum ceruloplasmin levels normally are low.

Normal ceruloplasmin concentrations are found in up to 15 percent of patients with Wilson's disease presenting with severe chronic active hepatitis, presumably secondary to increased hepatic synthesis or release of the glycoprotein. Estrogen administration and pregnancy may increase ceruloplasmin levels.

Thus, in the absence of Kayser-Fleischer rings, a liver biopsy for quantitative copper determination is essential. It is necessary for the biopsy needle and container to be free from copper contamination. Normal hepatic copper concentration is 15 to 55 μg/gm dry liver, whereas in untreated patients with Wilson's disease, concentrations range between 250 and 3,000 μg/gm dry liver. Elevated hepatic copper levels may be found in chronic cholestasis (e.g., primary biliary cirrhosis, biliary atresia) in addition to Wilson's disease, although diagnostic confusion is unlikely.

Urinary copper excretion, normally about 40 µg/day, is in excess of 100 µg/day in most patients with Wilson's disease beyond Stage I. However, patients with other liver diseases frequently manifest increased urinary copper levels, diminishing greatly the specificity of urinary copper excretion as a diagnostic test.

Rarely, a diagnostic dilemma may arise in patients with a normal ceruloplasmin level or in whom a liver biopsy is contraindicated. In this situation, the incorporation of orally administered radio-copper into ceruloplasmin may be a useful test. In normal subjects or in patients with hepatic disorders that mimic Wilson's disease, the plasma concentration of radiocopper (nonceruloplasmin bound) rises rapidly and peaks at 1 to 2 hours. Plasma radioactivity then falls and rises again over the ensuing 48 hours as radiocopper is incorporated into ceruloplasmin and released into the circulation. In contrast, patients with Wilson's disease incorporate little or no radiocopper into newly synthesized ceruloplasmin and hence do not exhibit the secondary rise.

Treatment

Once the diagnosis of Wilson's disease is made, lifelong therapy with the chelating agent D-penicillamine is indicated. In asymptomatic patients, a daily dose of 1 gm D-penicillamine can prevent indefinitely the development of clinical disease. Complete reversal or improvement of hepatic, neurologic, and psychiatric abnormalities can be expected in most patients, although some may take many months to respond to D-penicillamine. A small proportion of patients develop serious toxic reactions to this drug (i.e., nephrotic syndrome, bone marrow suppression) and may require administration of an alternative chelating agent, triethylene tetramine dihydrochloride (trien). It is prudent for patients to avoid the few foods that contain substantial quantities of copper (vide supra). In a few selected patients with advanced cirrhotic liver disease or fulminant hepatic failure, orthotopic liver transplantation may be lifesaving. Following successful transplantation, the clinical signs of liver disease abate, the biochemical findings in serum and urine normalize, and the copper content of the grafted liver remains normal.

Primary Biliary Cirrhosis

Definition

Primary biliary cirrhosis is a chronic cholestatic disease of unknown etiology that is characterized by slowly progressive destruction of medium-sized intrahepatic bile ducts. Middle-aged women are most frequently afflicted by primary biliary cirrhosis. In recent years, it has become apparent that the disease may progress very slowly over many years and often remains asymptomatic until late in the course of the disease.

Pathogenesis

Although the pathogenesis of primary biliary cirrhosis is unknown, there is considerable evidence suggesting that an autoimmune mechanism is involved. Clinically, most patients have circulating autoantibodies and high IgM levels, and many patients have associated autoimmune diseases (vide infra). The histopathology of primary biliary cirrhosis frequently includes granulomas and may resemble graft-versus-host disease. The presence of immune complexes, complement abnormalities, defects in Kupffer cell–mediated clearance function, and both quantitative and qualitative alterations in T-cell function have been described in primary biliary cirrhosis. In addition, several hypotheses involving abnormalities of cytotoxic lymphocyte function have been proposed. Whether these diverse abnormalities of immune function are etiologic or secondary to an initiating agent such as a virus or drug or are simply a result of the disease itself remains to be determined.

Clinical
Manifestations

Primary biliary cirrhosis is widespread throughout the world, with a female to male ratio of about 9 : 1. Most commonly, primary biliary cirrhosis is recognized during the third to sixth decades of life, although it may be diagnosed in patients as young as 20 years or in those 70 years of age. In England, the prevalence has been estimated to be between 40 and 54 cases per million population. There are no recognized HLA associations, nor does the disease appear to be inherited.

The clinical presentation of the illness is usually insidious, with pruritus and fatigue being the most common symptoms. The pruritus may be intermittent, is often worse at night, and may become disabling. Elevated serum and tissue bile salts, owing to cholestasis, may account for the pruritus. Jaundice is usually a late and persistent symptom, but it may occur transiently during pregnancy or while the patient is receiving estrogen-containing medications such as birth control pills. Skin pigmentation, weight loss, hepatomegaly, and ultimately splenomegaly and signs and symptoms of portal hypertension and liver failure may be present. Some patients with high serum cholesterol levels, as a result of defective hepatic excretion, will develop xanthelasma and xanthomas, which rarely may be associated with peripheral neuropathy. Pathological fractures are a common problem in advanced cases of primary biliary cirrhosis, owing to both osteomalacia and osteoporosis, with the latter occurring more frequently. Depressed osteoblast function, diminished intake of vitamin D and calcium, malabsorption of vitamin D, and exposure to medications such as cholestyramine may contribute to osteopenia. Decreased hepatic secretion of bile salts may result in steatorrhea and malabsorption of fat-soluble vitamins.

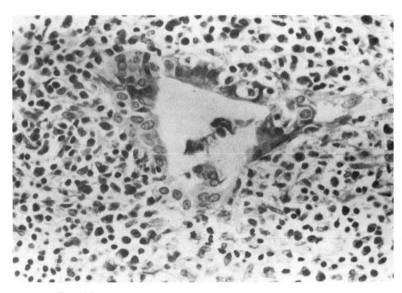

Fig. 16-4
Liver biopsy from a patient with primary biliary cirrhosis, depicting characteristic florid duct lesion. The damaged bile duct epithelium contains inflammatory cells and exhibits degenerative changes.

Associated
Disorders

A variety of autoimmune disorders have been associated with
primary biliary cirrhosis. More than half of all patients manifest
keratoconjunctivitis sicca, and nearly 20 percent of patients will
be found to have a polyarthritis, often rheumatoid in nature,
scleroderma and its variants, or thyroid disorders, particularly
Hashimoto's hypothyroidism. Cutaneous disorders, including
lichen planus and discoid lupus erythematosus, pernicious
anemia, distal renal tubular acidosis, and interstitial pneumonitis have also been reported. Some of these associated disorders, such as hypothyroidism, may not be clinically apparent
and require routine biochemical evaluation.

Pathology

The pathologic process in primary biliary cirrhosis initially affects the small septal and interlobular bile ducts (45–100 μM in
diameter) with destruction of the biliary epithelial cells. Chronic
mononuclear inflammatory cells surround and destroy these
bile ducts in a focal, patchy manner, often with the formation of
granulomas, which occasionally may exhibit germinal centers.
The initial pattern (stage 1), known as the florid duct lesion (Fig.
16-4), is characteristic of primary biliary cirrhosis. At this stage,
inflammation is limited to the portal tracks, with or without
piecemeal necrosis (i.e., inflammation involving the limiting
plate of the portal tracts). In stage II, bile ducts in the portal

tracts are diminished in number with the appearance of bile ductular proliferation. Mild portal fibrosis and cholestasis may be evident during this stage. Stage III is characterized by portal fibrosis, which extends into the lobule, with increasing cholestatic changes, and stage IV is characterized by macronodular cirrhosis, marked cholestasis, and absent bile ducts. All four stages may be present simultaneously in liver biopsies from the same patient and, except for the florid duct lesion (stage I), are nondiagnostic. Extrahepatic bile duct obstruction, sclerosing cholangitis, pericholangitis, cholestatic cases of chronic active hepatitis, and sarcoidosis are important diseases to consider in the differential diagnosis. Patients with graft-versus-host disease and fungal and cytomegalic inclusion virus infections and those exposed to drugs and chemicals such as paraquat, chlorazepate, tolbutamide, thiobendazole, organic arsenicals, and sex steroids may occasionally present with similar clinical and histopathologic findings.

Diagnosis

The clinical diagnosis of primary biliary cirrhosis is rarely made on the basis of a single test. The clinical history, biochemical and serologic tests, liver biopsy, and, in some cases, visualization of the biliary tree (ERCP) may be required to make the diagnosis. Asymptomatic patients with primary biliary cirrhosis are frequently discovered on the basis of elevated hepatic alkaline phosphatase and serum antimitochondrial antibody (AMA) levels. It is now recognized that many of these patients may remain symptom-free for more than a decade. Patients complaining of chronic fatigue or pruritus may also be found to have an elevated hepatic alkaline phosphatase and a positive antimitochondrial antibody, consistent with the diagnosis of primary biliary cirrhosis. An elevated AMA level is a fairly sensitive diagnostic test for primary biliary cirrhosis, being present in more than 90 percent of patients. However, in a minority of patients with chronic active hepatitis and other autoimmune disorders, serum AMA levels may be elevated to a low titer (<1:40). Serum cholesterol, IgM, sedimentation rate, and serum transaminases are frequently elevated but of little specific diagnostic value. The serum bilirubin level is usually elevated in the terminal phase and implies a poor prognosis in patients with primary biliary cirrhosis. Those with serum bilirubin levels persistently greater than 2 mg/dl survive an average of 4 years, whereas those with levels over 10 mg/dl live only 1 to 2 years.

As discussed previously, the histology may suggest primary biliary cirrhosis, but apart from the infrequently observed florid duct lesion, the diagnosis can be based on the clinical history, biochemistry, serology, or liver biopsy alone. Treatable causes of extrahepatic obstruction (i.e., common duct stones) should be excluded by abdominal ultrasound. In atypical cases (e.g., male patients or patients with a negative AMA), endoscopic retrograde cholangiography should be performed. Because many cirrhotic patients develop gallstones and because common duct stones can cause secondary biliary cirrhosis, it is important to consider this possibility. Sclerosing cholangitis and cholangiocarcinoma will also be ruled out by the appropriate cholangiographic studies. A careful history and studies such as chest x-ray and liver biopsy should rule out diagnoses such as drug- or toxin-induced cholestasis, sarcoidosis, and chronic active hepatitis.

Treatment

An array of medications have been used in an attempt to arrest the progression of primary biliary cirrhosis. It should be appreciated that most patients are asymptomatic or only mildly symptomatic for many years, and, in order to treat this disease, the potential risks of serious drug side effects must be considered. The agents that have been tried unsuccessfully include corticosteroids, azathioprine, and D-penicillamine. None of these agents have been found to alter the natural course of the disease and may be accompanied by serious side effects. At present, there is no established treatment for primary biliary cirrhosis itself, although initial results with colchicine appear promising. Cholestyramine may be required for pruritis or to lower serum cholesterol levels in the presence of advanced cutaneous xanthomas. Xanthomatous neuropathy and, at times, severe pruritus, may regress after plasmapheresis. Fat-soluble vitamins (i.e., vitamins A, D, E, and K), particularly vitamin D and calcium supplements, are recommended in patients with advanced disease. Finally, liver transplantation is now an option for some patients who have reached the stage of progressive terminal disease.

Alpha$_1$-Antitrypsin Deficiency

Alpha$_1$-antitrypsin is a low-molecular weight glycoprotein that is synthesized primarily in the liver and exported to the serum, where it functions as an important protease inhibitor. A diminished serum concentration of alpha$_1$-antitrypsin is often associated with panacinar emphysema. Compared to emphysema in general, this disorder exhibits lower lobe predominance and an early age of onset (third to fourth decade). It is believed that lack of inactivation of elastase results in destruction of the connective tissue framework of alveoli. Significant liver disease occurs in only a small proportion of patients with alpha$_1$-antitrypsin deficiency.

Genetics

A pair of codominant alleles located on chromosome 14 is responsible for the ultimate synthesis of alpha$_1$-antitrypsin. Hepatocytes are the principal source of the 52 to 54 Kd glycoprotein, with much smaller amounts being synthesized by mononuclear phagocytes. More than 25 distinct alleles or Pi (protease inhibitor) types have been identified by the technique of isoelectric focusing. In normal individuals, the Pi type is PiMM, and serum alpha$_1$-antitrypsin levels are 130 to 350 mg/dl. The most common abnormal Pi type is PiZZ, in which serum antitrypsin levels are only 10 to 15 percent of normal. In this situation, abnormal alpha$_1$-antitrypsin glycoproteins are synthesized, and there is little secretion into serum. Individuals with PiMZ, or heterozygotes, have serum levels of approximately 60 percent of normal. Rare cases of Pi null null have been reported, in whom no alpha$_1$-antitrypsin mRNA or glycoprotein is synthesized.

Pathophysiology

Patients with abnormal phenotypes (PiZZ, PiMZ, PiMS) synthesize glycoproteins with a single amino acid substitution in the polypeptide chain. This point mutation results in a product that cannot be transported out of the hepatocyte endoplasmic reticulum into the Golgi complex and subsequently into blood. This nontransportable glycoprotein thus lacks the terminal sugars normally added to it in the Golgi complex (i.e., sialic acid and galactose). Immunocytochemistry readily demonstrates the retained alpha$_1$-antitrypsin in the endoplasmic reticulum of hepatocytes. It is unknown whether liver dysfunction is secondary to the accumulated, nonexportable alpha$_1$-antitrypsin in hepatocytes or is due to the decreased antiprotease activity per se. The critical importance of a single amino acid substitution is further illustrated by the unique alpha$_1$-antitrypsin Pittsburgh, in which methionine in the reactive center is replaced by an arginine residue. The resulting glycoprotein binds to thrombin rather than elastase, resulting in antithrombin (anticoagulant) activity. Alpha$_1$-antitrypsin and antithrombin III apparently evolved from a common ancestral protein.

Clinical Manifestations

Nearly 10 percent of all persons with the PiZZ phenotype, as well as some individuals with other Pi types characterized by diminished serum alpha$_1$-antitrypsin levels, will present with neonatal cholestatic jaundice. Some cases closely resemble extrahepatic bile duct obstruction or other types of neonatal hepatitis. The cholestatic jaundice is often accompanied by hepatomegaly, splenomegaly, and liver function test abnormalities. In most cases, the jaundice resolves by the age of 6 months, with persistent hepatosplenomegaly and elevated liver function tests. Some of these jaundiced neonates will die as infants, and others will go on to develop cirrhosis and die of complications of their liver disease as children or adolescents. Approximately 90 percent of PiZZ persons who do not have a history of neonatal jaundice appear to have a better prognosis; some of these patients have abnormal liver function tests as infants and may go on to develop cirrhosis and its complications over a period of many years. Prospective studies of the natural history of PiZZ individuals with and without neonatal jaundice with serial liver biopsies will be necessary to better understand this disease. It appears likely that 10 to 20 percent of all PiZZ individuals will eventually develop cirrhosis and, consequently, in adults presenting with cryptogenic cirrhosis over the age of 50 years, especially males, it is not uncommon to find alpha₁-antitrypsin deficiency. The reputed association of liver disease (chronic active hepatitis and cirrhosis) with the heterozygous PiMZ phenotype is even less clear, and not all studies support this association. Finally, there is some evidence suggesting an association between alpha₁-antitrypsin deficiency and hepatocellular carcinoma in cirrhotic male patients.

Diagnosis and Treatment

The diagnosis of alpha₁-antitrypsin deficiency is best made by measuring serum alpha₁-antitrypsin levels and by determining the Pi type by isoelectric focusing. Serum protein electrophoresis may be inaccurate, and measurement of serum alpha₁-antitrypsin levels alone may miss heterozygotes with normal serum levels owing to associated liver disease or hormonal therapy. Liver biopsy will determine whether chronic active hepatitis or cirrhosis is present and will rule out other causes of liver disease. In the majority of PiZZ homozygotes as well as in occasional heterozygotes, periodic acid–Schiff (PAS)-positive diastase-resistant globules may be found focally in hepatocytes, particularly in the periportal areas (Fig. 16-5). These globules may also be seen in other diseases, such as hepatocellular carcinoma, and thus do not always represent alpha₁-antitrypsin (which requires immunocytochemistry).

Prenatal diagnosis is possible with the use of fetoscopy, although the risk of fetal mortality with this procedure limits its feasibility. Newer methods are in the process of development, using specific synthesized oligonucleotide probes for hybridization with DNA isolated from cultured amniotic fluid cells. One must consider the diagnosis of alpha₁-antitrypsin deficiency as an etiology for neonatal hepatitis or cholestatic jaundice and for chronic liver disease in general in both pediatric and adult age groups.

Treatment of liver disease secondary to alpha₁-antitrypsin deficiency is supportive and nonspecific. The only definitive therapy is liver transplantation; following a successful transplant, the Pi type of the patient converts to that of the donor, and serum

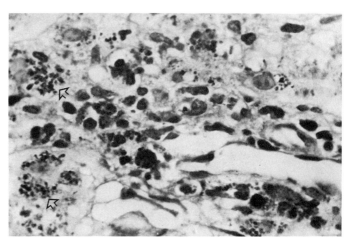

Fig. 16-5
Black-and-white photograph of liver biopsy stained with periodic acid Schiff (PAS) from a patient with alpha$_1$-antitrypsin deficiency. Arrowheads demonstrate intracellular PAS-positive granules in hepatocytes.

alpha$_1$-antitrypsin levels increase. The long-term effects of liver transplantation, including those in patients with pulmonary disease, have yet to be determined.

Study Questions
1. A 25-year-old man with thalassemia who has received over 80 units of transfused blood complains of progressive and severe fatigue. Which of the following disorders are likely to explain his symptoms?
   a. Progressive renal failure
   b. Diabetes mellitus
   c. Cirrhosis
   d. Congestive cardiomyopathy
   e. Adrenal insufficiency
   f. Pulmonary fibrosis

   Answer: b, c, d
   The patient most likely is suffering from iron storage disease or secondary hemochromatosis, due to the considerable number of blood transfusions he has received. Diabetes mellitus, cirrhosis, or congestive cardiomyopathy could explain his symptoms, and all may occur. Note that a, e, and f are not associated with secondary hemochromatosis.

2. A 14-year-old girl from a remote rural school system is referred to a university-based neurologist for evaluation of a persistent tremor. Which of the following are likely to be true?
   a. Her handwriting is illegible.
   b. She has not been doing well in school.
   c. Her mother had the same problem(s) as a child.

d. Her speech is slurred.

e. She has an older brother with cirrhosis.

f. Her urine contains glucose and amino acids.

Answer: a, b, d, e, f

A teenager with persistent tremor may have Wilson's disease. Therefore, all but c are true. Her mother is most unlikely to have the same disorder (Wilson's disease), as the inheritance is autosomal recessive. Her brother could have cirrhosis due to Wilson's disease. Problems with speech and handwriting, declining school performance, and renal tubular defects are all associated with Wilson's disease.

References

Idiopathic Hemochromatosis

Bacon, B. R., and Tavill, A. S. Role of the liver in normal iron metabolism. *Sem. Liver Dis.* 4:181, 1984.

Bassett, M. L., Halliday, J. W., and Powell, L. W. Genetic hemochromatosis. *Sem. Liver Dis.* 4:217, 1984.

Gollan, J. L. Diagnosis of hemochromatosis. *Gastroenterology* 84:418, 1983.

Milder, M. S., Cook, J. D., Stray, S., and Finch, C. A. Idiopathic hemochromatosis, an interim report. *Medicine* 59:34, 1980.

Wilson's Disease

Gollan, J. L. Copper Metabolism, Wilson's Disease and Hepatic Copper Toxicosis. In D. Zakim and T. D. Boyer (eds.), *Hepatology: A Textbook of Liver Disease.* Philadelphia: Saunders, 1982.

Scheinberg, I. H., and Sternlieb, I. *Wilson's Disease.* Philadelphia: Saunders, 1984.

Walshe, J. M. Copper: Its role in the pathogenesis of liver disease. *Sem. Liver Dis.* 4:252, 1984.

Winge, D. R. Normal physiology of copper metabolism. *Sem. Liver Dis.* 4:239, 1984.

Primary Biliary Cirrhosis

Beswick, D. R., Klatskin, G., and Boyer, J. L. Asymptomatic primary biliary cirrhosis: A progress report on long-term follow-up and natural history. *Gastroenterology* 89:267, 1985.

James, S. P., Hoofnagle, J. H., Strober, W., and Jones, E. A. Primary biliary cirrhosis: A model autoimmune disease. *Sem. Liver Dis.* 99:500, 1983.

MacSween, R. N. M., and Sumithran, E. Histopathology of primary biliary cirrhosis. *Sem. Liver Dis.* 1:282, 1981.

Warnes, T. W. Treatment of primary biliary cirrhosis. *Sem. Liver Dis.* 5:228, 1985.

Alpha$_1$-Antitrypsin Deficiency

Eriksson, S. G. Liver disease in alpha$_1$-antitrypsin deficiency: Aspects of incidence and prognosis. *Scand. J. Gastroenterol.* 20:907, 1985.

Eriksson, S., Carlson, J., and Velez, R. Role of cirrhosis and primary liver cancer in alpha$_1$-antitrypsin deficiency. *N. Engl. J. Med.* 314:736, 1986.

Hood, J. M., Koep, L. J., Peters, R. L., Schroter, G. P. J., et al. Liver transplantation for advanced liver disease with alpha$_1$-antitrypsin deficiency. *N. Engl. J. Med.* 302:272, 1980.

Sveger, T. Prospective study of children with alpha$_1$-antitrypsin deficiency: Eight-year-old follow-up. *J. Pediatr.* 104:91, 1984.

17 : Complications of Severe Liver Disease

Sanjeev Arora
Karim A. Fawaz

In the preceding chapters, liver diseases of varying etiologies have been described. Irrespective of the etiology of the liver diseases, they have similar complications, such as portal hypertension, ascites, spontaneous bacterial peritonitis, hepatorenal syndrome, hepatic encephalopathy, and coagulopathy.

Portal Hypertension

Portal hypertension is a diseased state characterized by a pathologic and sustained elevation in portal venous pressure. There is formation of portosystemic collaterals that shunt part of the blood from the splanchnic circulation to the systemic circulation bypassing the liver. The most common cause of portal hypertension is cirrhosis of the liver, and its main complication is gastrointestinal bleeding from esophageal varices.

The portal vein drains blood from the spleen and from the splanchnic vessels in the pancreas, stomach, and intestine (Fig. 17-1). After entering the liver, the portal vein divides and subdivides into progressively smaller branches and finally empties into the hepatic sinusoids. The sinusoids are intercommunicating spaces in the liver lined by endothelium and separated from each other by cords of liver cells that are one cell thick. After numerous subdivisions, the hepatic artery also empties into the sinusoids. From the sinusoids, the blood goes by way of the central veins of the hepatic lobules to the hepatic vein and finally empties into the inferior vena cava.

The pressure in the portal vein is raised in patients with portal hypertension. However, patients with an increased intraabdominal pressure from other causes such as ascites or gaseous distention may also have an elevated pressure. To get a meaningful assessment of portal hypertension, it is important to measure the portal vein pressure gradient (PVPG). There is normally a pressure gradient of 2 to 6 mm Hg between the portal vein and the inferior vena cava. This gradient is more than 10 mm Hg in patients with clinically significant portal hypertension. It is rare for a patient to bleed from esophageal varices unless the PVPG is at least 12 mm Hg.

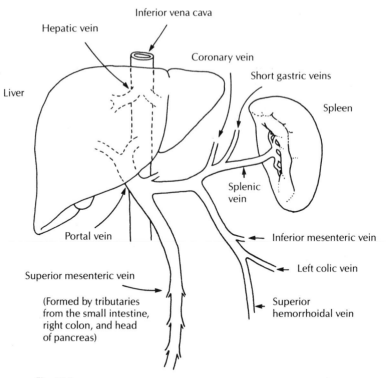

Fig. 17-1
Diagram of portal circulation.

Portal hypertension leads to the development of a collateral circulation. This develops in all sites where there is a communication between the portal and systemic circulation. There is dilatation of the periumbilical veins on the abdominal wall (caput medusa). The flow of blood in these veins is in a direction away from the umbilicus. There is also formation of esophageal and gastric varices that carry blood from the portal circulation to the azygous venous system. Other less common sites of development of varices are the duodenum, ileum, and colon.

In some patients, hemorrhoidal bleeding may be a prominent complaint. By far, the most clinically significant are esophageal varices, which are dilated submucosal veins in the distal esophagus. Esophageal varices receive blood from the lesser curvature of the stomach by way of the coronary vein and then drain into the azygous system. These veins have little perivascular support, do not have any valves, and protrude into the lumen of the esophagus. All the aforementioned factors render them prone to bleeding. Ascites and splenomegaly are other important clinical features of portal hypertension.

Table 17-1
Classification of portal hypertension

I. Presinusoidal
   A. Prehepatic
      1. Portal vein thrombosis
   B. Intrahepatic
      1. Schistosomiasis
      2. Congenital hepatic fibrosis
      3. Neoplastic diseases
      4. Infiltrative diseases
         a. Sarcoidosis
         b. Hodgkin's disease
         c. Non-Hodgkin's lymphoma
         d. Myeloid metaplasia

II. Sinusoidal
   A. Cirrhosis of liver

III. Postsinusoidal
   A. Intrahepatic
      1. Cirrhosis of liver
      2. Veno-occlusive disease
   B Extrahepatic
      1. Budd-Chiari syndrome
      2. Congestive heart failure
      3. Constrictive pericarditis
      4. Inferior vena caval obstruction above entry of hepatic vein

Classification

Although a variety of etiologies can cause portal hypertension, cirrhosis of the liver is the most common. These causes can be classified according to the site of obstruction to flow (Table 17-1).

Pathophysiology

The pressure in the portal circulation is determined by the resistance to blood flow and the rate of blood flow.

In cirrhosis of the liver, the regenerating nodules and contracting scar tissue distort the architecture and compress the hepatic veins causing a postsinusoidal resistance to flow. Portal hypertension is the result. Not only is there increased resistance to flow, there is also a hyperdynamic splanchnic circulation. Chronic portal hypertension results in an increased cardiac output and decreased peripheral vascular resistance. There is increased blood flow to the gastrointestinal tract and skeletal muscle. This increased blood flow is necessary for there to be sustained portal hypertension.

There are two probable mechanisms to explain the hyperdynamic circulation that is seen in chronic portal hypertension. First, there is an elevated level of vasodilators in the serum that lowers splanchnic resistance and therefore increases flow. Second, the vasculature has diminished sensitivity to endogenous vasoconstriction. The gradual increase in hepatic outflow resis-

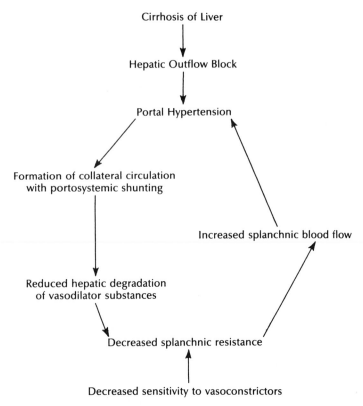

Fig. 17-2
Hypothesis for increased splanchnic blood flow and maintenance of sustained portal hypertension.

tance results in formation of collaterals. This leads to progressively increasing amounts of portal blood flow being diverted from the liver. Because of the portosystemic shunting, the liver is unable to degrade the vasoactive substances — for example, glucagon — that are released from the pancreas, stomach, or intestines. This leads to an increased circulating level of vasodilator substances, which, in turn, cause splanchnic hyperemia (Fig. 17-2).

In experimental models of portal hypertension, the pancreatic glucagon levels are found to be elevated. Glucagon is a potent splanchnic vasodilator, and infusions of glucagon in rats with portal hypertension cause a significant decrease in resistance to intestinal blood flow. Use of antiserum to glucagon in rats with portal hypertension results in a 30 percent decrease in portal blood flow. All this evidence suggests that glucagon is probably an important vasodilator responsible for the increased blood flow seen in portal hypertension.

Rats with portal hypertension show reduced vascular sensitivity to the vasoconstrictive effects of norepinephrine. There is also decreased receptor affinity to angiotensin II, a potent vasoconstrictor, in the mesenteric artery of cirrhotic rats. This may be another factor contributing to the hyperdynamic circulation.

Assessment

As mentioned previously, the most meaningful measure of portal hypertension in cirrhosis of the liver is the portal vein pressure gradient. To measure this directly, it is necessary to do two simultaneous invasive procedures — one to measure the portal pressure, and the other to measure the pressure in the inferior vena cava. To circumvent these difficulties, an indirect method to measure the PVPG has been used. This technique, the preferred method to assess portal pressure, measures the wedged and free hepatic venous pressure. A catheter is advanced in a hepatic vein until it is wedged and until flow in that vessel is occluded. Wedged hepatic venous pressure (WHVP) is measured. This is a measure of the hepatic sinusoidal pressure, since the fluid in the catheter is continuous with the blood in the sinusoid. In alcoholic liver disease and in other forms of micronodular cirrhosis, the hepatic sinusoidal pressure closely reflects portal pressure. The hepatic venous pressure gradient (HVPG), which is a good reflection of the PVPG, can be derived by subtracting the free hepatic vein pressure from the WHVP.

In conditions where the site of resistance to portal flow is presinusoidal (e.g., schistosomiasis) or prehepatic (e.g., portal vein thrombosis), the WHVP will greatly underestimate the portal pressure. Since the WHVP reflects the sinusoidal pressure, it may be normal in the presinusoidal and prehepatic forms of portal hypertension. In these conditions, the portal pressure, measured by direct route (e.g., by umbilical vein cannulation or percutaneous portal vein pressure measurement with a skinny Chiba needle), will be high.

Another method used to assess portal hypertension is the measurement of azygous blood flow by thermodilution technique. This is an index of the blood flow through gastroesophageal collaterals. Clinical studies have shown that azygous blood flow correlates well with portal pressure and also with the size of esophageal varices. Other procedures that are being evaluated are the measurement of pressure in esophageal varices by direct variceal puncture or noninvasively by endoscopic pressure gauges. These pressure gauges are covered by latex membranes and are perfused by a constant flow of air or nitrogen. They work on the principle that the pressure inside a varix is the same as that required to compress it.

Another promising new investigational technique is the completely noninvasive measurement of portal blood flow by a pulsed Doppler flow-meter technique in combination with real-time ultrasonography. The development of a safe, noninvasive method to assess portal blood flow would be extremely useful in future research for development of drugs to treat portal hypertension.

Variceal Bleeding Upper gastrointestinal bleeding from esophagogastric varices is one of the most catastrophic events in the life of a patient with cirrhosis. It is potentially lethal and may be associated with a mortality rate as high as 50 percent.

For patients who survive, it is often the beginning of a steady downhill course. Variceal bleeding can also precipitate hepatic encephalopathy and progressive hepatic failure. Esophageal varices are thin-walled veins, which become progressively dilated as the pressure and portal flow steadily increases. This dilatation causes increased wall tension until the wall ultimately ruptures, leading to hemorrhage.

$$\text{Wall tension} = \frac{\text{(Intravariceal pressure)} - \text{(Pressure outside varix in esophageal lumen)}}{\text{Wall thickness}} \times \text{Radius of varix}$$

The wall tension in a varix increases out of proportion to increases in intravariceal pressure. This is because an increase in intravariceal pressure also results in an increase in the radius of the varix and a decrease in the wall thickness.

At equal pressures, a large varix has a greater risk of bleeding than a small varix, since there is greater wall stress. Reducing variceal pressure by pharmacologic or other means would result in a decreased risk of bleeding. Endoscopy is a useful technique to evaluate the risk of variceal bleeding. Varices can be classified on a scale of I to IV, depending on their size.

Grade I Varices <2 mm in diameter (visible only during valsalva)
Grade II Varices 2–5 mm in diameter
Grade III Varices 5–10 mm in diameter
Grade IV Varices occupying almost the entire lumen of the esophagus

In a large study of patients with alcoholic cirrhosis, it was found that patients with grade I varices had a prevalence of bleeding of zero percent compared with 75 to 85 percent in patients with grades III and IV varices. The presence of telangiectasis, cherry red spots, varix over a varix (bulges), and a thin blue variceal wall all indicate a high risk of bleeding.

Management

The aims of management are:

1. Stop acute variceal bleeding
2. Prevent recurrent variceal bleeding
3. Prolong survival

Vasopressin

Several controlled trials have shown that vasopressin is effective in stopping acute variceal bleeding. The studies have had varying success rates, but overall approximately 52 percent of patients stopped bleeding when treated with vasopressin. In comparison, only 18 percent of control patients stopped bleeding.

The preferred method of using this is by constant intravenous infusion starting at a dose of 0.4 units/minute and increasing to 0.6 units/minute. Vasopressin produces generalized vasoconstriction but has more pronounced effects on the splanchnic circulation. This causes a decrease in portal pressure and often stops bleeding. The drug, however, has numerous side effects. It increases peripheral vascular resistance and also produces bradycardia by stimulating baroreceptors and thus reduces cardiac output. Vasopressin can cause coronary vasoconstriction and may precipitate myocardial infarction in patients with coronary artery disease. Bowel ischemia and infarction have been reported. Because of these serious side effects, vasopressin should be used only in an intensive care setting with close cardiac monitoring. Recent studies have shown that combining vasopressin with nitroglycerin may enhance its efficacy and also reduce the side effects.

Sengstaken-Blakemore Tube

Inserting a Sengstaken-Blakemore tube into the stomach and tamponading the bleeding varices by inflating a balloon has a high rate of success in stopping bleeding but is associated with a high risk of rebleeding and numerous complications.

Sclerotherapy

Sclerotherapy involves injection of a sclerosing agent (e.g., sodium morrhuate) in or around a varix. This induces an inflammatory reaction and thrombosis in the varix, with the aim of eventually obliterating the varices. Once this goal is achieved, the rebleeding rate is markedly reduced. There is still some controversy as to whether sclerotherapy prolongs the life of the patient. Sclerotherapy is associated with minor complications in about 12 percent of cases and major complications in about 3 percent. These include pleural effusion, esophageal stricture, esophageal necrosis, and perforation.

Surgery

Surgery for portal hypertension is based on reducing the portal pressure by creating a shunt between the portal circulation and the systemic circulation. These shunts are divided into two types: (1) nonselective shunt (e.g., portocaval shunt, which diverts the entire portal blood flow to the systemic circulation) and (2) selective shunts (e.g., distal splenorenal shunt, which decompresses a segment of the portal circulation while preserving antegrade portal vein blood flow).

These shunts are highly effective in preventing rebleeding. There is, however, a high rate of postoperative encephalopathy and hepatic failure. These complications are more frequent with the nonselective shunts than with the selective shunts. The procedure of choice in patients requiring elective shunt surgery who do not have much ascites is the distal splenorenal shunt.

In summary, when a patient presents with variceal bleeding he or she should be treated with intravenous vasopressin under careful monitoring. If bleeding does not stop or recurs, sclerotherapy should be used. If bleeding does not cease, balloon tamponade may be added as a temporizing measure. Only rarely is an emergency shunt necessary.

Once cessation of bleeding has been achieved by nonsurgical means, the patient should be put on a sclerotherapy program until obliteration of varices is achieved. If the patient continues to bleed in spite of a completed program of sclerotherapy, a distal splenorenal shunt should be considered.

Inderal, a nonselective beta-blocker, reduces cardiac output and hence splanchnic blood flow and portal pressure. It was found to dramatically reduce the incidence of rebleeding in one study but not in another.

Ascites

Ascites is defined as the accumulation of fluid in the peritoneal space. Most patients with advanced chronic liver disease develop ascites. The most common cause in North America is alcoholic liver disease, although there are numerous other causes of ascites. Some of the more common etiologies are listed in Table 17-2.

Clinical Features

The patient may present with increasing abdominal girth. The belt or clothing may become tight. There is often weight gain despite the protein wasting that accompanies advanced cir-

Table 17-2
Etiology of ascites

I. Cirrhosis of Liver

II. Cardiac Causes
   A. Congestive heart failure
   B. Constrictive pericarditis
   C. Tricuspid insufficiency

III. Malignant Causes
   A. Peritoneal carcinomatosis
   B. Lymphoma with lymphatic obstruction

IV. Infectious Causes
   A. Peritoneal tuberculosis

V. Pancreatic Causes
   A. Ruptured duct secondary to trauma
   B. Leakage from pseudocyst

VI. Miscellaneous Causes
   A. Lymphatic telangiectasia
   B. Nephrotic syndrome
   C. Meig's syndrome
   D. Dialysis-related ascites
   E. Hypothyroidism
   F. Budd-Chiari syndrome

rhosis. The arms and legs are thin because of loss of muscle mass, and the abdomen is protuberant because of ascites, giving the patient a malnourished appearance. Symptoms of gastroesophageal reflux, if present, may be exacerbated. The patient occasionally develops umbilical hernias owing to separation of the rectus muscle. Tense ascites can cause respiratory embarrassment by splinting the diaphragm and predispose to atelectasis and pneumonia. A patient with ascites can present for the first time with spontaneous bacterial peritonitis. This complication occurs exclusively in patients with ascites. The physical examination can detect the presence of ascites by noting bulging flanks or eliciting shifting dullness. When a patient with ascites is in the supine position, the fluid settles in the flanks and the bowel loops rise to the midabdomen. On percussion of the abdomen, the examiner finds a tympanitic note in the midabdomen because of underlying bowel loops and dullness in the flanks owing to the underlying fluid. A mark is made on the abdomen on both sides, indicating the transition from tympanitic note to a dull note. The patient is then rolled onto his or her right side. This results in movement of the ascitic fluid into the dependent right flank. Percussion in this position reveals that the left flank is tympanitic because of the presence of bowel loops. The zone of dullness, previously found in the left abdomen, has shifted to the right.

Another physical sign that indicates the presence of ascitic fluid is the fluid wave. To elicit the fluid wave, the patient should be in a supine position. The patient or an assistant is asked to place the ulnar edge of the hand on the midabdomen longitudinally to prevent the transmission of an impulse through the tissues of the abdominal wall. The examiner then places his or her right hand on the left flank of the patient and taps the left flank gently. Simultaneously, he or she puts his or her left hand on the right flank. If there is a sufficient volume of fluid in the abdomen, the examiner should then be able to sense a sharp wave with his or her left hand. The bedside examination is an insensitive technique for detection of ascitic fluid. Bilateral flank dullness can be elicited only if greater than 1.5 to 2 liters of fluid is present in the abdomen. In one study, clinicians could correctly diagnose the presence or absence of ascites in only 56 percent of patients in whom the diagnosis of ascites was in doubt. In contrast, abdominal ultrasonography is an extremely sensitive test and can detect as little as 100 to 200 ml of peritoneal fluid. It is, however, not necessary to do an ultrasound on every patient in whom ascites is suspected. It should be performed only if the information would influence the decision-making process in a patient's care. An ultrasound examination may also aid in performing a diagnostic paracentesis on a patient with minimal ascites.

Evaluation
All patients should have a detailed history and physical examination. Special emphasis should be placed on a history of alcohol intake, previous incidence of hepatitis, and symptoms suggestive of cardiac disease. Physical signs of importance are the presence of icterus, spider nevi, gynecomastia, and splenomegaly, all of which would suggest severe liver disease as an etiologic factor. The presence of distended neck veins and pulsus paradoxus (a fall of systolic blood pressure greater than 10 mm Hg with inspiration) suggest constrictive pericarditis. A heart murmur may indicate tricuspid insufficiency. All female patients with new onset ascites should have a pelvic examination to rule out the presence of an ovarian mass. Carcinoma of the ovary is the most common cause of peritoneal carcinomatosis. The presence of a myeloproliferative disorder — for example, polycythemia vera — should lead the physician to suspect Budd-Chiari syndrome (hepatic vein thrombosis).

Most patients with new onset of moderate ascites should have a diagnostic paracentesis. If a patient with ascites develops abdominal pain and fever, a diagnostic paracentesis should be performed, since early diagnosis of spontaneous bacterial peritonitis is important.

A cell count, gram stain, and pH should be done on the ascitic fluid. The presence of an absolute neutrophil count over 250 cells/μl usually indicates infection. The fluid should always be sent for bacterial culture. Acid fast stain, culture, and cytology should be done if indicated. Patients with cirrhosis of the liver usually have ascitic fluid, which is a transudate, that is, ascitic fluid protein to serum protein concentration less than 0.5 gm/dl, and ascitic fluid LDH (lactate dehydrogenase) to serum LDH concentration of less than 0.6 gm/dl. This is not always true, however, and approximately 20 percent of patients with cirrhosis have an ascitic fluid protein concentration greater than 2.5 gm/dl. A very high amylase level in ascitic fluid suggests pancreatic ascites.

Pathophysiology For ascitic fluid to accumulate in the abdomen, the rate of formation of lymphatic fluid must exceed the rate of its removal by the lymphatics. Ascitic fluid is derived both from the surface of the liver and the intestines. There is a considerable amount of evidence to suggest that at least in alcoholic cirrhosis, the majority of the fluid seeps out of the surface of the liver rather than the intestine.

In normal individuals, the hepatic sinusoidal pressure is very low, approximately 2 mm Hg. This is because of a very high ratio (50:1) of presinusoidal to postsinusoidal resistance in the hepatic microcirculation. In other body tissues (e.g., muscle), the ratio of a pre- to postcapillary resistance is about 5:1 in the baseline state. Therefore, intracapillary pressures in the musculature may be 20 mm Hg.

Because of this unique characteristic of the hepatic microcirculation, the hepatic sinusoidal pressure is very susceptible to changes in hepatic venous outflow. In alcoholic liver disease, there is inflammation and necrosis of hepatocytes along with fibrosis. Regenerative nodules develop, leading to distortion of the hepatic architecture. These changes lead to a partial hepatic venous outflow block. The hepatic sinusoidal pressure can increase seven- to tenfold, thus leading to a marked increase in transudation of lymph across the sinusoidal wall. Since the hepatic sinusoid is highly permeable to protein, this leads to a similar concentration of protein inside and outside the hepatic sinusoid. There is, therefore, almost no oncotic gradient across the hepatic sinusoidal wall, and fluid transudation across the hepatic sinusoidal wall is minimally influenced by changes in serum protein or albumin concentration. Consequently, the only factor that can increase the transudation of fluid across the hepatic sinusoid is an increase in the hydrostatic pressure. This is easily done by a hepatic venous outflow block as occurs in alcoholic cirrhosis.

Although the splanchnic capillaries are another source of ascites, the contribution of splanchnic circulation is small compared with that from the liver. The splanchnic capillary is not very permeable to protein; thus, there exists a considerable transcapillary oncotic gradient that counteracts the transudation of lymph. The colloid osmotic pressure in the capillary, however, continues to fall as the plasma level of albumin gets lower, thus increasing the formation of lymph.

Lymph is removed from the peritoneal cavity by the regional lymphatics and thoracic duct. Normally, about 800 ml of lymph flows through the thoracic duct. In response to formation of ascitic fluid, there is increased lymph flow, and, in severe cirrhosis, the lymph flow in the thoracic duct may increase 10- to 20-fold over normal levels. Therefore, for ascitic fluid to accumulate, the rate of formation of lymph in the peritoneal cavity should be markedly increased so as to overwhelm even the increased ability of the lymphatics to remove it.

Because ascitic fluid is derived from the vascular space, continued formation of ascitic fluid can only occur if there is simultaneous replenishment of the intravascular space. In cirrhotics, this occurs by urinary salt and water retention. The most important renal abnormality in cirrhosis with ascites is the inability of the kidney to excrete sodium. Normal subjects can increase urinary sodium to high levels in order to closely match salt intake. Patients with cirrhosis of the liver are unable to do this and retain sodium, leading to an expanded extracellular fluid volume. The majority of patients with alcoholic cirrhosis have very low values of urine sodium. It has also been shown that this defect is present in patients who have no evidence of ascites or edema, indicating that this defect may occur early in cirrhosis. Patients with early-stage primary biliary cirrhosis do not appear to have the same abnormality of sodium retention. This may explain the observation that ascites and edema are less common in primary biliary cirrhosis even when there is a comparable amount of portal hypertension.

Underfill Versus Overfill
The underfill theory of ascites formation is the traditional theory and has been considered for many years to be the true explanation for ascites formation (Fig. 17-3).

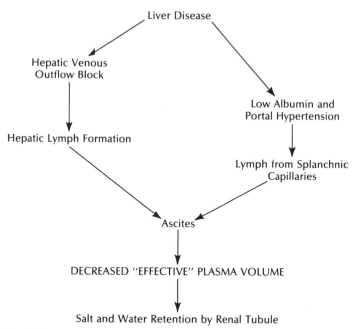

Fig. 17-3
Underfill hypothesis of formation of ascites.

Simply stated, the underfill theory states that the primary event in ascites formation is the accumulation of lymph in the peritoneal cavity. This causes a reduction in the plasma volume, which, in turn, triggers salt and water retention by the kidney to restore plasma volume.

Evidence to support the underfill hypothesis is that volume expansion in a cirrhotic patient may suppress the renin-angiotensin-aldosterone axis and increase the glomerular filtration rate. This is often associated with a marked increase in salt and water excretion by the kidney. This volume expansion can be attained by reinfusion of ascitic fluid intravenously either acutely or chronically by introduction of a LeVeen shunt (peritoneovenous shunt). This form of volume expansion usually results in marked sodium excretion and a negative salt balance.

Epstein and co-workers have used a novel technique to study the effect of volume expansion. They have studied the effect of water immersion on renal salt and water handling. A patient with cirrhosis and ascites is immersed in a water tank with his or her head outside the water. The physiologic effect of water immersion is an increase in central blood volume, which occurs

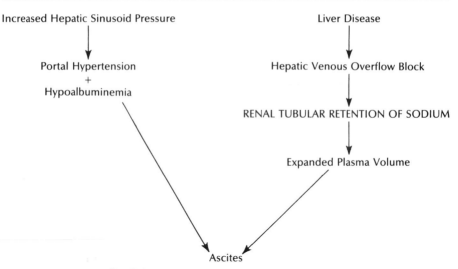

Fig. 17-4
Overflow hypothesis of formation of ascites.

because of redistribution. The major advantage of this maneuver is its easy reversibility. The investigators found that water immersion in 32 patients with cirrhosis and ascites resulted in a marked increase in sodium excretion in the majority of patients. During the final hour of water immersion, sodium excretion was 20 times greater than before immersion. All the aforementioned experimental evidence provides strong support that diminished effective blood volume is probably the major factor causing increased sodium retention by the renal tubule.

During the last several years, several investigators have cited observations that are against the underfill hypothesis. Actual measurements of plasma volume have shown that in cirrhosis with ascites, the plasma volume is increased rather than decreased. It is possible, however, that although the total plasma volume is high, the "effective plasma" volume is low. This may be due to redistribution of blood or an increase in size of the intravascular compartment that is in excess of the increase in plasma volume (Fig. 17-4).

In a series of careful experiments by Levy and co-workers, cirrhosis was induced in dogs by administration of dimethylnitrosamine. The investigators carefully studied sodium balance and showed that renal sodium retention and volume expansion occurred several days before the actual development of ascites. The overflow hypothesis thus states that the primary event in ascites formation is the inappropriate retention of salt and water by the kidney. This results in plasma volume expansion. The hypervolemia superimposed on the altered Starling forces leads to the formation of ascites. There is now considerable evidence to suggest that there are hepatic baroreceptors that are sensitive to increased intrasinusoidal pressure. These baroreceptors send signals to the kidney and the heart and may control sodium excretion. The overflow theory and underflow theory are probably not mutually exclusive. It is possible that different stimuli may be the predominant impetus for salt retention in different stages of the disease.

Efferent Factors   There are several mediators that may direct the kidney to retain salt and water. The relative importance of these efferent factors is not well defined as yet. A large number of patients with alcoholic cirrhosis have elevated aldosterone levels. These elevated levels can result from increased production secondary to "activation" of the renin-angiotensin system or from decreased degradation by a damaged liver. Although raised aldosterone levels certainly contribute to salt and water retention, they do not appear to be the sole explanation. The role for other factors is supported by the observation that the renin-angiotensin-aldosterone system is "activated" in only one third to one half of patients with cirrhotic ascites. Other probable mediators controlling renal sodium excretion are prostaglandins, humoral natriuretic factor, atrial-natriuretic factor, and the kallikrein kinin system. An increase in efferent sympathetic nerve activity to the kidney may also cause sodium retention.

Management   The presence of ascites alone does not constitute an indication for treatment. If a patient has stable mild to moderate ascites, no therapeutic intervention is needed. Moderate sodium restriction should be used to prevent continued accumulation. Some authors recommend rigid sodium restriction (250 mg/day [i.e., 10 mEq/day]). This modality of treatment is effective but may not be well tolerated. A diet with only 250 mg sodium per day may be unpalatable and may exacerbate the malnutrition that is often seen in cirrhotics. It appears reasonable, however, to impose modest sodium restriction. If the response to dietary sodium restriction is inadequate, diuretics should be used.

Indications
1. Tense ascites causing discomfort or eventration of umbilicus
2. Ascites causing respiratory embarrassment
3. Significant pedal edema accompanying ascites
4. Limitation of physical activity

The most important principle in diuretic therapy is to remove fluid slowly. Diuresis reduces ascites by reducing the intravascular volume, which, in turn, results in the absorption of ascitic fluid into the intravascular compartment. Unlike edema fluid, which can be absorbed almost immediately, ascitic fluid can be reabsorbed into the intravascular compartment only at a maximum rate of 900 ml/day with an average of 400 to 500 ml/day. If a patient with cirrhosis has ascites alone, diuretics should be used cautiously so that the daily weight loss does not exceed about 400 gm. If edema is also present, the patient can safely lose about 900 gm of weight per day. Large amounts of diuresis in patients with ascites alone occurs at the expense of the intravascular compartment with significant risk of hypovolemia and renal failure.

The drug of choice is spironolactone, which is an aldosterone antagonist. It acts by antagonism of the effect of aldosterone on the renal tubule and also by actively inhibiting the release of aldosterone from the adrenal glands. The site of action is the distal tubule, where it prevents the absorption of sodium. The drug should be started in a small dosage of 50 to 100 mg/day and should be increased in a stepwise fashion until the desired effect is obtained or a dosage of 400 mg/day is reached. This drug has been shown to be more effective than furosemide for the treatment of ascites. Side effects of spironolactone are hyperkalemia, metabolic acidosis, and gynecomastia. If spironolactone alone is ineffective, small doses of furosemide should be added to the regimen. Furosemide alone is not a very effective diuretic in this clinical setting, since it prevents salt and water reabsorption only in the loop of Henle. In cirrhosis of the liver, the sodium gets reabsorbed in the distal tubule, probably because of the hyperaldosteronism. Occasionally, one may see a patient who is unresponsive to both of these drugs because of a markedly increased proximal tubular absorption of sodium. In this setting, spironolactone and furosemide are not very effective, since very small amounts of sodium reach the loop of Henle and distal convoluted tubule. In this situation, metolazone should be used, since its site of action is the proximal tubule.

Major side effects of concern with furosemide and thiazides are hypokalemia, volume depletion, azotemia, and contraction alkalosis. With modern pharmacotherapy, it is uncommon to see a patient who is truly unresponsive to medical management. However, there is a small percentage of patients in whom ascitic fluid can be removed only at the expense of intravascular volume or renal function. This subgroup of patients should be considered for a LeVeen shunt (peritoneovenous shunt). Placement of this device corrects the maldistribution of fluid while simultaneously decreasing the ascites. This operation involves inserting a device that transports fluid from the peritoneal cavity to the superior vena cava when a pressure gradient exists between the peritoneal cavity and intrathoracic cavity. Although this operation is effective in relieving the ascites, it has many complications, including shunt occlusion, shunt infection, sepsis, and coagulopathy, and is associated with considerable morbidity and mortality. It should be used only if the physician is convinced that disease (i.e., ascites) is worse than the cure (i.e., shunt).

Spontaneous Bacterial Peritonitis

One of the major life-threatening complications of ascites is spontaneous bacterial peritonitis (SBP) (i.e., infection of the ascitic fluid). It has been observed that the frequency of this infection in hospitalized patients with ascites has been steadily increasing over the last 30 years. Most likely, this represents a true increase in the frequency of occurrence of SBP; however, another contributing factor may be the enhanced awareness and diagnosis of asymptomatic or minimally symptomatic infections.

Clinical Features

Spontaneous bacterial peritonitis occurs exclusively in patients with ascites. Most patients with SBP have advanced liver disease as attested to by the presence of jaundice and esophageal varices. The onset of SBP is usually characterized by fever and abdominal pain. Physical examination may reveal rebound tenderness and hypoactive bowel sounds; however, not all patients will have these findings. Nausea, vomiting, and diarrhea are common complaints. Approximately one third of patients with SBP will have no symptoms and signs referable to the abdomen. Such patients may present with hypothermia, hypotension, hepatic encephalopathy, or worsening renal function. A rising serum creatinine or resistance to diuretics may be an early sign in such patients. Sixty-five to 80 percent of patients have peripheral blood leukocytosis, and approximately 40 to 60 percent of patients have bacteremia diagnosed by positive blood cultures. Diagnosis is established by an abdominal paracentesis. All patients with clinical features suggestive of SBP or unexplained deterioration of hepatic or renal function should be considered for this procedure. Since SBP has an in-hospital mortality rate ranging from 48 to 70 percent, early diagnosis and prompt therapy are crucial.

The protein LDH and glucose concentration in the ascitic fluid are not reliable distinguishing factors between patients with SBP and those with uninfected ascites. The protein concentration in both conditions is low. Some investigators have found that SBP can be reliably diagnosed if the ascitic fluid pH is reduced and the pH gradient between blood and ascitic fluid is greater than 0.1. A Gram's stain for organisms is positive in only 22 to 60 percent of the patients, who eventually have a positive culture. The results of bacterial culture of ascitic fluid are not available before 24 to 48 hours. Thus, waiting for the results would delay treatment. The most reliable test to make the diagnosis of SBP before the results of culture are available is a polymorphonuclear cell count greater than 250/μl.

Sterile ascitic fluid has small numbers of leukocytes, usually less than 300/μl, and most of them are mononuclear cells. Thus, the absolute number of polymorphonuclear leukocytes is very low. Some patients who have been on diuretics may have higher counts. All patients with ascitic fluid polymorphonuclear cell counts greater than 250/μl should be treated for SBP pending results of culture.

Bacteriology and Pathogenesis

In about 90 percent of patients, a single organism is isolated from the ascitic fluid, and in approximately 75 percent of all patients, SBP is caused by gram-negative bacilli of enteric origin. *Escherichia coli* is the most common of these. Other enteric organisms such as *Pseudomonas* and *Streptococcus fecalis* may also be found. Pneumococcus is responsible for an additional 10 to 20 percent of cases. Surprisingly, anaerobes are isolated in only 6 to 14 percent of cases and are often found as one of multiple organisms. This suggests that patients with anaerobic infection may have a different pathogenetic mechanism.

There are several possible mechanisms by which ascitic fluid may become infected:

1. A patient with cirrhosis may have bacteremia, which then secondarily infects the ascitic fluid.
2. In cirrhosis, there may be an alteration in the permeability of the intestinal wall, thus allowing bacteria to traverse the intestinal wall and infect ascitic fluid.
3. The bacteria could enter the intestinal lymphatics, reach the liver, and then secondarily enter the peritoneal cavity when ascitic fluid is formed.

Since about 50 percent of patients with SBP have bacteremia, it seems that blood-borne infection is a likely route. In addition, some patients with pneumonia or urinary tract infection develop SBP with the same organisms, suggesting hematogenous spread. There is also evidence to suggest that destruction of blood-borne bacteria by the Kupffer's cells of the liver is deficient in cirrhosis of the liver. In addition, more than three fourths of the portal blood may bypass the liver by means of portosystemic collaterals, thus allowing the bacteria to bypass the hepatic reticuloendothelial filter. Several invasive procedures, such as liver biopsy, sigmoidoscopy, colonoscopy, and rectal examination, have been shown to cause bacteremia. Fiberoptic endoscopy and balloon tamponade may also be potential vehicles of infection by the same mechanism. Many patients with SBP have had one or more of these procedures in a relatively short period of time preceding the diagnosis of SBP. Blood-borne infection appears to be the most likely mechanism for the spontaneous infection of ascitic fluid. However, there is no direct evidence to prove that bacteremia is a cause rather than just an associated finding in patients with SBP. Also, several studies have failed to demonstrate the presence of bacteria in the portal blood of cirrhotic patients.

Another hypothesized mechanism is the direct passage of bacteria through the intestinal wall. For unknown reasons, patients with cirrhosis may have colonization of the upper small bowel with colonic flora. Other experiments in dogs have shown that C_{14}-labeled *E. coli* could pass from the bowel lumen to the peritoneal cavity if a hypertonic solution was introduced into the peritoneal cavity. There is also experimental evidence to indicate that in the presence of gastrointestinal bleeding and hypovolemia, the permeability of the intestinal wall to enteric bacteria is increased. This is supported by clinical data showing an increased incidence of SBP in patients with gastrointestinal bleeding and the efficacy of nonabsorbable antibiotics in preventing it. Vasopressin infusions can produce mesenteric ischemia, compromising the intestinal barrier, and have been implicated in precipitating SBP. One clinical observation argues against this hypothesis. If increased intestinal permeability were a major pathogenetic mechanism, one would expect a much higher incidence of infections with anaerobes and multiple organisms. This has not been found to be the case. Evidence to support the spread of bacteria by intestinal lymphatics is scant.

Recent evidence suggests that there are several other factors impairing the host defenses of a cirrhotic patient against bacterial infection. Malnutrition and alcoholism have been independently shown to reduce immunity to infection. In a patient with cirrhosis, both of these conditions commonly coexist. Patients with severe liver disease also have defects in serum bactericidal function, opsonization, chemoattraction, and impaired function of polymorphonuclear leukocytes and monocytes. In other studies, ascitic fluid from patients with cirrhosis was found to have impaired antimicrobial activity against *E. coli, S. fecalis,* and pneumococci — organisms commonly implicated in SBP. It is interesting to note that the ascitic fluid had good bacteriostatic activity against bacteroides.

Treatment

The mainstay of treatment is the early use of efficacious systemic antibiotic treatment. The conventional regimen is the combination of a first-generation cephalosporin such as cephalothin, or ampicillin in combination with an aminoglycoside. A recent randomized controlled trial has shown that cefotaxime, a third-generation cephalosporin, is more effective than a combination of ampicillin and tobramycin. One major advantage of this therapy is the avoidance of aminoglycoside nephrotoxicity to which a cirrhotic is more susceptible than the normal population. In spite of effective antimicrobial therapy, the mortality rate of patients with SBP is high. This probably reflects the nature of the serious underlying disease.

Hepatorenal Syndrome

The use of the term *hepatorenal syndrome* (HRS) has generated considerable controversy. In the past, some authors have used this term to encompass all forms of renal failure that occur in a patient with liver disease. Such a broad or imprecise use of the term did not give any insight into the pathophysiology of these disorders. In the last two to three decades, most investigators in the field have agreed to restrict the use of this term and establish more rigid diagnostic criteria.

HRS has been defined as progressive impairment in renal function, occurring in patients with liver disease, in the absence of clinical or anatomic evidence of other causes to explain the degree or persistence of renal failure. Thus, it is mandatory to rule out other factors such as hypovolemia or drug nephrotoxicity as a cause of renal failure.

Although alcoholic liver disease is the most common cause, other forms of chonic liver disease such as postnecrotic cirrhosis and primary biliary cirrhosis are also associated with the development of HRS. Other liver diseases that may predispose the patient to develop HRS are fulminant hepatitis, Reye's syndrome, fatty liver of pregnancy, and neoplasms of the liver.

Clinical Features and Diagnosis

Almost all patients who develop HRS have ascites. Most of them also have some degree of jaundice, hypoalbuminemia, and portal hypertension. Most of the patients are admitted to a hospital when they develop the syndrome. This has led investigators to suspect that some intervention in a hospital setting may be responsible to trigger the development of HRS. Others have even speculated that withdrawal of some substance — for example, alcohol — may be causative. The onset of this disorder is often preceded by SBP, gastrointestinal bleeding, induced diuresis, or abdominal paracentesis. In one study of 200 patients, approximately half of the patients had these predisposing factors. In the same study, about 80 percent of patients had some degree of

Table 17-3
Forms of renal failure in cirrhosis

Laboratory findings	Hepatorenal syndrome	Pre-renal azotemia	Acute tubular necrosis
Urine sodium	<10 mEq/liter, often 1–2 mEq/liter	<10 mEq/liter	>40 mEq/liter
Fractional excretion of sodium	<1	<1	>2
Urine osmolality/ plasma osmolality	>1.5	>1.5	1 isosthenuria
Urine sediment	Inactive	Inactive	"Active" with leukocytes and casts

hepatic encephalopathy. Most patients have a modest fall in blood pressure in comparison with values that have been recorded before the development of the syndrome. The onset of HRS may be acute over the course of 2 to 3 days or may be gradual over several weeks.

Patients have marked oliguria with the urine output usually between 100 and 200 ml/24 hours. Rarely, patients have a nonoliguric form of renal failure. The urinary sodium concentration is very low, usually less than 10 mEq/liter and can be as low as 1 to 2 mEq/liter. In the early stages of HRS, the urine is concentrated, with the urine osmolality more than 450 mOsm/liter and the urine osm/plasma osm greater than 1.5. The urine sediment is usually inactive with minimal proteinuria. Occasionally, cells and casts may be present, possibly owing to the presence of jaundice. These findings are in marked contrast to those seen in acute tubular necrosis (ATN). In ATN, the urine sodium is more than 40 mEq/liter, the kidney loses concentrating ability, and the urine is isoosmotic with the serum. In addition, the urine sediment is "active," containing numerous leukocytes and casts. Patients with cirrhosis of the liver without renal impairment often have low serum blood urea nitrogen (BUN) levels. In contrast, patients with HRS usually have a disproportionate elevation of the serum BUN in spite of the presence of severe liver disease. The serum creatinine rarely rises to the very high levels that are seen in ATN. The serum sodium concentration is often low, indicating a defect in free water clearance (Table 17-3).

HRS is associated with a grave prognosis. Less than 5 percent of the patients survive. Most patients die *in* renal failure rather than *of* renal failure. Uremia is rarely the cause of death. Most patients die of hemorrhage infection, hypotension, or hepatic failure. Gastrointestinal bleeding is the most common cause of death. The diagnosis of HRS should be one of exclusion. The physician should be certain that all treatable causes of renal failure have been ruled out. As is obvious from the clinical features, it is difficult to distinguish HRS from renal impairment owing to hypovolemia (pre-renal azotemia). In addition, as mentioned in the previous section, a patient may have marked ascites and yet have diminished effective blood volume. The first step in establishing the diagnosis is to rule out volume depletion. This is usually done by a therapeutic trial of volume expansion with intravenous crystalloids or colloids, until a central venous pressure of 8 to 10 cm of water is achieved. Overly vigorous expansion of the intravascular compartment should be avoided, since it may precipitate variceal hemorrhage by increasing intravariceal pressure. Patients with HRS do not show any sustained improvement in urine volume or renal function with volume expansion. In contrast, patients with pre-renal azotemia will recover with volume expansion.

Pathophysiology   There is a large body of evidence to suggest that the renal failure is due to functional impairment of the kidney by circulatory disturbances rather than intrinsic renal parenchymal damage. There appears to be a disturbance in the environment of the kidney rather than the kidney itself. This is supported by the evidence that when the kidney from a patient with HRS is transplanted into a patient with a normal liver, it functions normally. Second, if a patient with HRS undergoes successful liver transplantation, the kidneys can resume normal function. Third, when the kidney of a patient with HRS is examined histologically at postmortem, it is either perfectly normal or has minimal changes that do not account for the renal failure. There is no histologic evidence of primary renal disease.

The circulatory nature of this disorder is evidenced by its striking resemblance to pre-renal azotemia, suggesting that there is a decrease in effective renal perfusion. Thus, the kidney produces a concentrated urine with low urine sodium to conserve intravascular volume. Second, HRS is often preceded by minor gastrointestinal hemorrhage, paracentesis, or diuresis, all of which produce some reduction in effective blood volume. This may imply that the kidneys in patients with HRS are exquisitely sensitive to minor decrements in effective blood volume. Other direct evidence has shown that patients with HRS have a marked reduction in glomerular filtration rate and renal blood flow and an increased renal vascular resistance. Epstein and co-workers conducted excellent studies of the renal circulation in HRS. Using Xe^{133} washout techniques and direct renal arterial angiography, they showed that patients had severe vasoconstriction in the outer segments of the renal cortex, whereas the blood flow to the deep cortex and renal medulla was preserved. In addition, there was a marked instability of the arterial tree, which was not seen in acute renal failure from causes other than HRS. In contrast, the entire renal arterial tree was normal when it was inspected postmortem.

Reviewing all the evidence, it is tempting to think of the HRS as an exaggerated physiologic response to a minor alteration in effective circulating blood volume. The major drawback in this hypothesis is the inability of volume expansion to reverse the sequence of events. This has led to the hypothesis that there are humoral agents that are either produced by or inadequately destroyed by a diseased liver that are responsible for the initiation and persistence of the intense vasoconstriction.

Numerous humoral substances have been considered, including conjugated bilirubin; false neurotransmitters, such as octopamine and phenylethanolamine; endotoxins; renin-angiotensin system; vasoactive intestinal peptide; vasodilator substance; and the kallikrein kinin system. Currently, the evidence to incriminate any of these substances is inconclusive.

It is also possible that the signal for renal vasoconstriction is a neural one as a reflex secondary to intrahepatic hypertension seen in liver disease.

In summary, HRS is a functional impairment of the kidney owing to a circulatory impairment that results in renal hypoperfusion. The exact nature of the factors that trigger and maintain this circulatory change is unknown.

Management

It cannot be overemphasized that the most important step in the management of a patient with HRS is to rule out other reversible causes of renal failure, most significantly pre-renal azotemia. Some patients have improved after a peritoneovenous shunt (LeVeen shunt); however, most experts are not convinced by the usefulness of this technique, and its use still remains investigational. Hemodialysis or peritoneal dialysis is usually not indicated except in patients with acute liver disease such as fatty liver of pregnancy, fulminant hepatitis, or Reye's syndrome, where regeneration of the liver may result in spontaneous improvement in renal function.

Although hepatic transplantation may reverse the HRS, most patients are extremely ill and at high risk of operative mortality.

Hepatic Encephalopathy

Hepatic encephalopathy is a clinical syndrome that encompasses all the changes in mental status that occur directly be-

Table 17-4
Stages of hepatic encephalopathy

Stage	Symptoms	Signs
I	Personality changes, loss of affect, euphoria, apathy, inappropriate behavior, altered sleep pattern, insomnia with daytime somnolence	Constructional apraxia, difficulty in writing
II	Mental confusion, disorientation to time and place	Asterixis, fetor hepaticus
III	Severe mental confusion, light coma, may appear comatosed but is arousable by stimuli	Asterixis, fetor hepaticus, rigidity, hyperreflexia, extensor planters, grasping reflexes
IV	Deep coma, unresponsive to stimuli	Fetor hepaticus, unarousable, diminished muscle tone, decreased reflexes

cause of hepatic dysfunction. The clinical manifestations range from very subtle personality changes to deep coma. The early changes may be loss of affect, euphoria, depression, mild intellectual impairment, or alteration in sleep pattern. These changes will usually be reported by the family of the patient and may not be apparent during the first visit to a physician. If the encephalopathy progresses, the patient becomes confused, drowsy, and disoriented. This can progress to light coma and even deep coma, in which the patient is nonresponsive to stimuli.

Neurologic examination during the early stages reveals constructional apraxia (inability to reproduce simple diagrams such as a star) and writing difficulty (Table 17-4). During the stage of light coma, the patient usually has asterixis (a flapping tremor elicited by having the patient extend his or her hands with the fingers apart), rigidity of limbs, hyperreflexia, extensor planters, grasping and sucking reflexes, and fetor hepaticus. Fetor hepaticus refers to a sweet, musty odor in the breath, which is due to sulphur-containing mercaptans exhaled in the breath. If the coma deepens, there is loss of muscle tone and the reflexes may become depressed.

Patients with hepatic coma usually have elevations in blood ammonia levels and cerebrospinal fluid (CSF) glutamine. Electroencephalography (EEG) reveals generalized high-amplitude, low-frequency waves without any focal changes. Triphasic waves in paroxysmal bursts are common. Paroxysms of delta waves (1.5–3 Hz) are also present. Although these EEG changes are characteristic, they are not diagnostic of hepatic encephalopathy. Patients with other metabolic encephalopathies, such as uremia and carbon dioxide narcosis, may occasionally have similar findings.

Pathophysiology There are several postulated mechanisms to explain the presence of encephalopathy in a patient with cirrhosis:

1. Hepatic insufficiency results in failure of the liver to detoxify potentially toxic products, which then accumulate in the extracellular fluid.
2. Abnormal neurotransmitter balance.
3. Altered brain energy metabolism.
4. Alteration in structure and function of neuronal and synaptic membranes.
5. Increased permeability of the blood-brain barrier.

These mechanisms are not mutually exclusive. The first two are discussed here in greater detail.

Accumulation of Toxic Products
Ammonia
Patients with hepatic encephalopathy often have an elevated level of ammonia in their blood, which can then enter the central nervous system. A high brain ammonia level is believed to be associated with encephalopathy. Ammonia is produced in the gastrointestinal tract by the ingestion of protein or by gastrointestinal blood loss. Bacterial ureases and amino acid oxidases of the colonic bacteria act on the protein to release ammonia. Mucosal enzymes also result in protein breakdown. A normal liver converts the ammonia to urea by way of the urea cycle. In the presence of severe liver disease or portal systemic shunting, this ammonia is not metabolized efficiently and spills into the systemic circulation.

Ammonia is also metabolized in skeletal muscle by the conversion of glutamate to glutamine by the action of glutamine synthetase. In chronic liver disease, however, the skeletal muscle mass is often decreased. In cirrhotics, the presence of hypokalemia may also enhance the release of ammonia from the kidneys into the blood. High blood levels of ammonia in cirrhotics have been shown to cause increased blood levels of glucagon, which, in turn, stimulate hepatic gluconeogenesis from amino acids and a further increase in ammonia production. In addition, cerebral metabolism of certain amino acids results in increased production of ammonia. A high blood ammonia level in hepatic failure results in greater uptake of ammonia by the gray matter. This ammonia is converted by the astrocytes to glutamine, resulting in high CSF levels of glutamine.

Ammonia is known to directly depress neuronal membrane activity, probably by altering electrolyte and water transport. In addition, ammonia can alter the malate-aspartate-hydrogen shuttle across the mitochondrial membrane. This may decrease the NADH/NAD ratio, resulting in accumulation of lactate in the cell. There are, however, several pieces of evidence to suggest that ammonia may not be the main culprit in production of encephalopathy. Some patients with encephalopathy have normal blood levels of ammonia. In patients who have hyperammonemia, the level of ammonia often does not correlate with the level of coma; thus, ammonia is probably one of several factors contributing to the development of encephalopathy.

Accumulation of Neurotoxic Amino Acids and False Neurotransmitters

Patients with decompensated cirrhosis have a decrease in the concentration of branched chain amino acids such as valine, leucine, and isoleucine. In contrast, the blood levels of aromatic amino acids such as aspartate, glutamate, tyrosine, methionine, phenylalanine, and free tryptophan are greatly increased. This imbalance of amino acids is also seen in the central nervous system. Most patients with hepatic encephalopathy have an elevated glutamine level in the CSF.

Tryptophan and its metabolite serotonin are found in high concentrations in the central nervous system of patients with hepatic encephalopathy. This high concentration of tryptophan results in increased synthesis of false neurotransmitters such as octopamine and serotonin.

In recent years, there has been much interest in the role of gamma-aminobutyric acid (GABA). Increased plasma GABA levels and an increase in the permeability of the blood-brain barrier to GABA have been documented in an animal model of fulminant hepatic failure and encephalopathy.

Precipitating Factors

Clinical onset of hepatic encephalopathy may be insidious owing to gradually worsening liver disease or may appear suddenly as a result of some precipitating factors. The usual precipitating factors follow:

1. *Azotemia.* Patients with cirrhosis are more susceptible to azotemia than is the general population. This can be induced by use of diuretics. Overzealous treatment of ascites can often lead to this complication. Another cause is the excessive use of laxatives. Nonsteroidal anti-inflammatory drugs such as indomethacin (Indocin) may also produce renal insufficiency. During azotemic states, there is increased intestinal secretion of urea, which is then broken down by colonic bacteria to ammonia.

2. *Sedatives.* Patients with chronic liver disease are very sensi-

tive to sedatives, and small doses may precipitate encephalopathy. Drugs such as Valium may have very long half-lives in patients with hepatic dysfunction.

3. *Gastrointestinal bleeding.* Presence of blood in the gastrointestinal tract can induce hepatic encephalopathy acutely. One hundred milliliters of blood provides about 15 gm of protein load to the gastrointestinal tract, which causes increased production of ammonia and nitrogenous breakdown products. Patients with gastrointestinal bleeding can also develop hypovolemia and azotemia, which exacerbates the encephalopathy.

4. *Acid base and electrolyte disturbances.* Use of diuretics is a common cause of this problem. In metabolic alkalosis, there is enhanced diffusion of un-ionized ammonia across the blood-brain barrier. If present, hypokalemia also exacerbates the encephalopathy.

5. *Excess dietary protein.* In patients with borderline compensated cirrhosis, hepatic encephalopathy may be caused by ingestion of a high-protein meal such as a large piece of steak.

6. *Infection.* Presence of infection causes increased tissue catabolism and may precipitate encephalopathy.

Treatment

The aims of treatment of hepatic encephalopathy are to prevent the absorption of protein breakdown products from the lumen of the intestines and to reverse the precipitating factors.

Prevention of Absorption of Protein Breakdown Products

The most commonly used drug is *lactulose* (1,4 galactosidofructose). This is a nonabsorbable synthetic disaccharide that is not digested in the upper gastrointestinal tract. It is metabolized by colonic bacteria to form lactic acid, formic acid, acetic acid, and carbon dioxide. These acids result in a fall in the pH of the colonic lumen to about 5.5, which in turn causes the conversion of ammonia to ammonium ion. The low pH also results in the movement of ammonia from the intracellular compartment to the gastrointestinal lumen, where it can be excreted as ammonium ion in the stool. Lactulose is also a laxative and thus causes evacuation of the colonic contents. The dose of lactulose should be adjusted so that the patient has two or three soft stools per day. Diarrhea should be avoided to prevent dehydration, hypernatremia, and azotemia.

Neomycin is also effective therapy. The drug acts by reducing the counts of urea splitting organisms in the colon and thus reducing the production of nitrogenous breakdown products that cause encephalopathy. One to 3 percent of the drug is absorbed and thus may be ototoxic and nephrotoxic in patients with previously existing renal disease.

Correction of Precipitating Factors

The patient should be put on a low-protein diet until the encephalopathy is reversed. Infection is an important precipitating factor and should be looked for and treated. A patient with ascites and new onset encephalopathy needs a diagnostic peritoneal tap to rule out the presence of spontaneous bacterial peritonitis. Sedatives should be avoided. Electrolyte imbalances such as hypokalemia and alkalosis must be corrected. Often, patients with hepatic encephalopathy are dehydrated and require intravenous rehydration with crystalloid solutions. Administration of sodium chloride solution may correct the contraction alkalosis that is often seen. If there is any evidence of acute gastrointestinal bleeding, it is imperative to evacuate the blood from the gastrointestinal tract with a nasogastric tube or high colonic enemas.

Coagulopathy in Liver Disease

Except for the von Willebrand factor (vWF), all the coagulation proteins and the inhibitors of coagulation are synthesized by the liver. Therefore, it is not surprising that as many as 85 percent of patients with liver disease exhibit some problem with hemostasis. Although many of these patients are asymptomatic, defective hemostasis can cause excessive blood loss if a patient starts to bleed from esophageal varices, gastritis, or peptic ulcer disease. These patients may also bleed excessively after a venipuncture or a liver biopsy. Less commonly, when the hemostatic defect is severe, spontaneous bleeding in the form of petechiae, ecchymosis, or epistaxis can be observed. The abnormalities of coagulation observed in liver disease are very complex. The net result is the sum total of the alterations in the levels of coagulation proteins and inhibitors, platelet function, and the presence or absence of disseminated intravascular coagulation (DIC).

Alteration in the Coagulation System

There are often reduced concentrations of factors I (fibrinogen), II (prothrombin), V, VII, IX, X, XI, and XII in patients with severe liver disease.

In early liver disease, the concentration of fibrinogen may be normal or increased, since it is an acute phase reactant. With advancing liver disease or fulminant hepatitis, hypofibrinogenemia develops. In addition to the quantitative changes, a qualitative abnormality of the fibrinogen molecule is seen in 50 to 78 percent of patients with chronic liver disease. This condition, called *acquired dysfibrinogenemia*, is diagnosed when one finds a prolonged thrombin time in spite of normal levels of fibrinogen and fibrinogen degradation products. This condition is characterized by a defect of fibrin monomer polymerization caused by an alteration in the sialic acid content of fibrinogen.

The vitamin K–dependent factors (i.e., II, VII, IX, and X) are synthesized by the liver in the precursor forms. Vitamin K is necessary for carboxylation of the glutamic acid residues to convert the factors into active forms. The carboxylation is a necessary step for the binding of these factors to phospholipid and for participating in the coagulation cascade. A deficiency of these factors results in a prolongation of the prothrombin time. Factor VII has the shortest half-life and is often reduced to the greatest extent in liver disease. The response to administration of vitamin K helps to distinguish between vitamin K deficiency as seen in patients with obstructive jaundice and that seen in patients with primary hepatocellular disease. In patients with obstructive jaundice, the prolonged prothrombin time can be corrected by parenteral administration of vitamin K. In contrast, vitamin K does not correct the coagulation abnormality in cirrhosis, since it does not affect the synthesis of the coagulation factors.

Factor VIII is found in normal or raised concentrations in the presence of liver disease. The concentration of vWF is also often elevated. There is a disproportionate elevation in the nonfunctional factor VIII and vWF antigens in comparison to the biologic activity of these coagulation proteins. The major clinical usefulness of the measurement of plasma concentration of factor VIII is to distinguish between the coagulopathy of fulminant hepatitis from that seen in DIC of liver disease. The factor VIII levels are high in patients with fulminant hepatitis but are low in patients with DIC, since coagulation factors are consumed in the process.

Alteration in Platelets

Patients with cirrhosis can have quantitative or qualitative defects in platelets. Thrombocytopenia is often observed with platelet counts in the range of 50,000 to 100,000. The most common cause of thrombocytopenia is pooling of the platelets in an enlarged congested spleen, often seen in patients with cirrhosis and portal hypertension. The platelet life span may also be reduced owing to IgG antibodies as seen in chronic active hepatitis. Alcohol consumption also produces thrombocytopenia by directly suppressing platelet production by the bone marrow. In addition to thrombocytopenia, patients with cirrhosis also have defects in platelet function. Platelet adhesion to glass beads and aggregation in response to adenosine diphosphate (ADP) is impaired.

Disseminated Intravascular Coagulation

Disseminated intravascular coagulation is a state characterized by a pathological stimulation of the coagulation mechanism that results in generation of excess thrombin and consumption of coagulation proteins and platelets. This is accompanied by a compensatory fibrinolysis, which, along with the deficiency of platelets and clotting factors, can result in a hemorrhagic state. The pathogenesis of DIC in liver disease is complex. Mechanisms that may contribute include:

1. Systemic endotoxemia owing to reduced hepatic clearance and portosystemic shunting
2. Reduced synthesis of inhibitors of coagulation such as antithrombin III and protein C
3. Release of tissue thromboplastin by injured liver cells
4. Reduced clearance of coagulation factors

The severity of DIC in a patient with liver disease may vary from an asymptomatic state to a severe hemorrhagic state resulting in a fatal outcome.

Management

The mainstay of treatment for the coagulopathy of liver disease is fresh frozen plasma. It is useful for patients who are actively bleeding or are being prepared for surgery, liver biopsy, angiography, or other invasive procedures. Fresh frozen plasma contains all the coagulation factors in inactive forms. It also contains components of the fibrinolytic and inhibitor systems. It has to be given in large doses, and the response is only temporary. Some patients may need platelet transfusions in addition to fresh frozen plasma. Two newer forms of treatment being investigated are antithrombin III and desmopressin (DDAVP). Antithrombin III concentrates have been found to be useful in patients with DIC, fulminant hepatitis, and fatty liver of pregnancy. Desmopressin is an analog of vasopressin that produces an increase in the plasma concentration of factor VIII and vWF. It may also decrease the prothrombin time and raise the levels of factors VII, IX, and XII.

Study Questions

A 50-year-old white man with a long-standing history of heavy ethanol ingestion is admitted to the hospital with the complaint of vomiting bright red blood. His past history is remarkable for biopsy-proven cirrhosis of the liver. His medications include furosemide, 40 mg per day, and spironolactone, 200 mg per day. Examination reveals a jaundiced man with peripheral stigmata of chronic liver disease. He has moderate ascites and splenomegaly. In addition, the patient is confused and disoriented and has asterixis.

1. The most likely cause of the patient's mental confusion is hepatic encephalopathy. Which of the factors below may be contributing to this condition?
   a. Volume overload
   b. Gastrointestinal bleeding
   c. Volume depletion
   d. Electrolyte imbalance
   e. Spontaneous bacterial peritonitis

   Answer
   b, c, d, e
   Gastrointestinal bleeding can rapidly bring on hepatic encephalopathy in patients with underlying liver disease since blood is a rich source of protein that is broken down by colonic bacteria with the resultant production of toxic nitrogenous products that precipitate encephalopathy. In addition, severe blood loss can cause hypovolemia, which can worsen the mental status. Other factors that may be contributing to the encephalopathy include electrolyte imbalances such as hypokalemia and alkalosis, both of which are frequently encountered in patients with cirrhotic ascites who are being treated with diuretic drugs. The diagnosis of spontaneous bacterial peritonitis should always be considered in patients with ascites who develop hepatic encephalopathy.

2. Which of the following statements is or are correct regarding this patient with ascites?
   a. Urinary sodium is high
   b. The flow of lymph in the thoracic duct is increased
   c. The majority of the fluid in the peritoneal cavity (ascites) is produced by transudation from splanchnic capillaries

   Answer
   b
   The major portion of ascitic fluid is produced via transudation of lymph from the surface of the liver rather than from the splanchnic capillaries. In addition, the most important renal abnormality in cirrhotic ascites is decreased urinary sodium excretion because of avid sodium retention. When ascites is present, the body attempts to compensate for it by increasing several-fold the rate of removal of lymph via the thoracic duct. Simply stated, ascites accumulates only when the body's ability to remove lymph is overwhelmed.

References

Better, O. S., and Schrier, R. W. Disturbed volume homeostasis in patients with cirrhosis of the liver. *Kidney International* 23:303, 1983.

Conn, H. O. Spontaneous Bacterial Peritonitis and Other Infections. In L. Schiff (ed.), *Disease of the Liver* (5th ed.). Philadelphia: Lippincott, 1982. Pp. 948–955.

Crossley, I. R., and Williams, R. Spontaneous bacterial peritonitis. *Gut* 26:325, 1985.

Epstein, M. Derangements of renal water handling in liver disease. *Gastroenterology* 89:1415, 1985.

Fraser, C. L., and Arieff, A. I. Hepatic encephalopathy. *N. Engl. J. Med.* 313:865, 1986.

Garcia-Tsao, G., et al. Portal pressure, presence of gastroesophageal varices and variceal bleeding. *Hepatology* 5:419, 1985.

Grace, N. D. Is sclerotherapy the treatment of choice for bleeding esophageal varices? *Mayo Clinic Proc.* 5:584, 1985.

Groszmann, R. J., and Atterbury, C. E. The pathophysiology of portal hypertension: A basis for classification. *Semin. Liver Dis.* 2:177, 1982.

Hoefs, J. C., et al. Spontaneous bacterial peritonitis. *Hepatology* 2:399, 1982.

Kandel, G., and Diamont, N. E. A clinical view of recent advances in ascites. *J. Clin. Gastroenterol.* 8:85–90, 1986.

Kelly, D. A., and Tuddenham, E. G. D. Hemostatic problems in liver disease. *Gut* 27:339, 1986.

Lebrec, D., et al. Portal hypertension, size of esophageal varices and risk of gastrointestinal bleeding in alcoholic cirrhosis. *Gastroenterology* 79:1139, 1980.

Levy, M. Pathophysiology of Ascites Formation. In *The Kidney in Liver Disease* (2nd ed.). New York: Elsevier, 1983.

Levy, M. Hepatorenal Syndrome. In D. N. Seldin and G. Giebisch (eds.), *The Kidney, Physiology and Pathophysiology* (vol. 2). New York: Raven, 1985. Pp. 1945–1962.

Levy, M., and Wexler, M. J. Salt and water balance in liver disease. *Hosp. Pract.* July 1984, Pp. 57–71.

Linas, S. L., et al. The Rational Use of Diuretics in Cirrhosis. In *The Kidney and Liver Disease* (2nd ed.). New York: Elsevier, 1983.

Martinez, J., and Palascak, J. E. Hemostatic alterations in liver disease. In Zakim and Boyer (eds.), *Hepatology*. Philadelphia: Saunders, 1982.

Ohnishi, K., et al. Pulsed doppler flow as a criterion of portal venous velocity: Comparison with cine angiographic measurements. *Radiology* 154:495, 1985.

Papper, S. Hepatorenal syndrome. In M. Epstein (ed.), *The Kidney in Liver Disease* (2nd ed.). New York: Elsevier, 1983.

Renal failure in the patient with cirrhosis: The role of active vasoconstriction. *Am. J. Med.* 49:175, 1970.

Schenker, S., and Hoyumpa, A. M., Jr. Pathophysiology of hepatic encephalopathy. *Hosp. Pract.*, September 1984, Pp. 99–121.

18 : Neoplasms of the Liver

Jerome B. Zeldis

It is not surprising that neoplasms in the liver are exceedingly common. The liver is the largest and one of the most metabolically active visceral organs, with a blood flow greater than one fourth of the cardiac output. It is constantly exposed to the portal circulation, with its effluent from the gastrointestinal tract containing environmental toxins, metabolic by-products of digestion, and compounds synthesized by the gastrointestinal flora. Furthermore, hepatocytes may become infected with a variety of viruses that injure and stimulate the cells to replicate and perhaps undergo oncogenic transformation (i.e., become cancerous). Despite this, the most common neoplasms in the liver in the Western world are metastatic disease of cancers of other organs. The rarity of primary tumors of the liver in nineteenth century Germany caused the pathologist Virchow to conclude that organs that are common sites for metastases rarely develop primary cancers. This "Virchow's dictum" was commonly believed until excellent epidemiologic studies in the mid-twentieth century demonstrated that primary cancer of the liver and bile ducts are the most common visceral cancers in the world, with more than 2 million cases a year.

Primary Malignant Tumors

Primary Hepatocellular Carcinoma

Primary hepatocellular carcinoma (PHCC) is the most common visceral cancer in the world. In the past three decades, major advances in the understanding of the etiology, epidemiology, and pathogenesis of PHCC have been made. It is now clear that PHCC arises in individuals who have continued hepatocyte injury and regeneration. Hepatocytes are long-lived and replicate only a few times during a lifetime. During cellular replication and repair, the hepatocyte's DNA becomes more vulnerable to mutations and rearrangements — cytogenetic events that may lead to malignant transformation. Whereas various factors to be described here are associated with hepatocellular carcinoma, the process by which any of these factors causes liver cancer has not yet been explained adequately.

Cirrhosis

Hepatocellular carcinoma often arises in the setting of a cirrhotic liver. Although the most common etiology of cirrhosis on
a worldwide basis is chronic hepatitis B infection, PHCC has
been noted to occur in cirrhotic livers as a result of almost any
etiology, including hemochromatosis, alcohol abuse, and
alpha$_1$-antitrypsin deficiency. PHCC occurs more often in the
presence of macronodular cirrhosis, presumably because the
hepatocytes are undergoing more DNA replication than in micronodular cirrhotic livers. Frequently, PHCC will develop in an
alcoholic cirrhotic who had micronodular cirrhosis, but, upon
prolonged abstinence from alcohol, subsequently developed
macronodular cirrhosis. The risk of developing malignancy in a
patient with macronodular cirrhosis in the West is approximately 10 percent; whereas in Africa and the Far East, it is as
high as 50 percent. This epidemiologic difference supports the
hypothesis that factors in addition to cirrhosis are involved in
the malignant transformation of the liver. Also supporting this
hypothesis is the observation that not all patients with
hepatocellular carcinoma have cirrhotic livers or chronic active
hepatitis. Even though most cases of PHCC in Southeast Asia
occur in the setting of a cirrhotic liver, more than half of the
patients in Africa with PHCC do not have cirrhosis. Furthermore, PHCC rarely, if ever, occurs in patients who have cirrhosis owing to primary biliary cirrhosis, Wilson's disease, and
Indian childhood cirrhosis.

Hepatitis Viruses

Please refer to Chap. 13 for the biology, pathophysiology, and
nomenclature of the hepatitis viruses. Approximately 200 million people are chronically infected with hepatitis B virus (HBV),
making it one of the most common viral illnesses in the world.
Recent epidemiologic studies have demonstrated a strong association between chronic HBV infection and hepatocellular carcinoma. It is therefore not surprising that PHCC is one of the most
common carcinomas in the world. A strong parallelism exists
between the frequency of HBV carrier rates and the incidence of
PHCC. Patients with PHCC who are HBsAg negative often have
other serum markers of present or past HBV infection. PHCC is
often clustered amongst closely related individuals who are
HBsAg positive. One of the best prospective studies into the
relationship between HBV and PHCC was performed in Taiwan,
where more than 22,000 male government employees were
studied. The incidence of PHCC in HBsAg-positive Taiwanese
males was greater than 200 times that of HBsAg-negative males.
The few HBsAg-negative patients who developed PHCC had
other serologic markers for HBV infection. Furthermore, the

incidence of PHCC correlated not only with HBV carriage but also with the severity of the liver disease. HBsAg-positive cirrhotics had a 900 times greater incidence of PHCC than did HBsAg-negative Taiwanese males. These data support the hypothesis that HBV serves as an agent for continued hepatocyte injury and regeneration that somehow leads to oncogenic transformation.

The highest incidence of PHCC occurs in sub-Saharan Africa and Southeast Asia, where usually at least 10 years elapse between initial HBV infection and the discovery of PHCC. In Southeast Asia, most afflicted individuals become infected with HBV during the first year of life. Hepatocellular carcinoma is rare, however, in children younger than ten years of age and usually occurs in the third and fourth decade in a cirrhotic liver. In Africa, hepatitis B virus infections occur during childhood, yet hepatocellular carcinoma occurs in the second and third decade, a younger age than that in most Southeast Asians. Half of the Africans do not have cirrhosis.

Most hepatocellular carcinomas contain HBV DNA insertions (Fig. 18-1). In areas of high endemic rates of HBV infection, greater than 80 percent of tumors contain HBV DNA sequences. Since these tumors have marked karyotypic changes (i.e., changes in chromosomal structure and number), it is intriguing to hypothesize that the 10 to 20 percent of tumors that lacked HBV DNA sequences lost their viral DNA sequences through the process of chromosomal rearrangement and deletion. On the other hand, not all hepatocellular carcinomas are associated with HBV infection. For example, infants born with tyrosinemia may develop hepatocellular carcinoma soon after birth. Patients with alpha$_1$-antitrypsin deficiency may also develop hepatocellular carcinoma. These conditions are not thought to involve HBV infections. On the other hand, HBV DNA sequences have been found in the tumors of patients who lacked any serologic evidence of a current or previous HBV infection. These individuals had cirrhosis that had been attributed to chronic alcoholism or hemochromatosis. Presumably, these individuals had an HBV infection for a long period of time before they developed PHCC and lost all serologic markers of the HBV infection. In light of these findings, it is clear that any possible association between putative oncogenic factors and hepatocellular carcinoma must be reevaluated from the perspective of whether HBV DNA sequences are present in the liver cancers.

The pathogenic mechanisms by which a chronic HBV infection causes hepatocellular carcinoma remains to be elucidated. The integrated HBV DNA sequences may have a direct role in the

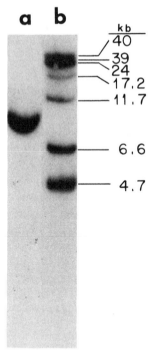

Fig. 18-1
HBV DNA integration patterns of two PHCCs. Chromosomal DNA was digested with a restriction enzyme that does not cut HBV DNA. Since the HBV DNA is integrated into the cellular chromosomes, the size of the DNA bands is greater than 3.2 kb, the length of the HBV genome. Tumor a had a single HBV DNA insertion approximately 10 kb in length after restriction digestion, and tumor b had at least seven HBV DNA insertions.

oncogenic process or may be nothing more than an epiphenomenon, a chromosomal marker of a chronic infection. Furthermore, some tumors contain episomal (nonintegrated HBV DNA) and maintain viral replication. Nude mice have been transplanted with such tumors, and the mouse sera have been found to contain viral particles and other markers of viral replication, a remarkable finding since HBV grows only in humans and primates.

Both epidemiologic and molecular biological studies into the association between PHCC and HBV suggest that hepatitis B virus behaves like a tumor virus that lacks oncogenes — genes that confer a malignant phenotype to cells. In experimental models of viral oncogenesis, viruses may be classified into those that lack or contain oncogenes. Oncogene-containing viruses often have a short incubation period between initial infection and tumor formation. Viruses that lack oncogenes usually induce tumors after a long period of time. The four possible gene products of HBV have not yet been shown to have any onco-genic properties. HBV does, however, contain a DNA sequence that "enhances" the transcription of neighboring genes. Many oncogenic viruses contain similar enhancing type sequences. One oncogenic virus in chickens has been demonstrated to cause malignant transformation by integrating near cellular on-cogenes (the "proto-oncogenes") and enhancing their tran-scription. Although it is tempting to believe that HBV may be-have similarly, only one instance of a HBV DNA integration near a known cellular oncogene has been described.

HBV DNA integrations have been found in every chromosome and are usually found in more than one chromosome of any particular tumor. In one case, the multiple HBV DNA inser-tions served as sites for "illegitimate" recombination between chromosomes. Whether this mechanism is the major cause of the karyotypic changes observed in PHCC tumors remains to be determined. Recent studies have demonstrated that PHCC tumors that contain HBV DNA often have chromosomal re-arrangements and deletions in sites independent of the viral DNA insertion. Whether HBV directly plays a role in these chromosomal rearrangements is not yet known.

Knowledge about the structure of the integrated HBV DNA se-quences in hepatocellular carcinomas has been limited; how-ever, in the few cases studied, none of these insertions con-tained an intact viral genome. Instead, the integrated viral chromosome had been scrambled with integrations, deletions, inversions, and duplications.

HBV is just one of a family of hepadna viruses known to infect the livers of various animals. In captivity, PHCC has been de-tected in Beechey ground squirrels, Eastern woodchucks, and Peking ducks chronically infected with their respective hepadna viruses. One hundred percent of woodchucks who are neona-tally infected with the woodchuck hepatitis virus who have chronic infections will develop hepatocellular carcinoma by the time they are 2 years old. Often, more than one tumor will occur simultaneously, and the chromosomal integration patterns of the woodchuck hepatitis virus DNA are different in the concur-rent tumors. As in humans, the tumor cells have multiple karyo-typic changes and multiple viral DNA integrations.

An association between PHCC and etiologies of viral hepati-tis other than HBV either does not exist or remains to be elucidated. There is no relationship between hepatitis A virus infection and liver cancer. Chronic hepatitis D virus infection (HDV, the delta agent) is negatively correlated with the inci-dence of primary hepatocellular carcinoma. Presumably, this is due to premature death from end-stage HDV-induced liver disease occurring before liver cancer has a chance to develop (see Chap. 13). PHCC following well-documented chronic active hepatitis owing to non-A, non-B hepatitis agents has been described. The difficulty with these studies is that there are no markers for non-A, non-B agents, so the viral etiology of the chronic hepatitis can only be surmised. Furthermore, in most reported cases, the liver cancer was not investigated to determine whether it contained HBV DNA sequences. As described previously, some patients with PHCC lack serologic evidence of HBV infection but have tumors containing HBV DNA. In Japan, despite the rising incidence of PHCC, the proportion of affected patients who have HBV serologic markers is declining. The rise in the rate of PHCC coincides with the introduction of post-transfusion non-A, non-B hepatitis to Japan. While it is tempting to attribute non-A, non-B hepatitis to the rise in cases of PHCC in Japan, this relationship remains to be firmly established. The intriguing aspect about post-transfusion non-A, non-B hepatitis is that approximately 10 percent of those persons infected will develop cirrhosis — a major predisposing condition for hepatic malignant transformation. Until markers for the non-A, non-B hepatitis agents are described and better prospective studies of patients chronically infected with post-transfusion non-A, non-B hepatitis are performed, a relationship between hepatocellular carcinoma and non-A, non-B hepatitis remains unestablished.

Chemical Carcinogenesis

Despite a large list of compounds that have been shown to be carcinogenic in animals, relatively few compounds have been demonstrated to induce tumors in humans. Even fewer have been unequivocally shown to cause hepatocellular carcinoma in higher primates or humans. Both rats and fish often form tumors of the liver in response to exposure to numerous chemical carcinogens. In fact, one way of monitoring water pollution is to determine the incidence of hepatocellular carcinoma in fish. Unfortunately, what has been learned about the pathogenesis of PHCC in these two animal models may not be applicable to humans.

Aflatoxin, AFB_1, is the most well-characterized chemical carcinogen that both induces liver cancer in humans and is found in foodstuffs. This mycotoxin is produced by the fungi, *Aspergillus flavus* and *Aspergillus parasiticus*. In addition to hepatocellular carcinoma, aflatoxin exposure is also associated with bile duct carcinoma, pancreatic carcinoma, hemangiomas, and osteogenic carcinoma in monkeys. Aflatoxin is metabolized to an active epoxide in the liver that reacts with DNA. This interaction may be the cause of aflatoxin's oncogenic action. Aflatoxin is produced by fungal contamination of food and is found in higher concentrations in grain that has been stored in dark and damp areas. The incidence of hepatocellular carcinoma in men roughly correlates with the daily intake of aflatoxin. In one study, the incidence of PHCC in men in the high altitudes of Kenya was 3.1 per 100,000 population, whereas the dietary intake of aflatoxin was 3 to 5 mg/kg body weight per day. In the more moist lowlands of Kenya, the incidence of PHCC was 12.9 per 100,000 population, and the dietary intake of aflatoxin was 6 to 8 mg/kg body weight per day. In Mozambique, where the dietary intake of aflatoxin is 222 mg/kg/day, the incidence of PHCC was 35 per 100,000 population. While ingestion of large amounts of aflatoxin can cause an acute hepatitis, it is thought that chronic exposure to aflatoxin is needed to cause cancer.

Other chemical compounds that cause liver tumors and hepatitis in laboratory animals and that are commonly ingested in foodstuffs include the mycotoxins, luteoskyrin and cyclochlorotrine; plant-derived carcinogens, including cycasin and saffrole (a constituent of sassafras root); nitrosamines; chlorinated hydrocarbons; organochlorine pesticides; androgenic anabolic steroids; and oral contraceptives. Although each is carcinogenic in experimental animals, none have yet been implicated as etiologies of human PHCC. Alcohol abuse increases the risk of PHCC in the setting of chronic HBV infection. Whether alcohol is by itself a carcinogen remains to be determined. Exposure to the radioactive dye thorotrast (thorium dioxide) and chronic arsenic exposure have also been associated with the induction of human liver tumors.

Other Associated Conditions

Numerous chronic liver diseases have been associated with increased incidence of PHCC. It is not known whether the metabolic abnormality causing the disease or the cirrhotic state induced by the condition is the oncogenic factor. Almost every metabolic cause of cirrhosis has been associated with PHCC, including hemochromatosis, alpha$_1$-antitrypsin deficiency, and tyrosinemia. Cases of PHCC have been associated with autoimmune chronic hepatitis, membranous Budd-Chiari syndrome, and hepatic syphilis. With the advent of molecular probes for HBV DNA, tumors that arise in individuals with these conditions must be evaluated to determine whether HBV was also involved with the pathogenesis of these tumors. In one small survey of liver cancers in patients with hemochromatosis, about half of the tumors contained integrated HBV DNA despite the absence of serologic markers consistent with active viral replication. Despite this, the incidence of PHCC in hemochromatosis with cirrhosis ranges from 10 to 40 percent in various surveys. HBV is probably not involved in the genesis of PHCC in most of these cancers.

Epidemiology

PHCC is found most frequently in sub-Sahara Africa and Southeast Asia — the areas of the world that have the highest incidence of HBV infection. The multifactorial etiology of the illness is illustrated by the correlation of the incidence of cancer to aflatoxin ingestion in populations where the frequency of HBV is uniform. Similarly, in the People's Republic of China, the annual incidence of PHCC was 6 to 10 times greater in those who drank water from ditches as opposed to those who drank well water. The brackish water from the ditches contained large concentrations of organochlorine pesticides and organic matter. After the population started drinking well water, the incidence of PHCC 5 years later was reduced by 20 to 35 percent in the same population.

Primary liver cancer is two to four times more frequent in men than in women. This relationship is true both in areas of high frequency of PHCC such as Mozambique and areas with low frequency such as Finland. Possible reasons for the sex difference include (1) chronic hepatitis B and non-A, non-B infections are more frequent in men than in women, and (2) men may have greater exposure to occupational and environmental carcinogens.

The annual incidence of PHCC increases with age. Furthermore, the average age of a population that develops liver cancer appears to be environmentally mediated. For example, the average age of developing PHCC has decreased by 10 years in South African blacks who have moved from rural environments to urban environments. The incidence of liver cancer is decreasing in some populations and increasing in others. In South Africa and the United States, the incidence of PHCC has declined. However, from 1959 to 1981, the incidence of liver cancer in Japan has increased from 1.7 to 5.4 percent of all autopsies. The reason for this disparity remains to be elucidated.

Pathology

Hepatocellular carcinoma has traditionally been classified into three types: nodular, diffuse, and massive. Nodular PHCC usually involves well-differentiated tumors that occur in the setting of a cirrhotic liver. If detected while small, the tumor may be completely resected. The massive type often occurs in a noncirrhotic liver and consists of a circumscribed mass occupying a large part of the liver, often with satellite nodules. This type of hepatocellular carcinoma is prone to rupture. The third type, diffuse PHCC, infiltrates the liver in a homogenous pattern and is difficult to distinguish from regenerating nodules. Recently, other classifications of the gross anatomy of PHCC have been defined. It is not clear whether any of these classifications help to distinguish the etiology or prognosis of one tumor from another.

On gross inspection, the tumors are often gray in appearance but may be bile stained if the hepatocytes are secreting bile (Fig. 18-2). Histologically, the tumors may be extremely well differentiated, resembling normal liver cells, or extremely anaplastic, resembling other undifferentiated cancers such as "oat cell carcinoma" at the light microscopic level. The well-differentiated tumors may form cords of cells similar to those seen in peliosis hepatis with intrasinusoidal mesenchymal cells resembling Kupffer's cells, or the cells form gland-like structures. In well-differentiated PHCC, the appearance of these cords may be difficult to distinguish from normal liver except for the absence of portal tracts and central veins and invasion of arteries and veins with tumor cells. A "skinny needle" biopsy of the liver often samples hepatocytes but spares architectural details such as portal tracts and central veins. Such a biopsy of a well-differentiated PHCC may be very difficult to distinguish from normal hepatic parenchyma if no architectural structures are seen. The tumor cells may secrete bile, depending on their stage of differentiation. Globules may be seen inside the cells if they are producing alpha-fetoprotein, alpha$_1$-antitrypsin, and other liver-specific proteins. Approximately 1 of 20 tumors will histologically resemble both hepatocellular carcinoma and cholangiocarcinoma.

Hepatocellular carcinoma frequently invades the vascular supply of the liver, resulting in portal vein thrombosis, hepatic artery occlusions, and obstruction of the inferior vena cava. Rarely, the tumor may spread from the liver into the right atrium by way of local invasion of the inferior vena cava. The most common site for metastases is the lung. Much less often, the tumor will spread to the adrenal gland, bone marrow, brain, pancreas, and kidney. PHCC also spreads to the lymphatic drainage of the liver and abdomen. In about 10 percent of cases in Africa, the tumor will rupture, resulting in hemoperitoneum.

Clinical Aspects
Most patients with early hepatocellular carcinoma are completely asymptomatic. Usually only after the tumor has grown to

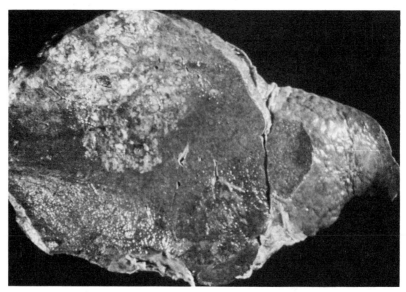

Fig. 18-2
Gross appearance of a PHCC arising from a cirrhotic liver with hemo-chromatosis. Note the nodular surface of the liver owing to cirrhosis. (Courtesy of Dr. Donald Antonioli.)

an advanced stage will a diagnosis be made. Most commonly, patients will describe an abdominal discomfort, a fullness in the right upper abdomen with or without a palpable mass. Less than 40 percent of patients will also complain of malaise, anorexia, fever, weight loss, and jaundice. None of these symptoms are specific for hepatocellular carcinoma. Infrequently, the tumor ruptures the liver and the patient presents in shock with bloody ascites. On physical examination, patients may appear normal or have hepatomegaly, cachexia, arterovenous bruits, and ascites. If the portal vein becomes obstructed, the cirrhotic patient with PHCC may present with bleeding esophageal varices and worsening ascites. PHCC must be considered in any cirrhotic who develops new or worsening complications such as jaundice, encephalopathy, ascites, and bleeding.

A variety of paraneoplastic syndromes have been associated with PHCC, including erythrocytosis, hypoglycemia, hypercalcemia, sexual precocity, dysfibrinogenemia, hypertrophic pulmonary osteoarthropathy, carcinoid syndrome, and porphyria cutanea tarda. The increase in erythrocytosis occurs in approximately 5 percent of patients with hepatocellular carcinoma. This is probably due to the release of an enzyme that converts a serum protein to erythropoietin rather than tumor production of erythropoietin. The hypoglycemia may be due to a combination of release of insulin-like hormones from the tumors, increased glucose utilization by the tumor, and decreased glucose production by the liver. Similarly, hypercalcemia is probably due to production of parathormone-like substances by the tumor. Sexual precocity results from production of gonadotropin. The other paraneoplastic syndromes are also directly related to products released by the neoplastic tissue.

Routine laboratory data are usually not diagnostic except for values related to the paraneoplastic syndromes just mentioned. The white count may be slightly elevated. Mild elevations of the alkaline phosphatase, AST, ALT (AST is usually greater than ALT), LDH, and GTT may occur. Large elevations of the serum alpha-fetoprotein (AFP) are virtually diagnostic for hepatocellular carcinoma. In Southeast Asia, more than 70 percent of patients with PHCC have elevated serum alpha-fetoprotein levels. In other parts of the world such as in the United States, a much smaller percentage of the afflicted patients will have elevations of this 70 kD protein. AFP is the major plasma oncotic protein in the fetus. During embryogenesis, the liver cells stop making AFP and begin to synthesize albumin. Hepatocytes also make AFP when they are injured, undergo regeneration, and take part in neoplastic transformation. The size of a PHCC tumor roughly correlates with the serum concentration of AFP; however, this relationship is not perfect. Small tumors may be associated with very high serum concentrations. Surveillance of AFP levels in patients at risk for developing PHCC has identified individuals who had minute tumors that were subsequently resected for cure. In addition to PHCC, malignant germ cell tumors may also cause elevated levels of AFP, but this is usually not a source of confusion. Individuals with regenerating liver and pregnant women will also have mildly elevated concentrations of AFP.

Isoenzymes of gamma-glutamyl transferase (GTT) and variants of alkaline phosphatase and of transcobalamin I have been identified in patients with hepatocellular carcinoma. These markers are not as specific as AFP. Patients may also have an elevated carcinoembryonic antigen (CEA).

Ultrasonography is excellent for identifying tumor masses, but this technique is unable to distinguish a small tumor from regenerating nodules in the cirrhotic liver. Furthermore, in the diffuse type of PHCC, sonograms may fail to distinguish the infiltrating tumor from normal hepatic parenchyma. Similar problems exist for computerized tomographic (CT) scans of the liver. The x-ray density of the tumors may resemble that of normal hepatic tissue and may not enhance with contrast. Despite this, the majority of primary hepatocellular carcinomas can be identified by either ultrasonography or CT scans. These techniques are usually unable to distinguish PHCC from metastatic lesions in the liver. During ultrasonography, Doppler determinations of the portal vein can be made. A tumor mass in the liver associated with a portal vein thrombosis in the appropriate epidemiologic setting is usually hepatocellular carcinoma. Liver/spleen radionuclide scanning is able to identify tumors greater than 2 to 3 cm in diameter; however, occasionally, the tumors will take up the radionuclide and appear invisible on the scan. Similarly, PHCC may take up gallium, but this is not specific. Short of performing a liver biopsy, hepatic angiography is the best means of making the diagnosis of hepatocellular carcinoma. Besides being a useful diagnostic adjunct, angiography allows for a determination of the possible resectability of the tumor. PHCC derives its circulation from the hepatic artery. The neovascularization associated with PHCC is fairly distinctive. "Vascular lakes" seen in angiography typical to PHCC also confirm the diagnosis. In one series of 170 cases of advanced PHCC, the correct diagnosis was made in 96 percent of cases by hepatic arteriography. Despite the tumor's vascularity, the diagnosis may be made safely by biopsy.

Prognosis, Prevention, and Treatment

Although the diagnosis of hepatocellular carcinoma is usually made prior to death, the size and metastatic spread of the tumor by the time diagnosis is established commonly precludes cure. Survival is usually measured in weeks, but occasionally, a patient lives for as long as 2 years. An exception to this is fibrolamellar carcinoma (see the following section). Patients who have minute PHCC will often survive 2 to 4 years before succumbing to the tumor. If the tumor is completely resected, most patients will have their AFP return to normal, and, for all intents and purposes, the tumor has been cured. The remaining liver in these resected patients, however, is still predisposed for developing other PHCC. Surgical cures of minute PHCC with subsequent development of a second or third minute tumor have been reported. Most clinicians who deal with PHCC therefore recommend frequent surveillance by ultrasound and AFP determinations in patients who are at risk for developing PHCC, including those who have had surgical resection of a minute PHCC. The 1-year survival rates of patients who have had liver transplantation for PHCC have been dismal except in those cases in which a minute cancer was incidentally found. Presumably, the poor survival rates are because the tumor had spread beyond the confines of the resected liver.

Nonsurgical therapies are ineffective. The tumors rarely respond to radiation and chemotherapy. Although tumors have been shown to shrink or become de-bulked by devascularization procedures using angiography, most patients will succumb in weeks to months. Recently, a number of experimental approaches have been developed to try to take advantage of differences between the tumor and normal hepatic tissues. These include the use of toxins linked to monoclonal antibodies directed against tumor-specific antigens and selective metabolic rescue schemes. The latter approach is based on the knowledge that some tumors lack receptors that are present on normal liver cells. These tumors still maintain some metabolic pathways that are distinct for the liver and are susceptible to the same hepatotoxins that affect normal liver. For example, both the liver and certain PHCC cells are killed by acetaminophen. This toxicity is reversed with N-acetyl-L-cysteine. If this antidote is linked to a protein that is taken up only by the liver and if the tumor lacks receptors for this protein, acetaminophen administration with the protein conjugated antidote will result in tumor killing but survival of normal liver that takes up the antidote. Both experimental approaches using monoclonal antibody–directed chemotherapy and selective metabolic rescue have been shown to prolong survival in animal models for hepatocellular carcinoma. The application of these strategies in humans awaits further refinements of these techniques.

Fibrolamellar Hepatocellular Carcinoma

Fibrolamellar hepatocellular carcinoma (FLC), or polygonal cell carcinoma, accounts for 20 to 40 percent of all cases of PHCC in young adults. There are no known etiologic associations for FLC. Unlike PHCC, fibrolamellar carcinoma is unassociated with HBV exposure, has an equal sex distribution, and usually occurs in the setting of a noncirrhotic liver. The tumor typically forms a large mass occupying either lobe and microscopically contains polygonal eosinophilic cells and large fibrous bands. The patient usually comes to attention because of abdominal swelling or discomfort. Laboratory findings are nonspecific, and the AFP is usually normal or only moderately increased. Of note is a marked elevation in the serum vitamin B_{12} binding capacity owing to an increase in a vitamin B_{12} binding protein that differs from transcobalamin I in that it contains more sialic acid residues. Diagnosis is made by biopsy but may be suggested by hepatic angiography. Unlike hepatocellular carcinoma, FLC has a favorable prognosis, with long-term survivals following surgical resection or liver transplantation. Survival as long as 21 years have been recorded after hepatic resection. In further contrast to PHCC, the overall mean survival is 5 years, with one patient living as long as 16 years after initial diagnosis of a nonresectable FLC.

Cholangio-
carcinoma

Carcinoma of the bile ducts, cholangiocarcinoma, may either arise in the intrahepatic or extrahepatic biliary systems. The incidence of cholangiocarcinoma is between one fifth and one twentieth that of PHCC, depending on the population studied. It usually occurs in people older than 40 years of age, being rare in those younger than 40 years. Although there is a male predominance to the disease, it is not as marked as in PHCC. Like hepatocellular carcinoma, the major underlying condition that appears to predispose patients to developing cancer of the bile ducts is chronic inflammation of the biliary tract. The only chemical agent that has been unequivocally demonstrated to cause cholangiocarcinoma in humans is the radioactive dye thorotrast that had formerly been used as a radionuclide for liver/spleen scans. In China and Korea, liver fluke infestations with *Clonorchis sinensis* and *Opisthorchis viverrini* are associated with cholangiocarcinoma. Other predisposing conditions for cholangiocarcinoma include chronic typhoid carrier state, longstanding inflammatory bowel disease with or without sclerosing cholangitis, congenital biliary atresia, and other developmental abnormalities of the bile ducts, including cystic dilatation of intrahepatic bile ducts (Caroli's disease). A relationship between gallstones and cancer of the bile ducts remains to be established. A few cases of alpha$_1$-antitrypsin deficiency have also been associated with cholangiocarcinoma.

The grayish white tumor forms either a single firm nodule or multiple nodules that are locally invasive and grow along the biliary tract. Lymphatic spread occurs in about one half the cases, but hematogenous spread is rare. Microscopically, the tumors are adenocarcinomas with a slightly granular eosinophilic cytoplasm. The tumors often evoke abundant scarring (desmoplastic reaction). This results is a very hard firm tumor that is difficult to biopsy.

Like hepatocellular carcinoma, most signs and symptoms of cholangiocarcinoma are not specific; malaise, weight loss, and right upper abdomen discomfort are often prominent. The extrahepatic tumors will eventually obstruct the biliary tree and result in jaundice. Since cholangiocarcinoma does not make AFP and is not associated with HBV infection, neither AFP nor HBsAg are helpful for making the diagnosis. Often, the alkaline phosphatase and 5'-nucleotidase will be markedly elevated. Ultrasound and CT scans will often reveal a mass in the liver, and the biliary tree may be dilated proximal to the tumor. Although hepatic angiography will distinguish this hypovascular tumor from PHCC, the diagnosis is best made by visualization of the biliary tree by percutaneous transhepatic cholangiography (PTC) or endoscopic retrograde cholangiopancreatography (ERCP).

Rarely, a tumor may obstruct the common bile duct early and be surgically resectable. In one series, cholangiocarcinomas of the distal common bile duct had a 15 percent 5-year survival after surgical resection. These tumors constitute only a minority of all cholangiocarcinomas. Most cancers of the common bile duct have a much more dismal prognosis. These adenocarcinomas are slow growing and will usually result in the patient dying of hepatic failure. Palliative procedures such as partial hepatic resection and passage of stents through the tumor to decompress an obstructed biliary tree may prolong the survival of afflicted patients. Unfortunately, most tumors have spread beyond the confines of the liver to be cured by liver transplantation.

Hemangio-sarcoma

Hemangiosarcoma is an extremely rare tumor and has also been called angiosarcoma or Kupffer's cell sarcoma. Although it is the most common malignant mesenchymal tumor of the liver, only 10 to 20 cases per year occur in the United States. Despite its rarity, the tumor is of special interest because of its strong association with a number of environmental toxins. Hemangiosarcomas result from exposure to thorotrast, chronic arsenic exposure, vinyl chloride resin (used in the synthesis of plastics), radium, anabolic steroids, phenethylhydrazine (an MAO inhibitor used as an antidepressant), and inorganic copper. Pathologically, the tumors usually form a single tumor mass with satellite lesions invading the entire liver. On cut section, large vascular cysts are revealed that are virtually diagnostic of the tumor (Fig. 18-3). Microscopically, the sinusoids may be dilated, resembling peliosis hepatis; however, vascular invasion of the tumor is also usually seen. Invasion of the portal veins and central veins occurs in the majority of cases. The tumor usually occurs in the elderly, with a peak incidence in the sixth and seventh decades. Like hepatocellular carcinoma, hemangiosarcoma has a male predominance of approximately four to one. Few signs and symptoms are specific for the tumor, with the majority of patients presenting with hepatomegaly. Diagnosis is made noninvasively by ultrasound, CT scan, or hepatic angiography. Because the tumor is so vascular, needle biopsy is hazardous and may result in a life-threatening hemorrhage. The tumors are rarely surgically resectable, and most patients succumb to the disease.

Hepatoblastoma

Embryonal hepatoblastoma is the most common hepatic malignancy of childhood. Although etiologic factors have not been associated with this tumor, affected individuals occasionally have other congenital malformations, including polycystic disease of the kidneys, abnormalities of the renal collecting system, Meckel's diverticulum, cardiac defects, congenital absence

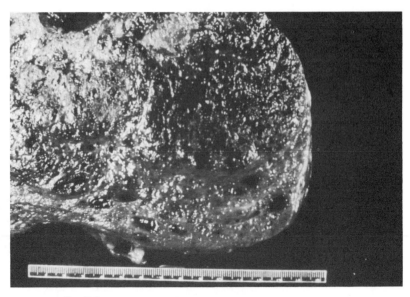

Fig. 18-3
Cut section of a hemangiosarcoma revealing large vascular cysts. (Courtesy of Dr. Donald Antonioli.)

of the right adrenal, and hydrocele. The tumors sometimes secrete human chorionic gonadotropin (HCG) and produce sexual precocity. Familial clustering of the tumor has also been described.

Hepatoblastoma usually presents as an encapsulated or well-circumscribed large solitary tumor, although occasionally, multiple masses are present. Grossly, the tumor is classified as an epithelial type composed of fetal-appearing hepatocytes and a mixed type that is often lobulated and composed of cells of mesenchymal and epithelial origin. As in the fetal liver, extramedullary hematopoiesis may be present in the fetal type of tumor. The mixed type also contains smooth muscle fibers, blood vessels, and cartilage. Patients usually present within the first 3 years of life with abdominal distention. Like most other hepatic malignancies, there is a male predominance. Plain films of the abdomen may reveal calcifications in the tumor. Blood tests are unremarkable except for an elevated AFP. Since the tumor is usually solitary and well circumscribed and metastasizes only late in its course, surgical resection for cure is possible. In those individuals whose tumors are so large that they are not immediately surgically resectable, palliation and cures have been achieved by chemotherapy to shrink the size of the tumor prior to surgical resection. In the absence of surgery, the prognosis is poor.

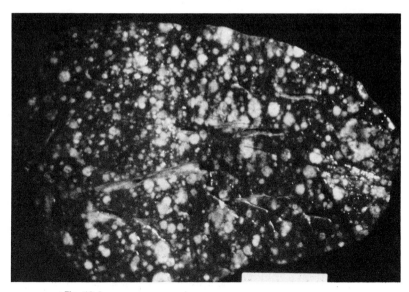

Fig. 18-4
Metastatic breast cancer. Note the buckshot distribution of the numerous breast cancer metastases. (Courtesy of Dr. Donald Antonioli.)

Neoplasms of Nonhepatic Origin

Metastatic carcinoma, leukemias, and lymphomas often affect the liver. In the United States, 40 percent of all patients dying of cancer have hepatic metastases, and 10 percent of these patients will die of liver failure.

Most metastatic disease probably reaches the liver by way of the circulation. The tumor cells usually behave and histologically resemble the tissue of origin. For example, neuroendocrine tumors often secrete hormones producing syndromes such as the carcinoid syndrome. Because the liver drains the portal system, carcinomas of the gastrointestinal tract often have metastatic involvement of the liver. Carcinomas of the lung and breast, two cancers that have early hematogenous spread, also frequently involve the liver (Fig. 18-4). With the exception of sarcomas and cancers of the head and neck, most cancers will metastasize to the liver. Metastases are usually multiple. If the tumors evoke scarring (e.g., a desmoplastic reaction) in their primary site, similar reactions will occur in the liver. Often, the tumor cells will grow in the sinusoids, crowding out hepatocytes and eventually will replace the hepatic parenchyma. Because only a small percentage of functioning liver is needed to maintain life, massive replacement of the hepatic parenchyma with tumor can occur by metastatic disease before this comes to the attention of the clinician. Rarely, metastatic disease will occur as a single or limited number of tumor nodules, which, if resected, can result in a cure.

Clinically, patients may complain of a discomfort in their right upper abdomen. The liver is found to be enlarged and may feel either hard or nodular, depending on the extent of metastases and whether a desmoplastic reaction is occurring. Occasionally, a bruit caused by neovascularization of the metastatic tumor is heard. The majority of patients with advanced disease will have anorexia and weight loss. Paraneoplastic syndromes such as flushing that occurs with carcinoids may become evident with hepatic metastases of certain tumors.

The diagnosis of metastatic carcinoma is usually suggested by ultrasound or CT and is confirmed by biopsy. Each technique can detect lesions as small as a few millimeters, although the accuracy of the technique depends on the skill of the radiologist and the technicians who perform the procedure. Radionuclide liver/spleen scanning will detect metastatic disease in lesions that are greater than 1 cm in diameter. Technetium sulfur colloid is taken up by Kupffer's cells. Areas of metastatic disease lack Kupffer's cells and appear as "cold spots" in the liver/spleen scan. Despite recent advances in the noninvasive imaging techniques, liver biopsy remains the definitive procedure for determining whether metastatic carcinoma in the liver is present. Often, the histologic appearance of the tumor will suggest its origin. In many patients with newly diagnosed metastatic adenocarcinoma to the liver, a primary tumor source cannot be determined despite extensive diagnostic studies. Angiography of the liver is rarely used to make the primary diagnosis of hepatic metastases because it is an invasive and morbid diagnostic procedure. However, angiography is used if surgical resection is contemplated, since it will elucidate the vascular supply of the metastases and the extent of disease.

Even though systemic chemotherapy, radiation therapy, and localized infusion of chemotherapeutic agents are common treatments for metastatic carcinoma, the results are dismal. Patients rarely survive 2 years after diagnosis. The exact prognosis depends on the biology of the tumor. For example, slow-growing neuroendocrine tumors (of the APUD type) have a reasonable 5-year survival. On the other hand, the rapidly growing tumors of the breast and lung are often associated with less than a 6-month prognosis.

Leukemias and lymphomas often have hepatic involvement but rarely produce symptoms referable to the liver. An exception is Hodgkin's disease, which occasionally causes a cholestatic syndrome probably by releasing uncharacterized substances that affect hepatocyte function. Rarely, jaundice will also be produced by enlarged lymph nodes near the porta hepatis, obstructing the common bile duct. The typical Reed-Sternberg cells of Hodgkin's disease are rarely present, but collections of abnormal mononuclear and lymphoid cells are often seen in Hodgkin's lymphoma. These collections may be misdiagnosed as being granulomas of the liver. This granulomatous appearance of Hodgkin's disease in the liver is associated with a better prognosis than other histologic appearances that may be seen in Stage IV Hodgkin's disease. Rarely, lymphomatous involvement of the liver has been associated with dilatation of the hepatic sinusoids, producing peliosis hepatis. The liver may or may not be enlarged and is usually smooth. Although 14 percent of all non-Hodgkin's lymphomas involve the liver, the diagnosis is rarely made unless diagnostic studies such as ultrasound, CT scan, and liver biopsy are initiated. In cases of agnogenic myeloid metaplasia and other myelophthisic processes of the bone marrow, the liver may become the major site of extramedullary hematopoiesis. This results in an enlarged liver that is smooth and nontender and that may be associated with signs of portal hypertension.

Rarely, lymphomas will form tumor masses in the liver. Primary lymphoma of the liver is rare but has been associated with chronic hepatitis, especially caused by HBV infection. Despite the lack of HBV DNA in the few primary lymphomas studied, it is believed that the continued antigenic stimulation of the immune system by chronic hepatitis eventually results in a lymphomatous transformation event.

Lymphomatous mass lesions of the liver (especially primary lymphoma of the liver) have usually been sensitive to radiation therapy. In addition, cure by surgical resection has been reported. Diffuse lymphomatous involvement of the liver usually responds to the systemic chemotherapy effective for the histologic type and stage of the tumor.

Benign Tumors

Almost every type of cell of which the liver is composed can be transformed into benign neoplasms. Although they do not invade the liver or metastasize, their recognition and treatment are important, because they can be confused with malignant disease and are often associated with various complications.

Liver Cell Adenoma

Liver cell adenoma is a rare tumor that is increasingly being recognized because of the widespread use of oral contraceptives and postmenopausal estrogen therapy. Most cases occur in women who have been taking a progesterone- or estrogen-containing medicine for more than 3 years. Liver cell adenomas are rare, despite the widespread use of estrogen- and progesterone-containing medicines, thus suggesting that other environ-

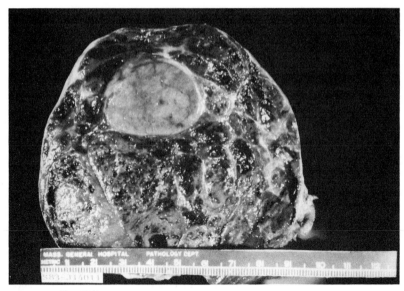

Fig. 18-5
Liver cell adenoma removed from a woman on oral contraceptives. (Courtesy of Dr. David Gang.)

mental or genetic factors are involved in the pathogenesis of these tumors. Estrogens have been shown to cause liver regeneration in rats, but its exact effect on human liver has yet to be identified. Rarely, liver cell adenoma occurs in patients using anabolic steroids or in patients with type I glycogen storage disease, diabetes mellitus, and beta thalassemia.

In the majority of cases, liver cell adenomas are single, well-encapsulated brown tumors that range from a few to 30 cm in diameter (Fig. 18-5). The right lobe is more often involved, and, in 30 percent of cases, there is more than one adenoma present. Microscopically, liver cell adenoma appears as sheets or cords of well-differentiated hepatocytes that often secrete bile. The tumors are usually asymptomatic but if large, may cause some upper abdominal discomfort.

Since more than half the tumors are near the liver surface, they are prone to rupture, and many of these come to medical attention in the setting of a woman in shock with a hemoperitoneum. Most cases of ruptured liver cell adenoma occur during menstruation, leading to the hypothesis that the tumor cells grow in response to the hormonal changes of the monthly menstrual cycle. Liver cell adenomas diminish in size upon withdrawal of estrogen therapy or at the termination of pregnancy. Ultrasound, CT scans, and liver/spleen scans rarely provide unequivocal identification of these benign tumors. The best nonin-

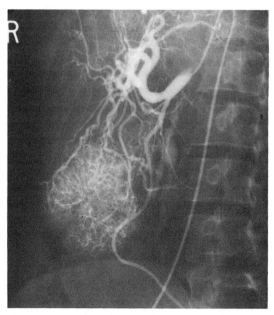

Fig. 18-6
Capillary phase of the angiogram of a liver cell adenoma. Note the hypervascularity of the tumor. (Courtesy of Dr. Ducksoo Kim.)

vasive means of making a diagnosis is hepatic angiography (Fig. 18-6). One half of liver cell adenomas are hypervascular, and one half are hypovascular. In both instances, the neovascularity that encircles the tumor is diagnostic. Because adenomas near the capsule of the liver are prone to rupture, these lesions should be surgically removed. Measures to prevent severe blood loss that occurs with the removal of these highly vascular tumors includes estrogen withdrawal and angiographic occlusion of the feeding arteries to the tumor prior to surgery. A thorough excision usually results in cure. PHCC has rarely been reported to occur in association with liver cell adenoma.

Hemangioma Cavernous hemangiomas are the most common benign tumors of the liver and consist of embryonic or mature vascular epithelium. These tumors, which are present in 5 to 7 percent of all livers, are mostly asymptomatic. Although most tumors are less than 1 cm in diameter, rare cases of giant hemangioma greater than 30 cm in diameter have been reported. Ten percent of patients have more than one hemangioma. Hemangiomas occur in women four to six times more often than in men. The symptomatic tumors usually occur in young women. The tumors are usually reddish purple or blue and soft. The cut surface is spongy and may contain clotted blood and central fibrosis. The thrombi may become calcified, which on plain x-rays of the abdomen apppears as a rim of calcification. Although small hemangiomas are usually asymptomatic, the larger tumors may present with a vascular hum in the liver. Enough shunting of blood may occur through large hemangiomas to induce high output congestive heart failure. The large cavernous hemangiomas may precipitate a chronic state of fibrinolysis, producing thrombocytopenia and hypofibrinogemia. With the increasing use of ultrasonography and CT scans in diagnostic medicine, benign hemangiomas are being found more frequently. The extremely vascular nature of hemangiomas contraindicates liver biopsy as a diagnostic maneuver. The diagnosis is suggested by performing a liver radionuclide scan that monitors dynamic hepatic blood flow and that reveals the tumor to be highly vascular. The diagnosis can also be confirmed by angiography. Some hemangiomas will grow and recede in relation to the use of estrogens or to pregnancy. Since most hemangiomas do not grow to significant size and are completely asymptomatic, they will not cause the patient any difficulty. Rarely, hemangiomas near the surface of the liver will rupture, causing shock resulting from hemorrhage. These highly vascular tumors are difficult to surgically resect with a minimum of blood loss. Large hemangiomas that cause symptoms can be treated with either radiation therapy or angiographic occlusion of the feeding arteries.

Other Benign Tumors

A number of exceedingly rare tumors involving the liver have been described. These consist of bile duct adenoma, cyst adenoma, teratoma, adrenal mass tumor, and pancreatic rests. These tumors are often found incidentally by ultrasound or CT scan or by causing symptoms of abdominal distention, cholangitis, or obstructive jaundice. The diagnosis is usually made in the surgically removed specimen. Most of these tumors are in the realm of medical curiosities, and, once removed, do not carry any other prognostic significance for the patient.

Tumor-like Lesions

Mesenchymal hamartomas, focal nodular hyperplasia (FNH), and microhamartomas (Von Meyenburg complexes) are probably not neoplastic growths but hyperplastic or regenerative tissue. Nodular transformation of the liver and FNH are discussed in the following paragraphs.

Nodular transformation of the liver consists of multiple nodules scattered throughout the hepatic parenchyma. Microscopically, the nodules consist of normal hepatic tissue that is compressed by surrounding areas of fibrosis and scarring. This condition occurs most often in elderly patients who have had chronic debilitating illnesses such as severe chronic rheumatoid arthritis. It is thought to result from a vasculitis of small arteries and veins of the liver that spares isolated areas of hepatic parenchyma that undergo hypertrophy. Although nodular transformation may rarely be associated with hepatic rupture, this lesion is usually an incidental finding at autopsy. Nodular transformation of the liver has been treated by portal decompression by either portal caval or mesocaval shunt surgery, although this is usually not necessary since portal hypertension is usually not clinically present.

FNH is a confusing entity that is probably not a tumor but an area of hypertrophic hepatic parenchyma. FNH usually consists of a single hard rubbery nodule that contains a central stellate scar with satellite lesions. Histologically, FNH appears similar to a macronodular cirrhotic liver with normal-appearing hepatocytes, Kupffer's cells, and sinusoidal architecture with fibrous bands and with polymorphonuclear leukocyte and lymphoid infiltrates. The etiology of FNH remains uncertain; however, recently, it has been noted that the central stellate scar tissue may be the remnant of a vascular abnormality in the liver. The diameter of arteries that feed the stellate body are larger than most in the liver. The hepatic parenchyma may hypertrophy in response to the hypervascular region generated by the vascular abnormality. Supporting this hypothesis is the observation that FNH is frequently found in patients with other vascular lesions such as hemangiomas and telangiectasias and in those with neuroendocrine disorders such as pheochromocytoma. It is controversial whether this lesion is stimulated by chronic ingestion of oral contraceptives; however, many patients with FNH are women of childbearing age who were taking these drugs. The majority of patients are asymptomatic. Only larger lesions cause symptoms of upper abdominal discomfort. If the tumor is pedunculated, it may undergo torsion and infarction. Rarely, the tumor will rupture. Although the lesion is benign and does not undergo malignant transformation, it is usually resected if at all possible. The diagnosis is usually made by hepatic arteriography that shows a dilated hepatic artery with one or more highly vascular lesions. FNH is not associated with elevated AFP.

Study Questions

1. A 25-year-old black man collapses while at work in the gold mines of South Africa. His co-workers have noticed that his abdomen has become protuberant over the last two weeks and they thought he had "the male pregnancy." The patient is in shock and has shifting dullness on abdominal examination. Which of the following are most likely to be true?
   a. The patient most likely has a ruptured liver cell adenoma.
   b. The peritoneal tap will yield blood.

c. The patient will probably have serological markers for hepatitis B virus in his blood.

d. The cancer will have hepatitis B virus sequences in its chromosomes.

e. The patient will probably be infected with hepatitis D virus (the delta agent).

Answers

b, c, d

The patient has a hepatocellular carcinoma (HCC) that has ruptured into the abdominal cavity, producing a hemoperitoneum. The peritoneal tap will yield blood. In South Africa, where the prevalence of hepatitis B virus (HBV) infection is quite high, a young man would have HCC on the basis of chronic HBV infection. Consequently the patient will have serological markers for HBV in his blood, and the cancer will have HBV sequences in its chromosomes. A hepatic adenoma would be quite uncommon in a male. Although hepatitis D virus may coexist with HBV, it plays no role in the pathogenesis of HCC and can actually decrease the incidence of this cancer by shortening the life expectancy of the infected individual.

2. A 25-year-old white woman from New Jersey in her second trimester of pregnancy notices a vague right upper quadrant dragging sensation. Her obstetrician obtains an ultrasound that reveals a 4-cm in diameter mass in the right lobe. The serum alpha-fetoprotein is elevated. The aminotransferases and alkaline phosphatase are normal. Of note, the patient took oral contraceptives since age 15 until six months prior to becoming pregnant. The patient refuses any diagnostic evaluation. Six months postpartum and without any birth control, a repeat ultrasound reveals a 1-cm mass that is subsequently removed surgically. The pathology revealed the mass to be a:

a. hepatoma

b. hepatoblastoma

c. hepatic adenoma

d. focal nodular hyperplasia

e. hemangioma

Answer

c

The most likely lesion is a hepatic adenoma. This tumor is more common in women, appears to be estrogen-sensitive, and occurs more commonly with oral contraceptive therapy. In the described patient, the fact that the tumor enlarged during pregnancy (when estrogen levels were rising) and then grew smaller in the postpartum period (when estrogen levels were falling) would argue strongly for this diagnosis. The other neoplasms listed would not display such marked estrogen sensitivity. The elevated serum alpha-fetoprotein is probably caused by the placenta and not by the hepatic adenoma.

3. What is true about focal nodular hyperplasia of the liver?
   a. It is a premalignant lesion.
   b. Oral contraceptives may be involved with its etiology.
   c. The lesion is related to hepatitis B virus.
   d. Alpha-fetoprotein concentrations in the serum are usually elevated.
   e. The tumor may be the remnant of a hepatic vascular abnormality.

Answers

b, e

Focal nodular hyperplasia (FNH) is an area of parenchymal hypertrophy rather than a true neoplasm. It is thought to be possibly the remnant of a hepatic vascular abnormality. The majority of patients with this lesion are women of child-bearing age taking oral contraceptives, and hence this medication is thought to play a role in the pathogenesis of the lesion. It is *not* related to HBV, is *not* a premalignant lesion, and is *not* associated with an elevated serum alpha-fetoprotein.

4. A 48-year-old Korean man immigrated to Boston six months ago. He has lost 25 pounds over the past four months. His alkaline phosphatase, 5'-nucleotidase, bilirubin, and ALT were elevated. Ultrasound revealed gallstones in both the gallbladder and common bile duct in addition to intrahepatic biliary dilatation in the left lobe. A 2-cm in diameter mass in the right lobe of the liver was noted. CT scan revealed other masses in the liver and positive perihepatic lymphadenopathy. Percutaneous liver biopsy revealed a cholangiocarcinoma. What is probably true about this case?
   a. Stools for ova and parasites may reveal *Clonorchis sinensis*.
   b. The alpha-fetoprotein is probably normal.
   c. The tumor will contain hepatitis B virus DNA.
   d. The tumor will be highly vascular with a major risk of rupturing.
   e. The tumor is responsive to estrogen therapy.

Answers

a, b

Cholangiocarcinoma often occurs in the setting of chronic inflammation of the biliary tree, such as occurs in sclerosing cholangitis and infestation with *Clonorchis sinensis*. *Clonor-*

chis is a liver fluke that commonly infects Oriental patients who ingest poorly cooked fish. With chronic infestations, the parasite and its ova would appear in the stool. The tumor is *not* related to HBV, is *not* responsive to estrogen therapy, and is usually *avascular*. The serum alpha-fetoprotein is usually normal.

References

Goodman, Z. D., and Ishak, K. G. Non-Parenchymal and Metastatic Malignant Tumors of the Liver. In J. E. Berk (ed.), *Bockus Gastroenterology* (4th ed.). Vol. 5. Philadelphia: Saunders, 1985. Pp. 3377–3387.

Hepatitis B virus, chronic liver disease, and primary hepatocellular carcinoma of the liver. *Hepatology* 2 supplement: 1S–133S, 1982.

Ishak, K. G., and Goodman, Z. D. Benign Tumors of the Liver. In J. E. Berk (ed.), *Bockus Gastroenterology* (4th ed.). Vol. 5. Philadelphia: Saunders, 1985. Pp. 3302–3314.

Kew, M. C. Tumors of the Liver. In D. Zakim and T. D. Boyer (eds.), *Hepatology. A Textbook of Liver Disease*. Philadelphia: Saunders, 1982. Pp. 1048–1083.

Okuda, K. Early recognition of hepatocellular carcinoma. *Hepatology* 6:729–738, 1986.

Okuda, K., and Nakashima, T. Primary Carcinomas of the Liver. In J. E. Berk (ed.), *Bockus Gastroenterology* (4th ed.). Vol. 5. Philadelphia: Saunders, 1985. Pp. 3315–3376.

Phillips, M. J., Langer, B., Stone, R., et al. Benign liver cell tumors. Classification and ultrastuctural pathology. *Cancer* 32:463–470, 1973.

Vyas, G. N., Dienstag, J. L., and Hoofnagle, J. H. *Viral Hepatitis and Liver Disease*. New York: Grune & Stratton, 1984. Pp. 201–274.

Wanless, I. R., Mawdsley, C., and Adams, R. On the pathogenesis of focal nodular hyperplasia of the liver. *Hepatology* 5:1194–1200, 1985.

Weiss, L., and Gilbert, H. A. *Liver Metastases*. Boston: GK Hall, 1982.

19 : Pathophysiology of Gallstones and Other Diseases of the Biliary Tract

Michael D. Apstein

In this chapter, we discuss the pathophysiology of diseases that primarily involve the gallbladder and bile ducts. In the West, more than 95 percent of biliary tract disease is caused by gallstones. Consequently, gallstone disease will be the focus of this chapter. Other topics discussed include acalculous cholecystitis, sclerosing cholangitis, and tumors of the gallbladder and bile ducts.

Gallstone Disease

Magnitude of the Problem

Gallstone disease is extremely prevalent in the United States. It affects 10 percent of the overall population, 33 percent of all women older than 40 years of age, and a staggering 70 percent of adult female American Indians. Approximately 500,000 cholecystectomies are performed annually in the United States, making it the third most common abdominal operation (after appendectomy and hysterectomy). The overall annual cost of gallbladder surgery is $4 to $5 billion, roughly equal to that of coronary artery bypass surgery.

Gallstone Composition

Gallstones can be categorized by their chemical composition as either cholesterol or pigment stones. Cholesterol gallstones are composed primarily of cholesterol, whereas pigment stones are composed primarily of bilirubin and its calcium salts (Fig. 19-1). Heretofore, this distinction was only of academic importance. However, now with efficacious medical treatment to dissolve cholesterol gallstones but not pigment gallstones, the particular stone type is clinically important.

Gallstones, either cholesterol or pigment, form because of abnormalities in the physical chemistry and secretion of bile. Therefore, to understand gallstone formation, a knowledge of the physical chemistry and secretion of normal bile is essential.

The Physical Chemistry of Bile
Bile is formed by the secretion of water and solutes across the canalicular membrane of the hepatocyte. Its composition is al-

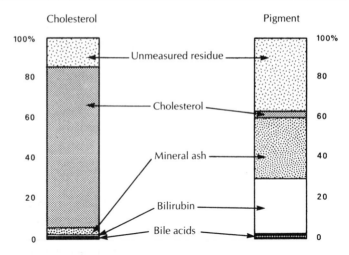

Fig. 19-1
Average composition of gallstones. Cholesterol gallstones are composed primarily of cholesterol, whereas pigment stones are composed primarily of bilirubin and its calcium salts. (Modified from *The Undergraduate Teaching Project in Gastroenterology Liver Disease,* American Gastroenterological Association, 1980.)

tered by the secretion and reabsorption of water and electrolytes by bile ductular and gallbladder epithelial cells.

Normal bile is a clear solution of lipids dissolved in water. The composition of normal human gallbladder bile is depicted in Fig. 19-2. Bile has two major functions: (1) It is the body's only excretory pathway for cholesterol, and (2) it delivers bile salts to the intestinal lumen to aid in fat digestion and absorption.

Cholesterol is very poorly soluble in water. However, its molecular association with the amphiphilic lipids in bile, lecithin (a phospholipid), and bile salts increases its solubility 2 million-fold. A perturbation of this molecular association can result in cholesterol gallstone formation.

An amphiphilic molecule is one that has functional groups that confer both lipid and water solubility. Bile salts (Fig. 19-3) have hydrophobic hydrocarbon rings that confer lipid solubility and hydrophilic hydroxy groups that confer water solubility. In addition, the conjugation of bile salts with the amino acids glycine or taurine increases their water solubility. Similarly, for lecithin, the major phospholipid in bile, the hydrophobic fatty acid portion of the molecule confers lipid solubility, whereas the polar phosphorylcholine group confers water solubility (Fig. 19-4).

There are two kinds of particles primarily responsible for cholesterol solubilization in bile: the mixed lipid vesicle and the mixed disc micelle (Fig. 19-5). Mixed lipid vesicles are spherical, uni-

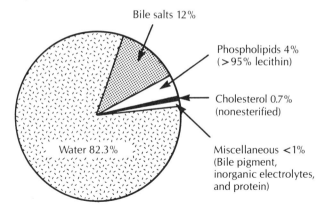

Percent by weight

Fig. 19-2
Average composition of normal gallbladder bile. Bile is primarily water. The small amount of cholesterol is normally kept in solution by its molecular association with bile salts and lecithin. (Modified from *The Undergraduate Teaching Project in Gastroenterology Liver Disease,* American Gastroenterological Association, 1980.)

lamellar vesicles 500 to 1,000 Å in diameter composed primarily of lecithin and cholesterol with lesser amounts of bile salt. Their molecular association results in a particle that, although thermodynamically unstable, is fully water soluble. These vesicles may be stabilized, in part, by apolipoproteins on their surface.

Mixed disc micelles, which are 50 Å in diameter, are composed of greater amounts of bile salts, with less lecithin, and cholesterol. In bile, mixed disc micelles can be formed by the addition of bile salts to the mixed lipid vesicle, and the two types of particles are in equilibrium with one another. The amount of cholesterol transported in bile as vesicles compared with mixed disc micelles varies, depending on the concentration of bile salts and cholesterol in bile. In dilute bile (lower concentration of bile salts), that is, hepatic bile, relatively more cholesterol is

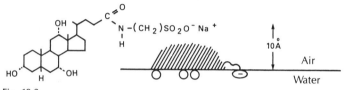

Fig. 19-3
The molecular structure and surface behavior of bile salts. The cross-hatched area represents the lipid-soluble hydrocarbon ring. The circles O and ⊖ represent the hydrophilic hydroxyl and taurine groups, respectively. (Modified from *The Undergraduate Teaching Project in Gastroenterology Liver Disease,* American Gastroenterological Association, 1980.)

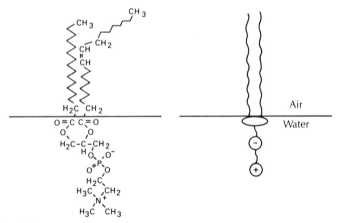

Fig. 19-4
The molecular structure and surface behavior of lecithin. The long wavy lines represent the hydrophobic fatty acid chains. The circles represent the hydrophilic phosphorylcholine portion. (Modified from *The Undergraduate Teaching Project in Gastroenterology Liver Disease,* American Gastroenterological Association, 1980.)

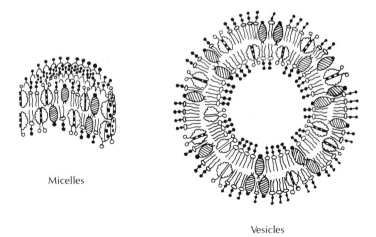

Micelles

Vesicles

Fig. 19-5
The particles responsible for cholesterol solubilization in bile, mixed lipid vesicle, and the mixed disc micelle. Bile salts are represented by ⟳, lecithin by ⎮, and cholesterol by ◖. (Modified from M. C. Carey and M. J. Cahalane. Enterohepatic Circulation. In I. M. Arias, W. B. Jakoloy, H. Popper, and D. Schacter, et al. [eds.], *The Liver: Biology and Pathobiology* [2nd ed.]. New York: Raven, 1988.)

carried in vesicles, whereas in concentrated bile, that is, gallbladder bile, mixed micelles are quantitatively more important. The initial step of cholesterol gallstone formation is the fusion of mixed lipid vesicles from which cholesterol crystallizes.

The amount of cholesterol that can be solubilized in bile can be predicted by knowing the relative amounts of the three bili-

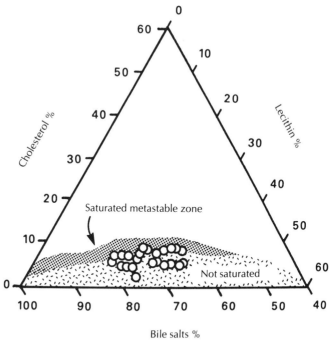

Fig. 19-6

The relative lipid composition of normal gallbladder bile plotted on triangular coordinates. Each circle represents one bile sample. Bile that has a composition that falls within the stippled area, the micellar zone, is not saturated with cholesterol. Cholesterol will not precipitate from these biles because it is all held in solution by adequate amounts of lecithin and bile salts. Such bile can solubilize additional cholesterol. Bile whose composition falls in the unshaded zone is composed of (1) liquid that is saturated with cholesterol and that cannot solubilize additional cholesterol, and (2) crystals (solid) of excess cholesterol that could not be solubilized and have therefore precipitated. Bile whose composition falls in the cross-hatched strip is termed *metastable*. Metastable bile carries more cholesterol than expected. It is supersaturated with cholesterol. Under appropriate circumstances, cholesterol can precipitate from these biles to form cholesterol gallstones. (Modified from *The Undergraduate Teaching Project in Gastroenterology Liver Disease*, American Gastroenterological Association, 1980.)

ary lipids — cholesterol, lecithin, and bile salts. The relative amounts of lipid (composition) of any bile sample can be plotted on triangular coordinates (Fig. 19-6). Bile that has a composition that falls within the shaded area, the micellar zone, can solubilize additional cholesterol. Cholesterol will not precipitate from these biles because it is all held in solution by adequate amounts of lecithin and bile salts. Such bile is unsaturated with cholesterol. Bile whose composition falls in the unshaded zone is composed of (1) liquid that is saturated with cholesterol and that cannot solubilize additional cholesterol, and (2) crystals (solid) of excess cholesterol that could not be solubilized and have, hence, precipitated.

Bile whose composition falls in the crosshatched strip is termed *metastable*. Metastable bile carries more cholesterol than expected. It is supersaturated with cholesterol. Under appropriate circumstances, cholesterol can precipitate from these biles to form cholesterol gallstones (see the section entitled Nucleation).

Bile Formation and Secretion

It is apparent from the previous discussion that alterations in biliary lipid composition are critically important in the pathogenesis of cholesterol gallstone formation. Biliary lipid composition is determined by the secretion of these lipids from the hepatocyte. The precise molecular mechanism of secretion is not known. One likely mechanism is that cholesterol and lecithin are secreted across the canalicular membrane as vesicles. An alternate hypothesis holds that cholesterol and lecithin are "pinched off" the canalicular membrane. Bile salt secretion probably occurs by way of a separate, specific membrane-bound carrier-mediated mechanism. Regardless of the precise mechanism of biliary cholesterol and lecithin secretion, their secretion is controlled, in large part, by biliary bile salt secretion.

The Enterohepatic Circulation of Bile Salts

Bile salts are synthesized from cholesterol in the hepatocyte and then conjugated at the carbonyl group with an amino acid, either glycine or taurine (Fig. 19-7). The conjugated bile salts are secreted into bile and stored in the gallbladder to be pumped into the intestinal lumen when the gallbladder contracts. At biliary and intestinal pH (6.0–8.5), bile salts are chiefly ionized (taurine conjugates are ionized more than glycine conjugates because of their lower pKa's). The ionized bile salts are not absorbed in the duodenum or jejunum but remain in the intestinal lumen to participate in fat absorption. A small fraction of unionized glycine conjugates are absorbed by passive diffusion in the duodenum and jejunum. The remainder and the ionized bile salts are selectively reabsorbed by a specific receptor-mediated process in the terminal ileum. This reabsorption is extremely efficient: about 2 percent of the conjugated bile salts pass into the colon and out into the feces. The reabsorbed bile salts return by way of the portal vein to the liver where they are efficiently cleared and resecreted into bile. Sixty to ninety percent of the bile salts in the portal vein are extracted during a single pass through the liver. As a result, in normal individuals, the concentration of bile salts in the portal vein is 40 to 70 μm, whereas it is only 2 μm in peripheral blood. This pathway of bile salt secretion, absorption, and resecretion is known as the en-

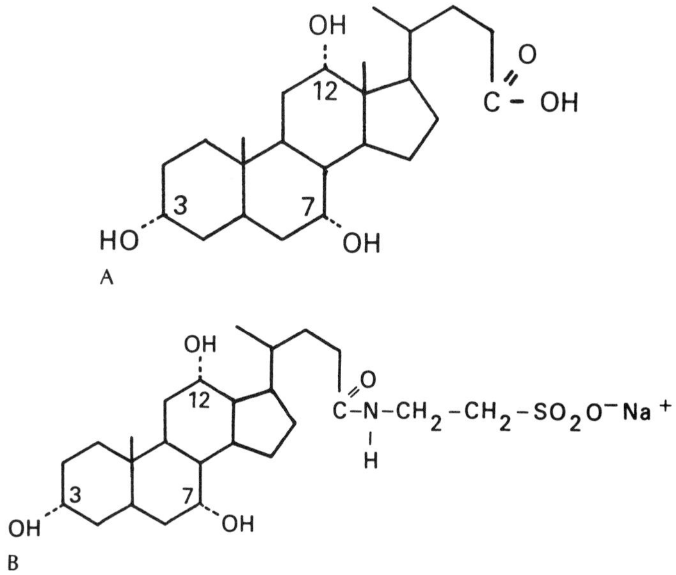

Fig. 19-7
A. The primary bile acid, cholic acid. A11 — OH's in α configuration. B. Cholic acid conjugated with taurine at the carbonyl group to form the bile salt taurocholate.

terohepatic circulation (EHC) (Fig. 19-8). In patients without liver disease, more than 99 percent of the bile salt pool is confined to the EHC. Diseases that interrupt the EHC can lead to a reduced bile salt pool size, decreased cholesterol holding capacity of bile, and subsequent cholesterol gallstone formation.

There are a variety of bile salts normally present in human bile. Cholic acid, chenodeoxycholic acid, and deoxycholic acid account for more than 90 percent of the bile salts of normal human bile (Fig. 19-9). Cholic acid and chenodeoxycholic acid are known as primary bile salts. They are synthesized in the liver from cholesterol. Their rate of synthesis is controlled by the amount of bile salts returning to the liver by way of the portal vein (feedback inhibition). The bile salt pool (total amount of bile salts) averages 3 to 4 gm and circulates two times with each meal. As a result, the terminal ileum "sees" 18 to 24 gm of bile salts per day. Under normal circumstances, the liver "senses" the quantity of bile salts lost in the feces (2%, or 500 mg/day) and synthesizes an equivalent amount. As a result, the size of the bile salt pool remains constant.

Deoxycholic acid and lithocholic acid are secondary bile salts because they are formed in the intestinal lumen by bacterial dehydroxylation of cholic acid and chenodeoxycholic acid, respectively. Deoxycholic acid constitutes about 35 percent of the

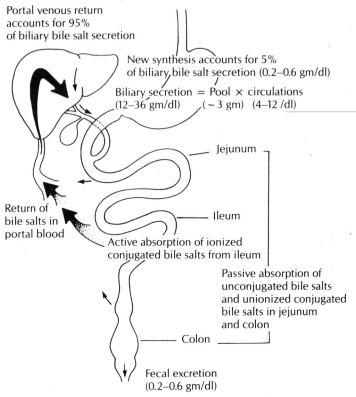

Portal venous return accounts for 95% of biliary bile salt secretion

New synthesis accounts for 5% of biliary bile salt secretion (0.2–0.6 gm/dl)

Biliary secretion = Pool × circulations
(12–36 gm/dl)   (~3 gm)   (4–12 /dl)

Jejunum

Return of bile salts in portal blood

Ileum

Active absorption of ionized conjugated bile salts from ileum

Passive absorption of unconjugated bile salts and unionized conjugated bile salts in jejunum and colon

Colon

Fecal excretion (0.2–0.6 gm/dl)

Fig. 19-8
The enterohepatic circulation of bile salts. See text for explanation. (Modified from M. C. Carey and M. J. Cahalane. Enterohepatic Circulation. In I. M. Arias, W. B. Jakoloy, H. Popper, and D. Schacter et al. [eds.], *The Liver: Biology and Pathobiology* [2nd ed.]. New York: Raven, 1988.)

human bile salt pool and has an enterohepatic circulation that is similar to that of cholic acid and chenodeoxycholic acid. In contrast, lithocholic acid does not undergo a significant enterohepatic circulation. After lithocholic acid is formed in the intestine, a smaller portion is reabsorbed in the ileum and colon and returned to the liver by way of the portal vein. In the liver, lithocholic acid is sulfated and excreted into bile. Sulfated lithocholic acid is not reabsorbed in the intestine but is excreted in the feces. Since lithocholic acid is toxic in humans, it is fortunate that this bile acid can be effectively excreted by the body.

The bile salt secretion rate, and, hence, the biliary cholesterol and phospholipid secretion, is determined by the amount of bile salts returning to the liver in the portal vein. For example, during an overnight fast, the bile salt pool is sequestered in the gallbladder. Very little bile salt is present in the ileum to be reabsorbed and returned to the liver for resecretion. Conse-

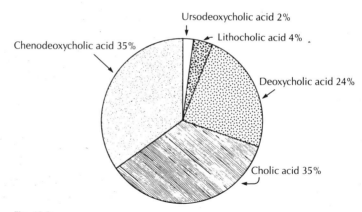

Fig. 19-9
Bile acids in normal human bile. The primary bile acids, chenodeoxycholic and cholic acid, each constitute about one third of the bile acid pool. The secondary bile acid, deoxycholic acid, accounts for about one fourth of the bile acid pool. (Modified from *The Undergraduate Teaching Project in Gastroenterology Liver Disease,* American Gastroenterological Association, 1980.)

quently, the bile salt secretion rate prior to breakfast is relatively low. In contrast, after a meal, the gallbladder contracts, delivering the bile salt pool to the intestine. Bile salts are reabsorbed, delivered to the liver, and resecreted into bile. As a result, after a meal, the bile salt secretion rate is relatively high.

The amount of cholesterol and lecithin secreted into bile depends primarily on the bile salt secretion rate (Fig. 19-10). At low bile salt secretion rates (during fasting), relatively more cholesterol is secreted into bile. At higher bile salt secretion rates (after a meal), relatively less cholesterol is secreted in bile. As a result of this normal variation in biliary lipid secretion, most individuals, even those without gallstones, secrete bile that is supersaturated with cholesterol during an overnight fast (Fig. 19-11).

Bile salts vary in their ability to control biliary lecithin and cholesterol secretion. Of the major bile salts — cholic acid, chenodeoxycholic acid, and deoxycholic acid — chenodeoxycholic acid stimulates biliary cholesterol secretion the least. As a result, individuals who have relatively more chenodeoxycholic acid (and less cholic acid and deoxycholic acid) in their bile salt pool will secrete bile with less cholesterol. Their bile will be less unsaturated with cholesterol.

Bile also contains small, but significant, amounts of proteins, including apolipoprotein AI and AII. They may stabilize mixed lipid vesicles by preventing their coalescence, and hence inhibit cholesterol precipitation.

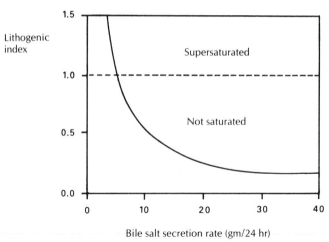

Fig. 19-10
The influence of bile salt secretion rate on biliary cholesterol saturation. At low bile salt secretion rates (i.e., during fasting), bile has a higher lithogenic index (is more saturated with cholesterol). As the bile salt secretion rate increases (i.e., after a meal), the lithogenic index (cholesterol saturation) falls. (Modified from *The Undergraduate Teaching Project in Gastroenterology Liver Disease*, American Gastroenterological Association, 1980.)

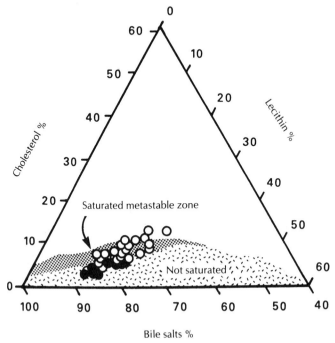

Fig. 19-11
Alteration in biliary lipid composition of normal hepatic bile before and after feeding. Closed circles represent bile samples obtained after feeding. Open circles represent bile samples obtained during fasting. During fasting, bile is more saturated with cholesterol. (Modified from *The Undergraduate Teaching Project in Gastroenterology Liver Disease*, American Gastroenterological Association, 1980.)

Cholesterol excretion from the body can take two pathways: (1) It can be excreted in the bile directly as unesterified (free) cholesterol, or (2) it can be metabolized in the liver to bile salts, which are then excreted in the bile. In humans, the conversion of cholesterol to bile salts is much less efficient than in all other animals. Consequently, a greater amount of free cholesterol is excreted directly into bile. As a result, no animals, except humans, form cholesterol gallstones spontaneously.

Cholesterol Gallstone Disease

Cholesterol gallstone formation is primarily a metabolic disease. The physical-chemical setting for cholesterol gallstone formation requires that there be an excess of cholesterol molecules compared to molecules of the solubilizing lipids, bile salts, and lecithin (Fig. 19-12). If this imbalance is not countered by other factors (see the following section: Nucleation), cholesterol molecules will not remain in micellar or vesicular solution but instead nucleate, crystallize, and precipitate. This imbalance between cholesterol and bile salts plus lecithin can be caused by an increase in biliary cholesterol secretion or a decrease in either biliary bile salt or biliary lecithin secretion. In humans, disorders involving "too much" biliary cholesterol or "too little" biliary bile salt have been described. However, a deficiency of biliary lecithin has not been identified.

Any condition associated with excessive biliary cholesterol secretion can result in bile that is supersaturated with cholesterol.

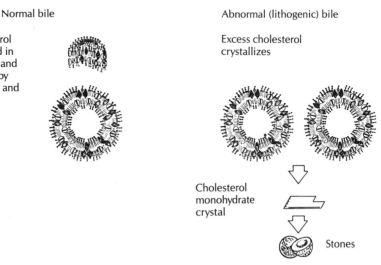

Normal bile

Cholesterol dissolved in micelles and vesicles by bile salts and lecithin

Abnormal (lithogenic) bile

Excess cholesterol crystallizes

Cholesterol monohydrate crystal

Stones

Fig. 19-12
Principles of cholesterol gallstone formation. In normal bile, cholesterol is dissolved in mixed disc micelles and mixed lipid vesicles by bile salts and lecithin. In lithogenic bile, excess cholesterol precipitates as vesicles fuse. Cholesterol crystals form and eventually grow, agglomerate, and form gallstones.

In addition, any condition that reduces the bile salt secretion rate places patients at risk for cholesterol gallstones. The bile salt secretion rate can be decreased by diseases that either interrupt the enterohepatic circulation or reduce hepatic bile salt synthesis.

Nucleation

It is now clear that bile that is supersaturated with cholesterol is not in itself a sufficient cause for cholesterol gallstone formation. Most humans have supersaturated bile for several hours each day, particularly during fasting, when biliary bile salt secretion rates are low. Factors that promote or inhibit nucleation and crystallization are critically important because many individuals with bile that is highly enriched with cholesterol do not form stones. In lithogenic (stone-forming) bile, cholesterol crystallizes from solution about five times faster than in control bile with the *same degree of supersaturation*. This observation can be explained by the presence of pronucleating factors, the absence of antinucleating factors, or both. Apolipoproteins AI and AII, present in bile at about 1 percent of their plasma levels, may be important antinucleating factors. On the other hand, gelled gallbladder mucin may accelerate cholesterol nucleation. Animal organ culture studies suggest that lithogenic bile stimulates gallbladder mucin synthesis and secretion. Furthermore, drugs that inhibit mucin production can prevent gallstone formation in an animal model of gallstone disease despite the persistence of supersaturated bile. It is obvious that much more work on the balance between pronucleating and antinucleating factors must be done to determine why only certain patients with supersaturated bile develop cholesterol gallstones.

Putative Risk Factors for Cholesterol Gallstone Formation

There are a number of putative risk factors of cholesterol gallstone formation (Table 19-1). The mechanism of increased risk can be attributed to an alteration of biliary lipid secretion and composition in at least one of the following three ways: (1) increase in biliary cholesterol secretion, (2) decrease in biliary bile salt secretion, or (3) decrease in the chenodeoxycholic acid fraction of the bile salt pool. Nonetheless, at least 80 percent of patients with cholesterol gallstones have no recognized risk factors.

Age

Increasing age is a risk factor for cholesterol gallstone formation — probably because of the increased secretion of cholesterol into bile associated with aging.

Table 19-1
Putative risk factors for cholesterol gallstone disease

Age	Drugs: estrogens, clofibrate
Female gender	Primary biliary cirrhosis
Pregnancy	Spinal cord injury
Obesity	Gallbladder stasis
Ileal disease	*Not* diabetes mellitus
Hypertriglyceridemia	

Sex

Women have twice the risk as men of developing cholesterol gallstones. This increased risk is probably due to endogenous estrogen secretion. Biliary cholesterol saturation correlates directly with urinary estrogen excretion, a marker of endogenous estrogen production. Women have smaller total bile salt pool sizes, smaller chenodeoxycholic acid pool sizes, and increased biliary cholesterol content. Additional evidence that the changes in bile salt pool sizes is a result of estrogen secretion is the observation that total bile and chenodeoxycholic acid pool sizes *increase* after oophorectomy in humans.

Pregnancy

Pregnancy is an independent risk factor for cholesterol gallstone formation. The risk increases with increasing parity. Hormonal changes during pregnancy affect both biliary lipid secretion and gallbladder motility. Biliary cholesterol saturation increases during the last two trimesters of pregnancy. This increased cholesterol saturation is probably due to increased biliary cholesterol secretion, which, in turn, may be a result of a decrease in the chenodeoxycholic acid pool size. Gallbladder motor function is also abnormal during pregnancy. The rate of gallbladder emptying is reduced, and the volume remaining in the gallbladder after contraction is increased. These changes may be a result of increased serum levels of progesterone, a smooth muscle relaxant. It is postulated that incomplete gallbladder emptying causes agglomeration of mixed lipid vesicles, nucleation and retention of cholesterol crystals, and stone growth.

Exogenous Estrogen Therapy

Most, but not all, studies suggest that estrogen therapy in either men or women is associated with an increased risk of developing cholesterol gallstones. Oral contraceptive steroids increase biliary cholesterol secretion and percentage of cholesterol saturation and decrease the chenodeoxycholic acid pool size. However, in contrast to pregnancy, oral contraceptive steroids have little effect on gallbladder motility.

Ileal Disease, Resection, or Bypass

Patients with ileal disease, resection, or bypass have a strikingly increased risk for developing cholesterol gallstones because of bile salt malabsorption. When bile salt malabsorption exceeds the liver's bile salt synthetic capacity, a reduction in the bile salt pool size occurs. Consequently, biliary bile salt secretion rates fall. Gallstones develop in approximately 30 percent of patients with Crohn's disease who have ileal involvement or resection. Since the enterohepatic cycling of the bile salt pool and, hence, bile salt secretion rates are critically dependent on active ileal transport, the risk of gallstone formation varies directly with the extent of ileal involvement with disease, resection, or bypass.

The development of gallstones immediately following an ileal bypass operation performed for treatment of obesity (itself a risk factor) is dramatic. Gallstones can develop in these patients within 6 months of the operation. By 2 to 4 years, the incidence of gallstones varies from 20 to 60 percent, in contrast to 4 percent in morbidly obese controls. These patients have a double metabolic defect. Following the operation, there is a marked bile salt malabsorption, decrease in the size of the bile salt pool, and decreased biliary bile salt secretion rates. In addition, biliary cholesterol secretion is markedly increased as cholesterol is mobilized from body stores and transported into bile.

Serum Lipids

There is an increased prevalence of gallstones in patients with certain forms of hyperlipidemia. Types IIb and IV hyperlipoproteinemia (elevated VLDL-triglyceride) are associated with increased biliary cholesterol content and increased biliary cholesterol saturation. Even in normolipemic subjects, there is a positive correlation between the biliary cholesterol saturation index, gallstone prevalence rates, and plasma triglyceride concentrations. In contrast, there appears to be an inverse correlation between serum HDL-cholesterol levels and both biliary cholesterol saturation index and gallstone disease. The link between serum lipids and gallstone disease is not known.

Obesity

Obesity of any magnitude increases the risk of cholesterol gallstone formation. Obese people secrete more cholesterol into their bile than people of normal weight and, as a result, have bile that is often greatly supersaturated with cholesterol. The increase in biliary cholesterol secretion is probably related to an increased total body cholesterol synthesis. Biliary cholesterol saturation reverts to normal after an obese subject achieves ideal body weight. When obese individuals begin to lose weight, biliary cholesterol saturation can increase acutely as a result of rapid mobilization of cholesterol from adipose tissue stores. With passage of time, caloric restriction eventually decreases total body cholesterol synthesis and reduces the amount of cholesterol destined for biliary secretion. However, bile salt synthesis is also reduced during prolonged caloric restriction, and the size of the bile salt pool decreases. Thus, whether obese patients on a weight-reducing diet will develop supersaturated bile depends on the delicate balance between increased mobilization of cholesterol from tissue stores, decreased bile salt synthesis, and decreased cholesterol synthesis.

Diet
There is much speculation but little reliable data concerning diet and cholesterol gallstone disease. A high intake of dietary fat or cholesterol may increase biliary cholesterol secretion and percent saturation. Although a diet high in polyunsaturated fats may be beneficial for lowering serum cholesterol, some individuals will increase their biliary cholesterol saturation. On the other hand, a diet high in bran has been reported to decrease biliary cholesterol saturation in patients with gallstones, possibly by increasing chenodeoxycholic acid pool size. Preliminary data suggest that decreased meal frequency may also be a risk factor for gallstone formation. However, there is no conclusive evidence that dietary habits, unless they result in obesity, influence cholesterol gallstone formation.

Primary Biliary Cirrhosis
Patients with primary biliary cirrhosis also probably have an increased risk of gallstone disease. Although stone composition has not been studied in these patients, biliary cholesterol saturation is increased, suggesting that these are cholesterol, not pigment, stones. Whether the increase in cholesterol saturation is due to increased biliary cholesterol secretion, decreased bile salt secretion, or a combination of both factors, is not known.

Drugs
Since bile is the major excretory route for cholesterol, drugs that alter cholesterol metabolism and serum cholesterol levels may influence the risk of forming cholesterol gallstones. Indeed, some agents that lower serum cholesterol, such as clofibrate, do so by increasing biliary cholesterol secretion. Long-term use of clofibrate may also decrease bile salt synthesis and pool size in some patients. It is not surprising, then, that an increased prevalence of symptomatic gallstones has been found among patients using clofibrate. Cholestyramine and other drugs that bind bile salts in the intestine cause bile salt malab-

sorption, stimulate the hepatic conversion of cholesterol to bile salts, and thereby lower serum cholesterol. Unlike extensive ileal disease or resection, sequestration of bile salts by drugs does *not* result in a smaller bile salt pool because the liver can compensate by increasing bile salt synthesis to maintain the size of the bile salt pool.

Stasis

Gallbladder stasis is a contributory factor to both cholesterol and pigment stone formation. Impaired gallbladder emptying is associated with gallstone formation in patients undergoing prolonged fasts, receiving total parenteral nutrition, and in women during pregnancy. Furthermore, decreased gallbladder emptying has been demonstrated in some patients with gallstones and in animals with lithogenic bile prior to gallstone formation. In cholesterol stone disease, gallbladder stasis could allow time for cholesterol crystal formation, aggregation, and stone growth.

Spinal Cord Injury

Patients with spinal cord injury have an increased prevalence of gallstones, possibly as a result of gallbladder stasis secondary to autonomic dysfunction.

Diabetes Mellitus

Diabetics have physiologic reasons to be at risk for cholesterol gallstone formation. They have increased total body cholesterol synthesis, independent of obesity. In addition, some diabetics have decreased gallbladder motility. Nevertheless, diabetes mellitus per se does not appear to be an independent risk factor for cholesterol gallstone disease. Most older epidemiologic and autopsy studies on diabetics that describe such a correlation fail to differentiate the effects of obesity and hypertriglyceridemia from the diabetes itself.

Pigment Gallstone Formation

There are two varieties of pigment gallstones: black or brown. Black pigment stones form principally in the gallbladder and are the more common pigment stones in the West. Brown ("earthy") pigment stones usually form de novo in the bile ducts following cholecystectomy. However, in the Orient, these brown stones are found in the bile ducts of patients who have not undergone a cholecystectomy. Little is known about the pathogenesis of either kind of pigment gallstone. The black pigment stone is composed of bilirubin polymers and inorganic salts of calcium (carbonate, phosphate), whereas the brown pigment stone is composed principally of calcium bilirubinate and organic fatty acid salts of calcium (usually palmitate and stearate). Because of this difference in chemical composition, most pigment stones formed in the gallbladder (black pigment stones) are radiopaque, whereas those found in the bile ducts (brown "earthy" stones) are radiolucent.

Bilirubin is secreted into bile primarily as water-soluble conjugates of glucuronic acid. Normal bile contains the diglucuronide conjugate (80%), monoglucuronide conjugates (18%), and only traces of unconjugated bilirubin. At normal biliary pH (6.5–8.5), the small concentrations of unconjugated bilirubin are soluble as a result of the detergent properties of bile salts. Under conditions of supersaturation of bile with unconjugated bilirubin, bilirubin can precipitate as calcium salts or polymerize to form pigment gallstones.

A likely mechanism for pigment stone formation in the Orient is that bacteria hydrolyze conjugated bilirubin in the bile to unconjugated bilirubin, which then precipitates. In the West, it is likely that gallbladder stasis is also an important factor. In fact, spontaneous or nonbacterial enzymatic hydrolysis of conjugated bilirubin occurs in sterile bile. This is consistent with the observation that in the West, pigment stones in the gallbladder are usually not associated with infection. In addition to elevated levels of unconjugated bilirubin in bile, Ca^{2+} levels, fluctuations in biliary pH, and bile salt secretion rates may also be important.

Biliary tract infection seems to be a prerequisite in the pathogenesis of brown pigment stone formation in intra- and extrahepatic bile ducts. These patients have high levels of unconjugated bilirubin in bile, probably secondary to bacterial deconjugation of conjugated bilirubin. Although glucaro-1-4-lactone, an inhibitor of bacterial β-glucuronidase, is normally present in bile, its activity is quickly overcome by bacterial infection.

In summary, biliary concentrations of unconjugated bilirubin, bile salts, free calcium ions, biliary pH, bacterial contamination, β-glucuronidase activity, and glucaro-1-4-lactone levels all appear to be important determinants of pigment gallstone formation. Little is known, however, about the regulation or interplay of these variables or why some patients acquire polymer (black) pigment stones and others acquire calcium bilirubinate (brown) stones.

Putative Risk Factors for Pigment Gallstones

As with cholesterol gallstone disease, the putative risk factors for pigment gallstone disease are not well understood (Table 19-2). The major identifiable physiologic derangements of importance in pigment gallstone formation are (1) increased bilirubin loads to the liver and bile, (2) stasis, and (3) bacterial invasion

Table 19-2
Putatitive risk factors for pigment gallstone disease

Age	Total parenteral nutrition
Hemolysis	Vagotomy
Alcoholism	Periampullary diverticula
Cirrhosis	Gallbladder stasis
Biliary infection	

of the biliary tree. Unlike cholesterol gallstone disease, the male : female ratio is the same for pigment gallstones. Women are *not* at increased risk for forming pigment gallstones.

Chronic Hemolysis
Inherited hemolytic anemias — that is, sickle-cell disease, spherocytosis, thalassemia — as well as chronic hemolysis associated with artificial heart valves and malaria dramatically increase the risk of pigment stone formation. The mechanism in all likelihood relates to an increased biliary excretion of unconjugated bilirubin.

Alcoholism or Alcoholic Cirrhosis
Patients with alcoholic cirrhosis or alcoholism alone have an increased prevalence of pigment gallstones. Autopsy and prospective studies indicate that 30 to 40 percent of alcoholic cirrhotics have gallstones; almost half of these are pigment stones. In contrast, the ratio of cholesterol to pigment stones in typical Western populations ranges from 3 to 9 : 1. The mechanism for this increased risk is unknown but may be related to (1) subclinical hemolysis, (2) defective bilirubin conjugation, or (3) alcohol-induced secretion of unconjugated bilirubin into bile.

Age
Increasing age is also a risk factor for pigment gallstone formation. Patients with pigment gallstones probably become symptomatic (as judged by cholecystectomy rates) at a later age than patients with cholesterol gallstones. Either pigment stones form later in life than cholesterol stones, or individuals with pigment stones remain asymptomatic for longer periods of time.

Infection or Infestation
In the Orient, pigment stones are frequently found in the intrahepatic bile ducts and are almost always associated with infection (usually *Escherichia coli*) or parasitic infestation (*Clonorchis sinensis, Ascaris lumbricoides*). In Western patients, intraductal stones that develop following cholecystectomy are almost invariably calcium bilirubinate stones, even in those pa-

tients whose original gallstones were cholesterol stones. These intraducted stones are invariably associated with stasis, biliary tree infection, or retained suture material.

Total Parenteral Nutrition
Total parenteral nutrition (TPN) dramatically increases the likelihood of pigment gallstone formation. Although TPN in and of itself promotes gallstone formation, the true frequency depends to a large degree on the underlying illness for which TPN was instituted. Routine ultrasonographic screening of adults on TPN for a mean of 23 months has shown a 35 percent incidence rate of gallstone formation. In a prospective study using ultrasonography, 43 percent of children on TPN for a mean of 21 months developed gallstones. Most patients in these studies had ileal disease, which explains, in part, these high prevalence rates. Nonetheless, even patients without ileal disease who are on long-term TPN have a 25 percent incidence rate of gallstone formation. In one study, 100 percent of patients on TPN for longer than 6 weeks developed sludge in their gallbladders.

Gallbladder sludge is composed of a mixture of mucin glycoproteins and microprecipitates, which can be composed of calcium bilirubinate, liquid crystals of bile lipids, and solid cholesterol monohydrate crystals. Mucin glycoproteins accumulate in the gallbladder during gallbladder stasis and in response to the presence of lithogenic bile. When the concentration of glycoproteins reaches a critical level, they polymerize to form a gel. Microprecipitates of calcium bilirubinate and cholesterol crystals can be trapped within this gel-matrix. In addition, the mucin may act to accelerate cholesterol crystallization. The relationship between biliary sludge and eventual gallstone formation is suspected but not yet clarified. It is likely that sludge represents an early but still reversible stage of gallstone formation in susceptible individuals.

The pathogenesis of gallstone formation during TPN is not clear. Decreased gallbladder motility during prolonged fasting may explain, in part, gallstone formation. At least in animals, gallstone formation during TPN can be prevented by the daily administration of CCK-octapeptide. It is not evident why patients at risk for cholesterol gallstone disease (i.e., ileal disease) should acquire pigment stones. In animal models of ileal resection, total calcium and bilirubin levels are elevated in gallbladder bile for unknown reasons.

Vagotomy
Although there are no rigorous prospective studies that examine the frequency of gallstones following truncal vagotomy,

available evidence suggests a four- to sixfold increase in gall-stone formation. Although stone composition in patients following vagotomy has not been studied, pathophysiologic evidence suggests that these stones should be pigment stones, rather than cholesterol stones. Biliary cholesterol saturation in man decreases after vagotomy, probably because of an increase in the size of the bile salt pool. In addition, in animals, gallbladder volume increases after vagotomy, which, by itself, could predispose to biliary stasis and pigment gallstone formation. Also, in an animal model, truncal vagotomy caused sludge and pigment stones to develop.

Periampullary Diverticula

There is a strong association between diverticula near the ampulla of Vater and the presence of pigment gallstones in the gallbladder. Patients with the former frequently have β-glucuronidase–producing bacteria in their biliary tract. An attractive working hypothesis is that decreased muscular tone and contractility of the sphincter of Oddi and the common bile duct secondary to the physical presence of the diverticulum allows the biliary tract to become infected with bacteria. In addition, the diverticulum itself may harbor bacteria and be the source of biliary tract seeding. The bacteria deconjugate bilirubin glucuronides in the gallbladder and biliary tree, liberating unconjugated bilirubin, which precipitates and produces calcium bilirubinate stones.

Cholelithiasis

Diagnosis

Recent epidemiologic data suggest that biliary pain, defined by one or more episodes of continuous pain in the right hypochondrium or epigastrium lasting at least 30 minutes, has a relatively low specificity (80%), sensitivity (35%), and predictive value (10%) for the diagnosis of gallstones. Since the physical examination of patients with gallstones is generally entirely normal, the physician must rely on one or more diagnostic tests for a definitive diagnosis of gallstones.

Oral cholecystography and real-time ultrasonography are both excellent methods for detecting cholelithiasis. Both have a specificity of approximately 98 percent, with a sensitivity of approximately 95 percent. Both of these tests have unique advantages; therefore, they are not mutually exclusive. Ultrasonography has now become the initial diagnostic procedure of choice, since it does not involve patient preparation or radiation and is simple to perform and interpret. Oral cholecystography has the small, but real, risk of administration of iodinated radiocontrast material and radiation. However, it has the advantage of demonstrating patency of the cystic duct, gallbladder function, and the apparent density of stones, all of which are crucial information when dissolution therapy with oral bile salts is contemplated.

Ultrasonography is superior to oral cholecystography in the diagnosis of cholelithiasis in unreliable patients, in patients with gastrointestinal disease, or in patients with abnormal liver function. For example, patients may not take the radiocontrast pills correctly or may vomit or malabsorb them. Even when absorbed in sufficient amounts, mild liver disease may prevent excretion of an adequate amount of contrast material into the biliary tree. Provided that these potential pitfalls are excluded, most (75%) gallbladders opacify following a single dose of the radiocontrast agent. Patients whose gallbladders do not visualize on the initial examination should be given a second dose of contrast agent that evening; this procedure is effective in opacifying the gallbladders of two thirds of these patients. If stones are observed or if the gallbladder does not opacify after the second dose of radiocontrast material, gallstones or gallbladder disease secondary to gallstones can be diagnosed with 95 percent certainty. Both oral cholecystography and ultrasonography are associated with a small percentage of false-negative examinations. Therefore, if one of these diagnostic tests is negative for stones and the clinical suspicion of gallstone disease is high, the other diagnostic test should be used.

The clinician is frequently faced with an abdominal ultrasonographic report that describes gallbladder sludge. This is the description of multiple weak echoes without acoustic shadowing in the dependent part of the gallbladder or, rarely, observed diffusely throughout the gallbladder. Sludge can form during normal pregnancy, prolonged fasting (7–10 days), or hyperalimentation and in debilitated, hospitalized patients, and in patients with extrahepatic biliary obstruction.

The natural history of biliary sludge is not fully known. In some patients, gallbladder sludge may be innocuous and disappear after pregnancy or oral refeeding. In others, however, sludge may cause biliary pain and acute cholecystitis. Approximately 10 percent of patients with sludge will develop gallstones.

Clinical Syndromes

Symptoms of cholelithiasis are unpredictable. They vary considerably and depend on movement of the stones. As many as two thirds of patients with gallstones remain asymptomatic all of their lives ("silent stones"). In other patients, stones once formed remain asymptomatic for 10 to 20 years. If the stones transiently block the cystic duct, biliary pain (misnamed "colic") occurs. A more prolonged obstruction of the cystic duct results in infection behind the obstruction, giving rise to the syndrome of acute cholecystitis. Stones migrating from the gallbladder through the cystic duct into the common bile duct may cause biliary pain, jaundice, cholangitis, or pancreatitis. More rarely, a gallstone erodes through the gallbladder directly into the stomach or small intestine to cause small bowel obstruction, "gallstone ileus."

Asymptomatic Gallstones

By definition, patients with asymptomatic (silent) stones have never had biliary pain. Their gallstones are discovered incidentally during radiographic (plain film) investigations or during abdominal surgery for other indications, or by oral cholecystography and ultrasonography performed in the setting of poorly defined abdominal complaints. Our understanding of the natural history of such patients has changed dramatically over the past 40 years.

Both retrospective and prospective studies indicate that (1) most gallstones, whether cholesterol or pigment in type, are asymptomatic; (2) once the diagnosis of asymptomatic gallstones has been made, such patients usually run a benign course, in that 70 to 90 percent will remain symptom-free for 10 to 25 years; (3) asymptomatic stones are probably more common in men than in women; and (4) patients who develop symptoms usually do so within the first 5 years of diagnosis. Moreover, in more than 90 percent of patients who develop symptoms, the initial symptom is biliary pain rather than a more serious complication, such as acute cholecystitis, cholangitis, or pancreatitis.

Treatment of Patients with Asymptomatic Gallstones

Because of the benign course of most patients with asymptomatic gallstones, expectant management only is the preferred treatment. Neither medical dissolution therapy nor elective cholecystectomy is warranted. These patients have a 10 to 30 percent chance of becoming symptomatic over the next 20 years. If they develop biliary pain, a reevaluation regarding the need for surgery or medical dissolution therapy is indicated.

The Role of Prophylactic Cholecystectomy

There are several groups of asymptomatic gallstone patients for whom prophylactic cholecystectomy (cholecystectomy in the absence of symptoms) is indicated. These include otherwise healthy patients who, because of their occupation, do not have easy access to high-quality medical care (e.g., crew members of nuclear submarines, missionaries or public health field workers in developing countries). In these patients, elective cholecystectomy at a convenient time might be preferable to the very small, but real, risk of developing symptoms or complications under inauspicious conditions. Medical dissolution therapy in these patients would not be advisable because of the necessity of continued close supervision.

A controversial issue is whether diabetics with asymptomatic gallstones should undergo prophylactic cholecystectomy. Since the precise natural history of gallstones in diabetic patients is not known, firm recommendations cannot be made. Once acute cholecystitis occurs, most older studies indicate that diabetics have a three- to fivefold increased mortality compared with non-diabetics. However, *elective* cholecystectomy is not more hazardous in diabetics than in non-diabetics. As a result, the recommendation of elective, prophylactic cholecystectomy was frequently made for all diabetics with stones, since it was not possible to predict which patients would develop cholecystitis. However, recent studies of patients undergoing surgery for acute cholecystitis over the last 15 years found little difference in age-adjusted operative mortality between diabetics and non-diabetics. Therefore, the blanket recommendation that all diabetics with gallstones undergo elective cholecystectomy may need to be revised.

Patients on Prolonged Total Parenteral Nutrition
As discussed earlier, patients receiving long-term TPN (i.e., for longer than 3 months) invariably develop sludge in their gallbladders. These patients have more complications — usually acute cholecystitis — than would be expected in conventional populations with cholelithiasis. It is the opinion of many experts that, if a patient is undergoing laparotomy for a condition that is likely to require long-term TPN — for example, massive small bowel resection or severe Crohn's disease — a prophylactic cholecystectomy should be performed *even though there are no stones* in the gallbladder.

Symptomatic Gallstone Patients
Traditionally, a group of vague, ill-defined "dyspeptic" symptoms have frequently been suggested to be associated with gallstones; these include particular food (usually fatty) intolerance, postprandial bloating, indigestion, flatulence, or abdominal discomfort. These symptoms occur periodically in the general population in the absence of organic disease. Since the general prevalence of gallstones in Western populations is high, it is not surprising to find these symptoms in many patients with gallstones. Large-scale prospective studies of ambulatory individuals and of hospitalized patients showed that these ill-defined "dyspeptic" symptoms occurred no more frequently in gallstone patients than in controls (34–50%). It is now clear that a

history of biliary pain is necessary to make the diagnosis of symptomatic cholelithiasis, even though its specificity is only about 80 percent.

Biliary Pain
Biliary tract pain (misnamed "colic") most often results when a gallstone transiently obstructs the cystic duct. One or more episodes of biliary pain usually precede the serious complication of gallstones such as cholecystitis, cholangitis, or pancreatitis. Biliary pain is not "colicky" (intermittent), but rather steady. Typically, the pain starts gradually, builds to a plateau of intensity over 15 to 30 minutes, remains constant for several hours, and gradually disappears. In a minority (<10%) of patients, both the onset and termination of biliary pain are abrupt. Biliary pain is most frequently localized to the epigastrium or the right upper quadrant, although rarely, pain can occur in the left upper quadrant, in the subxiphoid region, or in the back. In approximately 50 percent of patients, biliary pain radiates to other parts of the abdomen or back, classically to the right shoulder or right subscapular region. Therefore, the physician should not dismiss the possibility of biliary tract disease in the patient whose biliary pain is not in a typical location. Nausea and vomiting may occur during an attack of biliary pain but are often absent.

The time intervals between attacks of biliary pain are highly variable, ranging from months to yearly intervals, or very rarely, daily. There are no predictable precipitants of biliary pain. For example, there is no evidence that ingestion of fatty or rich food, overeating, exercise, straining, or stress induces biliary pain. Nevertheless, patients who have experienced frequent attacks of biliary pain should expect frequent attacks in the future.

The natural history of patients with biliary pain is less benign than that of patients with asymptomatic gallstones. Thirty to sixty percent of patients will develop recurrent pain over a 5- to 20-year period. The incidence of biliary complications also increases with time. Ten percent of patients with biliary pain will develop acute cholecystitis within the next 5 years. When followed for 20 years, 20 to 50 percent of patients with biliary pain will develop biliary complications — principally acute cholecystitis, cholangitis, or pancreatitis. The risk of recurrent pain or complications is greater in women.

Physical examination of a patient during an acute attack of biliary pain is usually normal. The patient frequently is restless, attempting to find a position that relieves the discomfort. Occasionally, tenderness is present in the right upper quadrant. More important, neither fever nor leukocytosis is observed during an attack of biliary pain. If the patient is or becomes febrile, with or without laboratory evidence of infection, progression to acute cholecystitis should be strongly suspected.

Treatment of Patients with Symptomatic Gallstones

The treatment of patients with biliary pain in the absence of biliary complications (acute cholecystitis, cholangitis, or pancreatitis) will vary depending on the severity of the symptoms and the patient's overall medical condition. Thus, the physician's approach to the patient should be individualized. It is controversial whether cholecystectomy should be performed after only a single attack of biliary pain or delayed until several attacks have occurred. It is also not clear what role medical dissolution therapy should play in the overall management of patients with symptomatic gallstones.

Patients with more than one attack of biliary pain should be treated definitively to prevent (1) repeated attacks of biliary pain, and (2) the complications of gallstones, acute cholecystitis, cholangitis, and pancreatitis. There are two drugs (both naturally occurring bile salts), chenodeoxycholic acid and ursodeoxycholic acid, approved for medical dissolution of cholesterol gallstones in selected patients. Thus, there are now potentially two choices available for treatment of symptomatic gallstone patients: medical dissolution therapy and cholecystectomy.

Medical Dissolution Therapy. Because the underlying metabolic abnormality in many patients with cholesterol gallstones is a contracted bile salt pool with a resulting decrease in bile salt secretion, the initial hypothesis was that the chronic ingestion of any bile salt would expand the bile salt pool, increase bile salt secretion rates, desaturate bile with cholesterol, and dissolve cholesterol gallstones. However, it has become apparent that bile salt feeding does not appreciably expand the total bile salt pool, nor does it increase bile salt secretion rates. Both chenodeoxycholic and ursodeoxycholic acid administration desaturate bile and dissolve cholesterol gallstones because they enrich the bile salt pool with their glycine and taurine conjugates. This change in pool composition despite constant total bile salt pool size markedly decreases the secretion rates of cholesterol into bile. Bile becomes desaturated with cholesterol. The newly unsaturated bile dissolves cholesterol molecules from gallstones and holds them in micellar or vesicular solution, and gallbladder contraction discharges the dispersed cholesterol into the duodenum.

Medical dissolution with cheno- or ursodeoxycholic acid dissolves gallstones completely in up to 50% of patients. The success rates depend critically on patient selection. With careful patient selection, successful dissolution rates are 50 to 70 percent. Only those patients who meet the following criteria should be considered for medical dissolution therapy:

1. Patients must have patent cystic ducts, since desaturated hepatic bile must reach the gallbladder and be in intimate contact with the cholesterol gallstones. The recommended method of assessing cystic duct patency is oral cholecystography.
2. Patients should have radiolucent gallstones, since most of them (86%) are composed of cholesterol. Cheno- and ursodeoxycholic acids are effective in dissolving only cholesterol stones. Radiopaque stones are usually (67%) pigment stones and are not amenable to medical dissolution therapy.
3. Female patients should be postmenopausal or using mechanical contraceptive techniques, because chenodeoxycholic acid in high doses has been shown to be harmful to developing fetal monkeys.
4. Patients with small stones (i.e., greater surface-to-volume ratios) respond to therapy better than do patients with larger stones, because stone dissolution is a physicochemical process. Stones larger than 15 mm in diameter dissolve extremely slowly.

Other relative contraindications to chenodeoxycholic acid but not ursodeoxycholic acid treatment include severe obesity (resistance to desaturation), chronic liver disease (liver toxicity), and inflammatory bowel disease (severe diarrhea).

Therapy must be continued until stones dissolve completely. Six to 24 months of treatment is usually necessary for complete dissolution. The bile acids are preferably given at bedtime, since this strategy reduces biliary cholesterol saturation during an overnight fast — a time when it would otherwise be maximal.

Adverse effects of chenodeoxycholic acid therapy are frequent. Hepatic toxicity with marked increases in transaminases is observed in 3 percent of patients. Diarrhea is dose-dependent and occurs in 40 to 50 percent of patients. Since bile secretion is the major route for cholesterol excretion, chenodeoxycholic acid treatment, even at low doses, increases serum LDL cholesterol by 10 percent above baseline in 85 percent of patients. Serum levels of HDL cholesterol are not altered. The potential risk of accelerating atherosclerotic cardiovascular disease in patients taking chenodeoxycholic acid for more than 2 years is unknown but may be appreciable.

After discontinuation of cholelitholytic therapy, all patients resume the secretion of lithogenic bile within 1 week, and 50 percent will reform gallstones within 5 years. It is unlikely that a low maintenance dose of cheno- or ursodeoxycholic acid will prevent gallstone recurrence after dissolution. Perhaps other regimens such as chenodeoxycholic acid plus ursodeoxycholic acid given at bedtime, or dietary manipulations (low cholesterol, high-fiber diet) might prevent gallstone recurrence. Once gallstones have dissolved, bile acid administration can be stopped and the patient reevaluated yearly with ultrasonography to determine whether new stones have formed. If new stones are found, a decision should then be made as to whether ursodeoxycholic acid should be reinstituted.

Ursodeoxycholic acid, the 7 OH epimer of chenodeoxycholic acid, is usually present in small amounts (<2%) in all human biles. Ursodeoxycholic acid, like chenodeoxycholic acid, decreases biliary cholesterol secretion, desaturates bile with cholesterol, and dissolves cholesterol gallstones. Whereas the criteria for patient selection are the same as those for patients taking chenodeoxycholic acid, ursodeoxycholic acid has a number of noteworthy advantages over chenodeoxycholic acid: (1) cholesterol gallstones dissolve faster; (2) the optimal dose is lower; (3) serum cholesterol does not increase; (4) it is not hepatotoxic; and (5) it does not cause diarrhea. Overall, gallstone dissolution and recurrence rates with ursodeoxycholic acid are not appreciably different from those observed with chenodeoxycholic acid.

A combination of extracorporeal shock wave lithotripsy (to shatter the gallstones) with ursodeoxycholic acid (to dissolve the fragments) appears to be a promising new alternative therapy.

Surgical Treatment of Symptomatic Gallstones. Despite the availability of drugs and lithotripsy, cholecystectomy remains the principal option for treatment of patients with symptomatic cholelithiasis. It is an extremely safe operation in young, otherwise healthy individuals and cures the patient's symptoms in more than 85 percent of cases.

Morbidity and mortality from cholecystectomy depend on the patient's age and sex and the presence or absence of acute cholecystitis, cholangitis, or pancreatitis. In all age groups, males have twice the operative mortality of females, probably because of the increased prevalence of cardiovascular disease. Operative mortality increases with age for elective cholecystectomy from an average of 0.2 percent in females at age 30 to 3 percent at age 75. This increase is probably due to concomitant medical problems associated with aging. Importantly, the operative mortality rate for both men and women in all age groups quadruples if a complication of gallstones is the indication for surgery. For example, the operative mortality of a 50-year-old male undergoing elective cholecystectomy is approximately 0.3 percent, but rises to 1 percent in the setting of acute cholecystitis. At 65 years of age, the operative mortality rate for emergency cholecystectomy for males and females increases to 1 and 4 percent, respectively. The latter operative mortality rate is comparable to that for coronary artery bypass surgery.

Older symptomatic patients present the most difficult therapeutic dilemma, because they are likely to have a concomitant medical problem that influences operative mortality and life expectancy. The physician needs to balance the risks of waiting and possibly being forced to perform surgery under adverse conditions, versus the chance that the patient will die of other causes before gallstones cause complications. For example, a male with his first attack of biliary pain at age 65 might be treated surgically if he were otherwise healthy and expected to live an additional 20 years. On the other hand, if the patient were a poor surgical risk, either symptomatic (expectant) treatment or a trial of medical therapy might be appropriate. Obviously, in those symptomatic patients who refuse surgery, expectant management or medical therapy are the only therapeutic possibilities.

Biliary Complications of Gallstones

Acute Cholecystitis

Acute cholecystitis is an acute inflammation of the gallbladder wall. More than ninety percent of cases are due to transient obstruction of the cystic duct by gallstones. Acalculous cholecystitis occurs occasionally, usually in otherwise severely ill hospitalized patients. The precise sequence of events from cystic duct obstruction to acute inflammation of the gallbladder is not fully understood. However, the earliest events (first 24–48 hours) are probably secondary to chemical inflammation of the gallbladder and are not bacterial in origin. Bacteria can be cultured from gallbladder bile in only 35 percent of cases during the first day of an attack. However, after 4 days of acute cholecystitis, cultures are positive in 80 percent of patients. Animal experiments have shown that stones in the gallbladder, with or without cystic duct obstruction, can cause the gallbladder wall to secrete fluid, resulting in a dramatic increase in intraluminal pressure. This secretion is thought to be mediated by prostaglandins.

Clinical Manifestations
The usual attack of acute cholecystitis begins in an identical fashion to an attack of biliary pain. The pain localizes rapidly to

the right hypochondrium and is associated with anorexia, nausea, and vomiting. The range of physical findings depends on the extent of the inflammatory process. Some patients have only mild direct, but no rebound, tenderness and a low-grade fever. Others will have marked tenderness and rebound with guarding and a fever to 102°F. In the first attack of acute cholecystitis, the gallbladder may become palpable, but this finding has no prognostic significance. Laboratory values are abnormal in all cases of acute cholecystitis. In the early stages, the white blood cell count is elevated to 10,000 to 15,000 cells/μl. Higher values suggest empyema or perforation of the gallbladder. Transaminases are usually less than 250 IU. Mild to moderate jaundice (serum bilirubin <7 mg/dl) occurs in roughly 20 percent of patients, even in the absence of common duct stones. The mechanism is unknown but may be a result of absorption of bilirubin across an inflamed gallbladder wall or secondary to transient obstruction of the common bile duct by edema and inflammation from the contiguous inflamed gallbladder. Nonetheless, hyperbilirubinemia of any magnitude in the setting of acute cholecystitis should raise the possibility that a gallstone is present in the common duct. Alkaline phosphatase or serum amylase often becomes elevated, even in the absence of common duct stones or pancreatitis. However, a marked elevation of serum amylase in this clinical setting should raise the suspicion of either a common bile duct stone or pancreatitis.

Diagnosis

The diagnosis of acute cholecystitis should always be considered in patients with abdominal pain, fever, and upper abdominal, especially right upper quadrant, tenderness. Radiographic studies are usually necessary to confirm the diagnosis. An abdominal flatplate and upright x-ray should be obtained and carefully examined for calcified gallstones, air in the biliary system, or free air in the peritoneal cavity.

Abdominal ultrasonography is the appropriate first diagnostic test. A thickened gallbladder wall or localized pericholecystic fluid collections demonstrated by ultrasonography is highly suggestive of acute cholecystitis. Because of the frequency of gallstones in the general population, the presence of stones alone in the gallbladder does not make the diagnosis of acute cholecystitis: Biliary scintigraphy with a ^{99}Tc-labeled iminodiacetic acid derivative (HIDA, PIPIDA, DISIDA) is the test of choice to confirm the diagnosis. These compounds, when injected intravenously, are excreted rapidly in high concentrations into bile even in patients whose serum bilirubin levels are

10 to 20 mg/dl. After injection, the radionuclide normally appears in the biliary tree within 15 to 30 minutes and in the duodenum within 45 minutes. Cholescintigraphy obtained at this time will outline the hepatic bile ducts, gallbladder, common bile duct, and duodenum. In patients with acute cholecystitis, radioactivity will outline the bile ducts and duodenum, but the gallbladder will not be visualized, since the cystic duct is occluded. Such a "positive scan" is consistent with, but not pathognomonic for, acute cholecystitis. However, a great deal of worldwide experience suggests that acute cholecystitis is extremely unlikely if the gallbladder is visualized during such a scan. Moreover, in patients with acalculous cholecystitis, cholescintigraphy is nearly always positive because the cystic duct, although not obstructed by a stone, becomes occluded by edema, viscous mucin, and inflammation. In some very jaundiced patients (serum bilirubin >20 mg/dl), sufficient radioactivity may not be excreted into the biliary tract to allow an adequate determination of gallbladder filling. Such a scan should be labeled "nondiagnostic." False-positive scans may occur in some alcoholics and in some patients receiving TPN. Additionally, some patients with healed, acute cholecystitis (misnamed "chronic cholecystitis") will have false-positive scans because the cystic duct is chronically occluded.

Treatment

The preferred treatment for acute cholecystitis is early cholecystectomy. Surgery should be performed within the first 72 hours of the onset of the attack rather than waiting 6 to 8 weeks after the patient has fully recovered from the acute episode. It is obvious that in acute cholecystitis, bile salt therapy has no role in management and is clearly contraindicated.

The acute treatment of some patients with severe concomitant medical illness (e.g., respiratory failure, myocardial ischemia, renal failure) will take priority over that of biliary surgery. Cholecystectomy should be delayed in these high-risk patients until they are reasonably stable following management by supportive measures. Occasionally, a patient in the high surgical risk category may still have a functioning gallbladder following recovery from acute cholecystitis. Chronic therapy with ursodeoxycholic acid might be tried in this situation. The natural history of patients with a prior episode of acute cholecystitis who do not have a cholecystectomy is poor. Recurrences of biliary colic and complications are common, occurring in 50 percent of patients within 5 years. A nonfunctioning gallbladder by oral cholecystography doubles the risk of future complications in these patients.

Gallstone Ileus

Small bowel obstruction secondary to an impacted gallstone is called gallstone ileus. It usually results from a large gallstone that has eroded through the gallbladder wall into the small bowel. In the nondiseased small bowel, the gallstone will become impacted at the ileocecal valve. However, in patients with small bowel disease or previous surgery, the gallstone can become impacted at any site. Clinically, gallstone ileus should be suspected in any elderly patient presenting with small bowel obstruction. The treatment of gallstone ileus is surgical removal of the impacted gallstone. Generally, the cholecystoduodenal fistula does not require repair, because it will rarely cause symptoms.

Although it often occurs in the setting of long-standing clinical gallbladder disease, 30 percent of patients give no antecedent clinical history of cholelithiasis. Most (85%) patients will experience vomiting, whereas only half will have right upper quadrant tenderness. The abdominal plain film is critical in making the diagnosis. Air in the biliary tree is present in at least 60 percent of patients. Additionally, a radiopaque gallstone outside the gallbladder will be seen in nearly half of these patients.

*Choledo-
cholithiasis
(Common Duct
Stones)*

Stones in the common bile duct originate in one of two ways. They either migrate from the gallbladder (95%) or form de novo in the common duct (5%). The migratory stones, having originated in the gallbladder, are usually cholesterol stones. In contrast, stones that originate de novo in the common bile duct are usually calcium bilirubinate stones. The frequency of coexisting stones in the common bile duct at the time of surgery for gallbladder stones increases with the age of the patient. In patients younger than 60 years of age, the prevalence of common duct stones in association with gallbladder stones is about 8 to 15 percent. This figure increases to nearly 50 percent in patients aged 80 years and older. These data suggest that the longer that stones are present in the gallbladder, the greater is the chance that they will migrate into the common bile duct. Even after careful surgical exploration and removal of common duct stones, one or more stones are left behind in 1 to 10 percent of cases.

The mechanisms by which stones form de novo in the common duct following cholecystectomy are poorly defined. Unabsorbed suture material clearly plays a role, being present in 30 percent of removed stones. Since the stones are composed chiefly of calcium bilirubinate plus calcium salts of long-chain fatty acids, it is likely that stasis and infection play a major role. Nevertheless, biliary strictures or other anatomic changes leading to stasis are usually not found in such patients: Intrinsic motor abnormalities of the sphincter of Oddi or in the common bile duct itself may be responsible.

With the widespread use of endoscopic papillotomy, the management of retained or newly formed common duct stones is now less hazardous. An endoscopic papillotomy or an attempt to remove a retained stone with a basket by the T-tube are acceptable methods of treatment.

Attempted dissolution of retained common duct stones with T-tube infusion of other cholesterol solvents, such as monooctanoin cholate, is not recommended. Sodium cholate is toxic to the biliary tree and should not be used. Use of monooctanoin is associated with a high incidence of side effects, including abdominal pain, nausea, vomiting, and diarrhea. Furthermore, it causes tissue damage in the biliary tree, stomach, and duodenum.

In patients with a retained common duct stone, but without a T-tube in place, the procedure of choice for removal is by endoscopic papillotomy. This procedure is safe and effective. It has a mortality rate of about 1 percent, and stones can be removed in more than 85 percent of cases. Relative contraindications include stones greater than 2 cm in size, bile duct stricture proximal to the ampulla, an ampulla situated in a duodenal diverticulum, and significant coagulopathy. If endoscopic papillotomy fails, medical dissolution therapy with ursodeoxycholic acid could be attempted provided that the following conditions are rigorously adhered to: (1) There is incomplete, not total, obstruction of the common duct; (2) there is no evidence of biliary tract infection; and (3) the patient's stones, removed at cholecystectomy, contain predominantly cholesterol. Surgical removal and exploration of the common bile duct should be considered the last resort. However, it should be done promptly if endoscopic papillotomy fails in the setting of a patient with an infected or obstructed biliary tree.

Clinical Syndromes of Choledocho- lithiasis

The clinical syndromes associated with common bile duct stones are highly variable. Ten percent of patients with stones in the gallbladder pass stones "silently" into the common duct and out into the intestines to be eliminated in the feces. The natural history of stones that remain lodged in the common bile duct is unpredictable. Some patients may remain asymptomatic for months to several years. Presenting features of the patient with common duct stones include (1) cholangitis, (2) intermittent or persistent obstructive jaundice with or without pain, (3) acute pancreatitis, and (4) biliary pain without other complications.

Cholangitis

Cholangitis is a bacterial infection of the bile ducts and bile. Whereas bile duct obstruction does not invariably produce cholangitis, cholangitis *cannot* occur without obstruction by either stone, stricture, or a neoplasm. The risk of cholangitis is related to the underlying cause, not to the degree of bile duct obstruction. For example, cultures of bile from jaundiced patients with a malignant obstruction are positive in 36 percent of cases, whereas they are positive in 72 percent of patients with calculi. The clinical correlate is that progressive high-grade obstruction from choledochal, pancreatic, or duodenal neoplasms is associated with only about a 10 percent risk of cholangitis in comparison to a 33 percent risk in patients with common duct stones. The clinical manifestations of cholangitis are protean. Some patients will have a mild, self-limited illness characterized by fever, chills, abdominal pain, and dark urine. Other patients present with sepsis and shock without specific signs of biliary tract disease. The usual patient presents with jaundice, chills, and fever (Charcot's triad) together with abdominal pain. Jaundice may be clinically absent in 20 percent of patients. Unlike biliary pain, the abdominal pain associated with cholangitis is generally mild; severe pain should raise the possibility that acute cholecystitis or acute pancreatitis is present.

The physical findings in patients with cholangitis are also variable. Abdominal tenderness is frequent but is not always present. Rebound tenderness or guarding is uncommon, because peritoneal irritation is not a prominent feature. Hypotension and mental confusion occur in about 15 percent of cases and forebode an ominous outcome.

In the diagnosis of cholangitis, laboratory tests are not pathognomonic. Leukocytosis, occasionally as high as 40,000/μl, often occurs. Elevations of serum bilirubin, alkaline phosphatase, transaminases, and amylase are common but will not distinguish cholangitis from acute cholecystitis or pancreatitis. However, cholangitis is extremely unlikely in the presence of normal liver function tests. Bacteremia occurs in 40 percent of patients: The organisms responsible are most commonly *Escherichia coli* and *Klebsiella*. In addition, in about 15 percent of patients, anaerobes are found in the biliary tract.

Radiographic studies are generally nondiagnostic. Abdominal plain films can show air in the biliary tree if gas-producing organisms are present but more often are normal or show a nonspecific small bowel ileus. Abdominal ultrasonography may show a dilated common bile duct with or without a stone. However, its specificity is low because cholangitis can occur without ductal dilatation. Furthermore, stones in the common duct are more difficult to visualize by ultrasonography than are stones in the gallbladder.

Cholangitis is a medical and surgical emergency. The patient should be quickly stabilized with intravenous hydration and antibiotics followed by prompt surgical or endoscopic decompression of the common bile duct. Medical dissolution therapy is obviously contraindicated in patients with gallstone-related cholangitis.

The options for emergency decompression include laparotomy and T-tube drainage of the common bile duct, endoscopic cannulation with catheter drainage or papillotomy, or percutaneous placement of a transhepatic catheter. Decompression should not be delayed because "the patient is too sick," since drainage of the biliary tree will produce immediately beneficial results.

The operative approach to definitive biliary decompression will depend on (1) the etiology of the ductal obstruction, and (2) whether the gallbladder is still present. Prior to definitive surgery, the anatomy of the biliary tree and the nature of the ductal obstruction should be delineated by direct cholangiography, either by percutaneous transhepatic cholangiography (PTC) or an endoscopic retrograde cholangiopancreatography (ERCP).

Intermittent or Persistent Jaundice

Common bile duct stones can also present with either intermittent or persistent jaundice, with or without pain. Common duct stones are the cause of obstruction in approximately 10 percent of patients presenting with "painless jaundice." Although a gallstone etiology of intermittent or persistent jaundice can often be inferred by history/physical examination, laboratory tests, or ultrasonography, the extrahepatic biliary tree should be visualized by PTC or ERCP preoperatively to confirm the diagnosis and to provide precise guidelines for surgical management. The degree of elevation of serum bilirubin is often proportional to the degree of biliary tract obstruction. Since common duct stones usually cause low-grade, intermittent obstruction, serum bilirubin levels rarely exceed 10 to 15 mg/dl. Elevation of alkaline phosphatase is less useful, although nearly always abnormal, varying from less than 400 (80% of patients) to more than 1000 IU.

The simplest and fastest method to initially evaluate the patient with suspected choledocholithiasis is abdominal ultrasonography. The ultrasonogram is extremely useful if a common duct dilatation or a gallstone is seen. However, a normal-sized common bile duct does not rule out the presence of common duct stones. Ductal dilatation may be absent if hepatic cirrhosis or sclerosing cholangitis is present. Moreover, ductal dilatation may not occur because of the low-grade, intermittent character of the obstruction.

Definitive diagnosis of common bile duct stones is made by direct visualization of the biliary tree by either PTC or ERCP.

Gallstone Pancreatitis

Alcohol abuse and gallstones are the leading causes of acute pancreatitis in industrialized societies. There is ample evidence that gallstones migrating from the gallbladder through the biliary tree and into the duodenum are the initial event in causing pancreatitis.

An acute attack of gallstone pancreatitis is indistinguishable from an episode of acute pancreatitis from any other cause. Gallstone pancreatitis rarely results in chronic pancreatitis or pancreatic insufficiency, even after recurrent attacks. In contrast, alcoholic pancreatitis is a chronic, progressive, or relapsing disease that often results in chronic pancreatitis and pancreatic insufficiency (see Chap. 20).

The diagnosis of gallstone pancreatitis can be difficult. An abdominal ultrasonogram or CT scan will only detect the common duct gallstone directly in 15 to 50 percent of patients, respectively. Lack of stones in the gallbladder is not helpful in excluding the diagnosis. A dilated common bile duct is also not that helpful in establishing that a stone is impacted, because dilatation of the bile ducts secondary to external compression can be seen in acute or chronic pancreatitis of any etiology.

The immediate medical treatment of acute gallstone pancreatitis is the same as that for acute pancreatitis of any other etiology. However, the definitive therapy is cholecystectomy and removal of ductal stones, particularly those impacted at the ampulla of Vater. If the patient with gallstone pancreatitis deteriorates or fails to improve with medical management, the stones must be removed urgently, usually within the first 48 hours. This is one of the few indications for emergency ERCP and papillotomy. If ERCP is not feasible, PTC should be performed to localize the obstruction, after which emergency surgery should be employed. After recovery from an acute attack of gallstone pancreatitis, the patient should have an elective cholecystectomy and common bile duct exploration as soon as possible. If cholecystectomy is delayed, 25 percent of patients will have another attack of potentially fatal acute pancreatitis within 30 days, and 50 percent will within 11 months.

Acalculous Cholecystitis

Acute cholecystitis occurring in the *absence* of gallstones is called acalculous cholecystitis. It is rare and usually occurs in patients in the postoperative period. It also occurs in patients already hospitalized for severe illnesses such as burns, trauma, or severe cardiovascular disease. Many of these patients have been receiving total parenteral nutrition. Because it is associated with prolonged fasting, gallbladder stasis may be responsible. Others have postulated the pathophysiology to be an ischemic injury to the gallbladder.

The signs, symptoms, and laboratory findings of acalculous cholecystitis are identical to those seen in calculous cholecystitis. The difficulty in diagnosis is that patients at risk for acalculous cholecystitis may be too ill to give an accurate history. Furthermore, the symptoms may be masked in the postoperative period by administration of narcotics. In contrast to the female predominance of calculous cholecystitis (reflecting the increased prevalence of gallstones in women), acalculous cholecystitis affects men more frequently (males : females 1.5 : 1).

The diagnosis of acalculous cholecystitis is made by abdominal ultrasonography and cholescintigraphy, just as is the case with calculous disease. Even though the cystic duct is not obstructed with a stone in acalculous cholecystitis, the radionuclide will not enter the gallbladder because of inflammation and edema of the cystic duct.

Acalculous cholecystitis is a serious disease with a mortality rate of 40 percent. This high mortality rate probably results from delay in diagnosis and concomitant, severe underlying disease.

Sclerosing
Cholangitis

Sclerosing cholangitis is a rare inflammatory disorder of the bile ducts of unknown etiology that results in multiple biliary strictures. The patient comes to clinical attention because of jaundice, pruritus, unexplained portal hypertension, or an unexplained elevation of alkaline phosphatase. Fever and chills characteristic of bacterial cholangitis are uncommon.

Jaundice results from progressive obliteration of the bile ducts. Pruritus presumably occurs because of the retention of bile salts and their metabolites. Portal hypertension can occur late in the disease secondary to long-standing biliary obstruction and secondary biliary cirrhosis. Serum alkaline phosphatase is invariably increased because, as with any disorder causing obstruction of bile ducts, biliary columnar epithelial cells increase their synthesis of this enzyme, which then refluxes into the serum.

More than 50 percent of patients with sclerosing cholangitis have ulcerative colitis. There is no relationship between extent or activity of the colonic disease and the sclerosing cholangitis. The treatment of ulcerative colitis, including colectomy, does not influence the course of sclerosing cholangitis. In recent years, as more patients with ulcerative colitis and subtle abnormalities of liver function (e.g., elevated alkaline phosphatase) are studied by ERCP, subclinical sclerosing cholangitis is being recognized more often.

The diagnosis of sclerosing cholangitis is made by direct visualization of the bile ducts. ERCP is preferred over PTC because of the difficulty in entering narrowed bile ducts with a needle.

Subclinical sclerosing cholangitis (i.e., abnormal liver function tests in the absence of symptoms) requires no treatment. Once pruritis occurs, it can be treated with bile salt binding agents such as cholestyramine. Surgery or endoscopic placement of biliary stents may be required to bypass tight strictures. Some patients with sclerosing cholangitis develop bile duct cancer.

Gallbladder Cancer

Gallbladder cancer is uncommon in the general population. However, there are certain groups of individuals who are at increased risk for developing carcinoma of the gallbladder.

All patients with gallstones have a slight increased risk of developing gallbladder cancer. In fact, more than 80 percent of patients with gallbladder cancer have gallstones. Four subgroups with gallstones have now been identified as having a four- to tenfold increased risk of developing gallbladder cancer: (1) Mexican-American women with strong American Indian heritage, (2) American Indian women, (3) patients with solitary stones that exceed 3.0 cm in diameter, and (4) patients with gallstones of very long duration.

There are two additional conditions associated with gallbladder cancer: (1) patients with "porcelain" gallbladders, and (2) *Salmonella typhosa* carriers. Porcelain gallbladder is a result of precipitation of salts of calcium phosphate in the gallbladder mucosa and, although rare, is associated with extremely high (20–60%) incidence of gallbladder cancer. The diagnosis is made on an abdominal flatplate x-ray by observing patchy calcification of the gallbladder wall.

Adenocarcinomas account for more than 80 percent of gallbladder cancer. Tumor growth is rapid, and extra mucosal and even local extension is common by the time that symptoms occur.

Symptoms and signs of gallbladder cancer mimic those of acute cholecystitis. Occasionally, a firm mass can be palpated in the right upper quadrant. Because the findings are nonspecific, the correct preoperative diagnosis is made infrequently (10% of cases).

Treatment is surgical resection. Cure is infrequent because of the frequency of local invasion or distant metastases at the time of operation.

Prophylactic cholecystectomy in *all* individuals with gallstones would reduce the incidence of gallbladder cancer. However, the risk for surgery for even elective prophylactic cholecystectomy far outweighs most patients' chances of developing gallbladder cancer. However, in the six groups at much higher risk for developing gallbladder cancer, prophylactic cholecystectomy is strongly indicated. Medical therapy to dissolve gallstones in these high-risk patients would not be appropriate, since the gallstones per se may not necessarily be the causative or even the promoting factor.

Bile Duct Cancer The etiology of bile duct cancer is unknown. Unlike gallbladder cancer, which is associated with gallstones in more than 80 percent of cases, bile duct cancer is associated with gallstones in only 30 percent of patients. Bile duct cancer is associated with ulcerative colitis and, like sclerosing cholangitis, is unrelated to the severity of the colitis.

Most bile duct cancers are adenocarcinomas. The location of the tumor will dictate the clinical presentation. Approximately 50 percent of bile duct cancers arise in the proximal one third of the bile ducts, 25 percent in the middle one third, and 25 percent in the distal third. Occasionally, they will arise diffusely or in the cystic duct.

Obstructive jaundice is the most common sign of bile duct cancer. In some patients, it may be preceded by pruritus. Cholangitis and biliary pain are rare. The gallbladder may be palpable if the tumor is distal to a patent cystic duct. The gallbladder will be contracted if the tumor is proximal to or involves the cystic duct.

The diagnosis of bile duct cancer must always be considered in patients with obstructive jaundice. Malignant obstruction of the biliary tree generally produces more severe jaundice (mean serum bilirubin 20 mg/dl) than obstruction caused by a gallstone (mean serum bilirubin 5 mg/dl).

The serum alkaline phosphatase is always elevated. Serum transaminases are normal or mildly elevated. Ultrasonography or CT scan of the abdomen may demonstrate a dilated biliary tree. Direct cholangiography either by ERCP or PTC is necessary to define the extent and exact location of the lesion and should always be performed preoperatively. The cholangiographic picture is usually diagnostic. Nonetheless, surgery for tissue conformation and attempted curative resection is generally indicated. In patients unfit for surgery, biliary stents can be placed either percutaneously or endoscopically for palliation.

Study Questions 1. A 30-year-old male with Crohn's disease limited to the ileum undergoes a resection of 150 cm of the distal ileum, the cecum, and the ascending colon with construction of an ileotransverse colostomy.

    A. How would this operation change the following:
       a. Fecal excretion of bile salts

  b. Bile salt synthesis
  c. Bile salt secretion rate and bile salt pool size
  d. Cholesterol saturation index of bile
  e. The relative amount of cholic, deoxycholic, and chenodeoxycholic acid in the bile salt pool
  f. Serum cholesterol

Answers

a. Fecal excretion of bile salts would increase because loss of 150 cm of distal ileum would lead to bile salt malabsorption.
b. Bile salt synthesis would increase in response to bile malabsorption and decreased return of bile salts to the liver.
c. The bile salt secretion rate would decrease because bile salt malabsorption would exceed the liver's capacity to increase bile salt synthesis.
d. The cholesterol saturation index of the bile would increase as the bile salt pool size decreases.
e. The amount of deoxycholic acid in the bile salt pool would increase while that of cholic and chenodeoxycholic acid would decrease because of increased bacterial conversion of the primary bile salts to secondary bile salts.
f. Serum cholesterol would fall. As a result of bile salt malabsorption the liver increases the synthesis of bile salts from cholesterol, eventually resulting in decreased serum cholesterol.

B. Would you expect this patient to develop gallstones? If so, what would their composition be?

Answer

This patient is at increased risk of developing cholesterol gallstones because his bile salt pool is markedly reduced. With less bile salt, the bile becomes supersaturated with cholesterol.

2. A 45-year-old woman comes to the emergency room with the complaint of two hours of severe, steady right upper quadrant pain accompanied by nausea. Her past medical history is unrevealing except for four uncomplicated pregnancies. A plain x-ray of the abdomen is unremarkable, but an abdominal ultrasound reveals several gallstones.

  A. Answer true or false:
    a. She is likely to have pigment gallstones.
    b. She is likely to have cholesterol gallstones.
    c. A risk factor for cholesterol gallstones in this patient is her previous pregnancies.

    d. The chance that a patient with biliary pain will develop a complication of gallstones such as acute cholecystitis, cholangitis, or pancreatitis within the next 20 years is in the range of 25 to 50 percent.

Answers
a. False
b. True
c. True
d. True

B. The patient is reluctant to undergo surgery and expresses a preference for oral dissolution therapy with ursodeoxycholic acid. Answer true or false:
    a. If the size of the largest gallstone exceeds 30 mm, she would not be a suitable candidate for oral dissolution therapy.
    b. The fact that the gallstones were not visible on a plain x-ray examination of the abdomen suggests that the stones are composed of cholesterol.
    c. Failure to visualize the gallbladder on an oral cholecystographic (OCG) study implies a high likelihood of success with oral dissolution therapy.

Answers
a. True
b. True
c. False

References

Apstein, M. D., and Carey, M. C. Gallstones. In W. T. Branch Jr. (ed.), *Office Practice of Medicine* (2nd ed.). Philadelphia: Saunders, 1987. Pp. 399–423.

Bachrach, W. H., and Hofmann, A. F. Ursodeoxycholic acid in the treatment of cholesterol cholelithiasis. *Dig. Dis. Sci.* 27:737–761, 833–856, 1982.

Carey, M. C., and Cahalane, M. J. Enterohepatic Circulation. In I. M. Arias, W. B. Jakoloy, H. Popper, D. Schachter, et al. (eds.), *The Liver: Biology and Pathobiology* (2nd ed.). New York: Raven Press, 1988.

Carey, M. C., and Cahalane, M. J. Whither biliary sludge? *Gastroenterology* 95:508, 1988.

Chalmers, T. C. (ed.). Gallstones. *Semin. Liver Dis.* 3:87, May 1983.

Fromm, H. Gallstone dissolution therapy. Current status and future prospects. *Gastroenterology* 91:1560, 1986.

Gracie, W. A., and Ransohoff, D. P. The natural history of silent gallstones. The innocent gallstone is not a myth. *N. Engl. J. Med.* 307:798, 1982.

Paumgartner, G. Fragmentation of gallstones by extracorporeal shock wave. *Sem. Liver Dis.* 7:317, 1987.

Somjien, G. J., and Gilat, T. Changing concepts of cholesterol solubility in bile. *Gastroenterology* 91:772–775, 1986.

20 : Disorders of the Pancreas

James M. Richter

Roger J. May

The pancreas is often neglected by students of digestive diseases because of its relatively inaccessible position in the retroperitoneum and the difficulty it poses for study, diagnosis, and effective treatment. Its importance in digestion and regulation of metabolism has stimulated much research to elucidate the biochemical pathways and mechanisms of pancreatic diseases. It is hoped that such investigations may offer a new understanding and opportunity for more effective treatments. In the last decade, ultrasonography, computed tomography (CT), needle aspiration biopsy, and endoscopic retrograde cholangiopancreatography (ERCP) have improved access to the pancreas and have allowed clinicians to assess the pathologic and physiologic changes that occur in pancreatic disease.

Embryology

The pancreas originates from outpouches of the primitive gastrointestinal tract in the fifth week of gestation. The dorsal bud forms the future body and tail of the gland. The ventral bud arises adjacent to the anlage of the gallbladder and bile ducts and later forms most of the head of the gland. Between the fifth and seventh week, the ventral pancreas and bile ducts rotate about the foregut and the two portions of the pancreas fuse. Usually the duct of the ventral bud grows and forms the major duct of the gland (duct of Wirsung). The duct of the dorsal bud, which joins the junction of the duct of Wirsung and the duodenum, develops to a lesser degree, forming the duct of Santorini.

Pancreas divisum occurs when the two ducts fail to fuse and the dorsal pancreas continues to drain into the duodenum through the duct of Santorini by way of the accessory papilla. Annular pancreas occurs when a second ventral bud develops and fails to rotate fully about the duodenum, resulting in pancreatic tissue encircling and possibly obstructing the duodenum.

Anatomy

The pancreas lies in a transverse position across the upper abdomen in the retroperitoneum (Fig. 20-1). The head rests in the curvature of the duodenum, and the body extends to the left so that the tail touches the hilum of the spleen. The gland is nor-

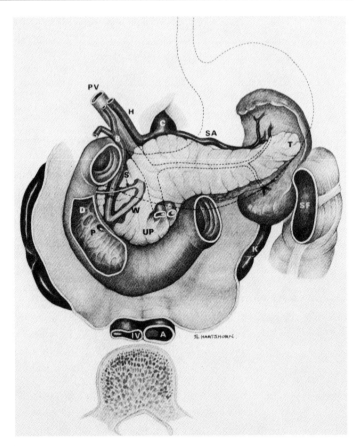

Fig. 20-1
Diagram of pancreas in situ and its major relations. (Key: A = abdominal aorta behind peritoneum on posterior abdominal wall; B = common bile duct; C = celiac trunk; D = second part of duodenum; H = hepatic artery; IV = inferior vena cava; K = lateral border of left kidney; P = major papilla; PV = portal vein; S = accessory pancreatic duct; SA = splenic artery; SF = splenic flexure of colon; T = tail of pancreas; UP = uncinate process passing behind superior mesenteric vessels; W = main pancreatic duct.) (From P. F. Harris. Anatomy. In H. Howat and H. Sarles [eds.], *The Exocrine Pancreas.* Philadelphia: Saunders, 1979.)

mally 10 to 15 cm in length and weighs from 60 to 100 gm. The head of the gland, which has the greatest mass, lies just anterior to the vena cava, renal veins, and right renal artery. The common bile duct usually passes through the head of the gland to the ampulla of Vater. The body and tail of the pancreas extend to the left, superiorly crossing the aorta, superior mesenteric vessels, left kidney, and left adrenal. The inferior surface of the pancreas is covered by peritoneum and the attachment of the transverse mesocolon.

The pancreas has a dual blood supply arising from the celiac axis and the superior mesenteric artery. The head of the gland is fed by the retroduodenal branch of the hepatic artery, the superior pancreaticoduodenal branch of the gastroduodenal artery, and the inferior pancreaticoduodenal branch of the superior mesenteric artery. The body and tail of the gland are perfused by branches of the celiac trunk and the splenic artery.

The pancreatic lymphatics drain into the pancreaticoduodenal and subpyloric lymph nodes on the right and to lymph nodes on the hilum of the spleen on the left. The pancreas is innervated by both sympathetic nerves, arising from the splanchnic nerves of the celiac ganglia and parasympathetic nerves, passing from the vagus also along the celiac axis. Pain from the pancreas is conducted along the visceral afferents to the splanchnic and sympathetic ganglia bilaterally.

The pancreas consists of units of exocrine cells clustered about a ductule forming acini (Fig. 20-2). The ductules successively merge into larger ducts and finally into the main collecting system. Digestive enzymes secreted by the exocrine cells are supplemented by bicarbonate-rich fluid produced by the ductular cells. This fluid then passes into the duodenum by way of the ductular drainage system. Islets of Langerhans are studded throughout the exocrine gland, separated from the acinar structures by a thin layer of reticular fibers. The islets have three types of granular cells: (1) alpha cells secreting glucagon, (2) beta cells secreting insulin, and (3) delta cells secreting somatostatin.

Physiology of the Exocrine Pancreas

The exocrine pancreas secretes a colorless, odorless alkaline fluid of low viscosity. The volume and composition of secretion varies considerably depending on diet and regulatory factors. On average, each human secretes about 20 ml per kg per day, which is about 1500 ml for the average adult male. The volume and secretion is substantially higher in the fully fed individual and lower in the fasting person. Pancreatic juice consists of water, inorganic salts, and proteins. The sodium content (145 mEq/liter) and potassium content (5 mEq/liter) of the liquid are similar to that of serum. There are usually 1.6 mEq/liter of calcium and 0.4 mEq/liter of magnesium. The concentrations of chloride and bicarbonate vary but together usually total 155 mEq/liter.

Under stimulation of secretin, pancreatic ductular cells secrete large volumes of a fluid rich in bicarbonate, raising the final concentration of bicarbonate in pancreatic fluid. At low rates of secretion, a fluid high in chloride and reciprocally lower in bicarbonate is produced. The pH of pancreatic fluid is generally 6.6 to 8.2. This alkaline buffer aids in the neutralization of the

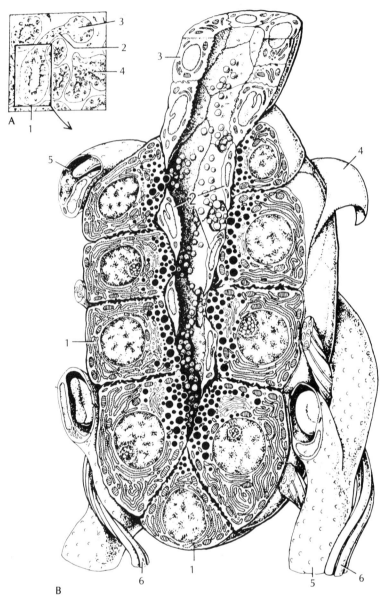

Fig. 20-2
Scheme of an acinus from the pancreas. A. 1, acinus; 2, intercalated duct; 3, intralobular duct; 4, centroacinar cell. B. 1, acinar cell; 2, centroacinar cells; 3, intercalated duct cell; 4, basement membrane; 5, blood capillaries; 6, nerve fibers × 3000. (From R. V. Krstic. *Die Gewebe dem Menschen und der Säugetiere.* © 1978 Springer-Verlag Berlin-Heidelberg-New York. Pp. 1–393.)

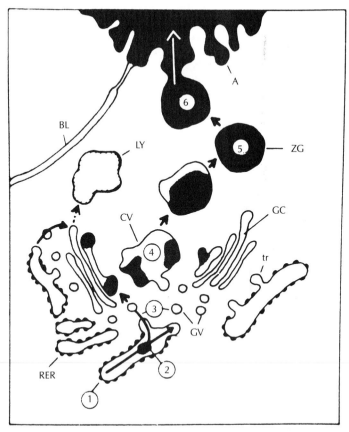

Fig. 20-3
Summary of primary steps in processing of a secretory protein. 1. Synthesis on polysomes and transfer into the rough endoplasmic reticulum (RER); 2. protein modification in the RER; 3. transfer by Golgi vesicles (GV) to the Golgi complex (GC); 4. further modification and concentration in the GC; 5. storage in the zymogen granule (ZG); 6. exocytosis. (Key: tr = transitional elements of RER; LY = lysosome; A = apical membrane; BL = basolateral membrane.) (From F. S. Gorelick and J. D. Jamieson. Structure-Function Relationships of the Pancreas. In L. R. Johnson [ed.], *Physiology of the Gastrointestinal Tract* [2nd ed.]. New York: Raven, 1987. P. 1099.)

hydrochloric acid from the stomach and adjusts the pH of the duodenal lumen to about 6.5 to 7, which is the optimal level for most pancreatic enzymes. Pancreatic acinar cells secrete fluid high in protein content. More than 90 percent of the proteins in pancreatic secretions consist of enzymes or proenzymes. The remainder are plasma proteins, proteolytic enzyme inhibitors, and mucoproteins. Enzymes are synthesized in the rough endoplasmic reticulum of the acinar cells and are then condensed by the Golgi apparatus into zymogen granules (Fig. 20-3). When the pancreas is stimulated either by the vagus nerve or by cholecystokinin, zymogen granules migrate to the apex of the exocrine

Table 20-1
Physiology of pancreatic enzymes

Zymogen	Enzyme	Activator	Catalytic function
Trypsinogen	Trypsin	Enerokinase, Ca^{2+}, trypsin	Cleaves peptide bonds adjacent to basic amino acids
Chymotrypsinogen	Chymotrypsin	Trypsin	Cleaves peptide bonds adjacent to aromatic amino acids
Procarboxy-peptidase A	Carboxypeptidase A	Trypsin	Cleaves carboxyterminal amino acids with aromatic or branched-chain alphatic side chains
Procarboxy-peptidase B	Carboxypeptidase B	Trypsin	Cleaves carboxyterminal amino acids with basic side chains
Proelastase	Elastase	Trypsin	Cleaves bonds adjacent to neutral amino acids, in elastin, other proteins
Proelastomucase	Elastomucase	Trypsin	A chymotryptic-like protease, complexed with proelastase, cleaves mucoproteins of elastin
	Prolinase		Cleaves dipeptides of proline, hydroxyproline
	Ribonuclease		Ribonucleic acids to nucleotides
	Deoxyribonuclease		Deoxynucleic acids to nucleotides
	Amylase	Chloride	Starch to dextrins and maltose
	Lipase	Colipase	Triglycerides to 1,2-diglycerides + fatty acids; 1,2-glycerides to 2-monoglycerides + fatty acids
	Esterase	Bile salts	Splits water-soluble esters of short-chain fatty acids
Prophospholipase A	Phospholipase A	Bile salts Trypsin	Phospholipid to fatty acids and γ^- lysophospholipids
	Phospholipase B	Bile salts	Lysophospholipids to fatty acids and glyceryl-phosphorylcholine, etc.

cell, their membrane fuses with the plasma membrane, and secretory proteins are released into the acinar space.

New enzyme synthesis proceeds at a very rapid rate, requiring only about 50 minutes for synthesis and secretion. The enzymes secreted by the pancreas include proteases, amylase, lipase, and phospholipase (Table 20-1). The proteases include trypsin, chymotrypsin, carboxypeptidases, and elastase, which cleave peptide bonds, yielding oligopeptides, and amino acids. Amylase hydrolyzes complex carbohydrates to oligosaccharides. Lipase hydrolyzes triglycerides to monoglycerides and fatty acids. Pancreatic phospholipase hydrolyzes phospholipids to lysophospholipids and fatty acids.

Most pancreatic enzymes are synthesized and stored as inactive precursors of enzymes or proenzymes. Activation in the duodenal lumen is catalyzed by a proteolytic enzyme called *enterokinase,* which is produced by duodenal epithelial cells. In addition, a trypsin inhibitor is present in pancreatic fluid, which decreases the small proteolytic activity of trypsinogen. When the enzymes are secreted into the gastrointestinal tract, the trypsin inhibitors are diluted and a critical amount of trypsin is formed, which further catalyzes the conversion of trypsinogen and other proenzymes into active enzymes. This complex mechanism of controlling the activation of pancreatic enzymes helps protect the pancreas from autodigestion.

Control of Pancreatic Secretion

Secretin is a polypeptide containing 27 amino acid residues that stimulates pancreatic secretion of relatively high volumes of fluid with low concentrations of enzymes and a high concentration of bicarbonate. The primary site of secretin-mediated stimulation appears to be the ductular epithelium, which results in secretion of fluid rich in bicarbonate. Secretin appears to be produced by mucosal epithelial "S" cells of the upper small intestine, and its release is stimulated by acidification of the duodenum and by hydrolyzed by-products of protein and fat.

Cholecystokinin is another hormone that stimulates pancreatic secretion. It causes the pancreas to produce small volumes of fluid containing high enzyme concentrations and relatively low bicarbonate concentrations. The fluid contains small amounts of sodium bicarbonate, suggesting that the primary effect of this hormone is on the acinar cell. The secretory effects of cholecystokinin are markedly potentiated by concomitant stimulation with secretin. The location of the synthesis of cholecystokinin is uncertain, but it appears to come from proximal intestinal mucosa. Its release is stimulated by the presence in the intestinal lumen of peptides, amino acids, and fatty acids.

Pancreatic secretion is also stimulated by parasympathetic neural stimulation, producing a fluid that is usually low in volume and rich in enzymes. Consequently, anticholinergic drugs or surgical interruption of the vagus nerve has an antisecretory effect.

Pancreatic secretion can be divided into three phases (Table 20-2). The cephalic phase begins 1 to 2 minutes after the sight of food and usually well before gastric secretion of hydrochloric acid. The initial fluid contains large amounts of bicarbonate and enzyme. The cephalic phase is largely mediated by vagal stimulation, but there is probably some secondary release of secretin or cholecystokinin owing to local vagal stimulation. The gastric phase of pancreatic secretion begins when food enters the stomach. Gastric distention and antral distention stimulate the

Table 20-2
Phases of pancreatic secretion

Phase	Stimulus	Mediator	Primary response
Cephalic	Sight or smell of food, chewing, swallowing	Cholinergic fibers from vagus	Enzyme secretion
Gastric	Distention	Vagus	Enzyme secretion
Intestinal	Fatty acids or amino acids in duodenum	Cholecystokinin	Enzyme synthesis and secretion
	H^+ in duodenum	Secretion	Bicarbonate and water secretion

pancreas by the vagus nerve and cholecystokinin. The third intestinal phase of pancreatic secretion begins when hydrochloric acid enters the duodenum and secretin release is stimulated. Amino acids and fat then further stimulate release of cholecystokinin.

The presence of high concentrations of active trypsin and chymotrypsin in the lumen of the duodenum and jejunum inhibits pancreatic acinar secretion of enzymes. The mechanism of this feedback is not known but may be used clinically by giving patients exogenous enzymes to decrease pancreatic stimulation and blunt the pain of chronic pancreatitis.

Hydrolysis of dietary proteins occurs mainly in the lumen of the duodenum and proximal jejunum. Trypsin, chymotrypsin, elastase, and carboxypeptidases are activated from their proenzymes and hydrolyze proteins to a mixture of free amino acids and short peptides of two to six residues in length. These peptides are further hydrolyzed and absorbed by the surface of the intestinal mucosa.

Fat is the most difficult nutrient for the digestive tract to assimilate. Ingested fat is disrupted by the mechanical activity of the stomach. Pancreatic procolipase is cleaved by trypsin to colipase, which binds to triglyceride in the duodenal lumen. Lipase complexes to colipase cleaving triglycerides to fatty acids and monoglycerides. Dietary phospholipids are also partially hydrolyzed by pancreatic phospholipase. The products of lipolysis are rendered soluble by bile salts forming mixed micelles, which are absorbed by the enterocyte. Deficiencies in pancreatic lipase, colipase, and phospholipase lead to incomplete hydrolysis and malabsorption of fat. This is the earliest and clinically most relevant manifestation of pancreatic exocrine insufficiency.

Starch, a principal dietary carbohydrate, is a glucose polymer containing multiple alpha 1-4 linkages. Pancreatic amylase hydrolyzes these linkages, yielding oligosaccharides, which may be absorbed or further hydrolyzed prior to mucosal absorption.

Acute Pancreatitis

A meaningful classification of pancreatitis has been problematic for decades. A pioneering symposium was held in Marseilles in 1963, where the disease was separated into four major groups: (1) acute pancreatitis, (2) relapsing acute pancreatitis (with the clinical and biological healing of the gland, (3) chronic relapsing pancreatitis, and (4) chronic pancreatitis. Clinicians, however, have had problems differentiating between chronic pancreatitis and relapsing acute pancreatitis because of the difficulty in obtaining accurate clinical data regarding gland structure and function. The following practical definitions are appropriate:

1. Acute pancreatitis is an acute condition presenting with abdominal pain and elevated pancreatic enzymes owing to inflammatory disease of the pancreas.
2. Recurrent acute pancreatitis is two or more attacks of pancreatitis with apparent intact gland function between attacks.
3. Chronic pancreatitis is a continuing inflammatory disease of the pancreas characterized by irreversible morphologic damage causing pain or permanent loss of function.

Precipitating factors of acute pancreatitis can be broadly classified into mechanical blockage of the pancreatic duct, toxic or metabolic insults, infection, and trauma (Table 20-3).

Oprie initially described pancreatitis resulting from gallstone impaction in the ampulla of Vater. He and other investigators suggested that obstruction of the pancreatic duct causes increased intraductal pressure and disruption of the ductal ar-

Table 20-3
Antecedents of acute pancreatitis

Mechanical block at ampulla
   Gallstones
   Accessory papilla stenosis (pancreas divisum)

Toxic and metabolic factors
   Alcohol
   Hypertriglyceridemia (endogenous, exogenous)
   Hypercalcemia (hyperparathyroidism, exogenous)

Infection
   Viruses (mumps, coxsackie, adenovirus)
   Worms (ascaris, clonorchis)

Trauma
   External
   Surgical
   Pancreatography

Ischemia
   Circulatory shock
   Cardiac surgery
   Vasculitis

Neoplasms
   Primary pancreatic
   Ampullary tumors

chitecture leading to pancreatitis. This explanation is not fully acceptable because obstruction of the pancreatic duct alone is insufficient to cause pancreatitis in most patients. For example, surgical ligature of the pancreatic duct causes atrophy of the pancreatic exocrine tissue rather than pancreatitis. This was demonstrated by Banting and Best and assisted them in isolating the islets of Langerhans 70 years ago. Nevertheless, evidence of impaction or passage of gallstones through the ampulla has frequently been found in patients with cholelithiasis and acute pancreatitis. It is not known what additional factors are necessary to produce acute pancreatitis.

An increased prevalence of pancreatitis has recently been postulated in persons with the congenital anomaly *pancreas divisum*. In this anomaly, failure of the dorsal and ventral anlage of the pancreas to fuse causes the major portion of the gland to drain by way of the smaller duct of Santorini and accessory papilla. Although clinical pancreatic disease is an uncommon sequela of this condition, there is a fourfold increased risk of the development of acute pancreatitis. Although there is a greater incidence in young women, it occurs in individuals in both sexes and of all ages. In most cases, the clinical pattern is recurrent acute pancreatitis, but chronic pancreatitis is found in some patients. It is hypothesized that this is due to long-term relative obstruction to the flow of pancreatic juice through an inadequate orifice at the accessory papilla. This hypothesis is supported by the observation that surgical sphincteroplasty of the accessory ampulla seems to prevent further attacks of acute pancreatitis in some but not all patients with this condition. Other anatomic anomalies such as stenosis of the ampulla of Vater or a duodenal diverticulum also seem to be associated with the development of pancreatitis.

Multiple toxic and metabolic factors are associated with the development of acute pancreatitis. Alcohol is the most common and best documented cause of chronic pancreatitis. Although the majority of patients with alcoholic pancreatitis initially develop acute pancreatitis, most already have histologic evidence of chronic pancreatitis and permanent injury to their gland. There may be exceptions, however, where complete clinical and histologic restitution is possible.

There is ample evidence that hyperlipoproteinemia (Frederickson types 1 and 5) can lead to the development of pancreatitis. Both of these abnormalities have periods of markedly elevated serum chylomicrons. Rarely, type 4, with very high levels of triglycerides and very low-density lipoproteinemia, can also lead to pancreatitis. It has been hypothesized that large lipid particles may embolize pancreatic capillaries or that high concentration of the pancreatic lipase in pancreatic capillaries may release large amounts of free fatty acids that subsequently damage capillary membranes with resulting pancreatitis. Relatively high serum levels of triglycerides may also predispose to recurrent pancreatitis in the previously damaged gland by similar means. Initial attacks are typically acute, and, rarely, multiple attacks over time can lead to chronic pancreatitis. It should be noted that transient hyperlipidemia may be a consequence of acute pancreatitis resulting from excessive lipolysis of pancreatic adipose tissue rather than the cause of the acute pancreatitis.

Some studies suggest that pancreatitis develops in up to 7 percent of patients with primary hyperparathyroidism and can be acute, severe, or chronic. The mechanism by which hyperparathyroidism or hypercalcemia causes pancreatitis is uncertain. An increased incidence of pancreatic calcification and intraductal stones has been found in patients with hyperparathyroidism and pancreatitis. It has been hypothesized that obstruction of the pancreatic duct by these stones or activation of trypsin by calcium within the gland leads to pancreatitis.

Multiple drugs have been implicated in the development of acute pancreatitis. In individual cases, however, a pathophysiologic relationship is often difficult to establish, and any relationship between the drug and pancreatitis may be strictly coincidental. Evidence for a relationship between glucocorticosteroid therapy and acute pancreatitis has been gleaned from laboratory and clinical study. In the experimental setting, glucocorticosteroids seem to increase the viscosity of pancreatic secretion, and there is histologic evidence of epithelial proliferation within the ductal system. However, even with widespread clinical use of steroid treatment, the incidence of acute pancreatitis is rare and the association less certain. Derivatives of sulfonamides, including sulfonamide antibiotics, thiazide diuretics, and sulfasalazine, have been observed to cause acute pancreatitis. Antitumor and immunosuppressive drugs, such as azathioprine, 6-mercaptopurine, and L-asparaginase, have also been associated with acute pancreatitis. Finally, elevated estrogens from administration of exogenous estrogens or increased endogenous estrogens during pregnancy may predispose to the development of acute pancreatitis.

Uncommonly, pancreatitis may also develop in association with acute viral infections. Mumps is the most widely recognized offender, but clinical signs of acute pancreatitis in patients with mumps are often not observed. Pancreatitis also develops in cases of acute Epstein-Barr, coxsackie, and adenovirus infections. It has also been observed that migration of *Ascaris lumbricoides* or *Clonorchis sinensis* into the pancreatic duct can precipitate acute pancreatitis.

Trauma resulting from external blunt injury, surgery, or endoscopic pancreatography can damage either the pancreatic parenchyma or ductular system and cause acute pancreatitis. This occurs in less than 1 percent of endoscopic pancreatograms but may be quite severe. Ischemia and vascular insult have also been associated with pancreatitis. This has been observed both experimentally and clinically in the setting of vasculitis, accidental hypothermia, and vascular surgery involving cardiopulmonary bypass. This is hypothesized to be due to relative inadequacy of blood flow in the pancreatic microcirculation leading to capillary and acinar damage.

Although many potential causes of acute pancreatitis are known, pancreatitis occasionally develops in the absence of a recognized precipitant and the etiology is uncertain. Traditionally, these have been denoted "idiopathic," but "agnogenic" is perhaps a more appropriate description, emphasizing the existence of a causative factor as well as our inability to identify it.

Pathophysiology   The pancreas produces large quantities of proteolytic enzymes, including trypsin, chymotrypsin, and elastase. These enzymes are normally stored within pancreatic cells and are secreted as inactive enzymes; they become active only after entry into the duodenum and conversion by enterokinase and activated trypsin. Premature activation of these enzymes in the pancreas is thought to be an important factor in the development of acute pancreatitis. Proteases not only activate one another but also activate phospholipase A, which may lead to membrane damage, parenchymal necrosis, and the disruption of glandular architecture. Although the initial precipitant of pancreatitis is unknown, an early step is the loss of integrity of the ductal system, allowing the release of activated enzymes into the tissue. Immediate local effects of these enzymes on the pancreas are inflammation, edema, and ischemia. Vascular damage reduces regional blood flow and causes leakage of fluid from capillaries. This may lead to capillary plugging by thrombi and disseminated vascular coagulation. Tissue damage continues to be propagated by the actions of escaped activated proteolytic enzymes. Ischemia and enzymatic injury combine to produce local tissue damage and sometimes widespread inflammation or necrosis. Free fatty acids released from lipolysis contribute to pancreatic injury in patients with underlying hypertriglyceridemia.

In addition to local effects in the pancreas, the activated enzymes damage the surrounding tissue and the peritoneal cavity. Vasoactive amines, including kallikrein and bradykinin, are released. These and other unidentified factors can produce profound effects on myocardial function, vascular endothelial integrity, and complement activation.

It is not understood why some cases of pancreatitis are relatively mild and self-limited, whereas others progress to major regional destruction of the pancreas and its surroundings. It can be postulated that the stimulus to development of pancreatitis is greater and more persistent in some cases, while the ability of the gland to resist injury to its architectural and metabolic integrity is stronger in others. Although proteolytic enzyme inhibitors, including alpha$_1$-antitrypsin and alpha macroglobulins, are present in the pancreas, little is known about their role in preventing or limiting pancreatitis.

Clinical
Presentation

Acute pancreatitis can occur at any age but is more common in adults of middle and older ages. The principal antecedents are chronic alcohol abuse and biliary tract disease. Pancreatitis occurs in men and women equally, with alcohol a more common insult in men and biliary tract disease more frequent in women. This probably represents the distribution of the etiologic features in the population.

The cardinal manifestation in acute pancreatitis is pain. The severity may vary from mild to extremely severe. It is characteristically sudden in onset and persists for hours to days, resisting conventional analgesics. Typically, it is located in the upper abdomen and radiates through to the back. Once the pain has reached its maximal severity, it tends to vary only slightly. Many patients feel some relief by sitting up and bending forward. Nausea and vomiting accompany pain in a majority of cases. It is important to note that, occasionally, a patient with severe, potentially complicated and fatal pancreatitis may present with little or no pain.

Abdominal tenderness is also a common clinical feature. It is usually limited to the upper abdomen and not accompanied by rebound tenderness or signs of peritonitis. Occasionally, the pain tends to be more generalized when there is sufficient intraperitoneal inflammation to produce signs of peritonitis. This may cause particular difficulty in distinguishing pancreatitis from other acute intraabdominal injuries. In severe complicated cases, an abdominal mass caused by pancreatic inflammation may be palpable. Later in the course of the illness a pseudocyst or pancreatic abscess can develop and can be detected as an abdominal mass.

Fever is commonly present but is often of low grade and rarely exceeds 102°F in the absence of complications. Shock or signs of intravascular volume depletion occur frequently in patients with severe pancreatitis or pancreatic necrosis. Jaundice may be observed, caused by coincident biliary tract disease or by compression of the bile duct by inflamed pancreatic tissue. Abdominal distention can be observed early, mimicking a paralytic ileus.

Mild pancreatitis is limited to abdominal manifestations as described previously and subsides within a few days. In more severe cases, cardiovascular function may be compromised by the loss of circulating plasma or volume, producing tachycardia and hypotension. Most commonly, these effects are due to alterations in capillary endothelial permeability, especially in the peritoneal cavity. This damage causes systemic loss of intravascular fluid into extravascular spaces. There also seem to be circulating substances that cause depression of myocardial contractility and decreased peripheral vascular resistance. Poor response to intravascular volume replacement with persistent shock is a major cause of death during the first week of severe acute pancreatitis.

Respiratory compromise can also develop during acute pancreatitis. Hypoxemia has been observed in 50 to 70 percent of patients. Although hypoxemia may be asymptomatic, it can cause tachypnea or progress to pulmonary edema. The early and mild hypoxemia seems to be due to increased right-to-left vascular shunting within the lung, whereas the more severe respiratory insufficiency seems to be due to alveolocapillary leakage and pulmonary edema. Circulating proteolytic enzymes, vasoactive amines, phospholipase A, or free fatty acids may damage the alveolar membranes. Poor respiratory function may also be exacerbated by elevation of the diaphragm, atelectasis, and pleural effusion caused by the subdiaphragmatic inflammatory process. Respiratory failure is most likely to occur in patients with severe pancreatitis and contributes significantly to mortality. Patients requiring intubation and mechanical ventilation have a very high risk of death.

Renal failure in pancreatitis is most often due to intravascular hypovolemia and acute tubular necrosis (ATN). It can also occur in patients without any discernible period of oliguria or hypotension. This may be mediated by circulating vasoactive substances causing intrarenal vasoconstriction and decreased glomerular filtration. Rarely, the circulating proteolytic enzymes can cause intravascular coagulation and renal cortical necrosis.

Fat necrosis often occurs in peripancreatic fatty tissue, presumably owing to local release of lipase and damage to local vascular tissues. Less commonly, it may be seen distant from the pancreas in subcutaneous tissue producing red nodules, and much less often in the synovial membrane of joints or in the pericardium. It is often hypothesized that these lesions are due to circulating serum lipases, although experimental evidence in favor of this is lacking. Subcutaneous fat necrosis alone is not associated with a poor prognosis.

Hyperglycemia is often observed in acute pancreatitis and, by itself, is of little prognostic significance. It is often due to increased release of glucagon rather than to insulin deficiency. Insulin levels are usually elevated or only slightly decreased. Most patients do not have sufficient destruction of islet cells to produce significant or permanent insulin deficiency. Hyperglycemia is usually transient, and glucose homeostasis returns to normal over a few days.

Many patients have a clinically insignificant depression of the serum calcium. Some patients with very severe pancreatitis develop hypocalcemia sufficient to cause tetany or abnormalities of cardiac conduction. It has been hypothesized that the fall in serum calcium is due to local deposition of calcium in areas of fat necrosis. Experimental data in support of this hypothesis is lacking, and it is most likely that hypocalcemia is due to multiple abnormalities, including decreased parathyroid secretion, decreased serum albumin levels, and decreased calcium mobilization from bone.

Laboratory Diagnosis

Clinical assessment and the interpretation of historical, physical, laboratory, and radiologic data are essential to the reliable diagnosis of acute pancreatitis. Although several laboratory studies have become quite important to the evaluation of the patient with acute pancreatitis, the serum amylase remains the single most valuable test.

In most cases of pancreatitis, the serum amylase level rises within several hours of the onset of symptoms and remains elevated throughout the course of acute pancreatic inflammation. Continued elevation of the serum amylase after 10 days to 2 weeks often suggests the presence of chronic pancreatitis or a complication such as pseudocyst. There is no correlation between the height of the serum amylase and the etiology, prognosis, or severity of the disease. Patients with severe pancreatitis, pancreatic necrosis, and hemorrhagic pancreatitis are more likely to have normal levels of serum amylase, perhaps because of the previous destruction of the gland. In addition, patients with acute exacerbations of chronic alcoholic pancreatitis can have normal serum amylase levels, which may also be due to previous destruction of the gland. Finally, patients with elevated serum triglyceride levels greater than 500 mg/dl can have "masked" hyperamylasemia, which may only be detected by performing serial dilutions of whole serum. The serum inhibitor of amylase in patients with hypertriglyceridemia and acute pancreatitis is unknown.

There are multiple diseases other than pancreatitis that can be associated with hyperamylasemia. Most important among these is choledocholithiasis, which can produce an elevation of the serum amylase level without acute pancreatitis. Presumably, mechanical blockage of the pancreatic duct by a stone impacted in the ampulla of Vater results in elevations of the serum amylase. The clinical presentation of abdominal pain and elevated serum amylase may make the clinical distinction difficult. The serum amylase can also be elevated by a perforated duodenal ulcer, which causes amylase-rich duodenal fluid to flow into the peritoneal cavity. Small intestinal obstruction or mesenteric infarction without acute pancreatitis can also cause hyperamylasemia, presumably resulting from leakage of intraluminal amylase through the compromised intestinal mucosa. Hyperamylasemia is often observed following intraabdominal surgery, particularly that of the biliary tree and stomach. Although in some cases this can be due to true pancreatitis caused by trauma to the pancreas, in many other cases, postoperative hyperamylasemia is of nonpancreatic origin.

Serum amylase may be separated into two isoenzyme fractions. One isoamylase is derived from the pancreas and the other from the salivary glands. Detection of elevated pancreatic isoamylase in the serum is more specific than total serum amylase in the detection of acute pancreatitis. In two studies of patients with suspected pancreatitis, approximately 25 percent of patients with hyperamylasemia had isoenzyme of extrapancreatic origin. In those cases, however, the clinical findings are sufficiently clear, making measurement of pancreatic isoamylase unnecessary.

The ratio of urinary clearance of amylase to creatinine clearance increases to about three times normal in 90 percent of patients with acute pancreatitis. The amylase-creatinine clearance ratio generally does not rise during chronic pancreatitis except during acute relapses. Because the amylase-creatinine ratio may be elevated in patients with renal failure and occasionally in other patients with intraabdominal inflammatory conditions, the major utility of the ratio is not the detection of pancreatitis but in distinguishing the hyperamylasemia of pancreatitis from that of other conditions.

An uncommon cause of persistent unexplained hyperamyl-asemia in patients with normal renal function can be macro-amylasemia. In this condition, serum amylase combines with a circulating macromolecule (e.g., immunoglobin), forming an amylase complex that is too large to be filtered through the glomerulus. In these patients, urinary amylase is either low or normal, and the renal amylase clearance is characteristically less than normal. Macroamylasemia occurs in 0.4 percent of the general population and is found in about 6 percent of patients with hyperamylasemia. In the majority of cases, macroamylasemia is a benign condition without evidence of pancreatic disease. Its major clinical importance lies in its recognition, so that needless testing or therapy is avoided.

Serum lipase is another pancreatic enzyme whose serum concentration is increased in pancreatic disease. With the development of rapid and precise assays for measurement of serum lipase, it has been recognized that, although less sensitive than serum amylase, this measurement is more specific than total serum amylase. With additional technical advances and experience, serum lipase may become the principal diagnostic test of acute pancreatitis.

Because the clinical and laboratory findings suggesting acute pancreatitis do not always rule out the possibility of another intraabdominal catastrophy, diagnostic laparotomy continues to be necessary in selected patients. Patients who progressively deteriorate despite supportive therapy, particularly those with peritonitis and atypical features for pancreatitis, should undergo laparotomy. Because exploratory laparotomy does not seem to increase the mortality of acute pancreatitis, some of the dangers of missing a surgically correctable intraabdominal disease outweigh the risk of laparotomy.

Radiographic Evaluation

Although radiographic tests are generally insensitive studies for the detection of acute pancreatitis, they do play a valuable role in (1) confirming the diagnosis, (2) determining its etiology, (3) identifying complications, and (4) ruling out other acute abdominal disease. Plain films of the abdomen and upper gastrointestinal radiography have been largely replaced by ultrasonography and computerized tomography (CT) but remain valuable in assessing the possibility of other intraabdominal diseases, such as small intestinal obstruction.

Ultrasonography has proven to be a valuable examination in many cases of suspected acute pancreatitis by demonstrating the presence of an edematous gland. Ultrasonography is abnormal in 30 to 50 percent of patients with acute pancreatitis but is limited because the pancreas is often obscured by increased intestinal gas. Ultrasonography is also the examination of choice for the detection of cholelithiasis. Ultrasonography can also detect pancreatic cysts as small as 2 cm and is a valuable technique for the early detection of true cysts, pseudocysts, or inflammatory masses.

Computed tomography demonstrates pancreatic edema and inflammation in approximately 70 percent of patients with acute pancreatitis. Because CT is not obscured by intestinal gas, better visualization of the pancreas and other retroperitoneal structures is obtained. Consequently, CT seems to be more useful than ultrasonography in the diagnosis of complications of acute pancreatitis such as pancreatic necrosis, pseudocysts, or abscess.

Most investigators agree that ERCP and transhepatic cholangiography have no role in the diagnosis of acute pancreatitis. Endoscopic pancreatography can substantially worsen the course of acute pancreatitis by increasing pancreatic duct pressure and causing further disruption of the granular architecture. In addition, the information derived from the study is often not useful in the acute phase of the disease. Endoscopic pancreatography is more valuable in assessing the status of the gland in resolving pancreatitis and detecting ductal abnormalities, such as tumor or stricture. Both the endoscopic cholangiogram and transhepatic cholangiogram can be valuable in the detection or documentation of biliary tract abnormalities that may be secondary to pancreatic disease or one of the causes of acute pancreatitis.

Assessment of Severity

Although serum measurements of amylase and lipase are valuable in the detection of acute pancreatitis, they are inaccurate measures of the severity of acute pancreatitis. The development of hypotension, hypoxemia, symptomatic hypocalcemia, or renal failure indicates the presence of severe pancreatitis and a poor prognosis.

Investigators have attempted to identify clinical and laboratory findings that are present in the early hospitalization and may predict a greater risk of complications later in the course of the disease. In one study, 11 factors were found to be significantly related to clinical outcome (Table 20-4). If three prognostic factors were present, the patient was considered to have severe pancreatitis. The greater the number of prognostic factors, the more severe the disease and the worse the outcome anticipated. This predictive rule has been modified by other investigators to improve the precision, but it remains most valuable as a measure for assessing the clinical severity of pancreatitis.

Table 20-4
Ranson's signs of severe acute pancreatitis

At admission:
  Age over 55 years
  Blood glucose >200 mg/dl
  Serum lactic dehydrogenase >300 IU/liter
  SGOT >250 IU/liter
  White blood count >16,000/μl

At 48 hours after admission:
  Hematocrit fall >10%
  Blood urea nitrogen rise >5 mg/dl
  Serum calcium <8 mg/dl
  Arterial PO_2 <60 mm Hg
  Base deficit >4 mEq/liter
  Estimated fluid sequestration >6000 ml

The analysis of peritoneal fluid obtained by aspiration or lavage may be used to assess the severity of acute pancreatitis. The presence of 20 ml of dark fluid that is high in amylase is indicative of severe pancreatitis. It must be noted that in other intraabdominal catastrophes, such as perforation of the small intestine, peritonitis can cause similar findings.

Patients with elevated serum ribonuclease pancreatic isoenzymes often have pancreatic necrosis and are much more likely to sustain serious complications than are patients with edematous pancreatitis only. This test is limited by its lack of availability and the fact that serum ribonuclease is also elevated in patients with renal failure. The measurement of methemalbumin in the serum and ascites has been used for the detection of hemorrhagic pancreatitis. Similar elevations have occurred in ruptured pregnancy, intestinal ischemia, and intestinal obstruction. These confounding variables make methemalbumin of limited clinical utility.

Complications   In the first 4 days of acute pancreatitis, inflammation of the pancreas can have many profound and important effects on diverse organ functions. Patients with severe pancreatitis have a large loss of plasma volume owing to leakage of fluid into the inflamed gland, peripancreatic spaces, and interstitial spaces throughout the body. Three to 5 liters of intravenous fluid are often required in the first 24 hours. Despite adequate fluid replacement, some patients remain hypotensive, owing to loss of peripheral vascular tone. Acute renal failure can occur as a result of decreased circulating volume. Hypoxemia develops in severe cases because of increased right-to-left shunting, injury to alveolar membranes, and subdiaphragmatic inflammation. Many of these systemic effects can be mitigated by the removal of the acute inflammatory ascites by peritoneal lavage.

Peritoneal lavage can be used as a treatment for acute pancreatitis with systemic complications. Although it reduces complications, such as circulatory instability, renal failure, or hypoxemia, increased patient survival has not been demonstrated.

After 4 or 5 days, the inflammation and edema of acute pancreatitis begin to subside in most patients. However, in a minority of patients with more severe pancreatitis, destruction of granular architecture or necrosis becomes apparent. Destruction of the pancreas or peripancreatic tissues can occur in defined small patches or in large segments of the gland and can extend into the retroperitoneum and mesentery. If the necrotic areas are small, physiologic absorption of the devitalized tissue may be successful. However, necrotic tissues not adequately resorbed can become infected and can present as pancreatic abscesses. CT is quite valuable in the detection of pancreatic abscess, showing irregular lucent areas suggestive of liquefactive necrosis. The CT can be used to direct a needle into liquified areas to aspirate fluid for bacterial culture.

Pancreatic hemorrhage occurs during the mid-stage of acute pancreatitis and is caused by injury to a major blood vessel by proteolytic enzymes. Intraabdominal bleeding usually occurs in the setting of pancreatic necrosis, damaging branches of the gastroduodenal, pancreatic, splenic, or superior mesenteric arteries and leading to life-threatening hemorrhage. Control of this bleeding usually requires urgent surgery, which can be assisted by the identification of the specific bleeding point through angiography and can sometimes be controlled by angiographic embolization.

Pseudocysts can also develop in the mid-phase of acute pancreatitis as a result of extravasated activated enzymes and fluid into areas of pancreatic necrosis. This type of acute pseudocyst may help perpetuate the inflammatory process as proteolytic enzymes dissect into adjacent structures. Although most acute pseudocysts are absorbed spontaneously or become thickly encapsulated, they appear to be much more problematic than pseudocysts found in patients with chronic pancreatitis. Ultrasonography or CT may show fluid collections; these must be distinguished from pancreatic abscess. If the collections appear to be large or if the distinction from an abscess cannot be made clearly, surgery is often indicated.

The expanding inflammatory process in the retroperitoneum can also impinge on adjacent structures. Mechanical compression of the gastric antrum or the duodenum owing to pancreatic swelling can cause gastric outlet obstruction. Compression of the intrapancreatic portion of the common bile duct frequently causes obstructive jaundice. Such jaundice is seldom severe but must be distinguished from that caused by choledocholithiasis. In addition, the inflammatory process may affect major blood vessels in the area of the pancreas, producing vascular thrombosis resulting in bowel ischemia.

In the late phase of pancreatitis (2 weeks after onset), pancreatic abscess is the most dangerous complication. Infection occurs in areas of necrotic pancreatic and peripancreatic tissues. Enteric gram-negative rods are the most common pathogens and seem to infect the necrotic areas by hematogenous spread. Overall, only 4 percent of patients with acute pancreatitis develop pancreatic abscess, but it is substantially more common in patients with severe acute pancreatitis. Predictably, patients who require surgical exploration or peritoneal lavage in the early phase of the disease have a substantial risk of pancreatic abscess. Therefore, patients who become febrile 2 weeks or more after the onset of pancreatitis must be evaluated for the possibility of a pancreatic abscess. Often, the clinical findings of abdominal mass, leukocytosis, and fever are present. Ultrasonography and CT are valuable tests for the identification of the abscess. Unless gas bubbles are present in the abscess, its distinction from sterile necrosis may be difficult. This distinction can often be supplemented by needle aspiration for examination and bacterial culture. When a pancreatic abscess is documented or is strongly suspected, surgery for the debridement and adequate drainage is mandatory.

Treatment

The principal treatment of acute pancreatitis is supportive care, which allows the patient's endogenous homeostatic mechanisms to control the pancreatitis. Blood pressure and urine output should be monitored and, in more seriously ill patients, arterial blood gas measurements, central venous pressure, pulmonary venous pressure, and cardiac output measurements can be valuable tools in assessment. Patients with dyspnea or hypoxemia should be treated with supplemental oxygen. Fasting appears to be the most important intervention, because it decreases stimulation of enzyme secretion. While the patient is fasted, the administration of intravenous fluids to maintain an adequate intravascular volume is a key factor.

Aspirating gastric secretions by nasogastric suction may further decrease the stimulation to the pancreas. Although it has not been shown to be a benefit in patients with mild pancreatitis, there is sufficient clinical experience to support this procedure for use in patients with moderate to severe pancreatitis, particularly those with vomiting or ileus. In addition, histamine H_2 antagonists, such as cimetidine or ranitidine, also seem to decrease stimulation to pancreatic secretion. The efficacy of these drugs has not yet been proved, but they can help to protect against gastritis or stress peptic ulceration. Controlled clinical trials have failed to show benefit for anticholinergic drugs, proteolytic enzyme inhibitors, glucagon, and antibiotics. Currently, there is interest in the use of somatostatin as an agent that can decrease pancreatic secretion and possibly limit the progression of pancreatitis, but the effectiveness of this agent has not been proved.

Surgery may be needed in a small number of patients with acute pancreatitis. Its principal role is to establish the diagnosis in patients in whom the diagnosis is otherwise uncertain and who may have another intraabdominal catastrophe. Early laparotomy for the debridement of the gland may also be needed for patients with severe necrotizing pancreatitis evidenced by circulatory and pulmonary instability. Later in the course of the disease, surgery may be needed for the management of pancreatic abscess, pseudocyst, or hemorrhage. If the pancreatitis is due to choledocholithiasis, cholecystectomy and common duct exploration are indicated, usually well after the acute phase of the pancreatitis.

Chronic Pancreatitis

Alcohol abuse predominates as the most common cause of chronic pancreatitis in the Western countries. Although there is substantial variation in the quantity of alcohol necessary to induce chronic pancreatitis, there is usually at least 10 years of heavy consumption. It has been estimated that alcohol ingestion averages 150 gm daily for 20 years. There is no relationship between the type of alcohol or the pattern of consumption and the development of alcoholic pancreatitis. Surprisingly, few alcoholic patients with chronic pancreatitis concomitantly develop cirrhosis. It is not known whether this reflects different toxic injuries, different susceptibilities, or an epidemiologic artifact.

Chronic alcohol ingestion causes an increase in the protein and bicarbonate concentrations of pancreatic secretions. Protein precipitates in secretions are found especially following a period of alcohol abuse. There are also increased levels of active trypsin and diminished levels of trypsin inhibition in such pancreatic secretions. Changes in the composition of pancreatic secretions appear to be due to a direct toxic effect of alcohol on the pancreatic parenchyma rather than to modifications of regulatory gastrointestinal hormones. At least one protein present in pancreatic secretion has a high affinity for calcium and can form a stable precipitate that remains within the smaller ducts. It has been hypothesized that this can cause occlusion of the lumen, leading to atrophy of the epithelium, followed by inflammation and scarring of the parenchyma. The "protein plug" theory, although widely accepted, remains unproved by available evidence; the precipitates may be harmless by-products rather than causative agents of the disease.

Gallstones have been implicated as a cause of acute pancreatitis but rarely of chronic pancreatitis. Pancreatitis secondary to gallstones can be recurrent, and residual fibrosis owing to necrosis, abscess, or pseudocyst from the acute inflammatory episode can result in chronic lesions; however, surgical removal of the gallstones will resolve or arrest the disease. Gallstone-induced ampullary stenosis has not been shown to lead to chronic pancreatitis.

Metabolic factors primarily produce acute pancreatitis. Although hypercalcemia, predominantly caused by hyperparathyroidism, can cause either acute or chronic pancreatitis, it accounts for less than 1 percent of all clinically recognized chronic cases. Similarly, hyperlipoproteinemia is a rare cause of chronic pancreatitis. Trauma is a common cause of acute pancreatic injury and can result in chronic disease if the major ductal system has been sufficiently disrupted.

There are several types of hereditary chronic pancreatitis. In affected families, onset typically occurs in adolescence, and males are affected slightly more frequently than females. The disease trait seems to be passed in an autosomal dominant fashion with incomplete penetrance. An aminoaciduria has been associated with the disease but is inconsistently found. Cystic fibrosis is an important cause of pancreatic insufficiency during childhood, but rarely causes clinically recognizable pancreatitis.

Chronic severe protein malnutrition can result in pancreatic insufficiency, especially in childhood. Steatorrhea is present, whereas clinical evidence of pain, inflammation, and endocrine insufficiency is absent. Presumably, the protein malnutrition results in inadequate enzyme synthesis. Pancreatic ducts are normal and fibrosis is uncommon, usually allowing a return of pancreatic function when nutrition is improved. A different form of pancreatitis associated with malnutrition occurs in some tropical regions. It is endemic on the Indian subcontinent, particularly in the state of Kerala, where a limited vegetarian diet is common. In this form, recurrent abdominal pain begins in childhood, and pancreatic insufficiency and calcification and diabetes are frequent findings and do not improve with adequate nutrition.

Other uncommon but identifiable causes of pancreatic insufficiency include hemochromatosis, sclerosing cholangitis, and biliary cirrhosis. An association with choledochal cysts, probably owing to a congenital malformation of the proximal pancreatic duct, has been identified in adults with chronic pancreatitis. A substantial number of cases in which no etiology can be identified are unsatisfactorily grouped and described as idiopathic.

Pathology

Initially, the gross appearance of the pancreas is normal. Episodes of pancreatitis cause swelling and inflammation, with eventual induration and scarring. End-stage atrophy creates a shrunken pancreas with a firm, hard texture and a relatively tubular, rather than flattened, configuration. The islets of Langerhans, encased in fibrous tissue, retain adequate function until late in the progression of the disease.

As the disease progresses, the pancreatic ducts become increasingly distorted. Dilatation of the duct sometimes punctuated by strictures is characteristic, but, instead, there can be diffuse fibrosis and uniform constriction. It has not been determined whether the changes are primary, associated directly with the pathogenesis of the disease, or secondary, caused by the scarring from chronic parenchymal inflammation or duct disruption during acute pancreatitis. Intraductal calculi are sometimes found in advanced pancreatitis and can be large enough to cause occlusion at the ampulla or at a stricture.

Clinical Presentation

Abdominal pain is the cardinal symptom of chronic pancreatitis. Although the inflammatory destruction of the gland may have evolved insidiously over many years, the initial manifestation generally mimics an attack of acute pancreatitis. Although in the course of disease, early episodes can vary in duration from several hours to several days, as attacks become more frequent and prolonged, pain-free intervals shorten and vanish. Constant pain eventually develops. Factors that precipitate or exacerbate attacks are difficult to identify. Alcohol intake tends to provoke the pain within 12 to 24 hours. The influence of meals is usually insignificant, although eating large amounts of fats can aggravate the discomfort, and prolonged fasting may relieve it. Antacids are ineffective. Some patients report relief with vomiting or sitting up and leaning slightly forward. The pain seems to worsen with fatigue.

The mechanism of the pain in chronic pancreatitis is not well understood. Inflammation of the pancreas and nearby parietal peritoneum is probably important in the early episodic form of the pain. Eventual entrapment of nerve fibers in scar tissue is thought to be a cause of fixed chronic pain. Obstruction of the

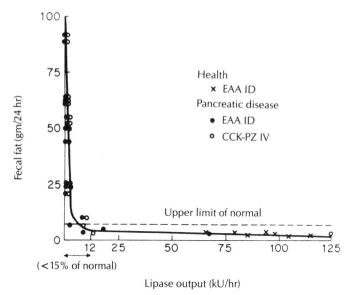

Fig. 20-4

Relationship of pancreatic lipase output in duodenal content to 24-hour fecal fat excretion in healthy subjects and patients with chronic pancreatitis. Values above the horizontal dashed line equal steatorrhea (7 gm fat per 24 hours). EAA ID represents perfusion of an essential amino acid mixture into the duodenum, which stimulates the release of endogenous cholecystokinin. CCK-PZ represents the intravenous infusion of exogenous cholecystokinin-pancreozymin. Note that steatorrhea occurs only when the output of pancreatic lipase into the duodenum falls below 15 percent of normal. (From E. P. DiMagno, V. L. W. Go, and W. H. J. Sumerskill. Relations between pancreatic enzyme output and malabsorption in severe pancreatic insufficiency. Reprinted with permission from *The New England Journal of Medicine*, 288:814, 1973.)

pancreatic ducts by strictures and intraluminal precipitates may contribute to the pain.

Although pain is the most common presenting symptom of chronic pancreatitis, it is not a sine qua non. Asymptomatic chronic pancreatitis can be revealed by the incidental finding of pancreatic calcifications on x-ray examination or as an incidental finding at laparotomy. Advanced disease can occasionally present as painless pancreatic insufficiency. Significant maldigestion of fat and protein with consequent malabsorption of these nutrients occurs when inflammation, atrophy, and fibrosis have reduced pancreatic secretion of enzymes to below 10 percent of normal (Fig. 20-4). The resultant steatorrhea causes frequent loose, oily, malodorous stools, along with bloating, cramping, and flatulence. Although there can be an initial compensatory hyperphagia, as the disease advances, weight loss becomes the rule, secondary to malabsorption and food avoidance caused by painful responses to eating. Despite the severe steatorrhea, clinically significant deficiencies of the fat-soluble vitamins are uncommon. Absorption of these vitamins (A, D, E, and K) depends on luminal bile salt concentration rather than lipase concentration; hence, in patients with chronic pancreatitis, their absorption may be diminished but is usually adequate. Vitamin B_{12} absorption can also be impaired, but clinical symptoms of deficiency are rare. Under physiologic conditions, vitamin B_{12} first binds with a salivary factor (R-factor) in the stomach. In the duodenum, pancreatic proteases cleave the R-factor, releasing vitamin B_{12} and allowing it to bind with intrinsic factor secreted by the stomach. In pancreatic insufficiency, luminal concentrations of proteases may be inadequate to achieve this transfer of vitamin B_{12} completely, and the remaining B_{12} R-factor complexes are poorly absorbed by the ileum. The pain-induced anorexia and reduction of oral intake can contribute to or cause deficiencies in either the fat-soluble vitamins or vitamin B_{12}.

Pancreatic insufficiency is also associated with a decrease in bicarbonate and a fall in duodenal pH. Some controversy exists as to whether this phenomenon increases the risk of duodenal ulcer disease in these patients.

Approximately one third of patients with chronic pancreatitis develop overt diabetes mellitus, and another third will exhibit abnormal glucose tolerance. The islets of Langerhans (beta cells) have a greater resistance to injury by inflammation and fibrosis than do the exocrine tissues; consequently, most patients who develop diabetes will already have pancreatic exocrine insufficiency and steatorrhea. The first manifestation will be transient hyperglycemia, most often associated with an episode of acute pancreatitis or an exacerbation of pain. In contrast to idiopathic diabetes mellitus, that associated with chronic pancreatitis is associated with decreased levels of glucagon owing to coincidental destruction of alpha cells. Overt diabetes mellitus usually evolves in the second decade of the disease, but it can be the presenting feature in painless chronic disease.

Rarely, chronic pancreatitis can present as a tender epigastric mass resulting from a pseudocyst. Other complications such as obstructive jaundice, gastric outlet obstruction, pancreatic ascites, or pleural effusions and upper gastrointestinal bleeding from varices are uncommon in the early stages.

Physical Examination

There are few pertinent physical findings in most patients with chronic pancreatitis. The most prevalent is weight loss proportional to the severity of anorexia and steatorrhea. Tenderness in the upper abdomen is common, especially in the setting of acute inflammation. An enlarged pancreas is occasionally palpable, especially in a thin person, and the finding of a mass may indicate a pseudocyst. Rare findings include (1) jaundice secondary to a stricture of the common bile duct, (2) an enlarged spleen secondary to thrombosis of the splenic vein, (3) ascites secondary to a pancreatic-peritoneal fistula, or (4) a succussion splash secondary to duodenal obstruction.

Laboratory Studies

The lack of a specific laboratory test makes the diagnosis of chronic pancreatitis, especially in earlier stages or milder forms, difficult. Serum amylase and lipase levels rise in acute pancreatitis and rise with exacerbations of chronic pancreatitis early in its course. Later in the course of chronic pancreatitis, serum amylase and lipase levels are usually normal or low, even in the setting of abdominal pain, presumably as a result of the extensive destruction of parenchymal tissue.

Tests reflecting the loss of exocrine pancreatic function have been used to detect chronic pancreatitis. Examination of the stool for neutral fat with the Sudan stain provides a crude qualitative test for pancreatic insufficiency. It is more precise to quantitate the fecal fat excretion over a 72-hour period on a standardized diet. If steatorrhea is found, the maldigestion of pancreatic insufficiency can be differentiated from that of intestinal disease by demonstrating normal D-xylose absorption or by reducing the magnitude of the steatorrhea with oral pancreatic enzyme replacement. Since steatorrhea will occur only late in the course of chronic pancreatitis after 90 percent of the acinar tissue is destroyed, a test for pancreatic insufficiency will be relatively insensitive and will fail to detect less-advanced stages of this disease.

An oral screening test, the bentiromide test, has recently been introduced that measures the ability of endogenous chymotrypsin to cleave a synthetic peptide, which includes a marker, para-aminobenzoic acid (PABA). In the presence of chymotrypsin, the PABA is liberated from the peptide, absorbed into the circulation, and finally excreted into the urine. Under the proper conditions, the test is reasonably sensitive and specific for exocrine pancreatic insufficiency, but its practical role in clinical practice remains to be determined. In the *Lundh test*, the patient consumes a standard meal designed to stimulate the production of endogenous secretin and cholecystokinin. In the *secretin test*, a standard dose of secretin is given intravenously. In these tests, a double-lumen tube is first passed by mouth and positioned under fluoroscopy so that the proximal aspiration port is in the gastric antrum and the distal port is in the duodenum beyond the ampulla of Vater. Through this tube, gastric and duodenal/pancreatic secretions are aspirated separately without cross-contamination. Following the collection of basal pancreatic secretions, a standard meal or an intravenous bolus of secretin is given, and timed specimens of pancreatic secretions are collected over an additional hour. Exocrine insufficiency owing to chronic pancreatitis is characterized by a decreased volume of pancreatic secretions with decreased concentrations of enzymes and bicarbonate. This test is a much more sensitive measure of exocrine insufficiency than the stool collection for quantitative fecal fat analysis and can detect pancreatic dysfunction prior to the appearance of steatorrhea.

Endocrine pancreatic function can be estimated using the fasting and 2-hour postprandial blood glucose levels or can be more precisely quantitated with a glucose tolerance test.

Liver function studies may suggest biliary obstruction caused by strictures of the lower common bile duct. Increased serum alkaline phosphatase occurs in up to one third of patients with chronic pancreatitis. A rise in the serum bilirubin level indicates increased bile duct obstruction or development of secondary biliary cirrhosis. Fluctuation in the serum bilirubin level occurs as well with superimposed bouts of pancreatic inflammation or with recurrent cholangitis.

Radiography   The value of plain films of the abdomen in the detection of chronic pancreatitis has not been diminished by the advent of complex radiographic techniques. Pancreatic calcifications are found in 30 percent of patients at relatively early stages and in 50 to 60 percent of patients with advanced disease. Barium contrast studies are helpful only when duodenal stenosis or coincident alimentary pathology such as duodenal ulcer is suspected. Ultrasonography is invaluable in the diagnosis of certain aspects of chronic pancreatitis, particularly the demonstration of pseudocysts. The gland is usually close to normal in size and configuration but can show swelling or even a mass when actively inflamed. The newer, real-time instruments can show dilatation of the pancreatic duct. The major limitation of ultrasonography is the frequent occurrence of incomplete imaging owing to overlying intestinal gas. Ultrasonography has largely replaced selenomethionine radionuclide scanning of the pancreas as a noninvasive test.

Computerized tomography offers better resolution than ultrasonography and is able to image through bowel gas. However, because CT relies on contrast of tissue density, particularly fat, good imaging can be difficult in emaciated patients. In both ultrasonography and CT procedures, there may occasionally be difficulty in differentiating chronic pancreatitis from pancreatic carcinoma. If cancer is suspected, percutaneous "skinny needle" aspiration offers cytologic proof of malignancy in nearly 90 percent of pancreatic cancers, and false-positive findings are rare.

In difficult diagnostic situations, direct opacification of the ducts with contrast material is accomplished by endoscopic retrograde pancreatography. In early stages, the duct appears normal. Abnormalities of moderate or advanced disease are irregular dilatation of the main pancreatic duct, occasional narrowing or diffuse constriction, and pruning of the ductal system. There can be segmental constrictions ("chain of lakes") or even complete obstruction, sometimes by an intraluminal stone. Often, the entire duct is narrowed with pruned secondary branches.

Extrinsic compression of the segment of common bile duct within the substance of the pancreas occurs in up to one third of patients with moderate or advanced chronic pancreatitis. Endoscopic or percutaneous transhepatic cholangiography (PTC) demonstrates the typically long, tapered, smooth stricture of the intrapancreatic portion of the bile duct. Jaundice or a persistently raised serum alkaline phosphatase are indications for cholangiography in patients with chronic pancreatitis.

Selective celiac angiography is used primarily when occlusion of the splenic or portal vein is suspected or to document vascular anatomy in preparation for major surgical resections.

Natural History   Chronic alcoholic pancreatitis becomes symptomatic in adulthood after 10 to 20 years of heavy alcohol abuse, most often presenting with acute abdominal pain and the clinical features of acute pancreatitis. Physiologic or histologic studies demonstrate established chronic pancreatitis even at presentation. Although the first attack of pain generally resolves completely, continued alcohol abuse leads to relapses of pain or acute pancreatitis. Successive attacks are less dependent on alcohol ingestion and are slower to resolve. Significantly elevated serum amylase levels are found only during early acute attacks. Later levels remain at normal concentrations during symptomatic exacerbations. After a mean of 5 to 8 years, discomfort diminishes in many patients; this may accompany the onset of pancreatic exocrine and endocrine insufficiency, indicative of "burning out" of the pancreas. Finally, pancreatic insufficiency progresses relentlessly even with faithful abstinence from alcohol.

Patients with diabetes caused by chronic pancreatitis have a much lower incidence of complications such as retinopathy, nephropathy, and peripheral arterial atherosclerosis than do patients with spontaneous diabetes. It is not known whether this is a function of the shorter duration of this form of diabetes, owing to its later onset and decreased patient longevity, or the absence of genetic factors that may be associated with idiopathic diabetes and may cause its complications.

Most patients survive at least two decades following the initial presentation of chronic pancreatitis. Most deaths are due to cardiovascular, malignant, or hepatic disease and are not directly related to pancreatitis or its complications. The incidence of cancer of the pancreas may be slightly increased in patients with chronic pancreatitis, with the exception of the rare kindreds of hereditary pancreatitis.

Complications At least 10 percent of patients with chronic pancreatitis develop clinically apparent pseudocysts. Pseudocysts are collections of pancreatic fluid and liquified tissue that form in pancreatic or peripancreatic tissues, encased by walls of granulation and fibrous tissue not lined by epithelium. Two kinds of pseudocysts are known: (1) those formed as sequelae of injury to the pancreas occurring during an acute episode of pancreatitis, and (2) those appearing in patients with chronic pancreatitis. In the latter, there is no identifiable antecedent attack of inflammation, and the pseudocyst may be due to ductal obstruction caused by a stricture or pancreatic calculus. Pseudocysts vary in size from 1 to 20 cm in diameter. The propensity of pseudocysts to track widely throughout the retroperitoneum and along fascial planes is thought to be caused by tissue erosion by the activated proteolytic enzymes in the cyst contents.

Pseudocysts commonly present with epigastric pain, which is frequently aggravated by eating. Impingement by the pseudocyst upon the stomach duodenum or bile duct can cause vomiting or jaundice, respectively. Asymptomatic pseudocysts may be discovered by palpation, an increased serum amylase, or even as an unanticipated finding from ultrasonography, CT, or endoscopic pancreatography.

Appreciation of the natural history of pseudocysts is changing in response to information gained by new diagnostic techniques, particularly ultrasonography and CT. An estimated 30 percent of pseudocysts resulting from an attack of acute pancreatitis will resolve spontaneously within 6 weeks, after which time the chances of resolution in larger cysts is markedly diminished. Spontaneous resolution rarely occurs with pseudocysts in chronic pancreatitis when there has been no identifiable superimposed acute attack.

The potentially serious complications of pancreatic pseudocysts are (1) rupture into the free peritoneal cavity or a viscus, (2) evolution into a pancreatic abscess, and (3) erosion of a major blood vessel with massive hemorrhage. The primary motivation behind the surgical treatment of symptomatic, persistent pseudocysts, especially those greater than 5 cm in diameter, is the avoidance of these complications. In a series of 93 patients with pseudocysts primarily caused by acute pancreatitis, the incidence of complications in medically treated patients was 41 percent, compared with a 20 percent incidence of complications in surgically treated patients. Pseudocysts arising in chronic pancreatitis are much less often associated with major signs of inflammation or spontaneous complications. The surgical treatment of chronic pseudocysts should be attended by a morbidity rate well under 5 percent.

Fibrotic pancreatic tissue, surrounding and encasing the distal several centimeters of the common bile duct, can cause a lengthy stricture of the duct in as many as one third of patients with chronic pancreatitis. Compression of the duct by an adjacent pseudocyst can also cause jaundice, but irreversible fibrosis of the duct is usually present. The earliest functional consequence is simple cholestasis, which, if untreated, can lead to secondary biliary cirrhosis. Although there is an initial, persistent increase of serum alkaline phosphatase followed by hyperbilirubinemia, bilirubin levels and clinical jaundice can fluctuate during periods of active pancreatic inflammation or low-grade cholangitis. Some patients with previously asymptomatic chronic pancreatitis can first present with obstructive jaundice, which can easily be misdiagnosed as cancer, especially in the absence of accompanying pain. Fibrotic strictures of the second portion of duodenum are less common than biliary obstruction.

Ascites in an alcoholic patient is correctly attributed to cirrhosis and portal hypertension in most cases. However, in patients with chronic pancreatitis, it can be due to a direct communication between the pancreatic duct system and the peritoneal cavity. This is usually the consequence of a ruptured pseudocyst, but it is sometimes caused by rupture and necrosis of a duct near the surface of the gland. These patients present with ascites, with or without chronic pain, but without an acute abdominal catastrophe. Paracentesis can establish the diagnosis of chronic pancreatic ascites by the presence of very high concentrations of amylase in the ascitic fluid, a protein concentration greater than 3 gm/dl, and a leukocyte count of greater than 1000/µl. Endoscopic pancreatography demonstrates the pancreaticoperitoneal fistula in most cases.

Chronic pleural effusions can develop by a similar mechanism. The pancreatic secretions from a ruptured pseudocyst or pancreatic duct leak into the retroperitoneum and then dissect cephalad through the esophageal foramen or behind the attachments of the diaphragm into the pleural space. There may also be a fistula into the pericardium. These patients present with dyspnea and cough owing to a large effusion, usually unilateral and more often on the left. In contrast to the pleural effusions that can follow an attack of acute pancreatitis, there is usually no precipitating recent acute episode. Chronic pancreatic pleural effusions do not resolve spontaneously and recur rapidly after thoracentesis. The diagnosis is established by a very high amylase concentration in the effusion and demonstration of the pancreaticopleural fistula by endoscopic retrograde pancreatography.

Obstruction of the portion of the splenic vein that lies within the pancreatic substance can occur as a result of fibrosis or thrombosis caused by contiguous inflammation. Splenomegaly usually develops slowly and remains asymptomatic as the gastric veins provide adequate collateral venous drainage. In some cases, however, hypersplenism or acute rupture of the spleen can occur. Localized portal hypertension in the gastric wall can lead to gastric varices, but these rarely rupture or bleed. Less commonly, the portal vein itself becomes obstructed either by propagation of thrombus from the splenic vein or by constriction of the portal and superior mesenteric veins as they course through the pancreas. This circumstance produces more generalized portal hypertension and is more likely to lead to bleeding esophageal varices.

Erosion and weakening of arterial walls by inflammation and enzymatic digestion can produce false aneurysms of the splenic, gastroduodenal, or pancreaticoduodenal arteries. In acute pancreatitis, this occurs during the active necrotizing phase or later in association with an abscess. In chronic pancreatitis, it occurs in the setting of a pseudocyst. Rupture of the aneurysm causes massive, but often intermittent, hemorrhage into the cyst cavity, and it may reach the intestinal tract by way of the pancreatic duct, presenting as gastrointestinal bleeding. Angiography can identify the bleeding vessel and facilitate control of hemorrhage by embolization; however, definitive treatment for the pseudocyst and ligation of the communicating artery must be accomplished surgically.

Medical Therapy   The treatment of chronic pancreatitis begins with the identification and correction when possible of etiologic factors to limit progression of the disease. Unfortunately, alcoholic pancreatitis can be particularly resistant to therapy because of the intractable nature of alcohol abuse. As the periods of pain become more frequent and evolve into continuous discomfort, the likelihood of significant improvement diminishes even with abstinence. Common sense dictates, however, that any patient with chronic pancreatitis should abstain from alcohol consumption completely.

After addressing the limitation of causal factors, treatment is directed to the manifestations and complications of chronic pancreatitis. At the present time, no means exist to relieve or even to halt the inflammation and scarring of the gland. Episodes of acute pancreatitis should be treated as previously discussed. In chronic pancreatitis, pain control is likely to be a major problem. It is often unresponsive to aspirin or nonsteroidal anti-inflammatory drugs and requires narcotics. Codeine or meperidine is suitable for intermittent use, but methadone is better for long-term maintenance analgesia. The effects of habituation or addiction become so closely entwined with those of the pain of the disease that they often become nearly indistinguishable. Decreased stimulation of the pancreas has been attempted with low-fat diets and anticholinergic medications, but there is little data supporting the premise that pancreatic secretion is lessened or pain decreased. Oral pancreatic enzymes may reduce pancreatic pain by feedback inhibition of pancreatic secretion. Splanchnic nerve block with alcohol has been effective in only 15 to 20 percent of patients with persistent severe abdominal pain, and the pain tends to return after several months. It is more useful in the short-term treatment of pancreatic cancer than for chronic pancreatitis. The possibility that the pain may be due to a treatable complication or coincident disease such as a pseudocyst or peptic ulcer should be explored.

Nutritional support is a critical element in the management of chronic pancreatitis. Pancreatic exocrine insufficiency and steatorrhea are preceded in many patients by periods of anorexia, nausea, and vomiting with a concomitant decrease in protein and calorie intake. This problem is magnified in alcoholic patients with irregular eating habits. A diet rich in carbohydrates and somewhat restricted in fat and protein is better tolerated, and vitamin deficiencies (e.g., B_2, B_{12}, and D) should be anticipated and treated.

When pancreatic exocrine capacity falls below 10 percent of normal, steatorrhea develops and malnutrition becomes significant. Initially, increased caloric intake can partially compensate, but further benefit is gained from oral replacement of pancreatic enzymes, especially those rich in pancreatic lipase, to limit steatorrhea. Treatment usually begins with two tablets of pancreatin with each meal and one tablet with each snack, increasing the dose until control of diarrhea and flatulence is achieved. Although malabsorption should be abolished by the replacement of 10 to 20 percent of normal enzyme activity in the duodenum, this rarely occurs, apparently because of inactivation of enzymes by gastric acid and insufficient mixing of food and pancreatic enzymes. The efficacy of enzymes is improved by the coincident administration of antacids, especially aluminum hydroxide or sodium bicarbonate, or H_2-receptor antagonist drugs. Microencapsulated, enteric-coated preparations of pancreatic enzymes are an effective but expensive alternative to adjuvant antacids.

Although the diabetes complicating chronic pancreatitis may initially be responsive to dietary control, oral hypoglycemic agents or insulin therapy are often ultimately required. There is a propensity to hypoglycemic attacks, owing, in part, perhaps, to irregular food intake during episodes of abdominal pain, anorexia, or impaired release of glucagon. Diabetic ketoacidosis is not often seen except as a sequela to major pancreatic resection.

Surgical Therapy

In more than 90 percent of cases requiring an operation, the indication for surgery is abdominal pain refractory to medical therapy. Complications of chronic pancreatitis, such as obstruction of the common bile duct or duodenum or the persistence of a pancreatic pseudocyst, are present in 35 to 40 percent of patients and occasionally occur without pain. Although the pain may "burn out" as the gland deteriorates, loses function, and calcifies, waiting years for possible spontaneous relief is unreasonable if an adequate surgical solution exists. Surgical procedures for the relief of pain in chronic pancreatitis include (1) exposure and drainage of the pancreatic duct into a Roux-en-Y pancreaticojejunostomy (Peustow procedure), (2) partial pancreatectomy, and (3) total pancreatectomy.

Tumors of the Pancreas

Tumors of the pancreas can arise from either the exocrine or endocrine components of the gland. Most tumors of the pancreas are malignant and arise from the exocrine portion. Ninety percent are mucinous adenocarcinomas of the pancreatic ductal origin. About 5 percent of carcinomas of the pancreas are of islet cell origin and manifest themselves by the production and secretion of hormones. Islet cell tumors are discussed in Chap. 21.

Cystadenomas

Cystadenomas are rare benign tumors of the pancreatic parenchyma, which principally occur in middle-aged women. Patients often complain of pain or mass similar to that of the pseudocyst but lack a history of previous pancreatitis. The speed of evolution of the symptoms is also slower than that of pseudocysts. Cystadenomas contain multiple small cysts with varying degrees of papillary budding in the walls of the cyst. Sometimes, the papillary buds contain malignant cells, suggesting that benign tumors may transform into malignancies. It is important to distinguish adenomas from the more common pancreatic retention cyst or pseudocyst. Pseudocysts usually follow discrete bouts of acute pancreatitis or abdominal trauma and are usually larger, unilocular, and surrounded by inflammatory tissue.

Carcinoma of the Pancreas

Epidemiology

There are approximately 25,000 cases of adenocarcinoma of the pancreas in the United States annually and nearly that number of deaths. Carcinoma of the pancreas may develop at any age in adulthood but is substantially more prevalent in later years. In Western societies, the incidence is nearly 10 per 100,000 persons per year and increases to 100 cases per 100,000 persons per year in individuals over the age of 75. Carcinoma of the pancreas is the fourth most common cause of cancer death in men, following lung, colon, and prostate cancers and is the fifth leading cause of cancer death in women, following carcinoma of the breast, colon, lung, and ovary and uterus. There seems to be an increase in the age-adjusted incidence over the past several decades in Western society. The reason for this increase in incidence is unknown but may be linked to cigarette smoking and coffee.

The cause of carcinoma of the pancreas is unknown. It can be induced in experimental animals by the administration of various chemical carcinogens, especially benzene, nitrosoamine, and cholanthrene. Industrial workers exposed to β-naphthylamine and benzidine had an increased frequency of adenocarcinoma of the pancreas. Specific chemical carcinogens, however, do not appear to be involved in the majority of patients with carcinoma of the pancreas. Carcinoma may be associated with chronic pancreatitis. Evidence of pancreatitis and fibrosis is frequently found at autopsy in patients with carcinoma of the pancreas. The temporal and possible etiologic relationship between these findings is controversial. Epidemiologic studies correlating the presence of clinical chronic pancreatitis and pancreatic carcinoma do not yield consistent results. A pathogenic relationship between diabetes mellitus and pancreatic cancer has also been postulated. It is possible that both conditions are secondary to chronic pancreatitis. In a large series of more than 20,000 diabetic patients, the risk ratio for pancreatic cancer is 1.5 in men and 2.09 in women, which suggests some link between the two conditions. This link, however, may not be etiologic.

There appears to be an increased risk of carcinoma of the pancreas in patients who smoke several packs of cigarettes per day. This risk is substantially less striking than the risk of lung cancer and cardiopulmonary disease in heavy smokers and has been difficult to substantiate. There has also been an interest in dietary factors, which may play a part in the pathogenesis of pancreatic cancer. Populations in which there is an increased incidence of pancreatic cancer also have a higher consumption of dietary fat, protein, and coffee. The importance of these epidemiologic observations remains incompletely defined.

Pathology

Approximately half of adenocarcinomas of the pancreas are located within the head of the gland, and half are situated in the body or in the tail. Many malignancies, however, have spread throughout the pancreas at the time of diagnosis. Carcinomas vary markedly in size and configuration. Small carcinomas are often difficult to identify at surgery and to distinguish from the nodularity of chronic pancreatitis. Larger tumors at later stages may be difficult to distinguish from other adenocarcinomas arising elsewhere within the digestive tract, such as carcinoma of the duodenum at the ampulla of Vater, or carcinoma of the stomach or bile ducts.

Microscopically, between 80 and 90 percent of adenocarcinomas of the pancreas arise from the ductular epithelium. The remainder arise from acinar cells or are indeterminant in origin.

A small number of carcinomas of the pancreas are cyst-adenocarcinomas. This classification is based on the presence of multiple small cystic cavities within an adenocarcinoma. These tumors seem to grow more slowly than their noncystic counterparts, have less distant metastases, and are more amenable to surgical resection. Rarely, squamous cell carcinoma can occur in the pancreas.

Less than 10 percent of pancreatic carcinomas are confined to the gland at the time of diagnosis. Initial spread is usually by direct extension along the lymphatics, blood vessels, and nerves. The most common sites of metastases are regional lymph nodes, liver, peritoneum, and lung. The tumor also grows by direct extension into the adrenals, duodenum, kidney, stomach, biliary tree, intestine, and spleen.

Clinical Manifestations

Clinical presentation can be categorized into three patterns. Initial symptoms can be jaundice secondary to obstruction of the extrahepatic bile ducts by tumor. Tumor can also spread along the perineural spaces in the retroperitoneum and cause severe constant pain. Third, there can be weight loss in the absence of pain or jaundice. The challenge for the clinician is to distinguish among the various causes of each of these presentations and identify patients with pancreatic carcinoma while there still is a possibility for cure or effective palliation.

Pancreatic cancer developing in the head of the gland frequently impinges on the common bile duct, producing jaundice. Characteristically, this is painless, although it may be accompanied by anorexia, dyspepsia, or epigastric discomfort. Jaundice in an elderly population at risk for pancreatic cancer always merits a careful evaluation. In very early stages, there may be no other physical findings. There can, however, be a distended nontender gallbladder (the Courvoisier's sign), which develops as the bile from the obstructed biliary tree distends a pliable gallbladder. A significantly enlarged or tender liver suggests metastases. Laboratory studies show elevated serum bilirubin and serum alkaline phosphatase levels with a slight elevation of the serum transaminases. The serum albumin is normal in early stages of the disease, but the prothrombin time may be prolonged because of malabsorption of vitamin K. Amylase or lipase levels may be slightly elevated but are usually normal.

Radiologic evaluation usually begins with ultrasonography to rule out the possibility of gallstones as an alternative explanation for the obstructive jaundice. Additionally, the ultrasound may show dilation of the bile ducts, confirming an obstructive process. Lastly, a mass in the head of the pancreas may be observed. In most cases, a cholangiogram should be performed when suspicion of obstructive jaundice exists or if dilated bile ducts are seen by ultrasonography. Endoscopic or transhepatic cholangiograms are preferred over intravenous or radionuclide scans because of the increased precision and the reliability of the information needed to plan surgical or nonsurgical palliative treatments. Endoscopic cholangiography is successful in 90 percent of cases and transhepatic cholangiography is successful in more than 90 percent of patients with dilated bile ducts.

If the presence of a neoplasm in the extrahepatic bile duct is confirmed by cholangiography, if there is no evidence of metastases, and if there is no contraindication to surgery, most patients undergo a laparotomy for possible resection of the tumor. Currently, surgery provides the only realistic hope for cure in patients who have carcinoma of the pancreas. In patients in whom the tumor is not resectable, the site of biliary obstruction is bypassed by anastomosis of the jejunum to the bile duct above the level of the obstruction.

Patients presenting with epigastric pain consistent with carcinoma of the pancreas are initially evaluated differently to consider the alternative diagnoses. Most patients who have carcinoma of the pancreas who present with pain have no physical findings apart from the discomfort and weight loss. Others with more advanced stages of pancreatic disease may have an abdominal mass, enlarged liver, or subcutaneous lymphadenopathy. Most patients have no abnormal blood tests early in their disease. Later, there may be an elevation of the serum alkaline phosphatase, serum 5′-nucleotidase, serum transaminases, and serum bilirubin. Elevated serum amylases are remarkably infrequent. Elevated carcinoembryonic antigen is also frequently seen but does not facilitate the diagnosis early enough for an opportunity for cure and does not distinguish between other intraabdominal carcinomas and pancreatic cancer.

The specific evaluation of the patient with suspected pancreatic carcinoma presenting with pain also begins with the abdominal ultrasound. A mass in the pancreas is identified in two thirds of the patients. In most patients, the presence of a neoplasm should be confirmed by needle aspiration biopsy, which yields diagnostic tissue in approximately 90 percent of cases. Laparotomy is usually not needed because the tissue diagnosis can be obtained without it, and palliative therapy involves chemotherapy and radiotherapy. Because the pain is produced by perineural spread of the tumor, most patients with pancreatic carcinoma who present with pain are not likely to be cured by surgery.

Computerized body tomography is helpful in evaluating those patients with nondiagnostic ultrasound or those with an unsatisfactory result owing to bowel gas obscuring the examination of the body and tail of the gland. CT detects approximately 80 percent of carcinomas of the pancreas presenting as pain and also serves as the guide for needle aspiration biopsy (Fig. 20-5). Endoscopic pancreatography may also be helpful in demonstrating stenosis of the pancreatic duct, because the majority of pancreatic neoplasms originate from the ductal epithelium (Fig. 20-6).

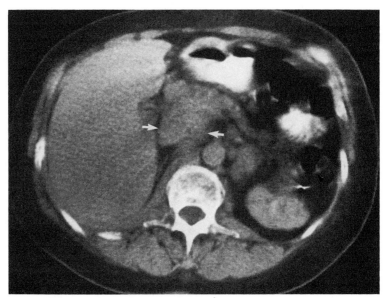

Fig. 20-5
Computerized tomography of the pancreas in a patient with pancreatic carcinoma. Arrows indicate the mass in the head of the pancreas caused by the
tumor. (Courtesy of Norman Joffe, M.D.)

The upper gastrointestinal radiography is not ordered initially to
investigate the pancreas but is often obtained in these patients
to rule out other potential causes of upper abdominal pain.
Occasionally, there is anterior impingement on the stomach or
displacement of the duodenal loop by a pancreatic mass.

Patients with pancreatic carcinoma also present with weight loss
in the absence of jaundice or pain. This occurs through two
mechanisms. First, the presence of liver metastases can occur
prior to the obstruction of the bile duct or the invasion of
peripancreatic nerves. These patients present with weight loss
primarily owing to anorexia and decreased caloric intake. Evaluation of these patients frequently shows a large nodular liver,
and liver function tests suggest an infiltrative disorder. Ultrasonography or radionuclide hepatic scanning confirm the presence of a nodular infiltrative process in liver, and biopsy is diagnostic for adenocarcinoma.

The second mechanism for weight loss is malabsorption. This
may be due to the concomitant presence of chronic pancreatitis
or obstruction of the pancreatic duct near the ampulla of Vater,
producing pancreatic insufficiency. These patients frequently
have a normal appetite and complain of frequent large bowel
movements caused by steatorrhea.

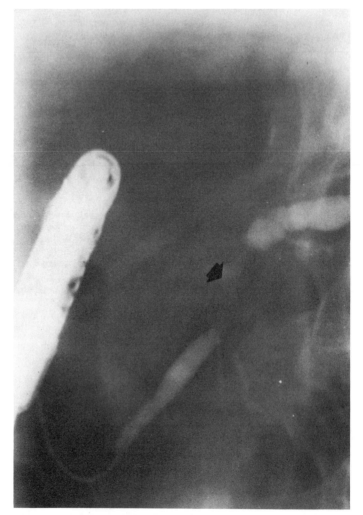

Fig. 20-6
Endoscopic retrograde pancreaticogram in a patient with pancreatic carcinoma. The head of the endoscope is seen on the left side of the figure with a
cannula entering the pancreatic duct. The contrast dye outlines the pancreatic duct. The arrow indicates the carcinoma obstructing the duct. (Courtesy
of Norman Joffe, M.D.)

Treatment

Treatment of carcinoma of the pancreas is difficult, and the results of all modes of therapy are poor. This tumor carries the
worst prognosis of any gastrointestinal tumor, with a 5-year survival rate of approximately 5 percent. This disappointing prognosis presumably results from the relatively "obscure" location
of the pancreas in the retroperitoneum, which allows the tumor
to reach an advanced stage before detection. For example, ab-

dominal pain, the most common symptom of this carcinoma, is usually caused by extrapancreatic spread of the tumor with perineural invasion; hence, the tumor is usually unresectable by the time it becomes symptomatic. An exception to this observation is ampullary carcinoma, since it typically produces common bile duct obstruction and is diagnosed earlier in its course. The earlier detection of ampullary carcinoma is associated with a 30 percent 5-year survival rate.

At the time of diagnosis, only 10 to 15 percent of patients with pancreatic carcinoma are candidates for surgery. Those with tumor apparently localized to the periampullary region or the head of the pancreas undergo the *Whipple procedure,* which consists of *proximal pancreatectomy, duodenectomy,* and *partial gastrectomy with gastrojejunostomy.* Despite this radical resection, the recurrence rate of tumor following the Whipple procedure is high. This poor result has prompted some investigators to favor the more radical *total pancreatectomy* with coincident resection of duodenum, spleen, lymph nodes, and distal stomach. More commonly, however, patients with carcinoma of the head of the pancreas present with obstructive jaundice owing to tumor encasement of the intrapancreatic segment of the common bile duct. Such patients are best managed by a palliative biliary bypass of the tumor, using either a gallbladder-to-duodenum anastomosis (cholecystoduodenostomy) or a common bile duct-to-jejunum anastomosis (choledochojejunostomy). Such a bypass affords a satisfactory reduction of the jaundice.

In general, chemotherapy with 5-fluorouracil, Adriamycin, or BCNU (bischloroethylnitrosourea) yields only a 10 to 15 percent response rate. Such agents are commonly used as palliative agents for metastatic carcinoma.

Although pancreatic carcinoma is not strikingly radiosensitive, in select patients with relatively localized disease, radiation therapy with high-voltage, small-volume treatment to a small target area has been relatively well tolerated and associated with a reduction in tumor size. In some series, this form of radiation therapy has even been associated with improvement in survival.

Study Questions

1. Which of the following are potential complications of acute pancreatitis?
   a. Shock
   b. Renal failure
   c. Respiratory failure
   d. Hypocalcemia
   e. Intra-abdominal hemorrhage

Answers
a, b, c, d, e
Severe hemorrhagic pancreatitis can produce catastrophic complications throughout the body and is associated with a 50 percent mortality rate. Shock is caused by both sequestration of plasma in the injured peritoneal cavity and the activation of bradykinin and other vasoactive factors. The resulting hypoperfusion of the kidney can produce acute tubular necrosis. Circulating pancreatic enzymes, such as phospholipase, damage the alveolar membrane and surfactant, resulting in varying degrees of respiratory failure. Hypocalcemia is caused in part by sequestration of calcium by free fatty acids produced by steatonecrosis. The extravasation of pancreatic enzymes in the peritoneal cavity damages blood vessels and results in varying degrees of intra-abdominal hemorrhage.

2. Which of the following statements regarding pancreatic carcinoma is or are correct?
   a. Abdominal pain is a universal finding in patients presenting with pancreatic carcinoma.
   b. The serum level of carcinoembryonic antigen (CEA) detects 90 percent of carcinoma still confined to the pancreas.
   c. Approximately 90 percent of pancreatic carcinomas arise from ductular epithelium.
   d. The majority of patients with pancreatic carcinoma are able to undergo successful surgical resection of the tumor.
   e. Endoscopic retrograde cholangiopancreatography (ERCP) has a 90 percent sensitivity for the detection of pancreatic carcinoma.

Answers
c, e
The vast majority of pancreatic carcinomas arise from ductular epithelium, hence the high sensitivity of ERCP in the detection of this cancer. Although the majority of patients presenting with pancreatic cancer have abdominal pain, many patients complain only of painless jaundice or weight loss. Neither CEA nor any other screening test is capable of detecting early pancreatic cancer. Only 10 to 15 percent of patients with pancreatic cancer are candidates for surgical resection.

References

Physiology of the Pancreas

Miller, L. J., Clain, J. E., Malagelada, J. R., and Go, V. L. W. Control of human postprandial exocrine secretion: A function of the gastroduodenal region. *Dig. Dis. Sci.* 24:150, 1979.

Singh, M., and Webster, P. D., III. Neurohormonal control of pancreatic secretion: A review. *Gastroenterology* 74:294, 1978.

Singh, M., and Webster, P. D., III. Pancreatic exocrine secretion. *Clin. Gastroenterol.* 10:555, 1981.

Solomon, T. E. Regulation of pancreatic secretion. *Clin. Gastroenterol.* 13:657, 1984.

Classification of Pancreatitis

Sarles, H. Revised classification of pancreatitis — Marseille 1984. *Dig. Dis. Sci.* 30:573, 1985.

Sarner, M., and Cotton, P. B. Classification of pancreatitis. *Gut* 25:756, 1984.

Acute Pancreatitis

Acosta, J. M., Pellergrini, C. A., and Skinner, D. B. Etiology and pathogenesis of acute biliary pancreatitis. *Surgery* 88:118, 1980.

Frey, C. F. Hemorrhagic pancreatitis. *Am. J. Surg.* 137:616, 1979.

Geokas, M. C., Baltaxe, H. A., Banks, P. A., et al. Acute pancreatitis. *Ann. Intern. Med.* 103:86, 1985.

Mallory, A., and Kern, F. Jr. Drug-induced pancreatitis: A critical review. *Gastroenterology* 78:813, 1980.

Ranson, J. H. C., Rifkind, R. M., and Turner, J. W. Prognostic signs and nonoperative peritoneal lavage in acute pancreatitis. *Surg. Gynecol. Obstet.* 143:209, 1976.

Ranson, J. H. C. Surgical treatment of acute pancreatitis. *Dig. Dis. Sci.* 25:453, 1980.

Ranson, J. H. C. Etiological and prognostic factors in human acute pancreatitis: A review. *Am. J. Gastroenterol.* 77:633, 1982.

Richter, J. M., Schapiro, R. H., Mulley, A. G., and Warshaw, A. L. Association of pancreas division and pancreatitis, and its treatment by sphincteroplasty. *Gastroenterology* 81:1104, 1981.

Salt, W. B., III, and Schenker, S. Amylase — its clinical significance: A review of the literature. *Medicine* 55:269, 1976.

Chronic Pancreatitis

Ammann, R. W., Akovbiantz, A., Largiader, F., et al. Course and outcome of chronic pancreatitis. Longitudinal study of a mix medical-surgical series of 245 patients. *Gastroenterology* 86:820, 1984.

Bradley, E. L., III, Clements, J. L., Jr., and Gonzalez, A. C. The natural history of pancreatic pseudocysts: A unified concept of management. *Am. J. Surg.* 137:135, 1979.

DiMagno, E. P., Go, V. L. W., and Sumersbill, W. H. J. Relations between pancreatic enzyme outputs and malabsorption in severe pancreatic insufficiency. *N. Engl. J. Med.* 288:813, 1973.

DiMagno, E. P., Malagelada, J. R., Go, V. L. W., et al. Fate of orally ingested enzymes in pancreatic insufficiency: Comparison of two dosage schedules. *N. Engl. J. Med.* 296:1318, 1977.

Niederau, C., and Grendell, J. H. Diagnosis of chronic pancreatitis. *Gastroenterology* 88:1973, 1985.

Pancreatic Cancer

Fitzgerald, P. J., Fortner, J. G., Watson, R. C., et al. The value of diagnostic aids in detecting pancreatic cancer. *Cancer* 41:868, 1978.

Gudjonsson, B., Livstone, E. M., and Spiro, H. M. Cancer of the pancreas: Diagnostic accuracy and survival statistics. *Cancer* 42:2494, 1978.

Longnecker, D. S. Carcinogenesis in the pancreas. *Arch. Pathol. Lab. Med.* 107:54, 1983.

21 : Endocrinology of the Gastrointestinal Tract

M. Michael Wolfe

In 1902, Bayliss and Starling prepared an extract of canine small intestinal mucosa, and following intravenous injection of this extract into a dog, secretion of pancreatic juice and bile flow were stimulated. They named the active substance *secretin*, and the discovery marked the development of a new concept of blood-borne chemical messengers that regulated physiologic function. It also ended nineteenth century thinking dominated by Pavlovian concepts in which digestive processes were controlled exclusively by the central nervous system. Bayliss and Starling theorized that secretin and other postulated chemical messengers were released by stimulation of the intestinal lumen and then were transported by blood to target organs, where their physiologic effects were exerted. At the suggestion of W. B. Hardy, they designated these messengers "hormones," from the Greek ορμαώ (to set in motion).

During the next 50 years, gastrointestinal peptide hormones were sought largely by reexamination of motor and secretory responses thought to be controlled by the central nervous system. However, progress was slow when compared with that made in "classical" endocrinology, largely because methods were not available for extraction and purification of the peptides, which originated from cells scattered throughout gastrointestinal mucosa, rather than being aggregated in glands. Following the discovery of secretin, other peptide hormones were described, including gastrin in 1905, cholecystokinin in 1928, and pancreozymin in 1943. Other hormones were postulated but not isolated and included "enterogastrone" and "incretin." After methods for isolation of these peptides were developed in the 1960s by Mutt and Jorpes, the field of gastrointestinal hormones became greatly expanded (Fig. 21-1).

However, for a peptide to qualify as a candidate hormone, it was agreed that certain rigid physiologic criteria had to be satisfied: (1) biological actions needed to be produced by very small quantities of the peptide; (2) release of the peptide into the blood had to follow physiological stimuli; and (3) normal blood levels of the peptide achieved in response to a stimulus needed

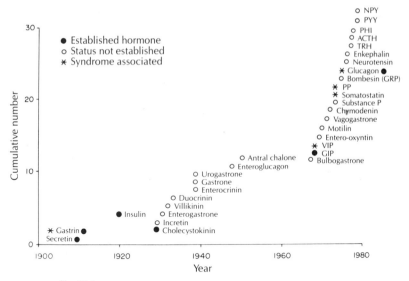

Fig. 21-1

Gastrointestinal regulatory peptides (adapted from J. F. Rehfeld). Figure denotes rapid proliferation of the field owing to the recent discovery of several peptides. (From T. M. O'Dorisio. Gut endocrinology: Clinical and therapeutic impact. *Am. J. Med.* 81 [Suppl. 6B]:1, 1986.)

to be comparable to those required to produce a biological action following its exogenous administration. Many of the peptides discovered did not, in fact, meet these criteria, but rather appeared to be neurotransmitters or local tissue factors. Therefore, it became evident that concepts regarding these chemical messengers were not completely understood and required reevaluation.

It is now recognized that coordination of biological activity among cells in living organisms involves various chemical messengers (usually peptides) that are secreted by one cell to interact with specific receptors on another. In response to binding at the receptor site, the target cell usually releases a second chemical messenger that interacts (by means of an aqueous environment) with the original secretory cell. Secretion of the initial messenger is then suppressed, thereby completing a negative feedback loop (Fig. 21-2). Simple multicellular, and even unicellular, organisms communicate among themselves by synthesizing and secreting such messengers, many of which are identical or remarkably similar to those found in humans and other vertebrates. In vertebrates, the principles remain the same, but, by necessity, the delivery systems became more complex. What began phylogenetically as a local tissue factor later developed into a hormone or neurotransmitter in developmentally advanced species. As a result, these protein messen-

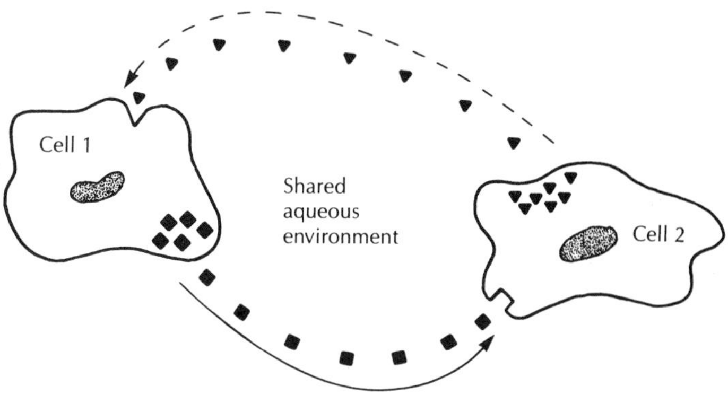

Fig. 21-2
Intercellular communication. Mechanism by which cells communicate with one another: Cell 1 releases a chemical messenger (generally a peptide) that travels by way of a shared aqueous environment to specific receptor sites on cell 2. In response to binding at the receptor site, the target cell releases a second chemical messenger, which communicates with the original secretory cell. Secretion of the initial messenger is suppressed, thereby completing a negative feedback loop.

gers are now often referred to as *regulatory peptides.* This concept provides an explanation for the finding that a classical hormone may also act physiologically as a neurotransmitter or paracrine agent (local tissue factor) in the same organism. Therefore, although the delivery system for chemical messengers appears to have undergone extensive evolution, the fundamental biochemistry of the system by which an agent carries its message from the secretory cell to the target cell has remained highly conserved.

Other attempts were made to classify the peptide-producing cells in the gastrointestinal tract in order to find a unifying theme behind their origin. In 1966, Pearse suggested that all peptide-producing cells of the gastrointestinal tract were derived from the embryonal neural crest and were synthesized within the cell by the process known as amine precursor uptake and decarboxylation. Thus, he coined the acronym APUD to classify this family of cells that possessed common ultrastructural and biochemical properties. Although APUD cells do appear to share these common cytochemical properties, recent experimental evidence has challenged the view that all APUD cells are of neural crest origin. Several studies performed in the developing embryos of various species have shown that normal migration and differentiation of APUD cells can occur even after the ectoderm has been removed, at a time when the neural crest has yet to be formed. Pearse and others now believe that these cells may arise from a discrete population of endodermal stem cells different from those that give rise to other epithelial cells. Therefore, although the precise etiology of APUD cells has yet

Table 21-1
Gastrointestinal regulatory peptide families

Gastrin/cholecystokinin (CCK)
  Gastrin
  CCK

Secretin
  Secretin
  Gastric inhibitory peptide (GIP)
  Vasoactive intestinal peptide (VIP)
  Peptide histidine isoleucine (PHI)
  Enteroglucagon

Pancreatic polypeptide
  Pancreatic polypeptide (PP)
  Peptide YY (PYY)
  Neuropeptide Y (NPY)

to be determined, their biochemical similarities provide a useful means for understanding and studying peptide-producing cells and the regulatory peptides they synthesize and secrete.

Gastrointestinal regulatory peptides are generally synthesized as precursors (prohormones), which are subsequently altered by enzymatic cleavage into their bioactive forms. Many of the peptides exist naturally in several molecular forms that vary by the length of the peptide chain, with the smaller form constituting an integral component of the larger molecule. Although the different forms of the peptide exhibit similar biological properties, their activities may differ with respect to potency or duration of action. In addition to multiple molecular forms of an individual regulatory peptide, many peptides are related, with variable degrees of structural homology in their amino acid sequence. Often, these structurally homologous peptides possess similar biological properties, and it has been postulated that such peptides may have been derived from a common ancestral form. These similarities in structure and biological properties form the basis for classifying such peptides into families (Table 21-1).

As stated previously, because gastrointestinal peptides originate from cells scattered throughout gastrointestinal mucosa, rather than being aggregated in glands as in "classical endocrinology," investigation aimed at determining the physiologic and pathophysiologic roles of these peptides has been delayed. As will be discussed in this chapter, several disease entities characterized by the overproduction of a gastrointestinal peptide have been well documented. However, in contrast to "classical endocrinology" in which disorders characterized by a deficiency of a hormone are frequently encountered (e.g., adrenal insufficiency, diabetes mellitus), clinical syndromes owing to a primary deficiency of a gastrointestinal peptide have not been firmly established.

Gastrin

The existence of a humoral substance involved in the stimulation of gastric acid secretion was first postulated in 1905 by Edkins, who characterized an antral mucosal extract that he termed *gastrin*. For many years, the activity of this substance was confused with histamine, casting serious doubt on the existence of gastrin. The studies of Komarov in 1938 verified gastrin as a hormone distinct from histamine. In 1964, Gregory and Tracy succeeded in isolating the peptide from porcine antral mucosa, identifying its amino acid composition in sequence, and then synthesizing it. The development of a specific radioimmunoassay permitted the detection and measurement of gastrin in both tissue extracts and body fluids. From such studies, substantial information has been acquired concerning the structure, localization, and physiology and pathophysiology of gastrin.

Gastrin is a heterogeneous peptide, existing in gastrointestinal mucosa in several molecular forms, the most prevalent being the gastrin heptadecapeptide (G17) (Figs. 21-3 and 21-4). In 1970, Yalow and Berson demonstrated a larger and more basic form, which they designated "big gastrin." Big gastrin was subsequently found to contain 34 amino acids (G34), including the G17 peptide covalently linked at its amino-terminus to a structurally distinct heptadecapeptide. Recent studies have demonstrated that these two forms are equipotent on a molar basis in their capacity to secrete gastric acid. Gastrin is found in highest concentration in antral mucosa, where G17 accounts for 90 percent of peptide immunoreactivity. However, the majority of circulating gastrin is G34, probably because of its substantially longer circulatory half-life. Other forms of gastrin have been described, which occur in low concentration and include the amino-terminal tridecapeptide (G13) and carboxyl-terminal tet-

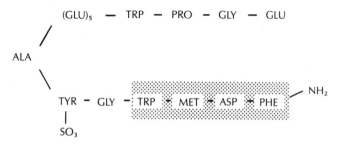

Fig. 21-3
Structure of human gastrin (G17). Stippled portion indicates the biologically active carboxyl-terminal portion. The tyrosine residue can be present in a sulfated (as shown) or nonsulfated form.

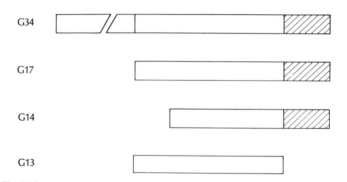

Fig. 21-4
Major molecular species of gastrin. All except G13 contain the biologically active carboxyl-terminal portion (indicated by the hatched portion).

radecapeptide (G14) of G17 (see Fig. 21-4). These have been referred to as *minigastrins,* and although no physiologic properties have been ascribed to G13, G14 appears to possess biological properties similar to those of G17 and G34. This observation is consistent with the finding that the carboxyl-terminal tetrapeptide of gastrin is the biologically active portion of the molecule and must be present for gastrin to stimulate acid secretion.

As stated previously, the principal physiologic property ascribed to gastrin is stimulation of the gastric parietal cell, where it acts in concert with histamine and acetylcholine to increase acid secretion. The major physiologic stimulus to the release of gastrin is feeding, particularly of meals containing protein. The presence of food in the stomach promotes gastrin release by at least three mechanisms: (1) elevation of intragastric pH, (2) antral distention, and (3) specific chemical stimulation by substances contained in food. Other biological properties for gastrin have been proposed, including a trophic effect on gastrointestinal mucosa, stimulation of pancreatic enzyme output, and stimulation of small intestinal water and electrolyte secretion. However, it has been difficult to classify these latter effects as physiologic, and they are probably pharmacologic in nature.

With the discovery of gastrin, it was predicted that the pathophysiology of duodenal ulcer (DU) disease would be explained on the basis of an increase in the number of gastrin cells and an elevation in circulating gastrin. Unfortunately, such has not been the case, although some abnormalities related to gastrin have been found in DU patients. For example, under normal conditions, when gastric acidity increases (pH <3), release of gastrin is inhibited. However, an autoregulatory defect in DU

Table 21-2
Conditions associated with hypergastrinemia

Achlorhydria or Hypochlorhydria
  Chronic atrophic gastritis
    Pernicious anemia
    Alopecia areata
    Vitiligo
    Rheumatoid arthritis*
    Thyrotoxicosis*
  Gastric ulcer
  Gastric carcinoma
  Postvagotomy
  Drug-induced

Normal Acid Output or Hyperchlorhydria
  Zollinger-Ellison syndrome (gastrinoma)
  Antral G-cell hyperfunction or hyperplasia
  Ordinary duodenal ulcer disease
  Excluded gastric antrum
  Pheochromocytoma
  Chronic renal failure
  Gastric outlet obstruction
  Massive small intestinal resection
  Diabetes mellitus

*May also be associated with normal acid secretion.

patients was detected by Walsh and co-workers, who found that acidification of a protein meal inhibited the acid secretory and serum gastrin responses to a lesser extent in DU patients than in normal controls. This may account for the observation that the average DU patient secretes more acid than do normals. It has also been observed that the parietal cells of DU patients appear to be more responsive to both endogenous circulating and exogenously administered gastrin. Increased responsiveness of parietal cells would explain the finding that DU patients secrete more gastric acid despite normal basal and postprandial serum gastrin levels.

Elevations in fasting serum gastrin levels (hypergastrinemia) are seen in several conditions (Table 21-2). It is most commonly seen in patients with chronic atrophic gastritis, a disorder in which patients are hypo- or achlorhydric (i.e., they secrete little or no acid). As stated previously, normally, when intragastric pH decreases to less than 3, the release of gastrin is inhibited. However, in patients who do not make gastric acid, the pH never falls below 3. As a result, the normal negative feedback mechanism for gastrin release is defective, and such patients develop hyperplasia of gastrin cells and secrete large amounts of the hormone. Many patients with chronic atrophic gastritis also have evidence of concomitant autoimmune disorders, such as pernicious anemia, vitiligo, alopecia areata, rheumatoid arthritis, and thyrotoxicosis (see Table 21-2). Hypergastrinemia may also be seen in conditions characterized by the secretion of normal or excessive amounts of gastric acid (see Table 21-2). These include patients with gastric outlet obstruction, chronic renal failure, pheochromocytoma, small intestinal resection, and diabetes mellitus (with or without diabetic gastropathy).

In addition to its rare occurrence in ordinary DU, hypergastrinemia is seen in two unusual disorders characterized by severe ulcer disease. The first of these is antral G-cell hyperfunction or hyperplasia, an entity characterized by mildly elevated fasting serum gastrin concentrations, but exaggerated postprandial increases in serum gastrin levels (>200%). These patients have no evidence of gastrinoma or gastrin-secreting tumor, but some studies have demonstrated an increase in the number of antral gastrin (G) cells. Other investigators have been unable to confirm this observation and, as an alternate theory, suggest that the normal number of G-cells is merely overly sensitive to physiologic stimuli — that is, they are in a "hyperfunctional" state. In some instances, antral G-cell hyperfunction is apparently familial in origin. In these cases, the mode of inheritance appears to be a pleiotropic autosomal dominant gene.

Gastrinoma

In 1955, Zollinger and Ellison described a syndrome characterized by a severe, often fatal, form of DU disease, accompanied by marked hypersecretion of gastric acid and non-beta islet cell tumors of the pancreas. The subsequent biochemical isolation and characterization of a potent gastric acid secretagogue in extracts of such tumors (gastrinomas) established gastrin as the hormone responsible for the clinical manifestations of this entity, subsequently named the Zollinger-Ellison syndrome (ZES). The demonstration of gastrin-secreting tumors in the pancreas, an organ that normally contains no gastrin, marked a new disease concept characterized by the ectopic production of a humoral substance. Although the precise incidence of the disease is not yet known, gastrinomas occur nearly as frequently as insulinomas and may account for up to 0.1 to 1 percent of all DU.

Approximately 90 percent of gastrinomas are localized to an area that has been designated the "gastrinoma triangle," defined by the junction of the cystic and common bile ducts superiorly, the junction of the second and third portions of the duodenum inferiorly, and the junction of the neck and body of the pancreas medially. Pancreatic islets, most commonly in the head of the organ, appear to be the primary site of most gastrinomas, but functionally identical syndromes occur with tumors located in the duodenal wall, as well as other extrapancreatic, extraintestinal locations. Gastrinomas vary enormously

Table 21-3
Pathophysiology of the Zollinger-Ellison syndrome

Peptic Ulcer Disease
    Gastric acid hypersecretion
    Increase in parietal cell mass
    Pepsin hypersecretion
    Paradoxical increase in rate of gastric emptying

Diarrhea
    Massive acid load delivered to small bowel
    Rapid intestinal transit
    Decrease in jejunal sodium and water absorption owing to hyper-
      gastrinemia

Steatorrhea
    Alterations in small bowel morphology owing to low pH and pepsin
      activation
    Denaturation of pancreatic lipase
    Precipitation of bile acids
    Reduction in intrinsic factor activity (vitamin B_{12} malabsorption)

Gastroesophageal Reflux
    Esophagitis and esophageal peptic ulceration
    Peptic esophageal stricture formation

in size, and neither the size nor histologic appearance accurately reflect the biological behavior of the tumors. Difficulty in interpretation is often encountered when initially performing histologic examination of gastrinomas. Both malignant and benign tumors may be encapsulated by fibrous connective tissue, but the capsule is often incomplete, leading to the misinterpretation of a malignant infiltrating growth. Additionally, both malignant and benign tumors may display nuclear pleomorphism and nucleolar prominence. Therefore, owing to these histologic ambiguities, the distinction between malignancy and benignity must be based on the presence or absence of gross metastatic disease at the time of diagnosis or, in retrospect, after the disease has been present for a period of time. Although the presence of hepatic metastases portends a poor prognosis, patients with gastrinoma metastatic to regional lymph nodes generally follow a clinically benign course. In general, gastrinomas, as well as other islet cell tumors, tend to be slow growing, and survival for several years, even in the presence of metastases, is not unusual.

The clinical manifestations of the ZES are due almost entirely to the effects of elevated levels of circulating gastrin (Table 21-3). During the course of their disease, 80 to 90 percent of patients develop ulcers as a result of massive hypersecretion of gastric acid and pepsin. In addition to direct secretory effects on the gastric parietal cell, prolonged gastrin stimulation markedly expands the parietal cell mass because of its trophic effect on gastrointestinal mucosa. This further enhances the maximum acid secretory capacity and contributes to the development of mucosal ulceration. In more dramatic cases, ulcers are giant, multiple, and distal to the first portion of the duodenum and are associated with complications, such as bleeding and perforation. However, more commonly, patients with the ZES present with ulcers indistinguishable from those seen in ordinary DU.

The second most common symptom in the ZES is diarrhea, which occurs in approximately one third to one half of all cases during the course of the disease and is the only symptom in 10 to 15 percent of patients. The pathogenesis of diarrhea is multifactorial and is principally due to the effects of massive quantities of acid secreted into the upper gastrointestinal tract. Rapid intestinal transit, owing to mechanical stimulation of intestinal motility by acid, may play a minor role in the development of diarrhea. As stated previously, pharmacologic serum concentrations of gastrin, as seen in the ZES, may increase electrolyte and water secretion into the intestinal lumen, thereby enhancing the diarrhea. Alterations in small intestinal morphology may occur; these are principally due to hypersecretion of gastric acid and lower than normal intestinal pH. In addition to the direct damaging effects of gastric acid on intestinal mucosa, the low pH also activates pepsin, which further contributes to ulceration and inflammation. These alterations in small intestinal morphology contribute to the development of steatorrhea, which is multifactorial. Steatorrhea is also caused by the irreversible denaturation of pancreatic lipase and precipitation of bile acids, both caused by the acidic milieu present in the intestinal lumen. Patients with the ZES may have vitamin B_{12} malabsorption, presumably resulting from a pH-dependent reduction in intrinsic factor activity. Reduction of gastric acid hypersecretion has been shown to correct vitamin B_{12} and fat malabsorption.

Although esophageal involvement was previously considered uncommon, approximately 10 percent of ZES patients may present with symptoms related to this problem. These symptoms include pyrosis and dysphagia owing to gastroesophageal reflux and its complications. Less commonly, patients have presented with pancreatitis, presumed to be a result of pancreatic duct obstruction by tumor. Symptoms owing to hypercalcemia can be observed in gastrinoma patients with evidence of parathyroid adenoma, as seen in the multiple endocrine neoplasia syndrome–type I (MEN–I). The MEN–I is inherited as an autosomal dominant trait and is associated with tumors of the pituitary and parathyroid glands, as well as tumors of the pancreas (e.g., gastrinoma, insulinoma, glucagonoma). In these patients, hypercalcemia also contributes to massive gastric acid hypersecretion, probably owing to calcium-stimulated gastrin release from tumors. Approximately 30 percent of cases of the ZES are associated with the MEN–I. Recently, investigators have reported the presence of Cushing's syndrome in patients with the ZES caused by either the presence of an ACTH-secreting pituitary adenoma when associated with the MEN–I, or the ectopic production of ACTH in sporadic (nonfamilial) gastrinoma.

The diagnosis of gastrinoma is best established by demonstration of marked hypergastrinemia (fasting serum gastrin >1000 pg/ml) and gastric acid hypersecretion in a patient with DU or other clinical features of the ZES, as described previously. When determining the acid secretory capacity of an individual suspected of having gastrinoma, it is often helpful to evaluate acid output in the basal state and in response to a stimulatory agent. Since the gastric parietal cell mass of the ZES patients is already maximally stimulated by endogenous circulating gastrin, following the administration of a parenteral exogenous secretagogue (e.g., subcutaneous pentagastrin), gastrinoma patients generally increase their acid output proportionally less than do patients with ordinary DU or antral G-cell hyperfunction. A ratio of basal- to pentagastrin-stimulated acid output of 0.6 or greater is virtually diagnostic of the ZES, although 15 to 20 percent of patients with proven gastrinoma will not meet this criterion.

Although the presence of elevated serum gastrin concentrations has been established as the sine qua non of the ZES, as stated previously, hypergastrinemia is not confined to patients with gastrinoma (see Table 21-2). Also, at least one half of all gastrinoma patients have less dramatic fasting serum gastrin values (<1000 pg/ml), and fluctuating, as well as persistently normal, gastrin levels have been observed. For this reason and because of the lack of specificity of the serum gastrin level, various provocative tests have been developed and used to help distinguish patients with the ZES from other patients with hypergastrinemia. The most reliable of these tests is the secretin injection test. As will be discussed, secretin is a gastrointestinal peptide found in the upper small intestine. When administered in pharmacologic quantities (and possibly in physiologic amounts), secretin normally suppresses serum gastrin levels. However, in patients with the ZES, a paradoxical increase in serum gastrin is seen. Although the mechanism accounting for this phenomenon remains unknown, the secretin injection test, if performed properly and interpreted accurately, is extremely useful in establishing the diagnosis of gastrinoma.

Historically, treatment of the ZES has been directed toward correction of gastric acid hypersecretion, and total gastrectomy was accepted uniformly as the treatment of choice. More recently, with the development of histamine H_2-receptor antagonists, effective medical therapeutic alternatives to surgery became available. However, neither total gastrectomy nor medical therapy prevent tumor progression, and, in contrast to early reports that emphasized mortality associated with ulcer complications (e.g., bleeding, perforation), patients with the ZES are now succumbing more frequently to metastatic disease. Therefore, at the present time, an aggressive surgical approach aimed at excising tumor is more often being advocated.

Cholecystokinin
As stated previously, cholecystokinin was discovered in 1928 by Ivy and Oldberg as a small intestinal extract that stimulated gallbladder contraction. In 1943, Harper and Raper isolated a small intestinal extract that stimulated pancreatic secretion, which they named *pancreozymin*. Subsequently, Jorpes and Mutt established that these activities were produced by the same substance, and, citing historical precedence, the term *cholecystokinin (CCK)* was adopted as the preferred name for the peptide. Analogous to the molecular heterogeneity of gastrin, CCK is known to exist in small intestinal mucosa in at least three recognized forms. The carboxyl-terminal octapeptide of CCK (CCK8) possesses all the biological activity attributable to the peptide, and the other two common forms, CCK33 and CCK39, represent amino-terminal extensions. In addition to being found in duodenal and jejunal mucosa, CCK is one of several regulatory peptides that are located in the central nervous system and that constitute the so-called brain–gut axis. Here, CCK8 appears to be the predominant form of the peptide and serves as a neurotransmitter in the cerebral cortex and hypothalamus.

The principal stimulants for CCK release are fat and products of fat digestion, although essential amino acids may also stimulate its secretion. The precise physiologic spectrum of CCK actions has yet to be fully defined, but, as originally suggested, it does appear that its primary biological effects are stimulation of gallbladder contraction and pancreatic enzyme secretion. All three forms appear to stimulate gallbladder contraction and pancreatic amylase secretion similarly on an equimolar basis. Although CCK has been proposed as a mediator of satiety, the mechanism by which satiety is induced and the relative importance of CCK in producing this effect have yet to be established. Other putative physiologic effects of CCK include the release of insulin from pancreatic islet cells and effects on gastrointestinal motility, including the regulation of gastric emptying. To date, no pathologic states characterized by excess secretion of CCK have been described.

Secretin Family

Various humoral regulatory peptides emanating from small intestinal mucosa have been shown to inhibit the secretion of gastrin from the antrum and thereby reduce gastric acid secretion. The existence of these peptides, which inhibit acid output, was first postulated by Ewald and Boas in 1886. They demonstrated that the addition of fat to a meal being fed to dogs decreased gastric acid and pepsin secretion. In 1930, Kosaka and Lim demonstrated that inhibition of both gastric secretion and gastric emptying could be induced by the intravenous infusion of a crude intestinal mucosal extract. They named this extract *enterogastrone* and believed that it represented a hormone located in the upper intestinal mucosa that was liberated by fat and the products of fat digestion. A broader interpretation of enterogastrone was later proposed, defining it as any substance released from the small bowel that would inhibit acid secretion. With the isolation of gastric inhibitory peptide, it was hoped that enterogastrone had finally been discovered. As discussed in the following paragraphs, all members of the secretin family (see Table 21-1) have at one time been proposed as candidate enterogastrones. These peptides are all structurally related, suggesting the possibility that they are derived from a common ancestral form, and they include both hormones and neuropeptides.

Secretin

As mentioned previously, secretin was the first substance to be classified as a hormone. Only one form of the hormone has been described, a linear 27-amino acid peptide. Secretin-containing cells are found in highest concentration in the duodenum, with smaller quantities found in the jejunum and ileum. As first demonstrated by Bayliss and Starling in 1902, the principal physiologic stimulus for the release of secretin appears to be acidification of the proximal duodenum, which releases the peptide into the circulation in quantities sufficient to stimulate pancreatic bicarbonate secretion. This property appears to be the main physiologic action of secretin and qualifies the peptide for hormonal status. Although alcohol and bile salts have also been shown to stimulate secretin release, studies examining peptide release in response to various foods have yielded conflicting results.

Other biological actions have been attributed to secretin, but whether or not these are physiologic in nature has yet to be determined with certainty. Secretin has been proposed as an enterogastrone, and, although it does appear to inhibit gastrin release, pepsin secretion, and gastric acid output in dogs, such an effect in humans has not been demonstrated unequivocally. Other potential actions of secretin include the potentiation of

CCK in stimulating pancreatic enzyme secretion, stimulation of hepatic bile flow, stimulation of other gastrointestinal and pancreatic cells, and an inhibitory effect on gastrointestinal motility. Motor actions include relaxation of the lower esophageal sphincter, a delay in gastric emptying, and a generalized decrease in duodenal and jejunal motility. These latter properties are considered by most investigators to be pharmacologic in nature.

Secretin is used extensively as a pharmacologic agent during diagnostic evaluations. As mentioned previously, in patients with the ZES (gastrinoma), intravenous infusion of the peptide produces a paradoxical increase in serum gastrin levels. Secretin infusion is also used to assess pancreatic exocrine function by measurement of bicarbonate output in patients suspected of having chronic pancreatitis. To date, no secretin-secreting tumors have been described; however, in patients with celiac sprue, intraduodenal acid does not stimulate secretin release. This impairment of secretion release may contribute to the associated reduction in pancreatic bicarbonate output observed in these patients.

Gastric Inhibitory Peptide

Gastric inhibitory peptide (GIP) was first isolated by Brown and Pederson in 1969 from a partially purified preparation of CCK. It is a linear 42-amino acid peptide that is found in the mucosa throughout the length of the small intestine. The primary site of GIP release following various stimuli is the duodenum and proximal jejunum. Release of GIP into the systemic circulation has been demonstrated after the ingestion of carbohydrates, fats, and protein meals. Acidification of the duodenum also provides a potent stimulus for the release of GIP.

Although originally named for its capacity to inhibit gastric acid secretion, pepsin secretion, and motor activity in dogs, the role of GIP as an enterogastrone in humans has been difficult to demonstrate. The peptide has, however, attained the status of a hormone by virtue of its insulinotropic action; recently, GIP has attracted substantial interest regarding its proposed metabolic function as "incretin," a theoretical peptide postulated to stimulate the release of insulin in response to food substances entering the small intestinal lumen. It has therefore been suggested that the acronym GIP may be used more appropriately to indicate glucose-dependent *insulinotropic peptide*. Other proposed biological actions of GIP include the inhibition of water and electrolyte absorption in the small intestine and inhibitory motor effects. The effects on gastrointestinal motility include a decrease in lower esophageal sphincter pressure, inhibition of gastric motor activity, and a delay in gastric emptying of liquids.

No GIP-producing tumors have been described; however, some reports of enhanced GIP release have been described. These studies include patients with obesity, chronic pancreatitis, and DU. Although it has been postulated that abnormalities in GIP release may contribute to the pathogenesis of diabetes mellitus, no unequivocal evidence has been obtained to date to confirm this notion.

Vasoactive Intestinal Peptide

Vasoactive intestinal peptide (VIP) is a 28-amino acid peptide, isolated from small intestinal mucosa by Said and Mutt in 1970. Of all the members of the secretin family, VIP (and peptide histidine isoleucine; see next section) contains the lowest degree of structural homology. Although originally identified as a vasodilator, VIP is now known to possess a wide spectrum of pharmacologic action and functions as a neurotransmitter both in the gastrointestinal tract and brain. It is distributed throughout the entire gastrointestinal tract, from esophagus to rectum, as well as in the central nervous system, autonomic ganglia, enteric nerve plexi, enteropancreatic ganglia, and in synaptic vesicles of nerve terminals. VIP release into the portal circulation has been demonstrated following various stimuli, including calcium, electrical stimulation of the vagus, acidification of the duodenum, and gastric distention and in response to ethanol, fat, and protein. However, VIP released into the portal circulation undergoes hepatic degradation and prevents the peptide from exerting peripheral effects, unless excessive amounts overwhelm the clearance capacity of the liver.

When given exogenously, VIP has been shown to have several biological actions, including a positive inotropic effect on the heart, smooth muscle relaxation, stimulation of small intestinal secretion of water and electrolytes, and inhibition of gastrin release and gastric acid secretion. VIP stimulates pancreatic bicarbonate secretion with approximately 20 percent of the potency of secretin, and it stimulates lipolysis, glycogenolysis, and both insulin and glucagon release. However, these actions are generally regarded as pharmacologic in nature, and, in all likelihood, its primary physiologic role is related to its effects on gastrointestinal motility. As mentioned previously, VIP relaxes smooth muscle and has been shown to produce graded decreases in lower esophageal sphincter pressure. It also inhibits the force of contraction of antral smooth muscle, relaxes the body of the stomach, inhibits contraction of intestinal circular muscle, and decreases gallbladder wall tension.

There have been recent reports of VIP deficiency in patients with diabetes mellitus, which may contribute to symptoms of autonomic dysfunction. A deficiency of VIP has also been postulated to contribute to the inability of the lower esophageal sphincter to relax in patients with achalasia. In patients with cirrhosis, VIP released from enteric nerves into the portal circulation may escape hepatic clearance and produce untoward effects. These include systemic hypotension, hyperventilation, and tachycardia, all of which are seen in patients with hepatic insufficiency and are also produced by the intravenous administration of VIP. Non-beta islet cell tumors of the pancreas containing VIP have been shown to produce the pancreatic cholera syndrome, also referred to as the WDHA (watery diarrhea hypokalemia achlorhydria) syndrome. This syndrome was first characterized by Verner and Morrison in 1958 in two patients with profuse and intractable watery diarrhea, resistant hypokalemia, dehydration, shock, and, ultimately, death. In addition to the pancreas, VIP-containing tumors producing severe diarrhea have been described in neuroblastomas, pheochromocytomas, and ganglioneuromas. The disease is characterized by elevated plasma levels of VIP. However, although "VIPomas" account for a large number of cases of WDHA, other peptide-secreting tumors can produce an identical clinical picture.

Although usually painless, the diarrhea in patients with VIPomas may be intermittent or constant, and it generally worsens with time. The diarrhea has been shown to be secretory in nature in that it persists despite the patient fasting. Owing to the capacity of VIP to produce peripheral vasodilation, some patients with these tumors complain of flushing, and because of hypovolemia and electrolyte depletion, patients may develop severe lethargy, muscle weakness, muscle cramping, nausea and vomiting, and a defect in renal concentrating ability. Patients with VIP-secreting tumors often have hypercalcemia, and although some patients may have the MEN–I syndrome, in others, the cause of the hypercalcemia is unknown. Hyperglycemia and impaired glucose tolerance is observed in nearly 50 percent of patients, which may be due either to the effects of VIP on glucagon release or to hypokalemia. VIPoma patients are either hypo- or achlorhydric, presumably because of the inhibitory effects of VIP on gastric acid secretion. However, in contrast to others with decreased acid output, these patients do not have hypergastrinemia, since VIP also inhibits gastrin release.

The treatment of VIPomas is surgical, with the aim being total resection of the tumor. In Verner and Morrison's review of 55 cases, approximately one third were malignant and nearly 50 percent were resectable. Although chemotherapy may be useful in treatment aimed at metastatic disease, it has recently been shown that the use of the somatostatin analog octreotide may drastically reduce the frequency and volume of diarrhea.

Peptide Histidine Isoleucine

Traditionally, new gastrointestinal regulatory peptides have been discovered on the basis of their biological activity. Tatemoto and Mutt proposed a chemical detection system based on fragmentation of peptides located in tissue extracts, followed by identification of distinct chemical features. Since most bioactive gastrointestinal peptides contain an amidated carboxyl-terminal amino acid, this chemical property was utilized to isolate several new peptides. One of the first of these was peptide histidine isoleucine (PHI), named for its amino-terminal and carboxyl-terminal amino acids, respectively. The human counterpart of PHI is PHM, based on a methionine substitution at the carboxyl-terminus.

Although the precise biological role of PHI has yet to be determined, it bears many remarkable similarities to its structural homologue VIP. The two peptides are co-localized in enteric neurons, have nearly an identical tissue distribution in both the gastrointestinal tract and central nervous system, and exhibit similar pharmacologic activities. Moreover, the two are derived from a common precursor polypeptide, and both are encoded from the same messenger RNA. Recent studies have demonstrated the presence of PHI in VIP-secreting tumors and have shown that PHI contributes to the clinical manifestations of the disease.

Enteroglucagon

It is now well recognized that peptides structurally similar to pancreatic glucagon are located in small intestinal mucosa, which are collectively referred to as enteroglucagon. Enteroglucagon-producing cells are localized primarily to the ileum and colon, with far fewer cells found in the duodenum and jejunum. Enteroglucagon release has been demonstrated experimentally in response to infusion of glucose into the ileum. The principal peptide in this group is glicentin, which is a 69-amino acid peptide similar in structure to the prohormone form of pancreatic glucagon. A second form of enteroglucagon is oxyntomodulin, a peptide consisting of the carboxy-terminal 37 amino acids of glicentin. Little is known regarding the physiology of these peptides. As its name implies, oxyntomodulin has been shown to inhibit acid secretion from oxyntic glands, and it has been suggested that it may also function as an incretin (stimulant of insulin release). Like oxyntomodulin and other members of the secretin family, glicentin is also a potent inhibitor of acid secretion, but whether it functions physiologically as an enterogastrone has not yet been determined.

Enteroglucagon appears to be an important trophic hormone, which stimulates intestinal epithelial cell proliferation and renewal. Although no pathologic states characterized by an enteroglucagon deficiency have been characterized, enhanced release of the peptide has been observed following massive intestinal resection. It is possible that enteroglucagon plays a role in intestinal mucosal cell proliferation seen in this clinical setting.

Somatostatin

Although originally identified in sheep hypothalamus as an inhibitor of growth hormone release, somatostatin is a potent physiologic inhibitor of several gastrointestinal regulatory peptides (e.g., gastrin, CCK, secretin), gastric acid secretion, gastrointestinal blood flow, small intestinal and gallbladder motility, and pancreatic enzyme secretion. Somatostatin exists naturally in both 14- and 28-amino acid forms, with the larger molecule representing an amino-terminal extension of the smaller form. In addition to being localized in several digestive organs, including the stomach, small intestine, and biliary tree, somatostatin has been demonstrated in the retina and hypothalamus, in close proximity to α- and β-islet cells of the pancreas, in the cardiac vagus, and in the glomerulus of the kidney. Somatostatin has been shown to function as a neurotransmitter, and some investigators have postulated an additional hormonal mode of action for the peptide. However, owing to its widespread distribution, somatostatin is a likely candidate for a local paracrine role in the regulation of various endocrine and exocrine cells (Fig. 21-5). Recent experiments have demonstrated that gastric somatostatin exerts inhibitory effects on gastrin release and H^+ ion secretion through paracrine pathways, accomplished by release of the peptide into the immediate interstitial environment of gas-

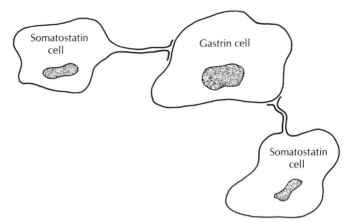

Fig. 21-5
Schematic diagram depicting the relationship between gastrin and somatostatin cells in the gastric antrum. Somatostatin cells contain long cytoplasmic processes that extend in close proximity to gastrin cells and that secrete somatostatin into the immediate interstitial environment of the gastrin cell.

trin and parietal cells, respectively. In these studies, somatostatin-containing cells were found to possess long cytoplasmic processes that extended in close proximity of their target cells. In addition, it appears that somatostatin may mediate the inhibitory properties of secretin and other candidate enterogastrones. Release of the peptide from somatostatin-containing cells can be demonstrated in response to mixed meals in both dogs and humans.

A deficiency of somatostatin has been implicated in the pathogenesis of both diabetes mellitus and DU disease. Recent studies in DU patients have demonstrated a decrease in the normal ratio of somatostatin- to gastrin-containing cells in the antrum, as well as a defect in the release of somatostatin in DU patients. These alterations may help explain the gastrin autoregulatory defect observed in patients with chronic DU disease. Somatostatin-containing tumors have been described and will be discussed here.

As is the case with all gastrointestinal regulatory peptides, somatostatin has a very short circulatory half-life (<5 minutes). However, analogs of the peptide have been synthesized that are not only far more potent than the naturally occurring peptide but that are also more resistant to proteolytic clearance. The delay in disappearance from the circulation and the enhanced potency permit the use of these analogs as pharmacologic agents. To date, the somatostatin analog octreotide has been used successfully in the treatment of clinical conditions caused by several peptide-secreting tumors, including gastrinoma, VIPoma, acromegaly (caused by increased circulating growth hormone levels), glucagonoma, and insulinoma. Although octreotide does not appear to prevent or impede the progression of metastatic disease, it lowers circulating concentrations of the tumor peptide by inhibiting its release, thereby producing symptomatic relief. For example, VIPoma patients treated with the analogs have had marked reductions in plasma VIP levels, as well as almost complete cessation of diarrhea. Because of its ability to decrease splanchnic blood flow, somatostatin has also been used, with variable success, to treat patients with gastrointestinal bleeding.

Other Regulatory Peptides

Pancreatic Polypeptide Family

Pancreatic polypeptide (PP) is a hormone that was discovered as a by-product during the biochemical purification of insulin. It is a 36-amino acid molecule located almost exclusively in the pancreas, in the periphery of the islets of Langerhans. Although PP secretion is stimulated by food intake, its release appears to be under vagal control and is cholinergic in nature. The principal physiologic role of PP appears to be regulation of pancreatic enzyme secretion and gallbladder contraction, with PP antagonizing the stimulatory effects of CCK.

Plasma PP concentrations are elevated in approximately 50 percent of patients with islet cell tumors, and it has been suggested that measurement of the peptide may be of value both for detecting the presence of these tumors and for monitoring their growth. Unfortunately, plasma PP levels are also elevated in alcoholism, chronic renal failure, diabetes, chronic relapsing pancreatitis, and after bowel resection, and levels tend to increase with advancing age. Recently, the use of cholinergic blockade with atropine has been advocated as a means of differentiating patients with islet cell tumors from others with elevated plasma PP concentrations. The rationale for the use of atropine is that normally PP release is under cholinergic control. However, PP release from tumors is usually autonomous, and, in contrast to normal cells, atropine does not suppress plasma PP elevations when associated with islet cell tumors.

Other members of the pancreatic polypeptide family (see Table 21-1) include peptide tyrosine tyrosine (PYY) and neuropeptide Y (NPY). PYY appears to function as a hormone, although a local regulatory (paracrine) role for the peptide has not been ruled out. Like members of the secretin family, PYY may inhibit gastric acid secretion under physiologic conditions, and a role for PYY as an inhibitor of pancreatic enzyme secretion has been postulated but not proved. As its name indicates, NPY is strictly a neurotransmitter, which appears to be distributed along adrenergic neurons. Its physiologic role is unknown.

Gastrin-Releasing Peptide

Gastrin-releasing peptide (GRP) is a neuropeptide that was isolated originally from porcine gastric mucosa. It exists naturally in both 14- and 27-amino acid forms, with the larger molecule representing an extension at the amino-terminus. GRP is regarded as the mammalian counterpart of bombesin, a decapeptide isolated from frog skin, which is structurally similar and possesses the same spectrum of biological activity. GRP is found in nerve fibers of the submucosal and myenteric plexus along the entire gastrointestinal tract, pancreatic acini, celiac ganglia, and brain. Although several studies have proposed GRP as a neurotransmitter of gastrin release, its precise role in the regulation of gastrin release and gastric acid secretion has yet to be fully defined. GRP does appear to produce a wide spectrum of biological effects; however, the physiologic significance of these actions is unclear. In addition to stimulating gastrin release, GRP stimulates the release of many peptides, including somatostatin, motilin, neurotensin, CCK, GIP, enteroglucagon, and PP. Other biological properties include stimulation of pancreatic enzyme secretion, gallbladder contraction, and gastric and intestinal motility. Although GRP stimulates acid output when administered intravenously, acid secretion is inhibited when GRP is injected into the brain of experimental animals. Owing to the ability of GRP to stimulate the release of other gastrointestinal regulatory peptides, it is unclear whether these actions are direct or mediated through other peptides. No disease states characterized by a deficiency of GRP have been described. However, GRP-like peptides have been isolated in a number of oat cell bronchogenic tumors and may contribute to the rapid growth of these malignancies.

Motilin

Motilin is a 22-amino acid peptide found primarily in small bowel mucosa, which is believed to be involved in the regulation of intestinal motility. Motilin accelerates the rate of gastric emptying of mixed meals, stimulates small intestinal peristaltic activity, and increases colonic myoelectric activity. Circulating levels of motilin fluctuate and correlate closely with intestinal motility events. The highest levels occur as fronts of activity pass through the stomach and upper small intestine. Other biological roles for motilin have been proposed and include stimulation of pepsin secretion, diminution of lower esophageal sphincter pressure, contraction of the gallbladder, and an increase in intestinal secretion of water and electrolytes. Increased circulating levels of motilin have been reported in several different conditions characterized by diarrhea.

Substance P

Substance P was the first peptide to be found in both the brain and gastrointestinal tract. It is an 11-amino acid peptide widely distributed to both endocrine cells and nerve fibers, but its physiologic role has yet to be defined. When given intravenously, substance P stimulates salivary gland secretion and inhibits pancreatic bicarbonate and enzyme secretion. Other proposed actions of the peptide include stimulation of intestinal motility and vasodilation of splanchnic and other vascular beds. Substance P has been identified in carcinoid tumors and may contribute to some of the clinical manifestations of the syndrome, such as flushing, hypotension, and diarrhea.

Neurotensin

Neurotensin, a tridecapeptide originally isolated from bovine hypothalamus, is present in high concentration in the distal small bowel, where it is found in specific mucosal endocrine cells. Increased plasma levels of neurotensin can be demonstrated in response to meals and GRP infusion, and somatostatin inhibits release of the peptide. Although initially found to produce systemic hypotension, neurotensin causes a wide range of pharmacologic actions, including hyperglycemia, inhibition of insulin release, stimulation of pancreatic glucagon release, inhibition of gastric acid secretion, and a delay in gastric emptying of liquids.

Other Secretory Tumors of the Pancreas

Insulinoma

Insulinomas were the first islet cell tumors to be described and, along with gastrinomas, occur with the greatest frequency of all these tumors. They are usually solitary benign tumors, although approximately 15 percent are multiple and an equal number are malignant. The clinical manifestations are due entirely to hypoglycemia and its consequences and are highly variable. Classically, patients present with diaphoresis, pallor, and palpitations, all of which are worse in the morning (after an overnight fast), and which are associated with secondary, excessive catecholamine release. However, symptoms are often subtle and can be masked by the tendency of patients to compensate for hypoglycemia by overeating. Moreover, patients with insulinoma often present initially with neuropsychiatric manifestations, which may further delay diagnosis. These range from subtle personality changes to confusion, coma, or a new seizure disorder.

The diagnosis of insulinoma can be established by detection of fasting hypoglycemia in the presence of hyperinsulinemia. Other conditions associated with hypoglycemia, such as liver failure, adrenal insufficiency, hypopituitarism, and alcoholic hypoglycemia, are characterized by diminished serum insulin levels. Measurement of elevated proinsulin and serum C-peptide levels aids in facilitating the correct diagnosis. Normal concentrations of these two peptides will help distinguish insulinoma patients from those taking insulin surreptitiously. The treatment of insulinoma is complete surgical extirpation, and the majority of these tumors are excisable. Patients with metastatic disease should receive chemotherapy, and long-acting somatostatin analogs can be used to ameliorate symptoms.

Glucagonoma

Glucagon-secreting tumors of the pancreas are far less common than both insulinomas and gastrinomas. The most characteristic clinical finding in this syndrome is migratory necrolytic erythema, an eczema-like dermatitis. These skin lesions have a characteristic evolution, progressing over 7 to 14 days from erythematous macules to large bullae, followed by central necrosis and scaly lesions with erythematous margins, and, finally, by central clearing and scaling. The pathophysiology of this lesion is unclear, and it does not appear to be related to plasma levels of glucagon. Because of the catabolic activity of glucagon, patients with these tumors often have profound weight loss and a normochromic, normocytic anemia. Mild diabetes mellitus is also generally present, which is usually treatable with diet and small doses of insulin.

The diagnosis of glucagonoma can be established in patients with the characteristic rash by measurement of plasma glucagon concentrations. Although surgical resection of these tumors is the treatment of choice, the majority of patients with glucagonoma will have metastatic disease at the time of diagnosis. Chemotherapy should be used in these latter patients and may result in objective tumor regression and symptomatic improvement. As with other islet cell tumors, octreotide has been used successfully to treat the rash and other symptoms of glucagonoma.

Somatostatinoma The classic clinical manifestations of somatostatinoma — diabetes, gallstones, and steatorrhea — represent the distinct consequences of the biological properties of somatostatin. In response to inhibition of both insulin and glucagon release by somatostatin, mild diabetes mellitus is often encountered. Somatostatin inhibits gallbladder contraction and may result in bile stasis and subsequent gallstone formation. The combination of bile stasis, impaired intestinal absorption, and decreased pancreatic enzyme secretion results in diarrhea with steatorrhea. Patients with somatostatinoma may also complain of early satiety and fullness caused by delayed gastric emptying as a result of the peptide. They may also be achlorhydric but do not have hypergastrinemia, since somatostatin also directly inhibits gastrin release.

The diagnosis of somatostatinoma is made by demonstration of elevated plasma levels of the peptide, but it is often delayed owing to the relatively mild and nonspecific clinical symptoms encountered. In all likelihood, this delay accounts for the presentation of most patients with advanced, metastatic disease. Therefore, surgical resection is generally unsuccessful in these patients.

Study Questions Questions 1–5 list clinical manifestations characteristic of the islet cell tumors listed below. More than one islet cell tumor may be responsible for the clinical feature described. Match the islet cell tumor(s) to the clinical manifestation listed below.

    a. Gastrinoma (Zollinger-Ellison syndrome)
    b. VIPoma

c. Glucagonoma
d. Somatostatinoma
e. None of the above

1. Diabetes mellitus treated either with insulin or diet alone
2. Migratory necrolytic erythema, a characteristic eczematous rash
3. Steatorrhea
4. Achlorhydria without coexistent hypergastrinemia
5. Gallstones

Answers
1. c, d
   Glucagonoma causes diabetes mellitus due to its hyperglycemic effects. Although somatostatin inhibits the release of both insulin and glucagon, it usually causes mild diabetes.
2. c
   This is the characteristic feature of glucagonoma, a rash whose pathogenesis is unknown.
3. a, d
   Gastrinoma causes steatorrhea due to small intestinal denudation by acid, lipase inactivation, and micellar precipitation. Somatostatinoma may cause mild steatorrhea due to inhibition of nutrient absorption and due to a decrease in pancreatic enzyme secretion. VIPoma causes a secretory diarrhea, not steatorrhea.
4. b, d
   Both VIP and somatostatin inhibit acid secretion. However, although achlorhydria generally produces enhanced gastrin release due to an interruption in the negative feedback produced by increasing acidity, both peptides inhibit gastrin release as well.
5. d
   Somatostatin inhibits gallbladder contractility, leading to gallstone formation.

6. Which of the following statements regarding somatostatin is not true?
   a. Regardless of the parameter examined, somatostatin appears to inhibit release or function.
   b. In humans somatostatin appears to function primarily as a hormone.
   c. Somatostatin has been localized to the heart, kidney, small intestine, and brain.
   d. Somatostatin exists in more than one molecular form.
   e. Despite its physiological function inhibiting both pancre-

atic glucagon and insulin, patients with somatostatin-secreting tumors generally have mild diabetes mellitus.

Answer

b

Somatostatin appears to function primarily as either a neuro-transmitter or paracrine mediator in most animal species, including humans. Although some feel it may function as a hormone, it does not work primarily through this route.

7. Which of the following statements regarding the Zollinger-Ellison syndrome (gastrinoma) is or are true (more than one choice may be correct):
   a. Diarrhea is due both to the secretory effects of gastrin and to fat malabsorption.
   b. Excluding those due to malignancy, all the clinical manifestations of the Zollinger-Ellison syndrome are due to gastrin.
   c. One third to one half of all gastrinoma patients have diarrhea.
   d. Patients with gastrinoma are now succumbing most commonly to the malignant nature of these tumors.
   e. All the above are correct.

Answer

e

All are true. As explained above, gastrinoma causes steatorrhea by several mechanisms, and gastrin may decrease water and electrolyte absorption, causing a secretory diarrhea. Moreover, one third to one half of all Zollinger-Ellison patients have diarrhea, with 10 to 15 percent having diarrhea only. Either directly or indirectly, gastrin causes all the clinical manifestations, and although gastric acid hypersecretion was formerly responsible for most deaths, acid output can be controlled both medically and surgically.

8. Which of the following gastrointestinal regulatory peptides is *not* located in the stomach?
   a. Secretin
   b. Gastrin
   c. VIP
   d. Somatostatin
   e. Gastrin-releasing peptide

Answer

a

VIP and gastrin-releasing peptide (GRP) are two neuropeptides found throughout the entire gastrointestinal tract, and somatostatin is closely linked to both antral gastrin cells and acid-producing parietal cells.

References

Andrew, A., Kramer, B., and Rawdon, B. B. Gut and pancreatic amine precursor uptake and decarboxylation cells are not neural crest derivatives. *Gastroenterology* 84:429, 1983.

Gorden, P., Comi, R. J., Maton, P. N., and Go, V. L. W. Somatostatin and somatostatin analogue (SMS 201-995) in treatment of hormone-secreting tumors of the pituitary and gastrointestinal tract and non-neoplastic diseases of the gut. *Ann. Intern. Med.* 110:35, 1989.

Kleibeuker, J. H., Eysselein, V. E., Maxwell, V. E., and Walsh, J. H. Role of endogenous secretin in acid-induced inhibition of human gastric function. *J. Clin. Invest.* 73:526, 1984.

Krejs, G. J., Orci, L., Conlon, J. M., Ravazzola, M., et al. Somatostatinoma syndrome: Biochemical, morphologic, and clinical features. *N. Engl. J. Med.* 301:285, 1979.

Pappas, T. N., Debas, H. T., and Taylor, I. L. Enterogastrone-like effect of peptide YY is vagally mediated in the dog. *J. Clin. Invest.* 77:49, 1986.

Pearse, A. G. E., Polak, J. M., and Bloom, S. R. The newer gut hormones: Cellular sources, physiology, pathology, and clinical aspects. *Gastroenterology* 72:746, 1977.

Roth, J., LeRoith, D., Shiloach, J., Rosenzweig, J. L., et al. The evolutionary origins of hormones, neurotransmitters, and other extracellular chemical messengers. *N. Engl. J. Med.* 306:523, 1982.

Solomon, T. E. Pancreatic polypeptide, peptide YY, and neuropeptide Y family of regulatory peptides. *Gastroenterology* 88:838, 1985.

Walsh, J. H. Gastrointestinal Peptide Hormones. In M. H. Sleisenger and J. S. Fordtran (eds.), *Gastrointestinal Disease* (4th ed.). Philadelphia: Saunders, 1989.

Wolfe, M. M., and Jensen, R. T. Zollinger-Ellison syndrome: Current concepts in diagnosis and treatment. *N. Engl. J. Med.* 317:1200, 1987.

Wolfe, M. M., Reel, G. M., and McGuigan, J. E. Inhibition of gastrin release by secretin is mediated by somatostatin in cultured rat antral mucosa. *J. Clin. Invest.* 72:1586, 1983.

Yamada, T. Secretory Tumors of the Pancreas. In M. H. Sleisenger and J. S. Fordtran (eds.), *Gastrointestinal Disease* (3rd ed.). Philadelphia: Saunders, 1983. Pp. 1527–1542.

22 : Gastrointestinal Immunology

Z. Myron Falchuk

The Gastrointestinal Mucosa

The mucosal surfaces of the intestine that are exposed to a hostile environment have evolved an elaborate system to protect themselves from the bacterial, viral, mechanical, and thermal onslaught unique to their position. Included in these protective systems are factors relating to the lumen, such as the flow of materials in the lumen (saliva, food, bile, and mucus), as well as certain peristaltic movements. These factors serve to cleanse the lumen by propelling the contents distally. Other factors relate to the physical barrier separating the lumen from the inside of the organism, that is, the epithelial cell and the other specialized cells of the mucosa, such as the goblet cell and the M cell. The epithelial cell is especially suited with its tight junctions to seal the external environment from the internal. Still another mechanism of protection at mucosal surfaces involves the system of local immunity, which has evolved into a very specialized set of effector cells and other cells as well as locally produced immunologic products, including immunoglobulins and other biologically active lymphoid cell products (lymphokines). Although most of the immunoglobulin classes are made in the intestinal tract, the IgA response has a special place in the gastrointestinal tract as in all externally positioned environments. It is probable that IgA is critical in limiting passage of immunogenic macromolecules through the mucosal barrier. Persons with isolated IgA deficiency may allow food antigens to enter the systemic circulation, eliciting immune responses to these antigens with possible pathogenic consequences.

The lamina propria of the gastrointestinal tract is populated by lymphoid and other cells, including so-called accessory cells, such as macrophages. Lymphocytes also migrate into the epithelial cell layer where they are known as intraepithelial lymphocytes (Fig. 22-1). Intraepithelial lymphocytes may have cytoeffector capability relevant to homeostatic as well as pathologic mechanisms. The intimate relation to epithelial cells places these lymphocytes, by virtue of their position, in a choice location to either protect against environmental factors or inflict damage in disease states such as gluten-sensitive enteropathy (celiac disease) or inflammatory bowel disease. In fact, in-

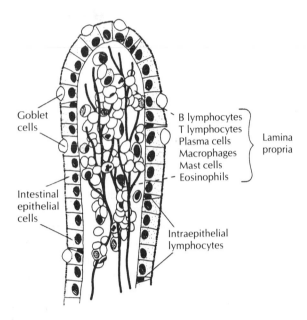

Fig. 22-1
A schematic representation of the intestinal villus with particular reference to the intimate relation among the intraepithelial lymphocytes, the lamina propria lymphocytes, and surface cells. (From M. F. Kagnoff. Immunology of the Digestive Tract. In L. R. Johnson [ed.], *Physiology of the Digestive Tract.* New York: Raven, 1981.)

traepithelial lymphocytes are increased in numbers in these diseases.

The Humoral Immune System

IgA is the predominant immunoglobulin present in external secretions such as saliva, tears, and intestinal secretions, in distinction to what occurs in the peripheral system where IgG and IgM are the predominant classes of immunoglobulin. IgA was first discovered as a serum protein in the 1950s, but it was not until the 1960s that the uniqueness of the external immune system and the role of IgA in that system was elucidated. Mucosal IgA is produced at all external mucosal sites, the greatest quantity being made in the gastrointestinal tract. In the serum, IgA constitutes some 10 percent of total serum immunoglobulin (100–200 mg/liter). Much of the IgA in serum is made in the periphery and differs from mucosal IgA in multiple respects. Serum IgA is monomeric, whereas mucosal IgA is dimeric and is composed of two molecules of IgA connected by a protein called secretory component (SC). SC confers certain properties on the molecule, including the ability to be transported across membranes and to resist proteolysis. There are also differences in the subclass distribution, with IgA1 constituting 85 percent of serum IgA but with IgA1 and 2 being equal in secretions. Monomeric IgA has a coefficient of sedimentation of 7S, and dimeric secretory IgA has a sedimentation coefficient of 11S.

Although IgA is the predominant mucosal immunoglobulin, all five immunoglobulin classes are represented in mucosal secretions. Serum IgA and secretory IgA belong to two separate metabolic pools and are made in different sites. Despite this, the presence of IgA in serum directed at antigens encountered at mucosal surfaces implies an interaction between the two systems. Thus, B cells exposed to antigens at mucosal surfaces may migrate to sites of systemic antibody production. B cells activated by antigen at Peyer's patches must circulate through the vascular system before terminal differentiation. B cell homing phenomena are not fully understood but appear to involve receptors on endothelial cell membranes of venules in lymphoid tissues such as Peyer's patches and cell surface sites on lymphocytes. These receptors allow gastrointestinal-associated lymphocytes to enter the systemic circulation and to mature and proliferate and selectively return to the gastrointestinal tract. Another explanation for the existence of serum IgA directed against antigens delivered to the mucosal immune system is that under some circumstances, disease or otherwise, these antigens penetrate the mucosal surfaces and are able to stimulate the peripheral immune system directly.

Regulation of Immunoglobulin Synthesis

Regulation of IgA synthesis occurs at multiple points. It is now clear that regulatory cells exist that allow changing of Ig class from IgM to IgA under the influence of so-called switch T cells. It also appears that factors produced by epithelial cells of the lamina propria may play a role in control of synthesis of secretory IgA. The ingestion of antigen may induce oral tolerance such that later parenteral immunization with the same antigen will not elicit an immune response. Tolerance is the specific ability *not* to develop an immune response to a specific antigen. Tolerance to oral immunogen is mediated by T cells that have been exposed to antigen at the gastrointestinal surface and have then migrated to the spleen where they suppress IgG and IgM production directed against the same antigen. The induction of tolerance to orally administered antigens is crucial to prevent the gross overburdening of the immune system by the myriads of antigens to which it is constantly exposed.

Study of the local immune system shows that SC and IgA are made at different sites, with the epithelial cell producing SC and the B cell producing IgA. It is also clear that development and maturation of the peripheral humoral immune system precedes development of the local immune system. It appears that ingestion of antigens is necessary for the secretory IgA system to develop, since animals maintained in germ-free environments exhibit little maturity in the local immune system. Mature levels of secretory IgA do not appear until the end of the first decade.

IgA antibodies do not activate the complement cascade. Their role in local homeostasis is likely to be mediated by antigen-antibody binding, limiting access of antigen to the circulation or inactivating viruses or bacteria by interfering with their access to the epithelial cell. Much study remains to fully elucidate the role of the local IgA system in health and disease.

The Cellular Mucosal Immune System

Until now, we have discussed the fact that antibodies are made at local tissue sites. We shall now consider the gastrointestinal tract as an immunologic organ. The barrier between the internal and external environment is populated by a structured immune apparatus collectively known as the *gut-associated lymphoid tissues* (GALT). The cells of this system are spread throughout the gastrointestinal tract as well as being aggregated in specialized areas called Peyer's patches. The Peyer's patches are composed of T and B cells and are covered by a specialized epithelial cell known as the M cell (Fig. 22-2). The M cell derives its name from the many small microfolds that form its surface. The cytoplasm of the M cell is very thinly stretched over the patch, allowing the underlying lymphoid cells to come into very intimate contact with particulate or soluble antigen, which makes its way through the cell by pinocytosis. This process involves the attachment of antigen to the cell membrane, which then surrounds the antigen, invaginates into the cell, and gets transported to the opposite side and released. The Peyer's patch contains macrophages that interact with antigen and "present" the antigen to T cells, allowing for an initiation of the immune response. The T cells involved in this initial phase of the immune response are the T4, or so-called helper cells, which interact with B cells in the course of events leading to antibody synthesis. It is also at this step that tolerance can be induced, again by the action of a specific T cell having suppressor function.

The Peyer's patch is also a site where the initial steps of amplification of the immune response occur. These events are facilitated by other lymphocyte products known as lymphokines and include growth factors such as interleukin 1 (IL-1) and 2 (IL-2). IL-1 is a macrophage-derived factor that amplifies the maturational response of T cells. IL-2 stimulates replication of T cell clones, which then become effective cytotoxic, helper, and suppressor cells. Once B cells are stimulated, there is a migration out of the Peyer's patch to the local mesenteric lymph node and

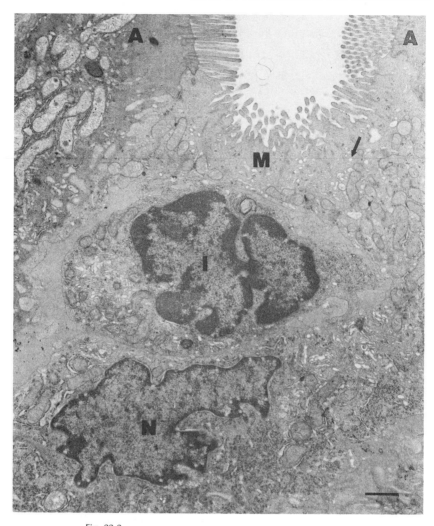

Fig. 22-2
Ileal epithelium overlying a Peyer's patch of an 8-week-old C₃H/Hej mouse. The M cell (M) has short, fat, irregular microvilli, a thin bridge of apical cytoplasm with many vesicles (*arrow*), and a basally oriented nucleus (N). Its cytoplasm envelops a mononuclear cell (I). The adjacent absorptive cells (A) have tall, thin microvilli. Bar equals 1 μm. (From J. L. Wolf and W. A. Bye. The membranous epithelial (M) cell and the mucosal immune system. Reproduced, with permission, from the *Annual Review of Medicine*, Vol. 35. © 1984 by Annual Reviews Inc.

then into the main lymphatics to the general circulation. These lymphocytes go to the spleen, expanding in number and recirculating to the GALT, Peyer's patch, and lamina propria. Just as specific stimulation of B-cell clones takes place in this system, specific stimulation and activation of T-cell clones also takes place. The GALT includes cells of both helper (T4) and suppressor/cytotoxic (T8) phenotype. About 70 percent of the lamina propria cells are T cells, and two thirds of these cells are T4.

Cells capable of mediating lectin-induced cytotoxicity, as well as natural killer (NK) cells, are found in this compartment.

The intraepithelial (IEL) compartment is somewhat different in that B cells are lacking. The IEL compartment is composed of T4 and T8 cells as defined by their surface and functional characteristics.

Cellular Cytotoxicity

The discussion of elements of the immune system has to this point only briefly touched on the effector cellular response to antigenic stimulation. A very important function of the cellular immune response deals with cells capable of mediating cytotoxicity. It is important to understand that target cells of cytotoxicity include allogeneic normal cells (cells from different hosts that differ at the major histocompatibility complex [MHC] and that are encountered in allogeneic grafts), virally infected autologous cells that are MHC identical, and tumor cells. T cells, in mediating T-cell-specific cytotoxicity, do not recognize antigen alone through their surface receptors but recognize antigen in molecular association with a membrane protein called a *restriction element*. The T-cell receptor can bind foreign antigen, which must also associate with the restriction element, which in turn is coded for by the MHC gene. The interaction must occur both with the T-cell receptor and the MHC restriction element to sensitize the T cell. The MHC gene-coded proteins are present either as class I (the classically defined histocompatibility markers HLA-A,B,C), which code for T8 suppressor/cytotoxic cells, or as class II, which are typed by means of mixed lymphocyte culture markers known as HLA-D. The class II proteins serve as restriction elements for the helper (T4) lymphocyte. Class I molecules are present on all nucleated cells, whereas class II molecules are present on B cells, macrophages, activated T cells, and certain other accessory cells. Regulation of certain responses is in part controlled by the ability or lack thereof of certain antigens to bind to the class I or II molecules and may form the basis of certain pathologic states. If a given antigen cannot make an effective union with any of the MHC antigens, the cascade of events required to initiate the immune response cannot occur, and, consequently, the generation of B-cell clones capable of making specific antibody, or of T-cell cytotoxic clones, capable of killing the specific target cell, cannot be generated. The relation between MHC class II molecules and certain diseases emphasizes the importance of these molecules to immune response characteristics and to the pathogenesis of specific cytotoxic phenomena in disease.

The types of lymphocytes capable of killing target cells are cytotoxic T-cell precursors activated by cell surface antigens such as viral molecules presented in conjunction with host class I or II molecules. This type of cytotoxicity is very specific for the initial sensitizing antigen. A second cytotoxic mechanism is mediated by a lymphocyte called NK cells. These cells recognize their target through the NK receptor and are not MHC restricted. This type of cytotoxicity does not require prior sensitization and is believed to represent a key element in the surveillance mechanism of the immune system against virally infected or tumor cells. A third type of cell-mediated cytotoxicity occurs when antibody directed against specific cell surface antigen bridges a target cell to an effector cell, which can be a lymphocyte, macrophage, or granulocyte. This bridging results in antibody-dependent, cell-mediated cytotoxicity (ADCC) and requires the prior sensitization to the antigen with formation of antibody to the antigen, but not a restriction molecule of the MHC class. The presence of NK cells, cytotoxic T cells, and cells capable of mediating ADCC has clearly been demonstrated in the immunocytes of the gastrointestinal tract, although the relative numbers of these cells and their efficiency in the GALT remains an unanswered question.

Immunologically Mediated Intestinal Disease

In the final portion of this chapter, we consider how the local immune system may relate to specific disease processes. Techniques are now available that allow one to isolate the cells of the lamina propria, the interepithelial lymphocytes, and the cells of the Peyer's patches. Study of isolated cell populations has allowed the definition of the cell types in each compartment and assessment of function of those cells. It is clear that diseases that affect the intestinal mucosa such as ulcerative colitis and gluten-sensitive enteropathy (celiac disease) are more likely to have as potential etiologies factors relating to the local immune system than to the systemic immune system. Study of many conditions has been complicated by the fact that the specific agents involved in the disease pathogenesis are unknown. A significant exception to this quandary is gluten-sensitive enteropathy, a disease in which the intestine is exquisitely sensitive to the dietary protein gluten. Gluten is a complex glycoprotein found in wheat, barley, rye, and oats, which, when ingested by patients with gluten-sensitive enteropathy, produces an intense inflammatory reaction in the lamina propria and is accompanied by great damage to the epithelial cells and by "flattening" of the intestinal villi. The intense inflammation with lymphocytes and plasma cells in the lamina propria has suggested for some time that these cells were important to the ongoing tissue damage in these patients. Isolation of the antibodies made by these plasma cells showed that there was a strong response to gluten with production of anti-gluten antibody of both IgA and IgM class. Secretion of these antibodies is greatly decreased by addition of cortisol to in vitro cultures of tissue explants; in fact, cortisol added to such cultures prevents the deleterious effect of gluten on the epithelial cell. These and other experiments showed that patients with gluten-sensitive enteropathy mount a specific B cell response to gluten. This response not only involves B cells but also includes T cells, as shown by local lymphokine production in response to gluten stimulation. Great insight into the possible mechanism of the disease is supplied by asking why patients with gluten-sensitive enteropathy make a specific immune response to the gluten molecule. It has been shown that gluten-sensitive enteropathy is associated with particular HLA types (HLA B8 and DR3). Since immune response genes are associated with the major histocompatibility locus, it seems reasonable to propose that an immune response gene defect in humans could manifest as an abnormal tendency to respond immunologically to oral challenge with gluten. In addition to HLA-MHC genes, it has also been shown that there is an association with certain allotype markers on the IgG heavy chain, which are termed *Gm markers*.

A most intriguing recent observation in this disease is the discovery of homology between a certain part of the gluten molecule and a virus that infects humans (adenovirus type 12). This observation suggests the following hypothesis: Infection with adenovirus type 12 in early life results in immunity to the virus because of the chance occurrence of a receptor on the epithelial cell surface for this virus. In later life, exposure to gluten results in binding of gluten to the same or similar cell surface receptors coded for by MHC genes. The bound antigen is "presented" to local macrophages and in turn to T cells, creating specific helper cells leading to a specific immune response to the gluten. Antigluten antibody and cytotoxic cells are generated in an anamnestic or secondary response created by the memory cells stored after the initial priming by the homologous viral antigen. The T cells and antibody can then kill the epithelial cell, rendered a target for specific immune lysis by attached gluten.

The understanding of the local immune response has come a long way. Definition of disease mechanisms — for example, in gluten-sensitive enteropathy — will one day be the end result of expanding insight and should enable us to offer new and better modes of treatment for patients with immunologic disorders of the gastrointestinal tract.

Study Questions   1. Discuss the evidence supporting the existence of an immune system unique to external mucosae of the body.

Answer

The external mucosae of the body are populated by immunocytes representing all the cells of the immune system — lymphocytes (both B and T), macrophages, granulocytes, and mast cells. These cells engage in specific traffic patterns, involving migration to the regional lymph glands, proliferation, travel to the systemic immune system, and return to the gut-associated lymphoid system (GALT). Homing back to the GALT is accomplished by means of specific receptors on endothelial cells, involving Peyer's patches and other special sites. In addition to unique cellular immune patterns, a specialized humoral immune system has evolved involving a dimeric IgA molecule, joined by a molecule known as secretory component (SC). SC confers special qualities on the IgA that allow it to exist in the harsh environments of the external milieu. In addition, it facilitates the transepithelial transport of IgA into the lumen. Dimeric IgA is confined, for the most part, to the mucosae of the body.

2. The intestinal mucosa is infected with salmonella. The patient's symptoms of severe diarrhea abate after five days. What are the immune mechanisms by which the infection is terminated?

Answer

The initial phase of the infection brings the bacteria into the intestinal lumen, where it proliferates and produces toxins. It may also become invasive, causing damage in this way. The interaction with the immune system likely occurs at the level of the M cell. The bacteria enter the epithelium, come into contact with the mucosal T cells, and an immune response is started. These cells, likely T4 helper cells, migrate to regional nodes, proliferate clonally, and interact with other cells including macrophages. Lymphokines are produced, further modulating the immune response. With homing responses, the T cells return to the lamina propria, stimulating B cells to produce specific antibody. The combination of humoral and cellular responses to the salmonella results in immune lysis of the bacteria. The process takes five days.

References

Bull, D. M., and Bookman, M. A. Isolation and functional characteristics of human intestinal lymphoid cells. *J. Clin. Invest.* 59:966, 1977.

Butcher, E. C., Scollay, R. G., and Weissman, I. L. Organ specificity of lymphocyte migration: Mediation by highly selective lymphocyte interaction with organ-specific determinants on high endothelial venules. *Eur. J. Immunol.* 10:556, 1980.

Delacroix, D. L., Dive, C., Rambaud, J. C., and Vaerman, J. P. IgA subclasses in various secretions and in serum. *Immunology* 47:383, 1982.

Ernst, P. B., Befus, A. D., and Bienenstock, J. Leukocytes in the intestinal epithelium: An unusual immunologic compartment. *Immunol. Today* 6:50, 1985.

Falchuk, Z. M., Rogentine, G. N., and Strober, W. Predominance of histocompatibility antigen HLA-B8 in patients with gluten sensitive enteropathy. *J. Clin. Invest.* 51:1601, 1972.

Falchuk, Z. M., and Strober, W. Gluten sensitive enteropathy: Intestinal synthesis of antigliadin antibody in vitro. *Gut* 15:947, 1974.

Henkart, P. A. Mechanisms of lymphocyte-mediated cytotoxicity. *Ann. Rev. Immunol.* 3:31, 1985.

Kagnoff, M. F., Austin, R. K., Hubert, J. J., and Kasarda, D. D. Possible role for a human adenovirus in the pathogenesis of celiac disease. *J. Exp. Med.* 160:1544, 1984.

Katz, A., Falchuk, Z. M., Strober, W., and Schwachman, H. Gluten sensitive enteropathy. Inhibition by cortisol of the effect of gluten protein in vitro. *N. Engl. J. Med.* 295:131, 1976.

Kawanishi, H., Saltzman, L., and Strober, W. Mechanisms regulating IgA class specific immunoglobulin production in gut associated lymphoid tissues. I. T cells derived from Peyer's patches that switch sIgM B cells in vitro. *J. Exp. Med.* 157:433, 1983.

Levenson, S. D., Austin, R. K., Dietler, M. D., Kasarda, D. D., et al. Specificity of antigliadin antibody in celiac disease. *Gastroenterology* 89:1, 1985.

Nossal, G. J. V. The basic components of the immune system. *N. Engl. J. Med.* 316:1320, 1987.

Selby, W. S., Janossy, G., Goldstein, G., and Jewell, D. P. T lymphocyte subsets in human intestinal mucosa. *Clin. Exp. Immunol.* 44:453, 1981.

Tomasi, T. B., Tan, E. M., Solomon, A., and Prendergast, R. A. Characteristics of an immune system common to certain external secretions. *J. Exp. Med.* 121:101, 1965.

Wolf, J. L., and Bye, W. A. The membranous epithelial (M) cell and the mucosal immune system. *Ann. Rev. Med.* 35:95, 1984.

Index